CLINICAL ELECTRO-CARDIOGRAPHY

A PRIMARY CARE APPROACH

CLINICAL ELECTRO-CARDIOGRAPHY
A PRIMARY CARE APPROACH

Ken Grauer, MD
Associate Professor

R. Whitney Curry Jr., MD
Associate Professor and Associate Chairman

Department of Community Health and Family Medicine
University of Florida College of Medicine
Gainesville, Florida

Medical Economics Books
Oradell, New Jersey 07649

Library of Congress Cataloging-in-Publication Data

Grauer, Ken.
Clinical electrocardiography.

Bibliography: p.
Includes index.
1. Electrocardiography. 2. Heart—Diseases—Diagnosis. I. Curry, R. Whitney. II. Title.
[DNLM: 1. Electrocardiography. 2. Heart Diseases—diagnosis. WG 140 G774c]
RC683.5.E5G66 1986 616.1'207547 86-8596
ISBN 0-87489-404-2

Cover design: Penina M. Wissner

Technical artwork by Janet Kroenke

ISBN 0-87489-404-2

Medical Economics Company Inc.
Oradell, New Jersey 07649

Printed in the United States of America

To my father, Samuel Grauer,
without whom this book would
not have been possible.

CONTENTS

PART THREE

FOREWORD

Robert Eliot, MD, chief of cardiology at the University of Nebraska, called the primary care physician in rural America the "front-line cardiologist." To provide comprehensive care, the physician must be proficient in electrocardiographic interpretation. Computers and machines have not replaced doctors. Individual reading of the ECG is necessary to the proper care of the patient. The primary care physician sees a cross section of patients, well and sick, male and female, young and old — not in a triage role but as a diagnostician or as a case manager referring to more narrow-based specialists when appropriate.

This book provides the "front-line cardiologist" with the tools and references needed to read an ECG. The systematic approach to ECG interpretations in Table 1-6 will guide you in perfecting your skills.

The authors combine theoretical knowledge with practical problem solving and even a little humor, the smiley and frowny faces of ST segment elevations in Chapter 1. The workbook format helps you acquire and retain the knowledge you need.

Written by practical, primary care physicians with superb backgrounds in cardiology and clinical experience, this book is a challenging, informative, and immediately useful key to electrocardiography.

Thomas L. Stern, MD

Clinical Professor of Community Health and Family Medicine,
University of Florida College of Medicine
Vice President for Professional and Corporate Affairs,
Family Health Foundation of America

FOREWORD

The first electrocardiograph arrived in this country in 1912. Although a primitive, cumbersome instrument that only recorded bipolar leads I, II, and III, it was a wonderful beginning. Subsequent developments brought additional leads and clarification of the early "patterns." Many of the empiricisms, based on clinical correlation, were found to be correct.

When I was a third year medical student, I learned electrocardiography from the superb lectures of Dr. Robert P. Grant, who brought to Georgetown University the concepts he and Dr. Harvey Estes had developed at Duke. My classmates and I were familiar with "Spatial Vector Electrocardiography" long before Dr. Grant's text was published. Subsequently, I have read many works on this subject, some excellent, others full of the same errors that appeared in ancient lore. I've learned a great deal from the writings of Drs. Sodi-Pallares, H.J.L. Marriott, Harold Friedman, Mervin Goldman, and many others.

So why another book on electrocardiography? And one by primary care physicians? My friend Dr. D.H. Davies said, "The learning of any subject is made much easier if the teacher's aim is to provide understanding, as well as to impart knowledge." In this Drs. Grauer and Curry are very successful. While my opinions may differ on some of the material in the text, I nevertheless find it stimulating, instructive, challenging, and up to date. No reader, beginner or advanced, should come away without new thoughts, concepts, and clarifications.

I wish I had written this book!

William P. Nelson, MD

Professor of Medicine
Division of Cardiology
College of Medicine
University of South Florida

PUBLISHER'S NOTES

Ken Grauer, MD, is an associate professor in the Department of Community Health and Family Medicine, College of Medicine, University of Florida and assistant director of the Family Practice Residency Program in Gainesville. Certified in family practice, he is on the editorial board of *Continuing Education for the Family Physician,* and is an ACLS affiliate faculty member for the state of Florida. He has written numerous articles on cardiology for family physicians and a book, *"Study Guide for Advanced Life Support: Problem Solving in Cardiac Arrest"* (C.V. Mosby, 1984). He has taught ECG and dysrhythmia workshops to physicians in practice, physicians in training, medical students, nurses, and other paramedical personnel, simplifying otherwise complicated topics into a concise, practical, and easy-to-remember format.

R. Whitney Curry Jr., MD, is an associate professor in the Department of Community Health and Family Medicine, College of Medicine, University of Florida, and director of the Family Practice Residency Program in Gainesville. He is the Medical Editor of *Data Centrum.* Board certified in both internal medicine and family practice, he has directed the family practice hospital service at Alachua General Hospital for 10 years. With Dr. Grauer, Dr. Curry has co-authored articles and taught ECG interpretation to physicians and medical students.

ACKNOWLEDGMENTS

We are particularly grateful to the American Academy of Family Physicians that allowed us to modify and reproduce the following figures from *Monograph #47, Interpreting ECGs: A Workbook 1983,* one of a continuing series of monographs from the AAFP Home Study Self-Assessment Program: Figures 2-1, 2-2, 2-11A, 3-2, 3-8, 4-3, 4-5, 4-6, 4-7, 4-13, 4-15, 5-3, 5-14, 5-21, 5-26, 7-2, 7-12, 7-13, 7-14, 7-15, 7-29, 8-1, 8-2, 8-11, 8-12, 8-13, 8-15, 8-16, C-9, D-2, and E-17; Tables 1-6, 3-2, 3-3, and 4-3.

We are also grateful to Continuing Education for the Family Physician for allowing us to modify and reproduce the following figures from articles and the "ECG of the Month" series that we write for their journal: Figure 2-14, 2-15A and B, 2-16, 2-18, 2-19, 3-25, 3-26, 3-27, 5-15, 5-27, 6-15, 7-27, 7-28, B-6, B-7, C-4, D-3, D-4, E-2, F-2, F-3, and F-4.

In addition, we are indebted to the following people whose contributions were instrumental in the preparation of this book:

Louis Kuritzky, MD, and Holly Jensen, RN, for their expertise and diligence in reviewing the majority of the manuscript.

Jack Bruggeman of Medical Economics Books, for his unlimited enthusiasm and skillful guidance of the project.

The Apple Macintosh Computer, without which I would still be typing the manuscript.

Michelle C. Grauer, for her patience, love and support during the seemingly endless hours of my "vacation" at the Macintosh.

The family practice residents, medical students, and physician assistant students of the College of Medicine, University of Florida, for allowing us to learn by teaching them.

Diane Hazen for mounting and remounting countless tracings for me over the years.

John Shelton, MD, Perry Hearn, MD, George Benchimol, MD, and Candy Blankenship for their constructive commentary on selected portions of the text.

The many excellent cardiologists from whom we have learned.

All those who have knowingly (and unknowingly) provided tracings for the book.

HOW TO USE THIS BOOK

A book on electrocardiography faces the inevitable variability in the knowledge base of the readers. Most texts suffer from being either too advanced for the beginner or too basic for the experienced electrocardiographer. Ours strives to accommodate both. Readers may select the portions most suitable for them.

Part One introduces basic concepts in electrocardiography, including terminology, electrophysiologic principles, and a systematic approach to interpretation of ECGs (Chapter 1), determination of rate and rhythm (Chapter 2), calculation of mean QRS axis (Chapter 3), and theoretical considerations on the coronary circulation and on derivation of standard waveforms for chamber enlargement, intraventricular conduction defects, and myocardial infarction (Chapter 4). Although introductory in nature, many advanced concepts have been integrated in this initial section to maintain the interest of the experienced interpreter. In addition, reference to those principles will be made throughout the text, so even the advanced reader may benefit from a review of this section *before* tackling the clinical examples of Part Two. Some readers may prefer to begin with the clinical examples and refer as needed back to basic principles of Part One.

Part Two addresses the ST segment in health and disease (Chapter 5), intraventricular conduction defects (Chapter 6), myocardial infarction (Chapter 7), and chamber enlargement (Chapter 8). Although the reader could cover this material much more rapidly by skipping ahead to the answers that follow each tracing, much benefit would be lost by doing so. It is far better to interpret each ECG systematically and take the extra moment to *write* that interpretation down.

Brief commentaries follow the interpretations of most tracings. Some involve subtleties that extend beyond the scope of the novice interpreter. Subtleties are usually clearly labeled as such. The beginner should not get hung up on these points, but rather should skip over them if they are confusing and proceed to the next example. Doing so will not disturb the flow of the book. Important concepts are reinforced. A point not initially understood will become clear later in the text, or during a second reading.

Part Three presents review exercises in ECG interpretation. These cases solidify the material presented in the text, and increase the reviewer's confidence in the ability to interpret. To enhance clinical relevance, exercise tracings have been arranged in common presentations: ECGs that suggest metabolic disturbances, atypical ECGs in healthy asymptomatic subjects, ECGs in patients with cardiomegaly on chest X-ray films, ECGs with a tall R wave in lead V_1, ECGs from patients with chest pain, and pseudoinfarction patterns.

Part Four offers references, including a key to abbreviations, a list of important figures and tables, a handy reference guide, a list of references and an index. The handy reference guide consolidates much of the important diagnostic information presented throughout the text. You may want to detach it for use as a pocket guide.

Ken Grauer, MD
R. Whitney Curry Jr., MD

PART ONE

Basic Principles

CHAPTER 1

INTRODUCTION

Man has known for well over a hundred years about the heart's ability to generate and transmit electric current. Willem Einthoven, in 1902, became the first to record this electric current in an accurate and reproducible form with his invention of the string galvanometer. His electrocardiograms comprised only the three bipolar limb leads (I, II, and III). In the 1930s, Frank N. Wilson and associates devised the unipolar lead system, which was later modified by Emmanual Goldberger to form the augmented lead system (employing leads aVR, aVL, and aVF). Finally, unipolar chest leads were added to complete the three-dimensional survey of the heart's electrical activity. The true art and science of electrocardiography, however, derives not from these theoretical origins, but rather from the correlation of theory with anatomic and pathologic findings, and application to clinical medicine. This work, begun by Wilson, is still ongoing today.

In this introductory chapter, we will trace the heart's electrical activity in its path through the conduction system. Basic concepts important to electrocardiography will be discussed, and an approach for systematic ECG interpretation that will be used for analysis of tracings throughout the text will be presented.

Conduction System of the Heart

An ECG is simply the graphic representation of electrical activity generated by the heart. In the standard ECG, this electrical activity is recorded from 12 different viewpoints called *leads.*

The electrical activity of the heart originates at a cellular level. During the resting state, individual myocardial cells are said to be "polarized"; they are negatively charged on the cell interior and positively charged on their surface. When electrical stimulation of the cell occurs, the inherent negativity of the interior becomes positively charged, and a wave of depolarization is propagated along the length of the cell. With the organized depolarization of the mass of cardiac cells, mechanical contraction of the myocardium occurs.

Conduction of the electrical impulse of depolarization is carried to individual myocardial cells by the specialized tissues of the heart's conduction system. This system is illustrated in Fig. 1-1A approximately as it occurs

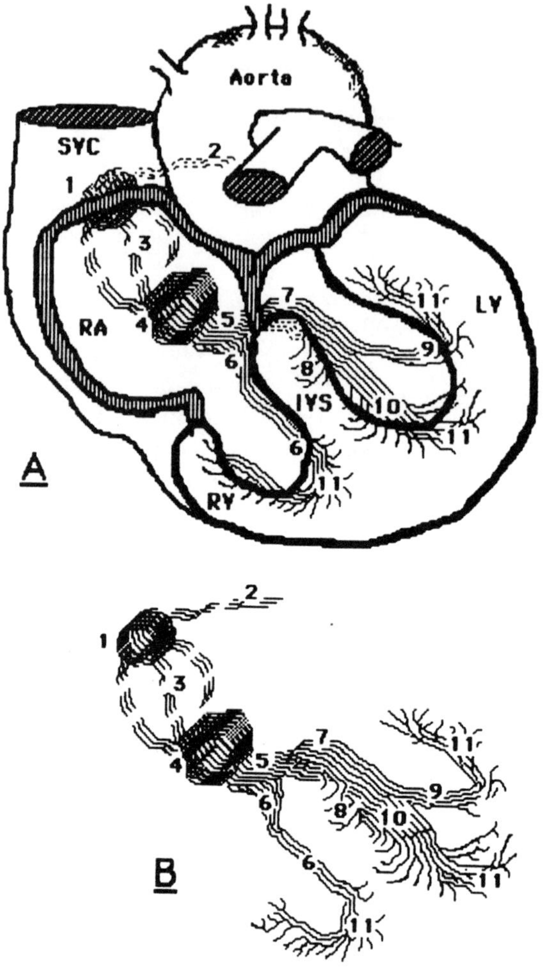

Figure 1-1. Conduction system of the heart. **A.** Anatomic position. **B.** Isolated outside the heart. SVC—Superior vena cava; RA—Right atrium; RV—Right ventricle; LV—Left ventricle; IVS—Interventricular septum; 1. SA node; 2. Bachmann's bundle; 3. Internodal tracts; 4. AV node; 5. Bundle of His; 6. Right bundle branch; 7. Left bundle branch; 8. Branches that activate the IVS; 9. Left anterior hemidivision of #7; 10. Left posterior hemidivision of #7; 11. Purkinje network.

anatomically within the heart. In Fig. 1-1B, the conduction system has been isolated for greater clarity.

Normal electrical activation of the heart begins in the *sinus* (sinoatrial or SA) *node,* located where the superior vena cava enters into the right atrium (#1 in Fig. 1-1). The SA node is the principal pacemaker of the heart. Whereas the majority of myocardial cells maintain their resting state of polarization, the pacemaker cells in the SA node undergo spontaneous depolarization and initiate an action potential. This electrical impulse is rapidly conducted through the atria via specialized conduction pathways. Bachmann's bundle (2) is the major interatrial tract, and conducts the impulse from the SA node in the right atrium over to the left atrium. Three internodal tracts (3) conduct the impulse to the atrioventricular (AV) node or junction (4). Conduction is rapid through the specialized atrial pathways, but is significantly delayed as it travels through the AV node. After emerging, conduction velocity accelerates dramatically as the electrical impulse now enters the bundle of His (5). This divides into the right bundle branch (6) and the common left bundle branch (7) on its way to spread the process of depolarization to the ventricles. The common left bundle branch gives off branches to activate the interventricular septum (8), and then splits into the left anterior hemidivision (9) and left posterior hemidivision (10). The right bundle branch continues as a slender fascicle until it reaches near the right ventricular apex. Finally, each bundle branch terminates by ramifying into the specialized Purkinje network (11) that carries the electrical impulse to the ventricular myocardium.

Following the above process of depolarization, repolarization of the heart occurs as individual myocardial cells regain the negativity of their interior. Mechanical counterparts of the cardiac cycle (atrial and ventricular contraction) follow shortly after completion of their corresponding electrical events (atrial depolarization and ventricular depolarization, respectively). Electrocardiographically, these electrical events are represented by the P wave (reflecting atrial depolarization), QRS complex (ventricular depolarization), and T wave (ventricular repolarization) (Fig. 1-2). Atrial repolarization also occurs, but is usually simultaneous with ventricular depolarization. Evidence of atrial repolarization (inscription of a Ta wave) is usually hidden within the QRS complex, so this phenomenon for all practical purposes can be ignored clinically. Finally, a U wave, thought to represent the terminal phase of ventricular repolarization, may sometimes be seen following the T wave.

On a historical note, it may be of interest to learn that the impetus for selecting the sequence of letters P—Q—R—S—T—U to denote various waveforms on the ECG has *nothing* to do with electrocardiography. Instead it dates back to the time of the great mathematician, René Descartes, who lived in the mid-1600s. At that time Descartes opted to choose the letter "P" as a convenient starting place in many of his mathematical series primarily because of its alliterative and mnemonic effects ("point P"). These effects operated in the Latin, French, Dutch, and German languages. Willem Einthoven (1860–1927), trained as a physician at the University of Utrecht in Holland, was heavily schooled in mathematics and physiology. It is felt that he adopted this sequence of letters as the nomenclature for electrocardiography as a result of his mathematical training.*

*Henson JR: Descartes and the ECG lettering series. *J Hist Med* 1971;26:181–186.

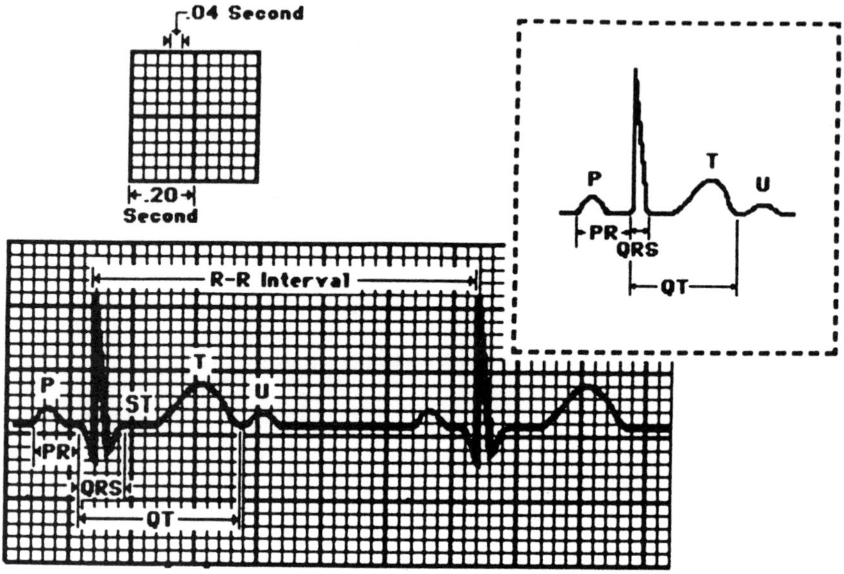

Figure 1-2. Components of the normal ECG.

The PR Interval

As indicated in the upper left-hand portion of Fig. 1-2, ECG paper is made up of a grid in which each little box represents 0.04 second and each large box (=5 little boxes) represents 0.20 second. A number of important ECG intervals are illustrated. The PR interval comprises the time period from the onset of atrial depolarization (the beginning of the P wave) until the onset of ventricular depolarization (the beginning of the QRS complex). This interval normally lasts 0.12 to 0.20 second (between 3 and 5 little boxes). A substantial portion of this time (up to 0.10 second!), is taken up by the delay that occurs at the AV node. A point commonly overlooked is that the PR interval includes not only the time period for the electrical impulse to activate the atria and travel to the AV node, but also the time for it to travel down the bundle of His, the bundle branches, and enter the Purkinje fibers—in short, everything up until ventricular myocardium itself is activated!

The inset in Fig. 1-2 (enclosed within the rectangle in dotted lines) indicates that should there be no negative component to the QRS complex (no Q wave), the PR interval would be calculated from the beginning of the P wave up to the onset of the first positive deflection of the QRS complex (the R wave).

As stated above, the normal PR interval is 0.12 to 0.20 second. These limits are not rigid, as they vary with factors such as age and heart rate. Whereas a PR interval of 0.17 second may be prolonged in a young child, one of 0.21 second may be normal in the elderly. Generally speaking, once conduction is delayed *beyond* 0.20 – 0.21 second in an adult, 1° AV block is said to be present. On the other hand, too short a PR interval (<0.12 second in an adult) may also be abnormal. In such cases, the depolarization impulse may either be accelerated in conduction through the AV node, the AV node itself may be anatomically smaller (hence, there being less nodal tissue resulting in less delay), or the impulse may simply bypass the AV node completely and be conducted to the ventricles via an accessory pathway. The point to remember is that a bell-curve distribution for PR intervals does exist, and 1 to 2% of all adults may have a slightly shortened or prolonged PR interval that is without clinical significance.

The QRS Complex

As previously mentioned, the QRS complex represents spread of the depolarization impulse through the ventricles. Fig. 1-2 indicates that the QRS interval is measured from onset of the first negative deflection (the Q wave) in the complex until the end of the S wave. If there is no Q wave (as illustrated in the dotted upper right-hand inset in this figure), the "QRS interval" is measured from onset of the R wave until completion of either this wave or of an S wave if it is present. Normal duration of the QRS complex in adults is not more than 0.10 second (2-1/2 little boxes). Prolongation beyond this usually suggests intraventricular conduction delay (bundle branch block), although at times uncomplicated left ventricular hypertrophy may slightly prolong QRS duration because it takes longer to activate the increased left ventricular mass.

As in calculation of the PR interval, it is usually *not* important to quibble about a few milliseconds if QRS duration is clearly normal. That is, it really doesn't matter if the QRS complex is 0.07, 0.08, or 0.09 second in duration. All of these are within normal limits. However, meticulous attention should be devoted to precise definition of the interval if QRS duration appears to be prolonged (*greater* than 0.10 second).

At times, a portion of the QRS complex may be isoelectric (lie on the baseline), giving the false impression in a particular lead that the QRS complex is shorter than it really is. To avoid this pitfall, one should always survey at least several leads of the ECG and select the QRS duration (and PR interval) that is of greatest duration.

Terminology for describing the appearance of the QRS complex is extremely important in verbal communication of morphologic characteristics. Although at first glance it may appear confusing, the system for terminology illustrated in Table 1-1 is easy to learn if one remembers a few guiding principles. Deflections are assigned lower-case letters or capital letters depending on their relative size. Smaller deflections receive lower-case denominations while larger deflections receive capital-letter denominations. (Al-

TABLE 1-1

Description of various QRS morphologies

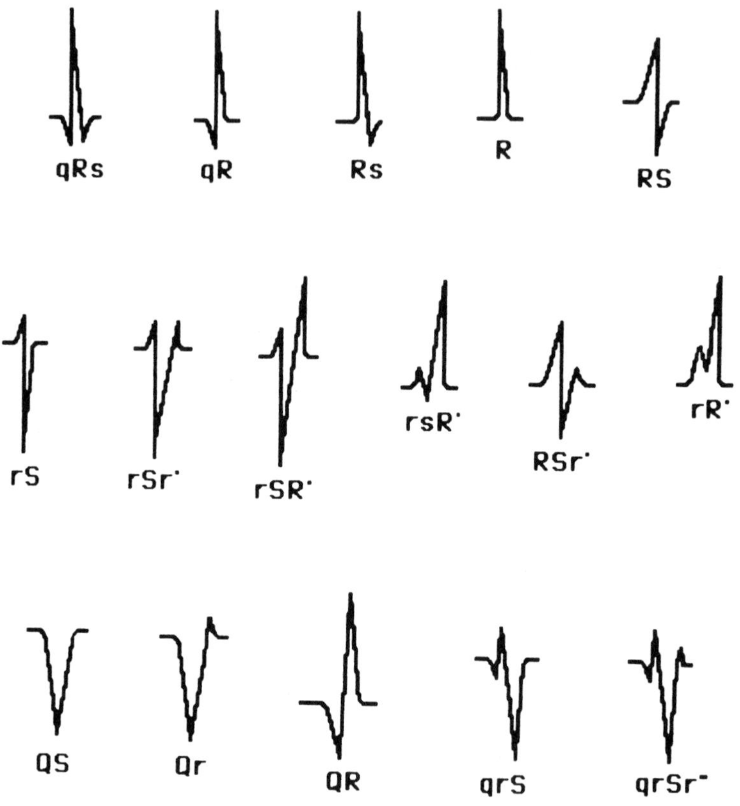

though subject to interobserver variability, capital-letter denomination should probably be assigned for deflections surpassing 3 mm in amplitude.)

The first negative deflection in a particular complex is called a Q wave. The first positive deflection, an R wave. A negative deflection that follows an R wave is called an S wave once it descends below the baseline. If a second positive deflection occurs, it is given a prime notation (an R′ wave). If there is no positive deflection at all and the QRS complex is completely negative, the deflection is called a QS wave (because without an R wave one can't be sure whether the negative deflection represents a Q wave or an S wave).

Q waves take on particular importance in electrocardiography. When sufficiently deep or wide, they often suggest myocardial infarction. The clinical signifiance of Q waves will be discussed in much greater detail later in this book.

Physiology of a Theoretical Myocardial Cell

Before going on further to discuss ST-segment and T-wave abnormalities, a brief review of cellular physiology will help our understanding of the effect of individual myocardial cells on the ECG. As discussed at the beginning of this chapter, an ECG is simply the graphic representation of electrical activity generated by the heart. This electrical activity originates at a cellular level. During the resting state, individual myocardial cells are said to be "polarized"; they are negatively charged on the cell interior and positively charged on their outer surface (Fig. 1-3A). When electrical stimulation of one end of the cell occurs (applied at point *x* in Fig. 1-3B), the inherent negativity of the interior becomes positively charged. As this occurs, a moving boundary of potential difference (between negative and positive charges) is established on the outer surface of the cell, and a wave of depolarization is propagated along the length of the cell. The direction of this wave of depolarization (arrow pointing to the right in Fig. 1-3B) is by convention from negative to positive charge. After the wave of depolarization has spread across the entire length of the cell (to reach point *y*), the entire cell interior will have become positive, and the cell will be "depolarized" (Fig. 1-3C).

It is important to emphasize that Fig. 1-3 illustrates the sequence of events that occur in *one* single theoretical myocardial cell. In reality, there are millions of myocardial cells, and events are *not* all occurring simultaneously in each cell.

Electrocardiographically, for the theoretical myocardial cell shown in Fig. 1-3B, a positive deflection will be inscribed by a recording electrode positioned at *y* since the wave of depolarization (arrow) is seen as directly approaching by this electrode. Once the cell is depolarized (Fig. 1-3C), no net ECG deflection occurs, and an isoelectric ST segment is recorded. This reflects the fact that no net potential difference exists at this moment along the outer cell surface—only negative charges line the cell exterior.

Following depolarization, repolarization of the heart occurs as individual myocardial cells regain the negativity of their interior. The process is complete in F, in which the resting polarized state of the myocardial cell (inherent negativity of the cell interior) has been restored.

Theoretically, repolarization of individual myocardial cells may proceed from either end of the cell. Thus, in Fig. 1-3D, repolarization begins on the left (at position *x*), which was also the first part of the cell to be depolarized. Orientation of the wave of electrical activity (arrow pointing to the left) will be *away* from the exploring electrode in this case, and a negative ECG deflection is recorded during repolarization. If, on the other hand, the last part of the myocardial cell to be depolarized is the first to be repolarized (if repolarization begins on the right at position *y* as in Fig. 1-3E), then the wave of electrical activity (arrow pointing to the right) will be seen as approaching the exploring electrode, and a positive deflection is recorded during repolarization.

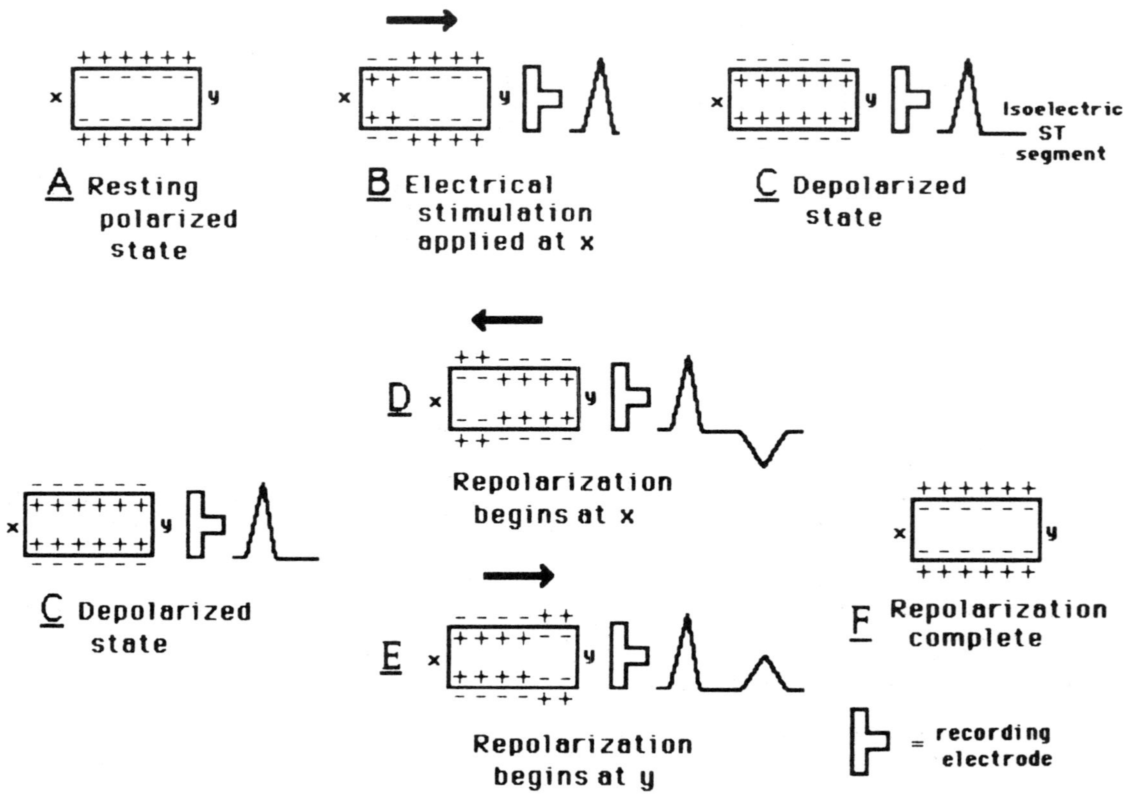

Figure 1-3. Theoretical myocardial cell electrical charges during the resting state, depolarization, and repolarization.

In the human heart, the process of ventricular depolarization proceeds from the inside of the ventricular cavity (the endocardium) to the outer surface of the heart (the epicardium). Ventricular repolarization in the human heart is in the opposite direction. Thus, the first part of the heart to be depolarized (the endocardium) is the last part to be repolarized. This sequence of activation is similar to the events illustrated in Fig. 1-3E where the last portion of the theoretical myocardial cell to be depolarized (y) was the first to be repolarized. As a result, T waves will usually be oriented in a similar direction as the QRS complex in most leads of a normal ECG. That is, if the QRS complex in a particular lead is upright, the T wave will also usually be upright in that lead. If on the other hand QRS complex is inverted in a particular lead, the T wave may normally be inverted.

The ST Segment

The ST segment represents that portion of the normal ECG that connects the QRS complex with the T wave (Fig. 1-2). It therefore represents the time period immediately following ventricular depolarization (which occurs during inscription of the QRS complex), but preceding ventricular repolarization (occurring during inscription of the T wave). Under normal conditions, during the ST segment (during the period immediately following depolarization), no significant regional differences in electric potential exist in the ventricle. As a result, the ST segment normally appears isoelectric and lies on the baseline of the ECG. This situation is similar to the one shown in Fig. 1-3C, in which an isoelectric segment is recorded from the theoretical myocardial cell during the period following depolarization, when no potential difference exists along the outer surface of the cell membrane. Should something happen to affect the relationship between ionic charges on either side of the myocardial cell membrane, deviations of the ST segment above or below the baseline may occur. For example, with injury to the myocardial cell (as takes place during myocardial infarction), negative ions may "leak" out of the cell membrane and change the polarity of the outer cell surface with respect to its interior.

Clinically, accurate interpretation of ST-segment deviations is of fundamental importance in electrocardiography. Yet accurate interpretation is not always easily accomplished. At times it may not even be obvious whether an ST segment is elevated above or depressed below the baseline! Critical in this decision is first to determine exactly what to use as "the baseline." The American Heart Association has recommended that the *PR segment* (that portion of the ECG connecting the end of the P wave with the beginning of the QRS complex) *be used as the baseline and reference point for judging ST-segment deviations.* Therefore, in Fig. 1-4 the ST segment in A is isoelectric (neither elevated above nor depressed below the baseline). Definite ST-segment elevation is seen in B, and definite ST-segment depression in D.

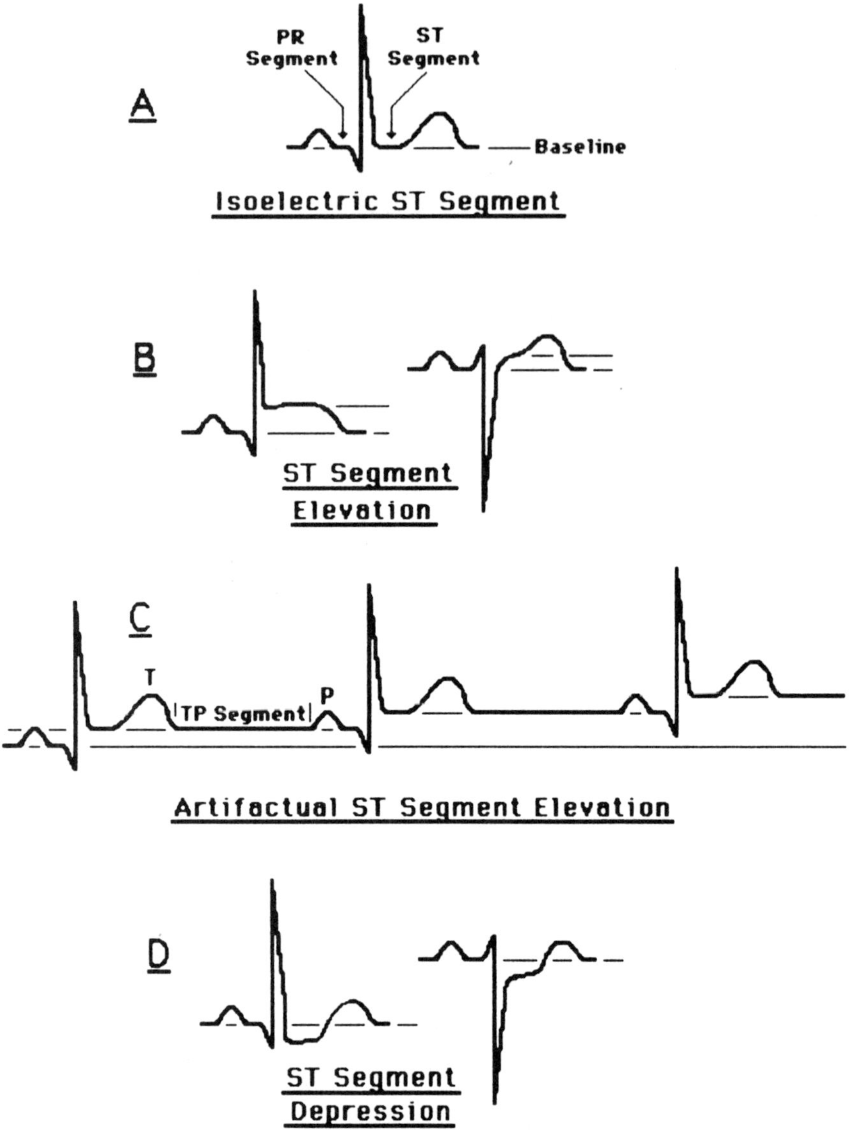

Figure 1-4. ST segment deviations.

At first glance, the ST segment appears to be elevated in C. Close inspection, however, reveals that wander of the TP segment has invalidated use of the PR baseline as a reference point and produced artifactual ST-segment elevation. Thus, there is no true ST-segment elevation in C. Other situations in which the TP segment may have to be used as the reference point for judging ST-segment deviations include when the PR interval is very short, when there is PR-segment deviation from the baseline (as may occur with atrial infarction or pericarditis), or if artifact distorts the PR segment. These situations are generally few and far between.

Equally important in assessing ST-segment deviations is interpretation of the *contour* of such deviations. With respect to ST-segment elevation, Fig. 1-5 illustrates the terminology we favor. The type of ST-segment elevation shown in A is often termed coved (or "convex up"). Note the abrupt "take-off" following the QRS complex, and the ST segment itself is very rounded in contour. Coved ST-segment elevation is commonly associated with the injury current seen with acute myocardial infarction. Contrast this to the appearance of the ST-segment elevation depicted in B that is said to have an "upward concavity." Here the takeoff is more gradual, and the ST segment describes a much gentler upward sloping curve on its way to the summit of the T wave. Finally in C, J-point ST-segment elevation is illustrated. The J point marks the *junction* of the end of the QRS complex with the beginning of the ST segment. In individuals with the normal variant known as *early repolarization,* a *notch* often occurs at the J point, and the ST segment may take off several millimeters above the baseline at this point. The contour of this ST-segment elevation is most often similar to that shown in B. Interpretation of ST-segment abnormalities will be discussed in much greater detail later in the book. For now, the "smiley" and "frowny" figures at the bottom of Fig. 1-5 should assist in recall of the *usual* clinical implications for each type of ST-segment elevation.

The T Wave

The T wave is the ECG representation of ventricular repolarization. During this period myocardial cells regain their initial polarized state.

As discussed above, the T-wave deflection in patients with a normal heart tends to be in the same direction as the QRS deflection in most leads. This is because the general orientation of the wave of electrical activity for ventricular depolarization and repolarization is in a similar direction. Therefore, in the normal standard ECG of an *adult,* T waves should be upright (positive) in most leads. This is the case in Fig. 1-6 in which both the QRS complex and the T waves are upright in most leads.

PROBLEM: In which leads of Fig. 1-6 is the T wave negative (inverted)?

ANSWER to Fig. 1-6: The T wave is negative in leads III, aVR, and V_1. While the T wave will usually be positive in most leads of a normal ECG, it may normally be inverted in several leads. These are indicated in Table 1-2.

Clinically, the ECG appearance of T waves is subject to a number of

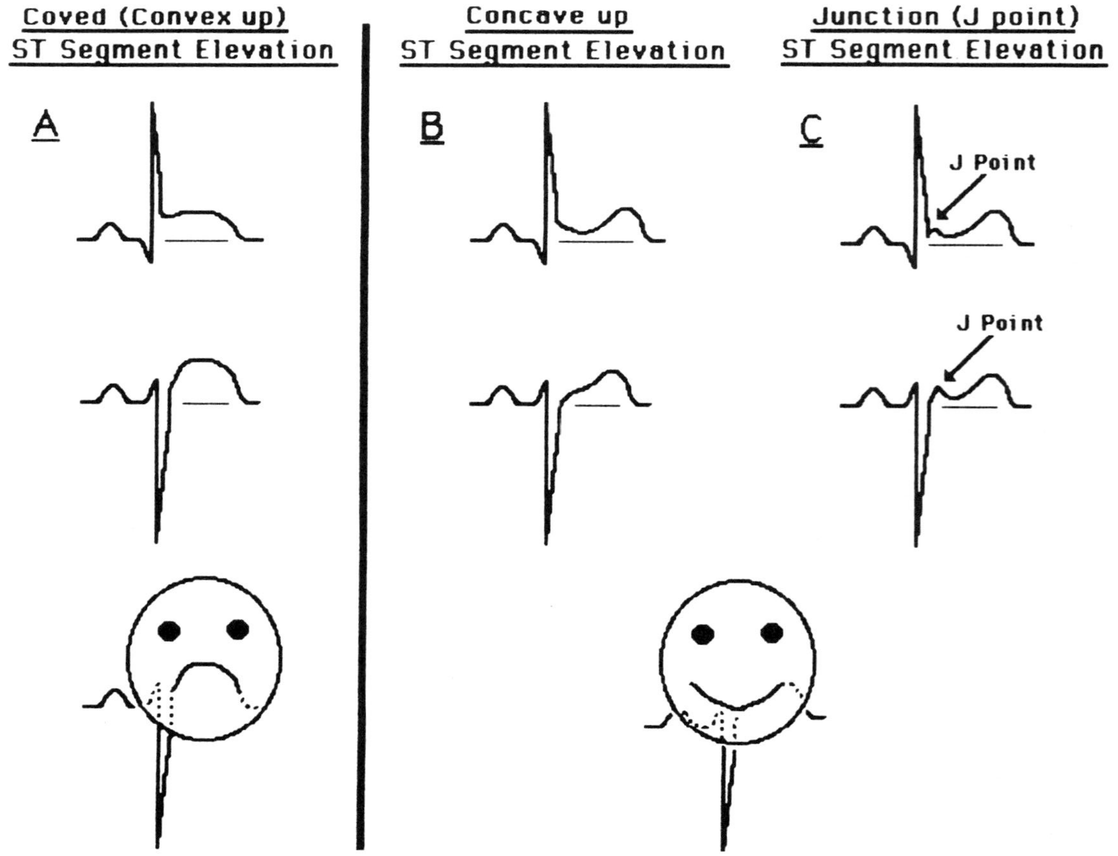

Figure 1-5. Description of ST segment elevations.

different configurations. Terminology used to describe these configurations is illustrated in Fig. 1-7.

T-wave changes result from alterations in the process of repolarization. There are two principal ways in which such alterations take place. The first produces "primary T-wave changes"—it is due to factors that affect the internal environment of the myocardial cell. Examples include ischemia or injury to the myocardial cell, in which negative charges may leak across the cell membrane. Typically, primary T-wave changes produce the symmetric T-wave inversion shown in Fig. 1-7F.

The other principal type of repolarization change is known as a "secondary T-wave change." This T-wave abnormality is the direct result of (it is *secondary* to) an altered sequence of ventricular activation. Since the order of ventricular depolarization is changed, the order of repolarization will also change. Clinically, secondary T-wave changes occur with conditions in which the sequence of ventricular activation is altered, such as in bundle branch block and ventricular hypertrophy. Electrocardiographically such changes tend to produce ST-segment depression and the asymmetric T-wave inversion shown in Fig. 1-7G.

When these repolarization changes occur with ventricular hypertrophy, they are commonly known as "strain." If causes of both primary and secondary T-wave changes occur simultaneously (if for example, left ventricular hypertrophy and ischemia coexist), either clear differentiation between primary and secondary T-wave morphology may not be possible, or one type of T-wave change may mask the other. It is important to emphasize that T-wave changes are often "nonspecific," and that any of the other T-wave morphologies illustrated in Fig. 1-7 may also occur as the result of primary and/or secondary alterations in the repolarization process.

Numerous clinical factors affect T waves. In addition to those discussed above, other factors affecting T waves are listed in Table 1-3. This list is *not* complete. Note that many of the causes of T-wave changes are *not* cardiac-related, and that even such seemingly benign actions as hyperventilating or having a drink of iced water may in certain individuals produce significant (and often dramatic) alteration in the appearance of T waves. Even though one must *always* assume that the patient with chest pain and an abnormal ECG has a cardiac etiology for his symptoms until proven otherwise, consideration of noncardiac causes of T-wave abnormalities remains extremely important. Thus, the anxious individual who presents to an emergency department complaining of chest pain may have T-wave abnormalities on ECG due to a variety of reasons *other* than coronary artery disease. These include anxiety (what person doesn't exhibit some anxiety in an emergency department?), hyperventilation (from anxiety), stress or other emotions (fear of or pain from venipuncture to obtain blood studies, especially when performed just before the ECG is taken), temperature extremes (what examination room is ever warm enough?), and oral ingestion (either from a recently eaten meal or a drink of iced water from the fountain in the waiting room). If one adds to this list the many types of normal repolarization variants that are so commonly found in the general population, the difficulty in interpreting T-wave changes becomes evident.

The U Wave

The U wave is the small upright deflection that may follow the T wave (Fig. 1-2). Although its exact significance is not known, it is thought to represent the final phase of ventricular repolarization during which time the

Figure 1-6. Normal ECG of an adult. Note that the T waves are upright in most leads.

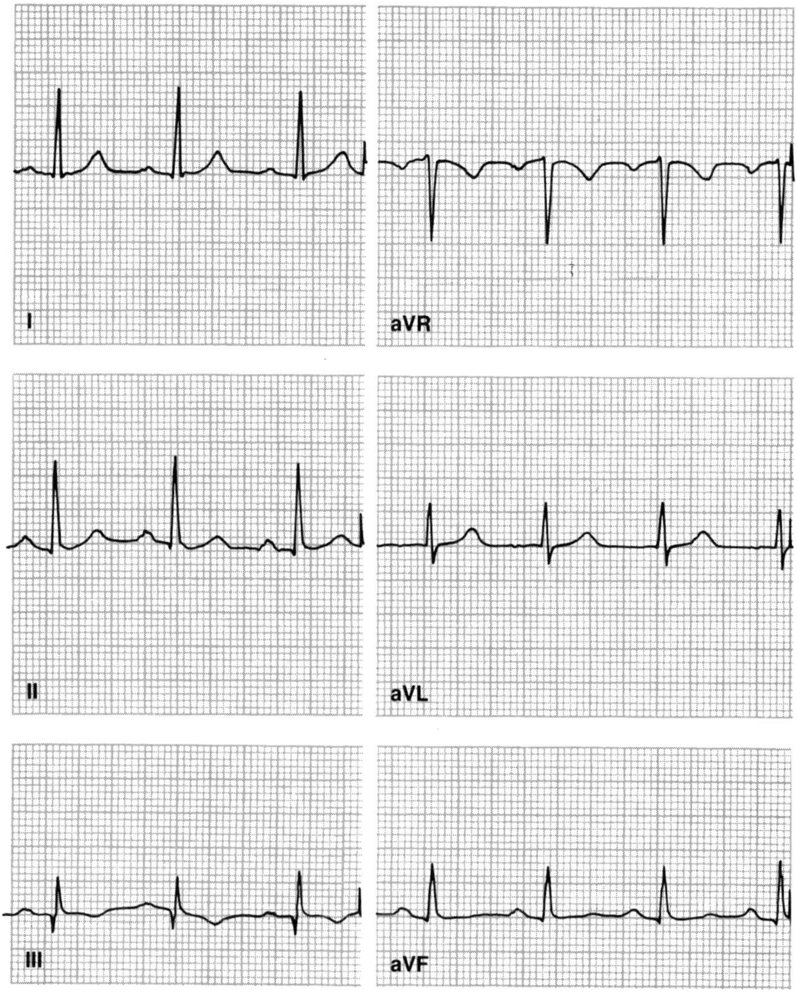

Purkinje system recovers. U waves are often not seen on the normal ECG. Even if present, they may be difficult to detect when they fuse with or are hidden by the terminal portion of the T wave. Leads in which U waves are usually most easily recognized are V_2 to V_4.

Clinically, U waves commonly occur in association with bradycardia, hypokalemia, use of certain drugs (quinidine, procainamide, phenothiazines), central nervous system disorders, and left ventricular hypertrophy. Hypokalemia, in particular, should be strongly suspected whenever the amplitude of the U wave exceeds that of the T wave in one or more leads.

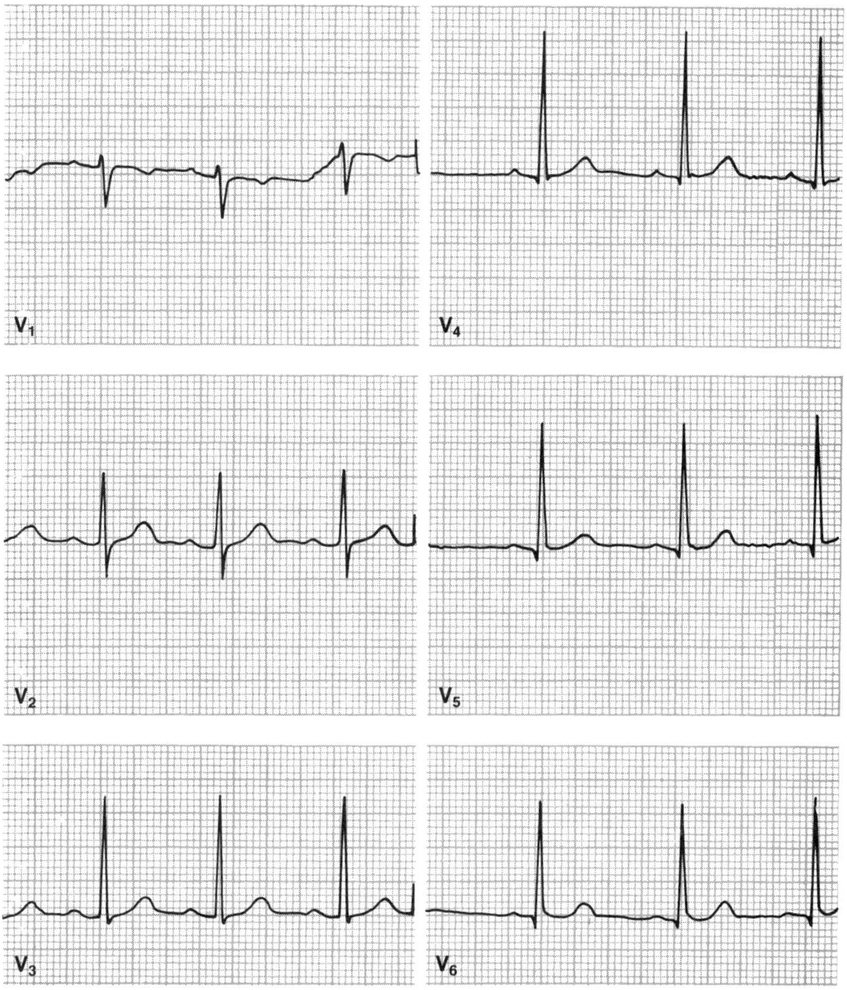

TABLE 1-2

Leads in which the T wave may be normally inverted in the adult ECG

ECG lead	Comments
III, aVF	Especially with a horizontal axis
aVL	Especially with a vertical axis
V_1	The T wave may normally be upright, isoelectric, or inverted in lead V_1. It usually is upright in adults by V_2, and should definitely be so by lead V_3.
aVR	Normally there is global negativity in this lead (the P wave, QRS complex, and T wave are all negative)

The QT Interval

The QT interval comprises the period from the onset of ventricular depolarization (Q wave) until ventricular repolarization is complete (end of the T wave). Clinically, it is important to recognize QT prolongation because this may sometimes be the only sign of metabolic disturbance, pharmacologic drug effect, or other ECG abnormality (Table 1-4).

Determination of the QT interval is illustrated in Fig. 1-8A. As shown, one should measure from the beginning of the QRS complex until the end of the T wave. A number of leads may need to be inspected to ensure accuracy. Use the longest QT interval measured from a lead in which you can *clearly* define the terminal portion of the T wave. Measurement of the QT interval is particularly difficult when there is diffuse ST-segment and T-wave flattening. Similarly, in hypokalemia, the presence of U waves that merge with the terminal portion of the T wave may make it impossible to differentiate between the QT interval and the QU interval.

It is difficult to define specific normal limits for duration of the QT interval because it varies with the heart rate, age, and sex of the patient. An inverse relationship exists between heart rate and QT-interval duration. The faster the heart rate, the shorter the QT interval. Conversely, the slower the heart rate, the longer the QT interval. With respect to the age and sex of the patient, the QT interval of women tends to be slightly longer than it is in men or children.

Practically speaking, the clinician is usually more concerned with determining whether the QT interval is prolonged than if it is shortened. Although QT interval shortening may be associated with digitalis effect or hypercalcemia, it is rare for either condition to be picked up solely on the basis of identifying a shortened QT interval. On the other hand, QT-interval prolongation occurs more commonly, is easier to recognize, and not infrequently is the only ECG clue to a number of medical conditions (Table 1-4).

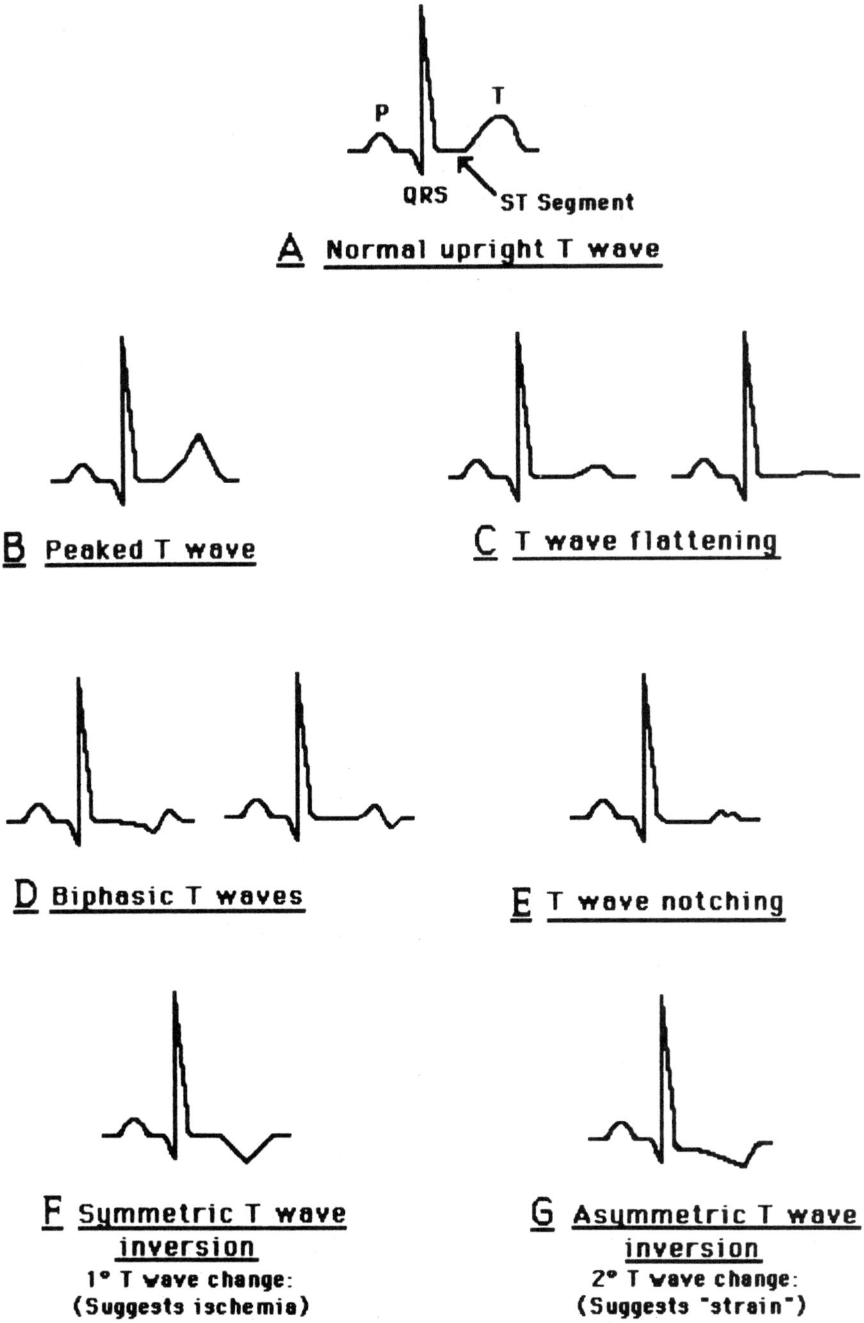

Figure 1-7. Description of T wave morphologies.

TABLE 1-3

Causes of T-wave changes

Physiologic and metabolic	Cardiac-related
Drugs	Myocardial infarction
Electrolyte disorders	Coronary artery disease/ischemia
Acid-base disturbance	Coronary spasm
Hypoxia	Pericarditis
Hyperventilation	Cardiomyopathy
Temperature extremes	Mitral valve prolapse
Exercise	Left or right ventricular hypertrophy
Sleep	Conduction defects
Oral ingestion (food, iced water, etc.)	Tachycardia
Position changes	
Emotions (anxiety, fear, etc.)	**Miscellaneous**
Uremia	Repolarization variants
Shock	Juvenile T-wave syndrome
Acute illness	Central nervous system disorders
Stress	(stroke, intracerebral bleed, etc.)

Detailed tables defining precise limits for short, normal, and prolonged QT intervals according to age, sex, and heart rate of the patient can be found in comprehensive books on electrocardiography. Table 1-5 illustrates a greatly simplified adaptation of such a table. For ease of recall, age and sex of the patient have been omitted, and only the approximate upper normal limit of the QT interval for a given heart rate is included.

For example, the QT interval in Fig. 1-8B is 0.44 second. This is less than the maximum QT interval (of 0.47 second) that is allowed for a heart rate of 50 beats/min. On the other hand, the QT interval of 0.70 second in Fig. 1-8C far exceeds the upper normal limit of 0.47 second.

TABLE 1-4

Common causes of QT-interval prolongation

Conditions in which QT prolongation may be the only ECG clue:

- Drugs (quinidine, procainamide, phenothiazines, tricyclic antidepressants, etc.)
- Electrolytes (hypokalemia, hypocalcemia)
- Central nervous system catastrophe (subarachnoid or subdural bleed, cerebrovascular accident, etc.)

Conditions in which QT prolongation is usually secondary to the underlying ECG disorder:

- Myocardial ischemia or infarction
- Intraventricular conduction abnormalities (left or right bundle branch block, nonspecific intraventricular conduction delay, etc.)

An alternative method that can be used to decide if the QT interval is prolonged is derived from the rule of thumb that states that *the QT interval is normally less than one half of the R-R interval.* When this determination cannot be easily made by simple inspection, one may "walk out" the QT interval with calipers. Position the calipers so that the legs span the QT interval. If the next advance of the calipers falls before the next QRS complex, the QT interval is probably normal for that heart rate.

Application of this method to Fig. 1-8B suggests that the QT interval is

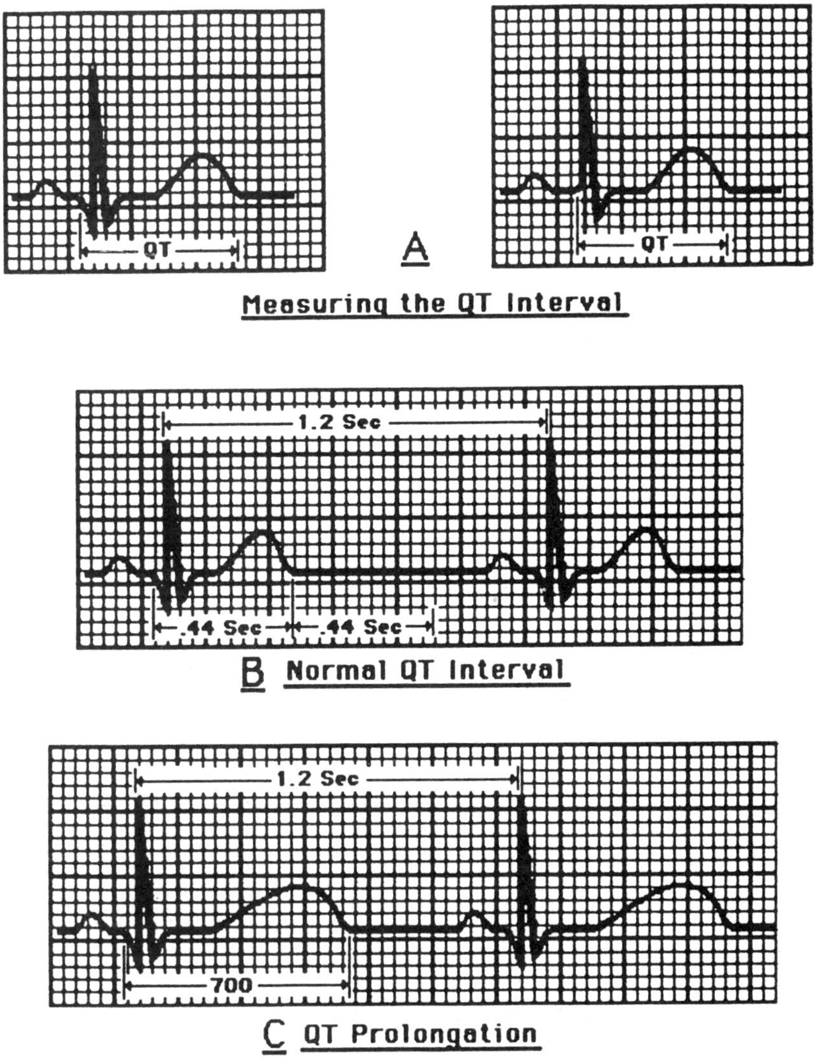

Figure 1-8. Determination of QT interval prolongation.

TABLE 1-5

Simplified table for determination of QT-interval prolongation

Heart rate (beats/min)	Approximate upper normal limit of the QT interval (sec)
50	0.47
60	0.43
70	0.41
80	0.39
90	0.37
100	0.35
110	0.33

probably normal for this heart rate (since it is definitely less than one half the R-R interval), whereas it is clearly prolonged for Fig. 1-8C. Although not nearly as precise as using a table to determine QT-interval prolongation, visual inspection as described above is easy to do and fairly accurate when the heart rate is under 100 beats per minute.

The Standard 12-Lead ECG

Now that we've introduced the various components of the normal electrocardiographic complex, let us discuss how they have been put together to make up the standard ECG. The first ECG machine was invented in 1902 by Willem Einthoven. Initially, only three monitoring leads (I, II, and III) were used. As a result, events could only be viewed in one plane, and an incomplete picture of the heart's electrical activity was obtained. However, since events really occur in three-dimensional space, monitoring leads from *all* three planes (the frontal, sagittal, and horizontal or transverse planes) are needed to view the heart's electrical activity adequately.

We can illustrate this concept by examining the sphere shown in Fig. 1-9. It would be virtually impossible to view an area from the undersurface of this sphere if observation points were only positioned in the frontal plane. Similarly, one would not be able to obtain adequate visualization of the lateral aspect of the sphere from a vantage point in the frontal plane. To visualize the sphere completely, one would have to position multiple observation points strategically in all three planes around the object. The more vantage points used, the more complete the visualization.

The same holds true in electrocardiography. To view every aspect of the heart's electrical activity completely as it unfolds during the normal cardiac cycle, hundreds of monitoring leads would have to be positioned in the frontal, sagittal, and transverse planes. Although an ECG recorded from

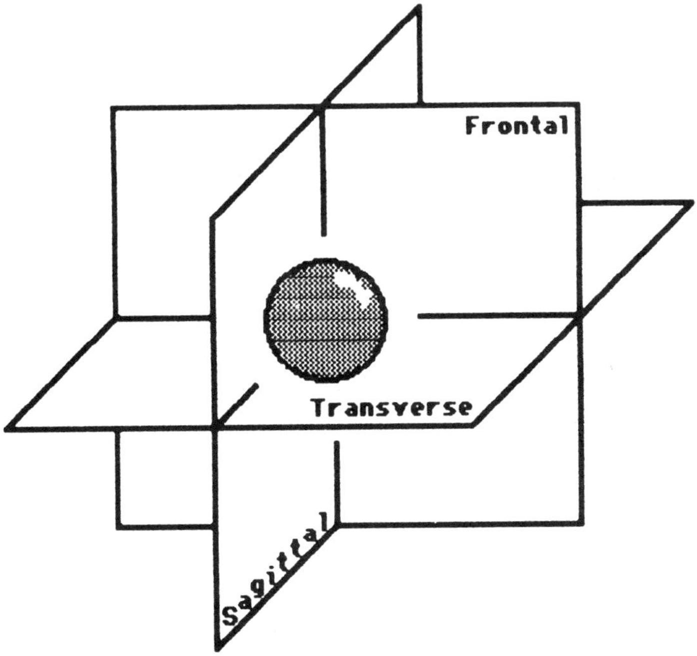

Figure 1-9. Three-dimensional perspective of sphere.

such a lead system would have the advantage of being extremely accurate, the task of setting up that number of electrodes would be so cumbersome and time-consuming as to make it impractical for clinical use.

As a compromise, we have limited the number of monitoring leads used in recording the standard ECG to 12. This number allows for adequate "three-dimensional" visualization of the heart's electrical activity in most adults, yet is not too cumbersome clinically to apply. Six monitoring leads view the heart's electrical activity from the frontal plane (leads I, II, III, aVR, aVL, and aVF), and six view it from the transverse plane (leads V_1, V_2, V_3, V_4, V_5, and V_6). However, despite general acceptance of this 12-lead monitoring system, certain areas of the heart are still not well visualized. In these instances, use of additional leads V_7, V_1R, V_2R, etc.) may be needed.

Systematic Approach to ECG Interpretation

The key to accurate ECG interpretation is to use a systematic approach. This clinical axiom has been borrowed from our radiology colleagues who long ago recognized that failure to be systematic in interpretation was the principal reason that subtle and sometimes even obvious X-ray findings were overlooked.

If one follows the eyes of a number of radiologists while a series of chest X-ray films are interpreted, it becomes immediately apparent that the sequence used for analysis of roentgenographic findings varies tremendously from one radiologist to another. While one radiologist might first survey the soft tissues before inspecting the heart, lungs, and mediastinal structures, a second may proceed with his examination in the reverse order. Still a third might begin with the heart, and proceed to examine remaining structures in a circumferential manner while making his way toward the periphery. Yet, were the eyes of any *one* particular radiologist followed as he consecutively interpreted a series of X-ray films, the observer would likely be struck by the repetitive pattern of analysis for the reading of each X-ray.

Thus, despite the fact that no two radiologists employ exactly the same systematic approach, *individual* radiologists tend to be very consistent in the application of their own personalized system. By contrast, most nonradiologists are decidedly less organized in their approach to interpreting X-rays, and consequently are much more likely to miss even obvious findings.

In a similar manner, both the accuracy and speed of ECG interpretation may be enhanced by incorporating a systematic approach. The approach we favor is illustrated in Table 1-6. With practice, you should be able to analyze most ECGs by this method within a minute or two. Whether you choose to adopt this system, or prefer to use your own, is not nearly as important as following a rigorous policy of self-discipline to become more

TABLE 1-6

Systematic approach to ECG interpretation

RATE

RHYTHM
- Regularity of rhythm?
- Presence of P waves?
  - Upright P wave in lead II?
- Width of QRS complex?
  - Intervals: PR/QRS/QT intervals
  - Is bundle branch block present?
- Relation of P waves to QRS complex?
  - Is each QRS "married" to a preceding P wave?

AXIS

CHAMBER ENLARGEMENT
- LAE/RAE?
- LVH/RVH?

QRST CHANGES
- Presence of **Q** waves?
- Is there normal **R**-wave progression?
- Is there **ST**-segment elevation or depression?
- Is there **T**-wave inversion?

systematic in interpretation. Only in this way can one hope to avoid prematurely jumping at obvious findings without having searched the rest of the tracing for more subtle clues.

Note in Table 1-6 that evaluation of "intervals" (the PR, QRS, and QT intervals) is included under Rhythm, and is assessed *before* evaluation of chamber enlargement and infarction (QRST changes). Analysis of intervals should be done early, because it will lead to detection of intraventricular conduction delays. Recognition of conditions such as bundle branch block will often *modify* how one interprets the remainder of the ECG for changes of infarction or of chamber enlargement.

The importance of a systematic approach is emphasized with analysis of Chamber Enlargement and QRST Changes. It is easy to overlook ECG diagnosis of enlargement of one or more of the cardiac chambers unless one consistently considers this possibility. Similarly, the presence of small q waves, abnormalities in R-wave progression, and/or ST-T wave abnormalities may also be easily overlooked unless regularly included in one's systematic approach. Thus when interpreting an ECG, each of the 12 leads should first be inspected for the presence of Q waves. Following this, R-wave progression should be analyzed. [With "normal R-wave progression," the height of the R wave progressively increases as one moves across the precordial (chest) leads until that lead is reached where R-wave amplitude exceeds S-wave amplitude. This normally occurs between leads V2 and V4, and is known as the *zone of transition.*] Finally, ST segments and T waves should be assessed in each of the 12 leads.

PROBLEM: Apply the systematic approach for analysis of intervals and QRST changes to the ECG shown in Fig. 1-10. For the moment, ignore determination of rate, rhythm, axis, and chamber enlargement; these items will be covered in detail in succeeding chapters.

INTERPRETATION of Fig. 1-10

Intervals

PR interval: Normal (≤0.20 second).

QRS interval: Normal (≤0.10 second).

QT interval: Prolonged (the QT interval exceeds one-half the R-R interval).

QRST changes

Q waves: Small q waves are present in leads I, II, aVL, and aVF. (An rSR′ complex is seen in lead III.)

R-wave progression: Normal. The R wave increases in amplitude from V_1 to V_3 until transition occurs between V_3 and V_4.

ST segments and T waves: Slight J-point ST-segment elevation with an upward concavity is present in leads I, II, aVL, V_5, and V_6. T waves are upright in most leads, although they are more prominent and peaked than usual. T-wave inversion is present in leads III, aVR, and V_1.

COMMENT: The principal abnormality in this ECG is QT prolongation. As previously indicated in Table 1-4, conditions in which QT prolongation may be the only ECG clue include drug effects, electrolyte imbalance, and

Figure 1-10. 12-lead ECG.

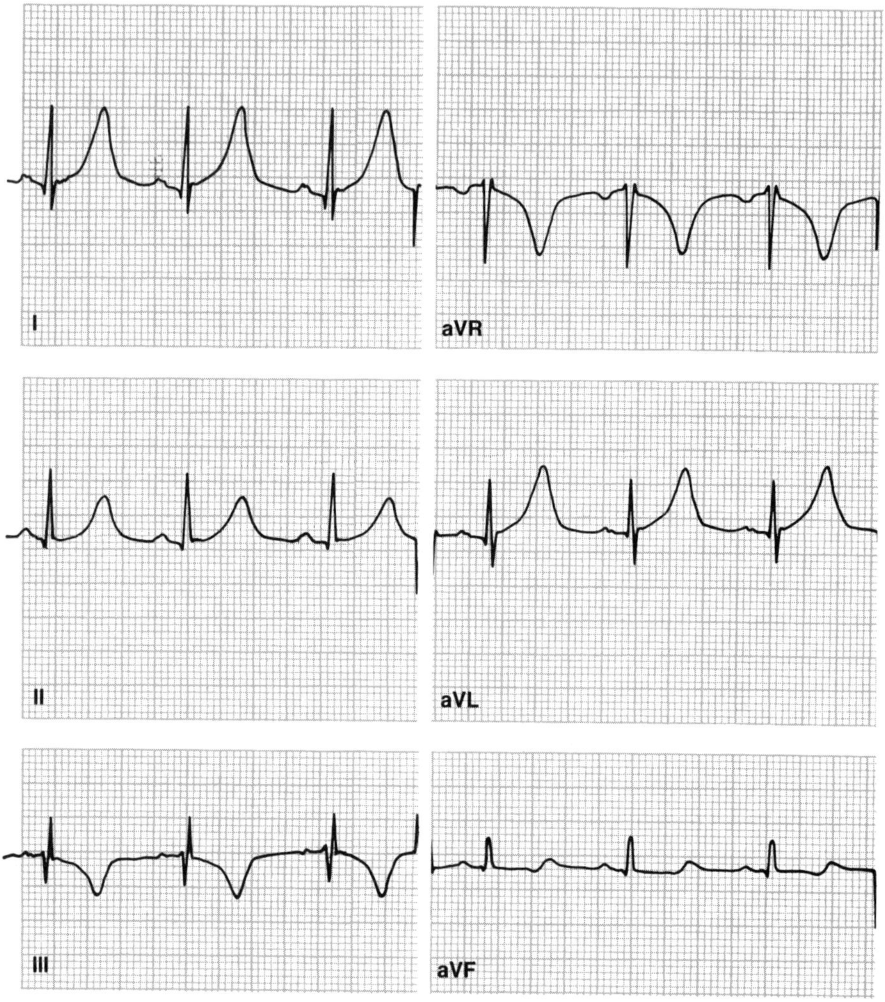

central nervous system catastrophes. This particular patient was being treated with too high a dose of quinidine. Detection of QT prolongation would have been easy to miss in this tracing without systematic evaluation.

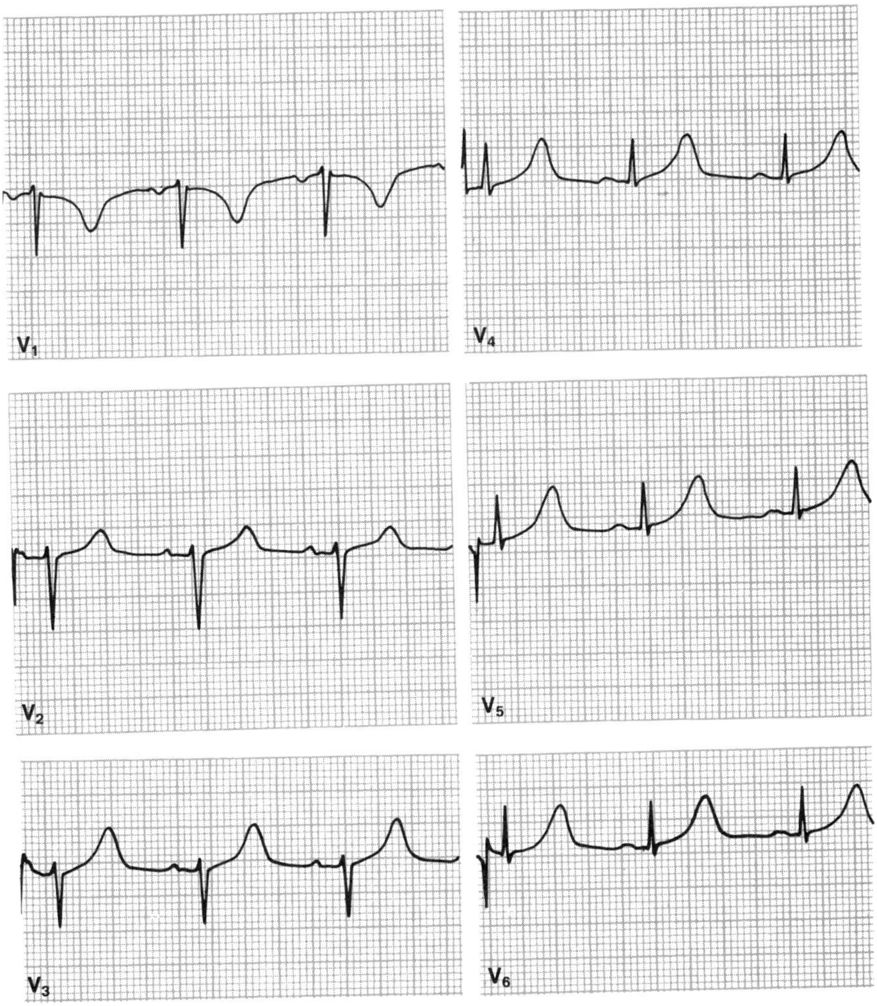

CHAPTER 2

RATE AND RHYTHM

The two initial steps in systematic interpretation of the standard 12-lead ECG are determination of rate and rhythm. Both will be addressed in this chapter. First we'll introduce a quick and easy method for calculating heart rate. Then we'll apply this method to the task of basic rhythm analysis. Evaluation of more complex dysrhythmias such as AV blocks and differentiation of ventricular ectopy from aberrancy is beyond the scope of this book.

Determination of Heart Rate

Many different methods exist for calculating heart rate. Perhaps the easiest to master is to simply *take 300 and divide it by the number of boxes in the R-R interval*. Explanation of this method is as follows. The dimensions of small and large boxes on ECG grid paper are 1 mm and 5 mm, respectively. Since the usual speed of recording is 25 mm/second, the amount of time needed to travel the distance represented by each small box (1 mm) is 1/25 (0.04) of a second (Fig. 2-1). Similarly, the amount of time needed to travel the distance represented by each large box (5 mm) is $5 \times 0.04 = 0.20$ second. If a QRS complex were to occur every large box (every 0.20 sec) as shown in Fig. 2-1, then five QRS complexes would occur in 1 second ($5 \times 0.20 = 1.0$ sec). Since there are 60 seconds in a minute, the heart rate would be 300 beats per minute (5 beats/sec $\times$ 60 sec = 300 beats/min).

Thus, if a QRS complex occurs every large box, the heart rate will be 300 beats/min. If the rate were only half as fast (if a QRS complex occurred every 2 large boxes), it would be 150 beats/min ($300 \div 2 = 150$ beats/min). A heart rate one third as fast (a QRS occurring every three large boxes) reflects a rate of 100 beats/min ($300 \div 3$); a QRS complex every four large boxes, a rate of 75 beats/min ($300 \div 4$); and so forth (Fig. 2-2).

PROBLEM: Apply this method in calculating the heart rate of the examples shown in Fig. 2-3.

ANSWER to Fig. 2-3A: A QRS complex occurs every 6 large boxes in this example. Therefore, the heart rate is $300 \div 6 = 50$ beats/min.

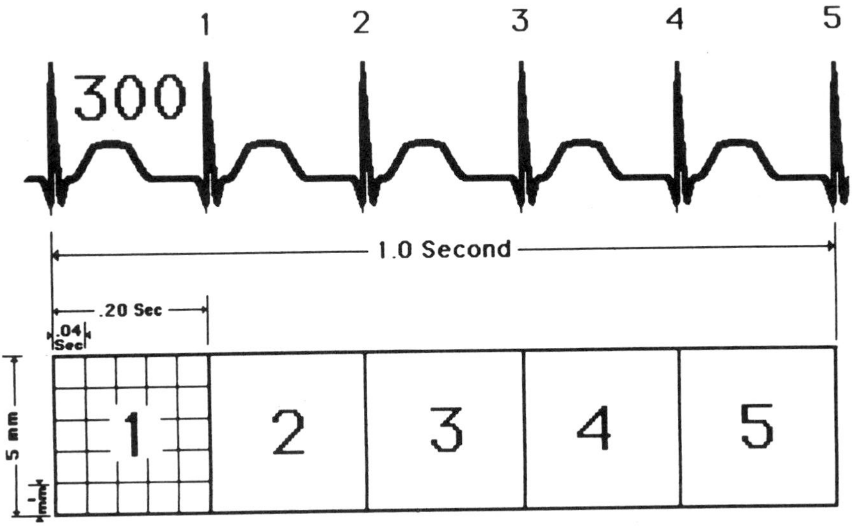

Figure 2-1. Since a QRS complex (a beat) occurs every large box (every 0.20 sec), 5 beats occur in 1.0 second. Since there are 60 seconds in a minute, the heart rate is 300 beats per minute (5 beats/sec × 60 sec = 300 beats/min).

ANSWER to Fig. 2-3B: The R-R interval in this example is 4 large boxes. Thus, the heart rate is 300 ÷ 4 = 75 beats/min.

ANSWER to Fig. 2-3C: This example shows that rhythms with very slow heart rates may also be calculated by this method. The R-R interval is 9 large boxes. If it were an even 10 large boxes, then the heart rate would be 300 ÷ 10, or 30 beats/min. Since it is a little faster than this, the heart rate is about 33 beats/min.

PROBLEM: Determine the heart rate of the two examples shown in Fig. 2-4. (Note that the R-R interval does *not* equal a precise number of large boxes in these two examples.)

ANSWER to Fig. 2-4A: The rhythm is regular. (When in doubt, regularity of a rhythm may be confirmed by measuring each R-R interval with a pair of calipers, or by marking down the R-R interval on a sheet of paper and checking to see if each beat is on time.)

When the rhythm is regular, the easiest way to determine the R-R interval is to select a QRS complex that begins on a *heavy* line, and to see when the next QRS complex occurs. In this example, the upstroke of the R wave of the first QRS complex occurs on a heavy line. The R-R interval is between 3 and 4 large boxes, and slightly closer to the former. If it were 3

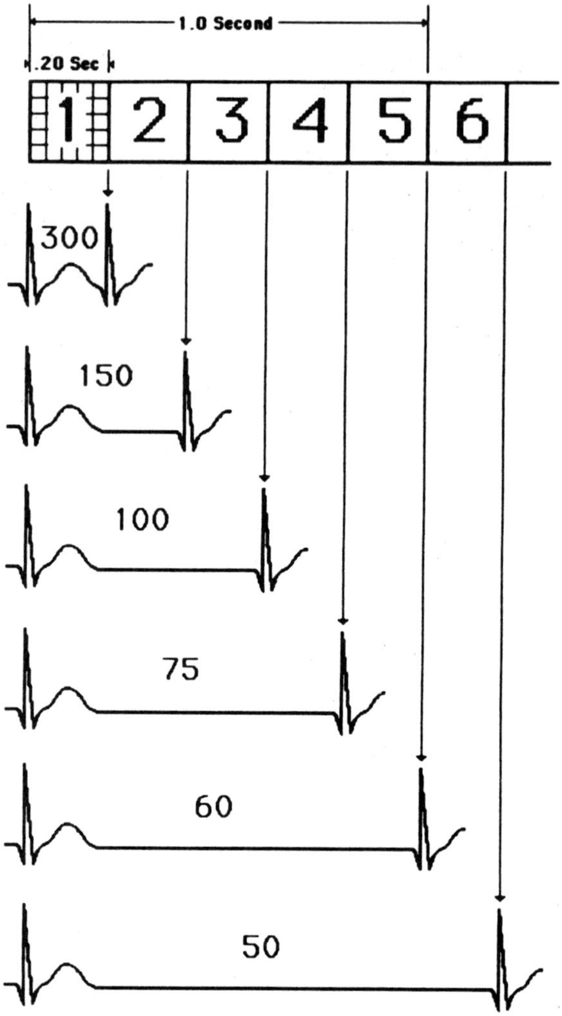

Figure 2-2. A quick and easy method of calculating heart rate is to divide 300 by the number of boxes in the R-R interval.

boxes, the rate would be 100 beats/min. If it were 4 boxes, the rate would be 75 beats/min. The rate is between 85 and 90 beats/min.

ANSWER to Fig. 2-4B: The rhythm is again regular, and the R-R interval is between 5 and 6 large boxes. If the R-R interval were 5 large boxes, the heart rate would be 60 beats/min. If it were 6 large boxes, the rate would be 50 beats/min. Since it is about $5\frac{1}{2}$ large boxes, the heart rate is about 55 beats/min.

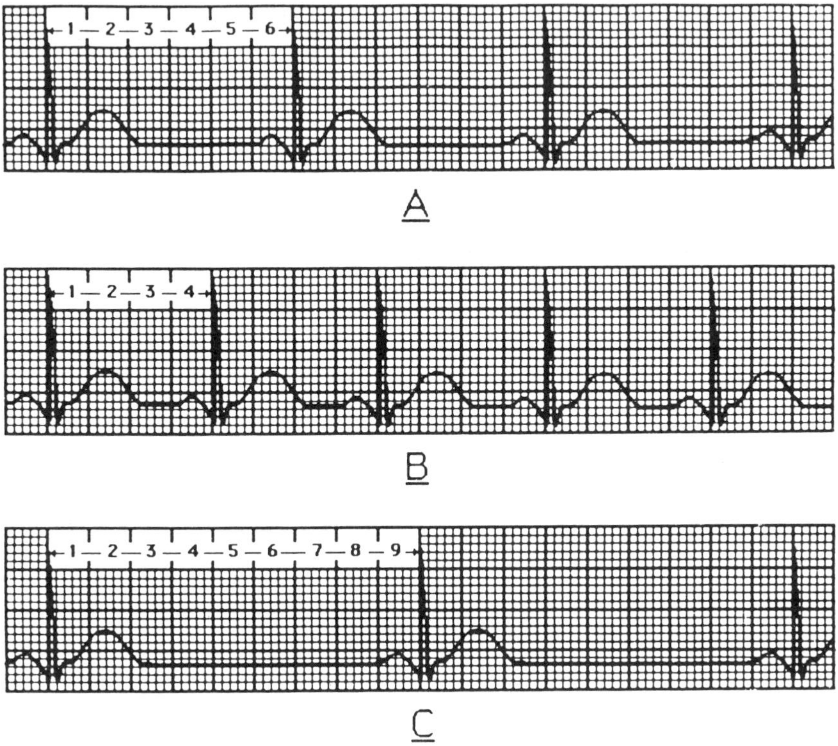

Figure 2-3

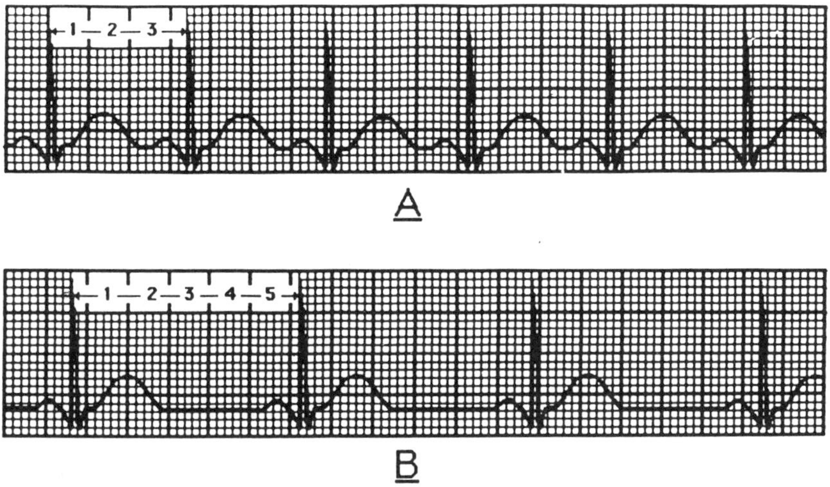

Figure 2-4

When the heart rate is extremely rapid (between 150 and 300 beats/min), accurate estimation becomes difficult, since minor discrepancies in how one measures the R-R interval may have a disproportionately large effect on the calculated rate. Not accounting for the thickness of one's calipers or even of the QRS complex itself may throw the estimate off by as much as 30 beats per minute!

PROBLEM: Calculate the heart rate in Fig. 2-5. Is it above or below 200 beats/min?

ANSWER to Fig. 2-5: Since the R-R interval is between 1 to 2 large boxes, the heart rate is between 150 and 300 beats/min. It would be hard to tell by the method just discussed whether the heart rate is above or below 200 beats/min.

Fig. 2-6 illustrates a handy trick for overcoming this difficulty. When the rate is fast and regular, one may simply measure the R-R interval of every two beats (or of one half the actual rate).

The R-R interval of every other beat in Fig. 2-6 is just over 3 large boxes. Thus, half of the rate is about 95 beats/min. The actual rate is 190 beats/min.

As stated above, the R-R interval of the rhythm in Fig. 2-5 is between 1 and 2 large boxes. If it were exactly 1 large box (= 5 little boxes), the heart rate would be 300 beats/min. If it were exactly 2 large boxes (= 10 little boxes), the rate would be 150 beats/min. One might reason that if an R-R interval of 5 little boxes reflects a heart rate of 300 beats/min, and one of 10 little boxes reflects a rate of 150 beats/min, each little box should represent an increment of 30 beats/min. Similarly, an R-R interval of 1-1/2 large boxes (7-1/2 little boxes) should represent a heart rate that is exactly between 300 and 150 beats/min, or 225 beats/min.

Unfortunately, calculation of heart rate is not quite so simple. The incremental increase in heart rate for each little box is *not* equal. This concept is illustrated in Fig. 2-7.

Note in Fig. 2-7 that there is a 50 beat/min decrement in heart rate (from 300 to 250 beats/min) when the R-R interval lengthens from 5 to 6 little boxes, but only a 17-beat/min decrement (from 167 to 150 beats/min)

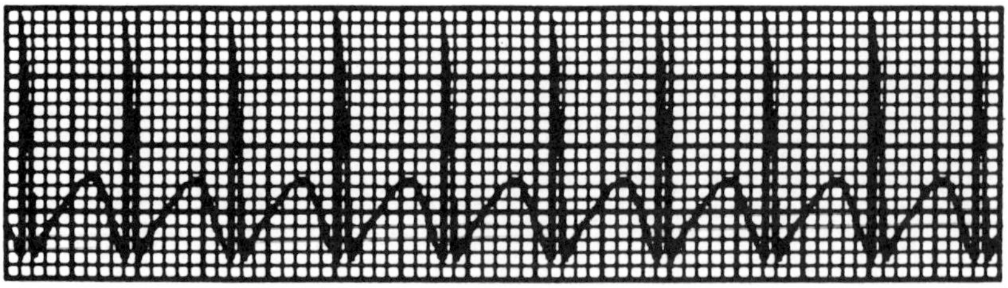

Figure 2-5

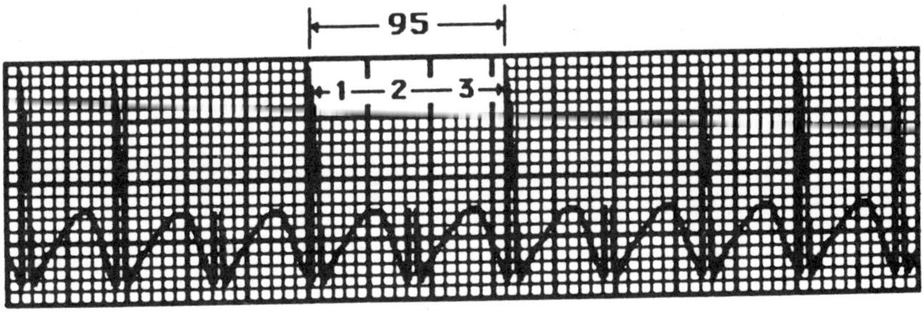

Figure 2-6

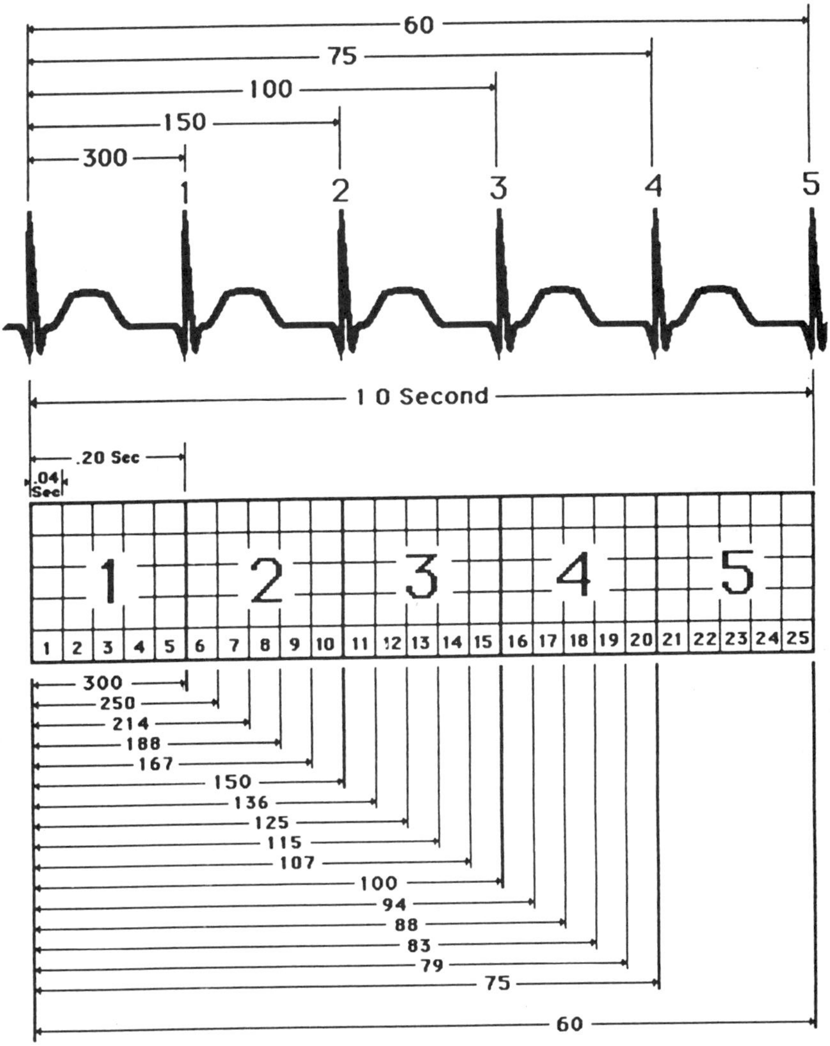

Figure 2-7

when it lengthens from 9 to 10 little boxes. Decrements become nearly equal once the heart rate drops below 100 beats/min.

PROBLEM: Return to Fig. 2-5 and determine the number of little boxes in the R-R interval. Refer to Fig. 2-7 to determine the heart rate.

ANSWER: The upstroke of the R wave of the fourth QRS complex in Fig. 2-5 occurs on a heavy line. Counting over, the R-R interval is 8 little boxes in duration. According to Fig. 2-7, the heart rate is 188 beats/min.

In practice, estimation of heart rate by dividing 300 by the number of large boxes in the R-R interval will *almost always* be accurate enough for our purposes. For those interested in more precise estimation, particularly in the presence of rapid heart rates, referral to Fig. 2-7 may be helpful.

Determination of Rhythm

As previously indicated in Table 1-5 cardiac rhythm is determined by answering four basic questions. These questions are repeated in a slightly modified form in Table 2-1, and are discussed below.

RATE: Calculation of heart rate is an important first step in rhythm analysis. The reasons for this will become obvious momentarily.

RHYTHM: When interpreting the rhythm of an ECG, it matters not in what order you consider the four basic questions listed in the table. What does matter is only that *each* of the points is considered.

1. ***Regularity of the rhythm*** is usually easy to assess from inspection. However, one should beware of the fact that slight irregularity may not be readily apparent with extremely rapid rhythms. In these cases, calipers should be used to verify regularity.

2. ***Detection of P waves*** is the cornerstone of rhythm analysis. By definition, the P wave should *always* be upright in standard lead II with sinus rhythm. This is because orientation of the electrical impulse as it travels from the sinoatrial node to the atrioventricular node is virtually parallel to this lead (Fig. 2-8). Under normal circumstances, *if the P wave is not upright in lead II, normal sinus rhythm cannot be be present!*

TABLE 2-1

Approach to rhythm analysis

RATE

RHYTHM

- Is the rhythm regular?
- Are there P waves?
- Is the QRS wide or narrow?
- Is there a relationship between P waves and the QRS complex?

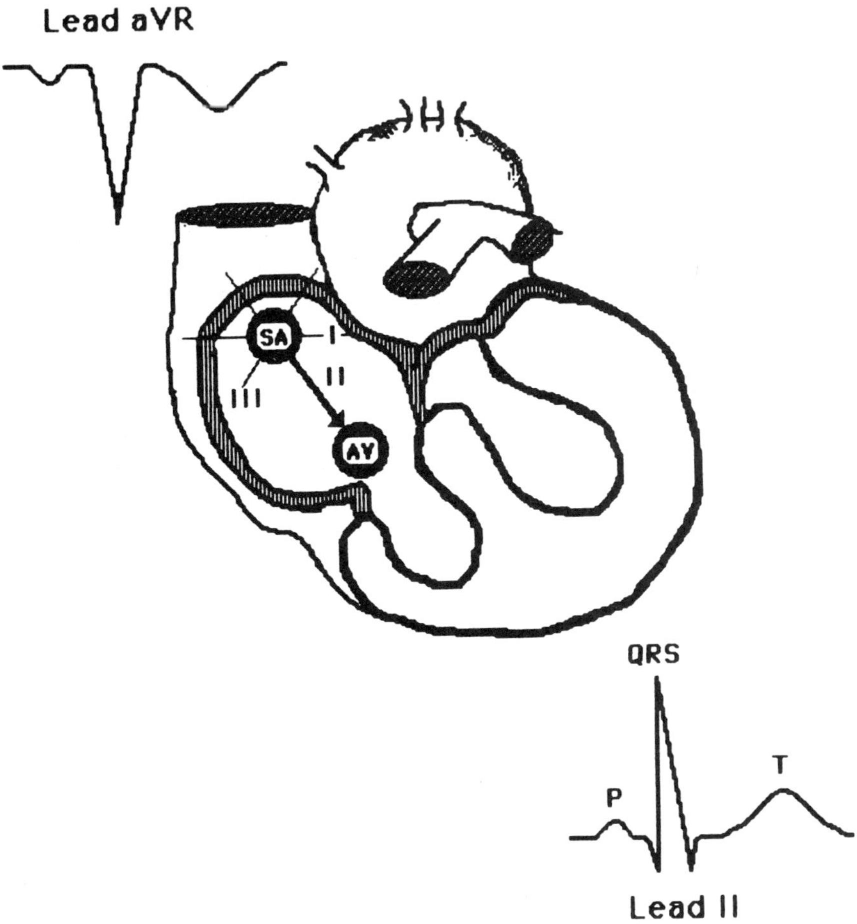

Figure 2-8. Since orientation of the electrical impulse as it travels from the SA (sinoatrial) node to the AV (atrioventricular) node is virtually parallel to lead II, the P wave *must* always be upright in this lead.

3. ***Width of the QRS complex*** is a most helpful determinant of the site of origination of the electrical impulse. As discussed in Chapter 1, the usual upper limit of normal for duration of the QRS complex in adults is 0.10 second. A QRS duration of 0.11 second is borderline, while one of 0.12 second or greater is definitely prolonged.

When the QRS complex is *narrow* (≤0.10 second), the electrical impulse almost certainly has a *supraventricular* origin. That is, the impulse originates from the sinoatrial (SA) node, the atrioventricular (AV) node, or from elsewhere in the atria (from anywhere above the dotted line in Fig. 2-9). On the other hand, when the QRS complex is *widened* (≥0.12 second), the site of origin may not be so certain. Although widening of the QRS complex

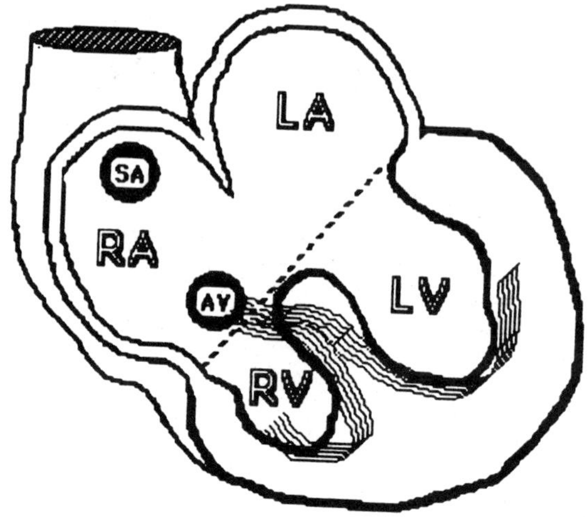

Figure 2-9. With normal sinus rhythm, the electrical impulse originates in the SA node and spreads through the atria on its way to the AV node. From there the impulse enters the ventricular conduction system to be carried to all parts of the ventricles. With supraventricular conduction (origin of the impulse above the dotted line) the QRS complex will be narrow unless something has happened to alter ventricular conduction. SA—Sinoatrial node; AV—Atrioventricular node; RA—Right atrium; LA—Left atrium; RV—Right ventricle; LV—Left ventricle.

suggests a ventricular site of origin, the impulse may still be supraventricular if something has happened to alter ventricular conduction.

With normal sinus rhythm, the electrical impulse originates in the SA node, the principal pacemaker of the heart. From there it spreads through the right and left atria on its way to the AV node. The impulse then enters the ventricular conduction system, from which it will be carried to all parts of the ventricles (Fig. 2-9).

When the ventricular conduction system is functioning normally, the time required for conduction of the electrical impulse from the SA node throughout the ventricular myocardium is short. Such conduction results in a narrow QRS complex. Should the impulse originate from another supraventricular site instead of the SA node (from either the right or left atrium, or from the AV node), it will still pass through the ventricular conduction system en route to activating the ventricles. Therefore, under normal circumstances the QRS complex will be narrow and of identical morphology for normal sinus beats, AV nodal beats, or beats originating from elsewhere in the atria, since the same conduction pathway through the ventricles will have been used.

Should there be a defect in ventricular conduction (bundle branch block), or should ventricular conduction be abnormal (aberrant) due to incomplete recovery of a portion of the conduction system following a premature beat, both the path and the time for the electrical impulse to travel through the ventricles will be altered. In such cases, the QRS complex may change in morphology and become *widened* despite a supraventricular origin.

A final caveat from Chapter 1 that should be kept in mind when assessing QRS duration is that occasionally a portion of the QRS complex may be isoelectric (lie on the baseline). When this happens one may get the false impression in a particular lead that the QRS complex is shorter than it really is. To avoid this pitfall, one should always survey a number of leads of the ECG, and select the QRS duration that is of greatest duration.

4. ***Determination of the relationship between P waves and QRS complexes*** is critical to rhythm analysis. One should first identify QRS complexes in a particular rhythm strip. Next, look to see if P waves precede each QRS. If P waves do come before each QRS complex, are they related (are P waves "married") to their respective QRS complex?

With normal sinus rhythm, every QRS complex is preceded by a P wave with a *constant* PR interval. That is, each atrial impulse is conducted to the ventricles. If atrioventricular (AV) conduction is normal, the PR interval will be ≤0.20 second. On the other hand, it each atrial impulse is conducted to the ventricles with a constant PR interval, but AV conduction is delayed (if the PR interval is ≥0.21 second), 1° AV block is said to be present. With more significant impairment of AV conduction (2° AV block), conduction of one or more atrial impulses to the ventricles is prevented *("blocked")*. P waves may precede and be related to at least some of the QRS complexes, but their relationship may not be readily apparent.

Finally, with complete block of AV conduction (3° or complete AV block), none of the atrial impulses is conducted to the ventricles. Both the atria and ventricles beat at their own inherent rate. P waves may precede QRS complexes, but they are totally unrelated to them, and the PR interval is continually changing.

Sinus Rhythm

In this and following chapters, we will concentrate on recognition of sinus rhythm and of basic dysrhythmias. Analysis of more complex rhythm disturbances is beyond the scope of this book. However, application of the approach to rhythm analysis suggested in Table 2-1 will prove invaluable to the reader regardless of the complexity of the rhythm disturbance.

PROBLEM: Apply this approach to analyze the cardiac rhythms shown in Fig. 2-10.

ANSWER to Fig. 2-10A: The rhythm is regular. The R-R interval is just over 4 large boxes, making the heart rate about 74 beats/min. The QRS complex is narrow. (≤0.10 sec). Each QRS is preceded by a P wave with a constant, normal (≤0.20 sec) PR interval. Thus, this is normal sinus rhythm.

By convention, we define normal sinus rhythm to have a rate between 60 and 100 beats/min. Sinus conduction with a faster ventricular rate is termed sinus tachycardia, while a slower rate is sinus bradycardia. Neither sinus bradycardia nor sinus tachycardia necessarily represent a disease state, and both are commonly found in normal subjects.

ANSWER to Fig. 2-10B: Once again, the rhythm is regular. The R-R interval is between two and three large boxes, making the rate 115 to 120 beats/min. The QRS complex is narrow, and each beat is preceded by a P wave with a constant PR interval. This is sinus tachycardia.

ANSWER to Fig. 2-10C: Although this rhythm may at first glance appear regular, measurement with calipers reveals a slight but definite irregularity.

Figure 2-10

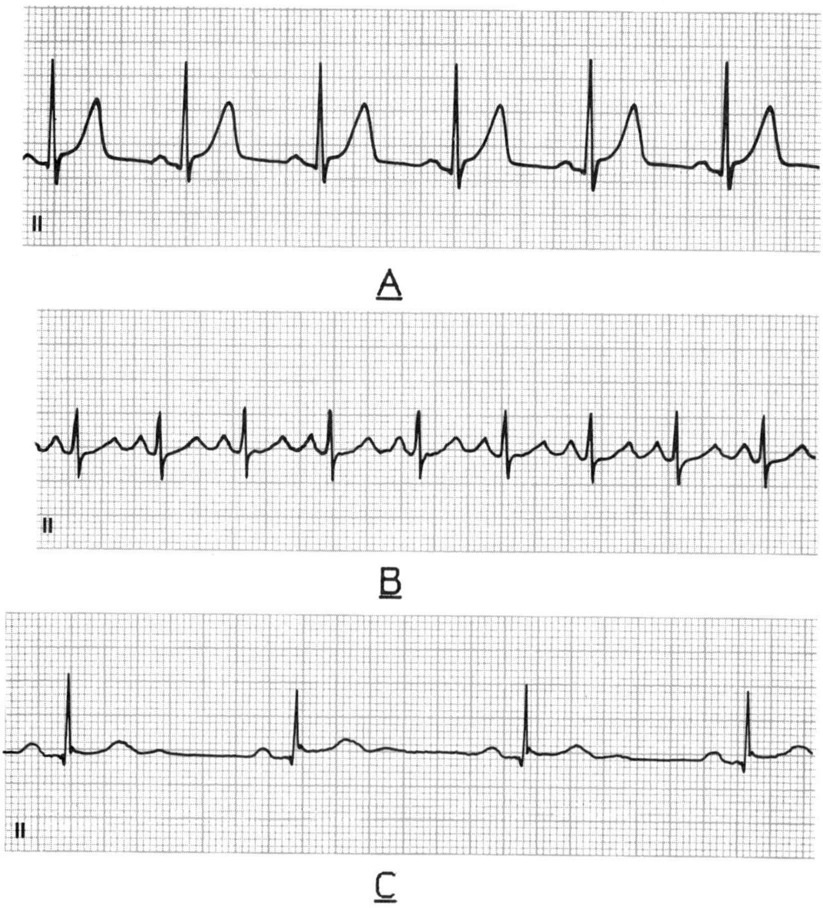

The R-R interval is between 6-1/2 and 7 large boxes, making the rate about 45 beats/min. Each QRS complex is preceded by a P wave with a fixed PR interval; however, the PR interval is *prolonged* (PR = 0.23 sec). This is sinus bradycardia and arrhythmia with 1° AV block.

Sinus Arrhythmia

Sinus arrhythmia is an extremely common finding among normal children and young adults, in whom heart rate often varies with respiration. Although sinus arrhythmia may also occur normally in the elderly, it is usually not related to respiration in this age group, and sometimes is the precursor of sick sinus syndrome.

The rate of even "normal sinus rhythm" will often vary slightly from beat to beat. In order to diagnose sinus *arrhythmia,* and to distinguish it from the slight normal variation in rate that occurs with normal sinus rhythm, there should be a difference of *at least* 0.08 second between the shortest and longest R-R intervals. Despite the existence of this criterion, in practice the presence of sinus arrhythmia is frequently not noted by the eletrocardiographer. This is because subtle differences in heart rate are easy to overlook unless one meticulously measures out each R-R interval on a tracing. While we will continue to apply the above criterion throughout this text, we recognize that minimal beat-to-beat variations are usually of little clinical significance, and need not necessarily be written as part of the interpretation. More marked variations (of perhaps $\geq$0.20 second), however, should probably be noted.

PROBLEM: Examine the three dysrhythmias shown in Fig. 2-11. Which of the three has (have) evidence of atrial activity?

ANSWER to Fig. 2-11A: The rhythm is fairly regular, and the R-R interval is between four and five large boxes. Thus, the heart rate is about 65 beats/min. The QRS complex is of normal duration, but there are no P waves. This is AV nodal (or junctional) rhythm.

AV Nodal (Junctional) Rhythm

We have already stated that the SA node is the principal pacemaker of the heart, and that with normal sinus rhythm, it usually fires at a rate of between 60 and 100 beats/min. Should something happen to the SA node's pacesetting ability, other areas of the heart with inherent automaticity may take over the pacemaking function. With an inherent rate of 40 to 60 beats/min, the AV node is usually next in line. Should the AV nodal pacemaker also fail, a ventricular pacemaker at a rate of between 30 and 40 beats/min may take over. In the event that no other area of the heart takes over the pacesetting function, asystole will result.

At a rate of 65 beats/min, the AV nodal rhythm in this example is slightly accelerated from its usual inherent rate.

A final point to be made about junctional rhythms deals with the atrial activity that one is likely to see with this rhythm. In Fig. 2-8, we discussed how with normal sinus rhythm the P wave must always be upright in lead II. This is because orientation of the electrical impulse as it travels from its origin in the SA node toward the AV node is virtually parallel to lead II.

PROBLEM: What would you expect P waves to look like in lead II if the electrical impulse originated from the AV node instead of the SA node?

Figure 2-11

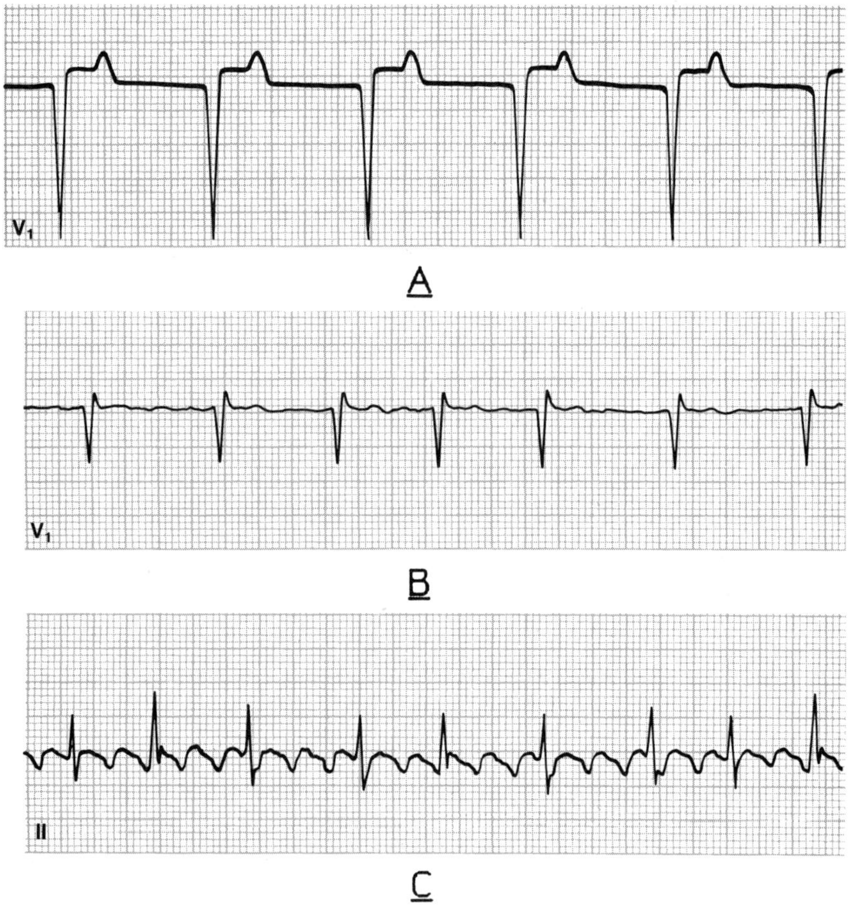

ANSWER: If the electrical impulse originated from the AV node (as it does with an AV nodal rhythm), P waves would be expected to travel in a backward *(retrograde)* direction from the AV node to the SA node. Consequently, one would expect the P wave to be negative (inverted) in lead II. If retrograde conduction is extremely rapid, then inverted P waves may *precede* the QRS complex. If retrograde conduction is slow, the atria will not be depolarized until *after* the ventricles, so that retrograde P waves *follow* the QRS complex. However, if the speed of retrograde conduction is about equal to the speed of forward *(antegrade)* conduction through the ventricular conduction system, the inverted P wave will occur *simultaneously* with the QRS complex, and be hidden by it. This is the case in Fig. 2-11A.

ANSWER to Fig. 2-11B: The QRS complex is narrow. The rhythm is irregularly irregular (each R-R interval is different). Although there are undulations in the baseline, no definite P waves are present. This is atrial fibrillation with a controlled ventricular response.

Atrial Fibrillation

In atrial fibrillation, multiple atrial foci are firing irregularly at an extremely rapid rate (up to 600 times/min). Only a fraction of these atrial impulses are conducted through the AV node. Untreated, atrial fibrillation characteristically manifests a *rapid* ventricular response (a rate greater than 120 beats/min). Following treatment with digitalis, the ventricular response becomes *controlled,* and usually falls into the range of 60 to 110 beats/min (as is seen in Fig. 2-11B). With too much digitalis, or in some cases of sick sinus syndrome or atrioventricular heart block, atrial fibrillation may manifest a *slow* ventricular response (a rate less than 60 beats/min).

ANSWER to Fig. 2-11C: Once again the QRS complex is narrow, and the rhythm is irregularly irregular. However, as opposed to Fig. 2-11B, more definite evidence of atrial activity is present. A repetitive negative deflection is seen at a rate of 280 beats/min. This is atrial flutter, in this case with a variable ventricular response. The negative deflections are flutter waves.

Atrial Flutter

The atrial rate in flutter most often hovers around 300 beats/min (with a range of 250 to 350 beats/min), except when it has been slowed by a medication such as quinidine. Fortunately, the AV node is unable to conduct each atrial impulse at this rapid a rate. If 1 : 1 AV conduction were possible, the ventricular response with atrial flutter would be about 300 beats/min, which is much too fast a rate to maintain effective cardiac pumping. As a protective mechanism, the AV node limits the number of atrial impulses that are conducted to the ventricles. Usually every other impulse is conducted, so that *the most common ventricular response in untreated atrial flutter is 2 : 1* (an atrial rate of 300 beats/min and a ventricular response of 150 beats/min). Less commonly there is 4 : 1 AV conduction or variable AV conduction (as in this example).

PROBLEM: The rhythm strip shown in Fig. 2-12 is taken from another patient in atrial flutter. How many flutter waves are present for every QRS complex?

ANSWER to Fig. 2-12: The QRS complex is narrow, and the ventricular response is regular at a rate of about 80 beats/min. Atrial flutter waves are regular and occur in this V_1 lead as upright deflections at a rate of about 320 beats/min. There are *four* flutter waves for each QRS complex (there is 4 : 1 AV conduction). If you had difficulty spotting the fourth flutter wave, it makes up the terminal r′ of the QRS complex (Fig. 2-13).

When the characteristic sawtooth pattern of atrial flutter (seen in Fig. 2-11C) or distinct atrial activity at a rate approximating 300 beats/min (seen in Fig. 2-12) is present, recognition of this dysrhythmia poses no problem. However, flutter waves are often much more subtle in their appearance.

PROBLEM: Consider Fig. 2-14. Focus for a moment on lead II. A regular supraventricular tachycardia at a rate of 160 beats/min is present. Could this be sinus tachycardia?

ANSWER to Fig. 2-14: No. Since normal, upright P waves are not present in lead II, sinus tachycardia can be ruled out. The rhythm in Fig. 2-14 is atrial flutter, although the diagnosis is not at all obvious from this tracing. Perhaps the only lead that even remotely hints at the presence of the characteristic sawtooth pattern of flutter is aVF. Note in particular that evidence of atrial activity is totally lacking from leads I, III, aVL, V_2, and V_6.

Because flutter waves are frequently not apparent in one or more leads

Figure 2-12

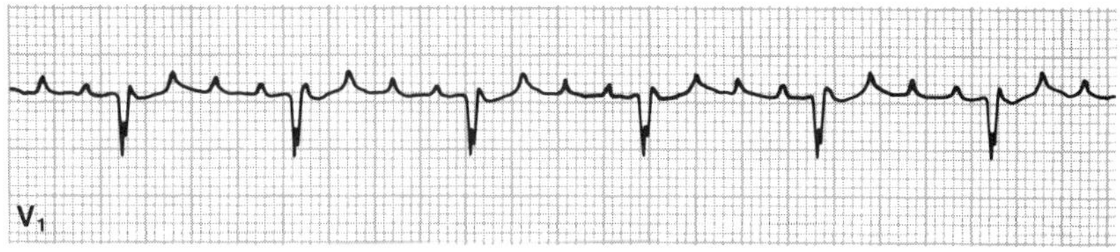

Figure 2-13

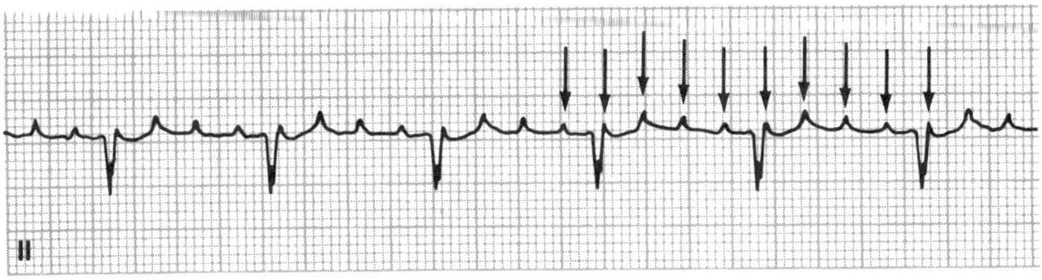

of the ECG, the diagnosis is often overlooked. In order to avoid this pitfall, one must always maintain a high index of suspicion and *strongly consider the possibility of atrial flutter in the presence of any regular supraventricular tachycardia with a rate of between 140 to 160 beats per minute when normal atrial activity cannot be identified.*

PROBLEM: Interpret the two dysrhythmias shown in Fig. 2-15. Is atrial flutter likely to be present in either tracing?

ANSWER to Fig. 2-15A: A regular supraventricular tachydysrhythmia at a rate of 150 beats/min is present. Although a seemingly normal P wave is seen preceding each QRS complex, notching on the upstroke of each T wave suggests that there may actually be two P waves for each QRS complex.

When definitive diagnosis of a tachydysrhythmia is not apparent from inspection of a tracing, it may sometimes be made clear by slowing the ventricular response with a vagal maneuver such as cartoid sinus massage. Fig. 2-16 shows the effect of cartoid massage on the rhythm in Fig. 2-15.

The degree of atrioventricular block has been increased by carotid massage, and atrial flutter waves at a rate of about 300 beats/min (arrows) are now evident.

ANSWER to Fig. 2-15B: Once again, a regular supraventricular tachydysrhythmia is seen. The rate, however, is significantly faster than it was for Fig. 2-15A. The R-R interval in this tracing is between 1 and 2 large boxes, making the rate between 150 and 300 beats/min. As suggested earlier, when the rate is regular and this rapid, a handy trick for calculating rate is to measure the R-R interval of every other beat. Here, the R-R interval for every other beat (half the rate) is a little less than 3 boxes. Therefore, half the rate is 110 beats/min, and the actual rate is 220 beats/min.

Atrial flutter with 1 : 1 AV conduction would be unlikely at this rate unless the patient were being treated with a medication (such as quinidine) that might slow the atrial response. Atrial flutter with 2 : 1 AV conduction would also be unlikely, since this would require an atrial rate of 440 beats per minute, which is well beyond the usual range for flutter.

PROBLEM: Does the upright deflection seen between QRS complexes in Fig. 2-15B represent atrial activity?

Figure 2-14

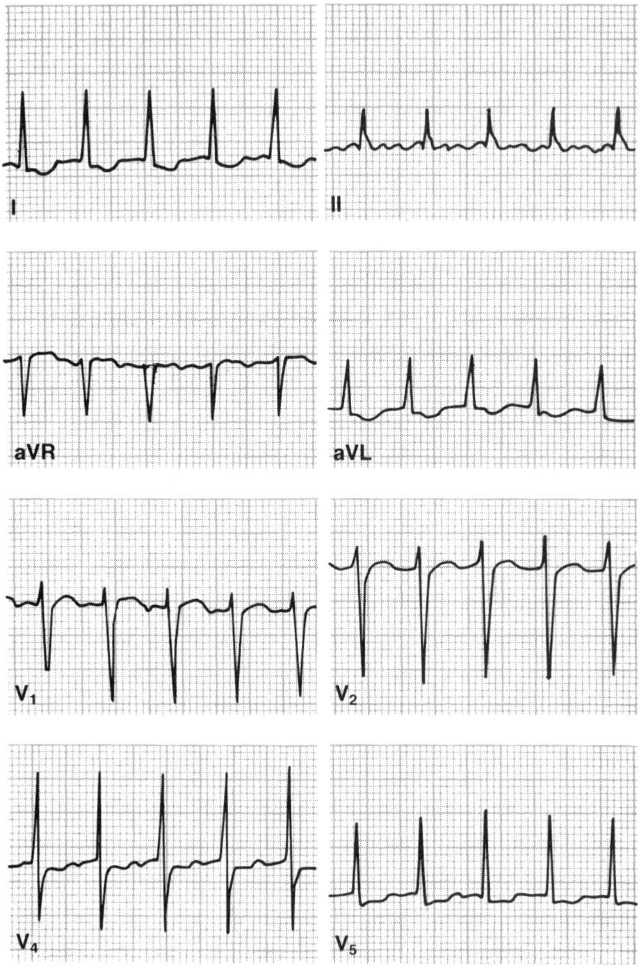

ANSWER: It is impossible to determine from Fig. 2-15B whether the upright deflection between QRS complexes represents the P wave, the T wave, or both. If it were the P wave, then the rhythm in Fig. 2-15B would be sinus tachycardia at a rate of 220 beats/min. Since sinus tachycardia rarely exceeds 160 beats/min in an adult, this diagnosis is unlikely. Thus, the upright deflection probably represents the T wave, and the rhythm is presumed to be paroxysmal supraventricular tachycardia (PSVT).

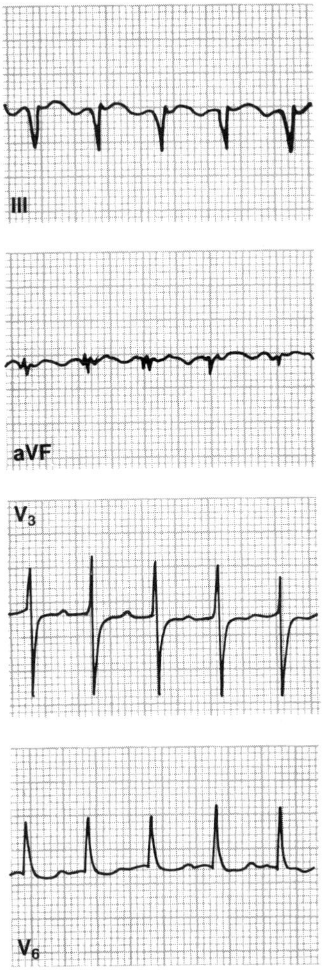

Paroxysmal Supraventricular Tachycardia

PSVT is a commonly seen, extremely regular tachydysrhythmia that usually has a rate of between 150 to 250 beats/min. In the past, distinction was made between two types of PSVT—paroxysmal atrial tachycardia (PAT) and paroxysmal junction tachycardia (PJT). Such differentiation was probably more of academic interest than of clinical utility, since both tachydysrhythmias are thought to be due to similar *reentry* mechanisms involving the AV node. In *reentry,* the impulse travels through the AV node, enters the ventricular conduction system, and then somehow is conducted back (*reenters*) the AV node. A continuous cycle in which the impulse is conducted down (to the ventricles) and back (to the AV node) is perpetuated, and rapid heart rates are attained.

The QRS complex is most often narrow with PSVT, unless bundle branch block or aberrant conduction exists. P waves are usually not evident. When present, they are frequently inverted and partially hidden in the terminal portion of the QRS complex.

One should not confuse PSVT with the more generally used term, supraventricular tachycardia. By definition, a *supraventricular tachycardia*

Figure 2-15

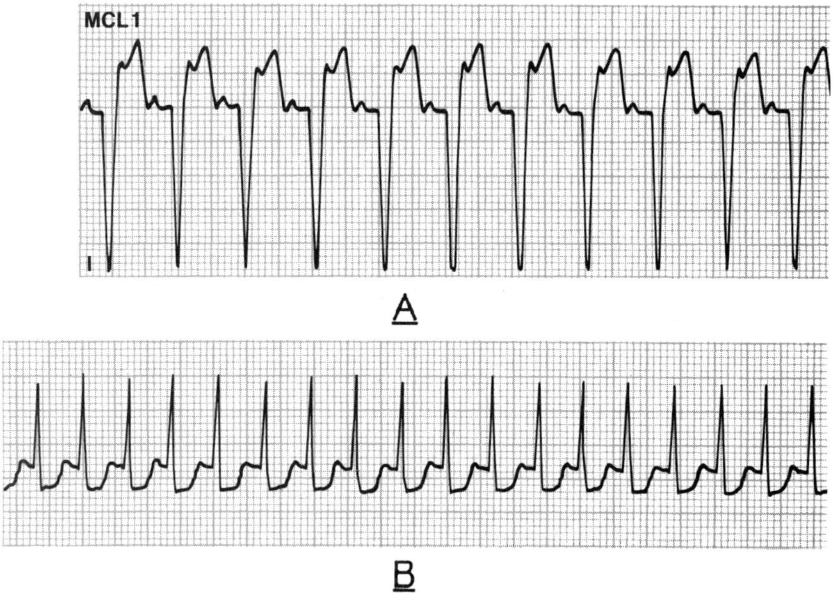

Figure 2-16

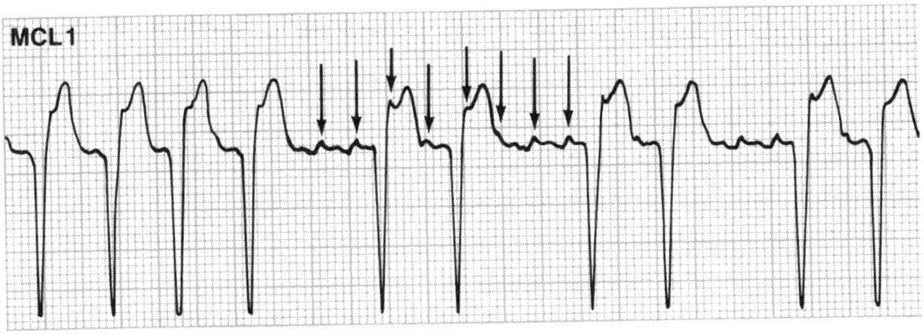

is any tachycardia in which the impulse originates at or above the AV node. Examples of supraventricular tachycardias are shown in Table 2-2.

On the other hand, the term PSVT implies that the mechanism of a particular tachydysrhythmia is reentry. A better term for these dysrhythmias might simply be to call them *re-entry tachycardias.* Thus, the rhythm in Fig. 2-15A is a *supraventricular* tachycardia, but it is not PSVT!

Premature Complexes

PROBLEM: Examine the tracings shown in Fig. 2-17. Beats #3, 6, and 10 all occur early. Are these premature beats likely to arise from the atria or the ventricles?

ANSWER to Fig. 2-17: The rhythm is sinus tachycardia at a rate of 100 beats/min. The QRS complex is narrow. Beats #3, 6, and 10 all occur early. QRS morphology of the latter two complexes is identical to that of the

TABLE 2-2

Supraventricular tachycardias
Sinus tachycardia
Junctional tachycardia
Atrial fibrillation
Atrial flutter
Multifocal atrial tachycardia
Ectopic atrial tachycardia
PSVT

normally conducted beats. In addition, these beats are preceded by premature P waves. Beats #6 and 10 are premature atrial contractions (PACs).

On the other hand, beat #3 is wide and bizarre in shape; it is not preceded by a premature P wave. Beat #3 is a premature ventricular contraction (PVC).

As discussed earlier in this chapter, when the QRS complex is narrow, it implies that the impulse is passing through the conduction system en route to activating the ventricles. Thus, a *premature supraventricular contraction*—either a PAC or a premature junctional contraction (PJC)—can be readily recognized as a beat that occurs *early* (is premature), and has a *narrow* QRS complex that is *identical* in morphology to the normal sinus beats. If such a beat is preceded by an upright premature P wave with a normal PR interval in lead II, it is a PAC. If it is preceded by an inverted P wave with a short PR interval, is not preceded by any P wave at all, or instead is followed by a P wave (if the P wave is *retrograde*), it is a PJC.

In the case where normal sinus rhythm is interrupted by a premature QRS complex that is wide but not preceded by any P wave at all, one should assume it is a PVC.

Exceptions to the above generalities exist. QRS complexes may be *wide* despite normal sinus rhythm if some type of intraventricular conduction delay (bundle branch block) is present. Even when sinus-conducted beats are narrow, premature supraventricular complexes (PACs or PJCs) may still be wide due to *aberrant conduction.* Finally, differentiation between PACs or PJCs that conduct with aberrancy and PVCs may be extremely difficult if the premature P wave is hidden within the preceding T wave. Many of these subtleties extend beyond the scope of this book.

Figure 2-17

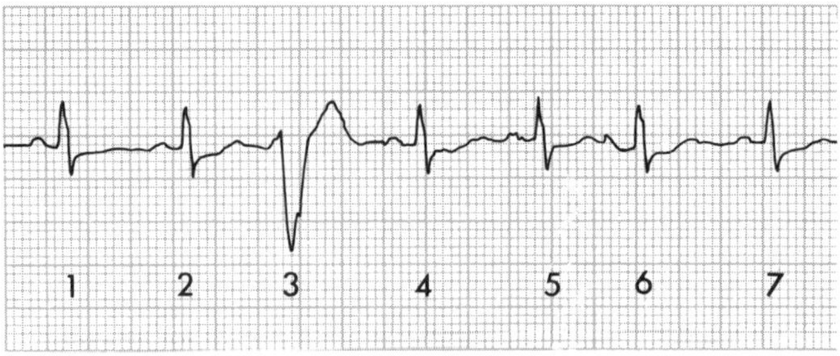

Tachydysrhythmias: Subtle Clues

PROBLEM: Put these concepts together and examine the three tracings shown in Fig. 2-18. Does the regularity of the rhythms and the width of the QRS complex supply clues to the etiology?

ANSWER to Fig. 2-18A: The rhythm is precisely regular at a rate of 190 beats/min. The QRS complex appears wide (at least 0.12 second in duration), and no atrial activity is evident. One has to assume that this is ventricular tachycardia.

PROBLEM: Could this tachydysrhythmia possibly be of supraventricular etiology?

ANSWER: Yes. Whenever one is confronted by a regular wide complex tachydysrhythmia, three entities should always be kept in mind in the differential:

- Ventricular tachycardia
- Supraventricular tachycardia with preexisting bundle branch block
- Supraventricular tachycardia with aberrant conduction

Unless there is strong evidence to the contrary, ventricular tachycardia *must* always be assumed until proven otherwise.

ANSWER to Fig. 2-18B: This rhythm is also precisely regular at 190 beats/min. The QRS complex appears to be narrow, and P waves seemingly precede each QRS complex. One might think that this was sinus tachycardia.

Actually, the rhythms shown in Figs. 2-18A and 2-18B were obtained *simultaneously* in the *same* patient! They emphasize the point previously stated that the QRS complex may appear deceptively narrow in certain leads

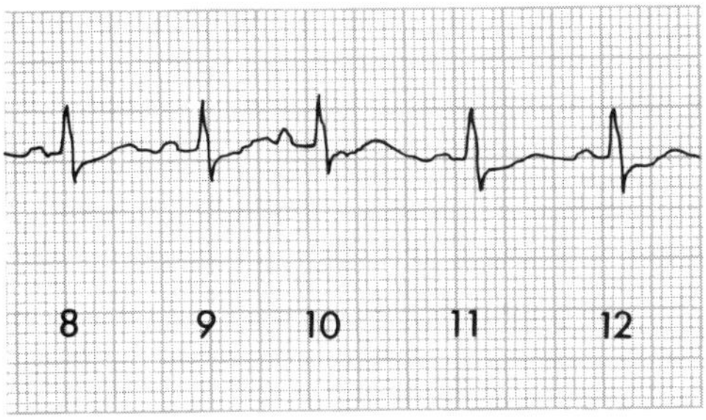

when a portion of the QRS is isoelectric with the baseline. This patient was in ventricular tachycardia! The rate is much faster than that which one usually sees with sinus tachycardia in adults, and the upright deflection seen between QRS complexes in Fig. 2-18B represents the T wave, *not* the P wave.

ANSWER to Fig. 2-18C: The QRS complex appears to be narrow in this lead, and no definite P waves are seen. At first glance, the rhythm appears to be regular. If this were the case, then the differential diagnosis for this dysrhythmia would be identical to that considered for the regular narrow com-

Figure 2-18

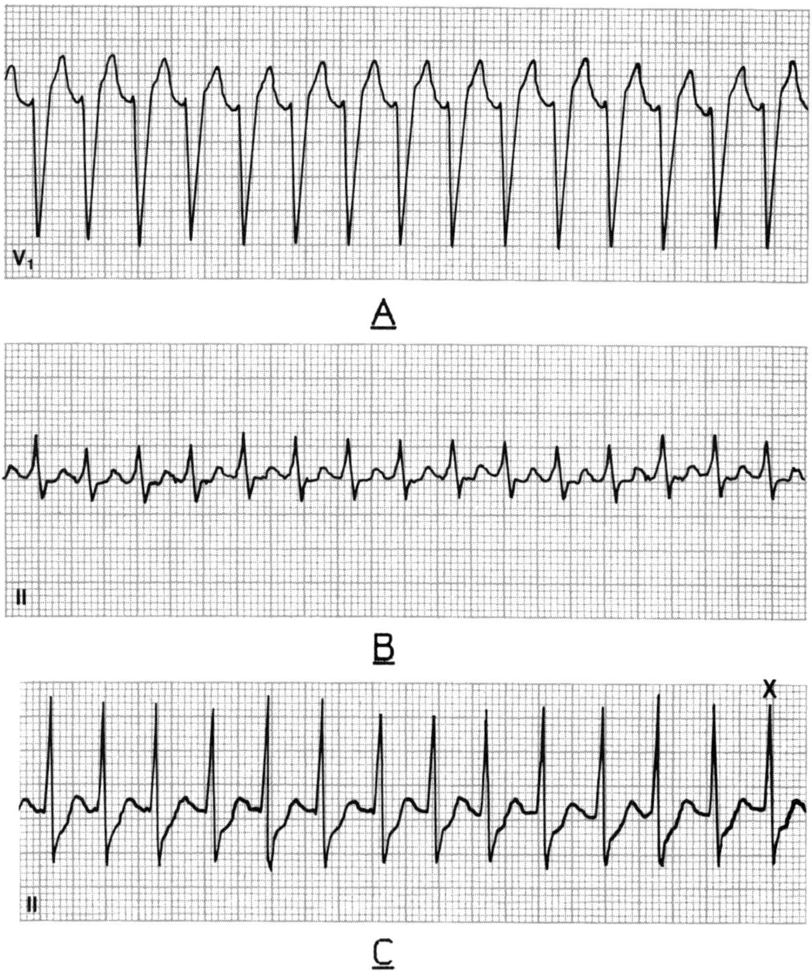

plex tachydysrhythmia shown in Fig. 2-15B—sinus tachycardia, atrial flutter, or PSVT.

PROBLEM: Is the rhythm in Fig. 2-18C really regular? (Be sure to verify your answer with calipers.)

ANSWER: Slight but definite irregularity of the R-R interval is present in Fig. 2-18C. Fig. 2-19 shows the continuation of this rhythm strip from the point marked X. The irregular irregularity of the rhythm becomes much more evident during the final beats of Fig. 2-19. Thus, the rhythm in Fig. 2-18C is *atrial fibrillation* with a rapid ventricular response.

Summary

Several points should be apparent from the examples presented in this chapter:

- Accurate estimation of heart rate may be very helpful in rhythm analysis. This is particularly true in the presence of supraventricular tachydysrhythmias for determining the likelihood of sinus tachycardia and atrial flutter.
- Systematic approach to rhythm analysis should always include assessment of the regularity of the rhythm, a search for P waves, determination of the width of the QRS complex, and establishment of the relationship between P waves and their respective QRS complex.
- Regularity of the rhythm may *not* always be reliably determined by simple inspection. This is especially true with rapid atrial fibrillation. When doubt exists, calipers should be used for measurement.
- Under normal circumstances, the P wave should *always* be upright in lead II with sinus rhythm. If the P wave is not upright in this lead, then sinus rhythm is not present.

Figure 2-19

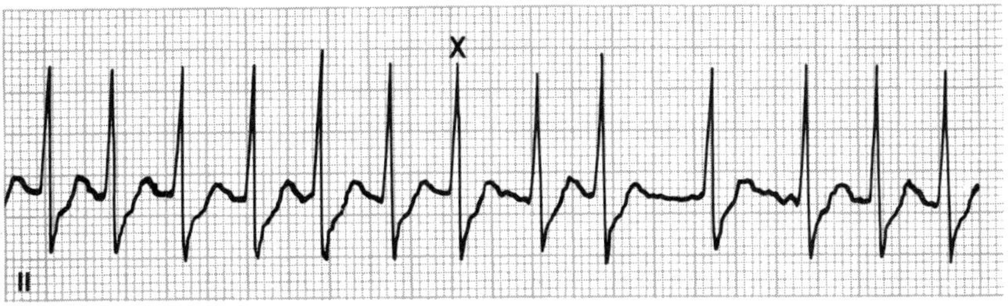

TABLE 2-3

Distinguishing characteristics of common dysrhythmias

Rhythm	Usual rate range	Regularity	Width of QRS	Atrial activity	P-QRS relationship
SINUS			Usually narrow (May be wide if bundle branch block or aberrant conduction is present)	Normal upright P waves are present in lead II.	1 : 1 Relationship (P waves precede each QRS with constant PR interval)
Sinus bradycardia	<60/min	Regular			
Sinus rhythm	60–100/min	Regular			
Sinus tachycardia	>100/min	Regular			
Sinus arrhythmia	Usually <100/min	Variable			
JUNCTIONAL (AV NODAL) RHYTHM	40–60/min (An accelerated junctional rhythm is said to be present when the rate is >60/min)	Regular	Usually narrow (May be wide if bundle branch block or aberrant conduction is present)	Inverted P wave in lead II [P waves may precede the QRS complex with a short PR interval; occur simultaneously with the QRS complex (and be hidden by it); or follow the QRS complex]	
ATRIAL FIBRILLATION	***Ventricular response:*** Slow: <60 Controlled (moderate): 70–110 Rapid: >120	Irregularly irregular	Usually narrow (May be wide if bundle branch block or aberrant conduction is present)	No P waves are present (The baseline may contain irregular undulations of small amplitude = fibrillation waves)	None

ATRIAL FLUTTER	Atrial rate is usually 250–350/min in adults (unless slowed by medication such as quinidine); Most commonly 2:1 AV conduction (vent. response ≈150/min) Less commonly 3:1, 4:1, or variable response	Usually regular ventricular response (May be variable)	Usually narrow (May be wide if bundle branch block or aberrant conduction is present)	Flutter waves are present	May not be apparent
PSVT	150–250/min	Precisely regular	Usually narrow (May be wide if bundle branch block or aberrant conduction is present)	Usually not evident (If present, P waves are not upright in lead II)	Usually not apparent
VENTRICULAR TACHYCARDIA	Usually >150/min	Usually fairly regular	Wide	Usually no atrial activity is apparent (If P waves are present, they are usually unrelated to the QRS complex)	

- The width of the QRS complex may appear deceptively narrow in certain leads if a portion of the QRS is isoelectric with the baseline. Whenever possible, QRS duration should be determined from inspection of *several* leads.
- Definitive diagnosis is *not* always possible for every dysrhythmia. This is particularly true when only one monitoring lead is available for interpretation.

Table 2-3 reviews the distinguishing characteristics of the more common dysrhythmias that the reader will encounter in clinical electrocardiography.

Although this short chapter could not possibly make the reader adept in complex rhythm analysis, application of the principles contained herein should provide a firm background for rhythm interpretation throughout the rest of the book.

Suggested Reading

Grauer K: *Study Guide for Advanced Life Support: Problem Solving in Cardiac Arrest.* C.V. Mosby, St. Louis:1984.

CHAPTER 3

AXIS

After determining rate and rhythm, one must establish the axis, simply defined as the spatial orientation of the heart's electrical activity. To do this we use the recordings of the six extremity leads and apply the laws of Einthoven, first described at the turn of the century.

Introduction — Einthoven's Triangle

Although the heart is really viewed spatially in three dimensions, we will discuss the axis in reference to the heart's electrical activity in the two dimensions of the frontal plane. The tranverse (or horizontal) plane views the heart's electrical activity in the third dimension, and will be discussed in the next chapter.

The process of ventricular activation will also be covered in detail in the next chapter. For now, suffice it to say that at any given moment during this process the heart's electrical activity can be represented by numerous small instantaneous vectors, each with its own magnitude and direction (see Fig. 3-1). Each instantaneous vector constantly changes its force (magnitude) and direction with time as depolarization spreads through the ventricles. Since the ECG is recorded at a distance from the heart, the 12 monitoring leads do not perceive each individual vector, but instead perceive their sum as the instantaneous resultant vector for that particular moment. Were one to add up all of the instantaneous resultant vectors that occur during one cycle, their sum would represent the average magnitude and direction of ventricular depolarization. The mean QRS axis that we determine on the standard ECG is the average direction of this sum.

Mean QRS axis can be calculated from the hexaxial lead system, which consists of the three standard bipolar limb leads (I, II, and III) and the three unipolar augmented leads (aVR, aVL, and aVF). These lead systems have been derived from the assumption that the heart electrically lies within the center of an equilateral triangle in which the sides of the triangle are formed by the standard limb leads (Fig. 3-2A). Each of these standard bipolar limb leads senses the potential difference in electrical activity passing between its corresponding extremity electrodes. Thus, standard lead I measures the potential difference between the left and right shoulder (lead I = LA − RA); lead II the potential difference between the groin (left leg) and right shoulder

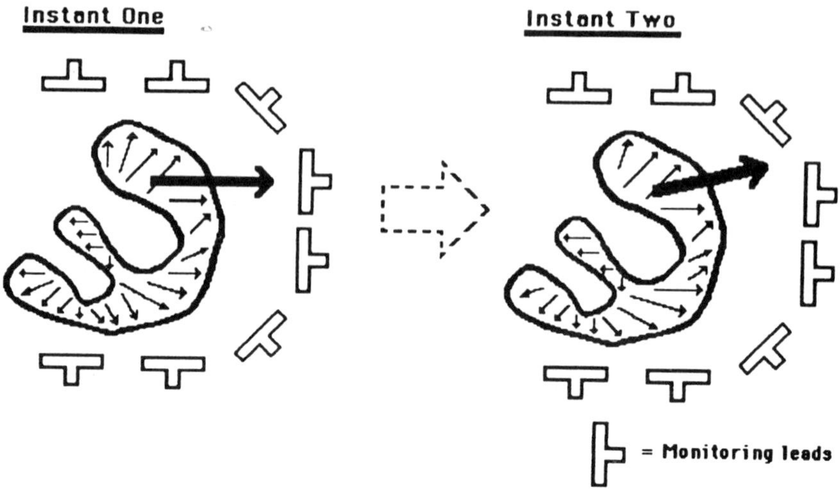

Figure 3-1. Representation of instantaneous vectors and their resultant sum as viewed by monitoring leads for successive instants in time during the spread of ventricular depolarization. The larger arrow in each figure represents the resultant vector for that instant.

(lead II = LL − RA); and lead III the potential difference between the groin and the left shoulder (lead III = LL − LA). Einthoven arbitrarily selected the left shoulder (LA, or left arm) electrode to be positive when recording lead I, and the groin (LL, or left leg) electrode to be positive when recording leads II and III. In this way, a majority of QRS complexes would be predominantly positive in the electrocardiograms of most individuals.

In reality, Einthoven's theory is *not* strictly true. The heart does not lie precisely in the center of Einthoven's equilateral triangle. In addition, the heart lies in a slightly different geometric plane than the standard limb leads. Finally, the body is not the uniform volume conductor of the heart's electrical activity that it was assumed to be. Yet despite these shortcomings, the basic concepts of Einthoven's theory are still extremely useful in electrocardiography. It is on the basis of Einthoven's triangle that we are able to construct the standard triaxial lead system simply by transposing lead III in space (Fig. 3-2B). When each side of the triangle is made to intersect at a common point (Fig. 3-2C), the system is complete. Note that standard lead I points horizontally and to the left—it views the heart's electrical activity from an axis of 0°.

PROBLEM: Where are leads II, III, and −III located (in degrees) on our triaxial lead system?

ANSWER: All three sides of Einthoven's triangle are equal by definition since they form an equilateral triangle. Consequently, each side must be separated by 60°. On our triaxial lead system, therefore, lead II must be located 60° from lead I, or at an axis of +60°. Lead III is 60° further away at an axis of $+120°$. Similarly, negative lead III ($-$III), which points upward and to the left, must also be located 60° away from lead I; it represents an axis of $-60°$. *Thus, an easy way to reconstruct the standard triaxial lead system shown in Fig. 3-2C is to begin with lead I, which is horizontal and located at 0°, and to remember that each succeeding limb lead must be located 60° farther away from this starting reference point.*

PROBLEM: Draw (without looking) the triaxial lead system.

ANSWER: As stated above, reconstruction of the triaxial lead system may be accomplished by beginning with lead I, which is horizontal and located at 0° (Fig. 3-3A and 3-3B), and by remembering that each succeeding standard limb lead is located at 60° intervals away from this point (Fig. 3-3C, 3-3D, and 3-3E).

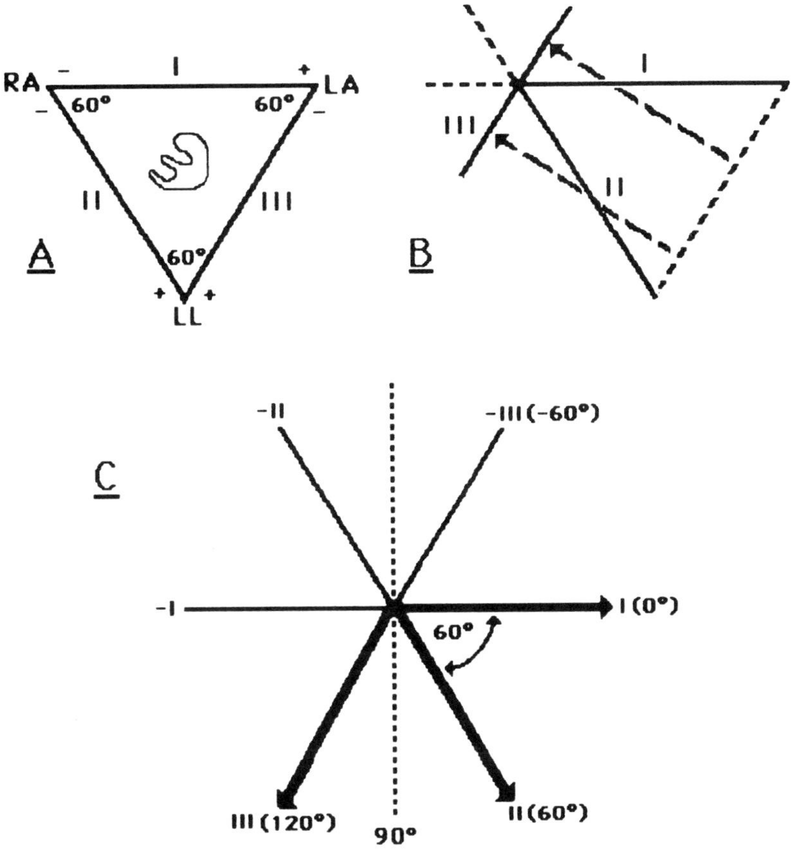

Figure 3-2. Construction of the standard triaxial lead system **(C)** from Einthoven's triangle **(A)** by transposition of lead III in space **(B)**. RA—Right arm; LA—Left arm; LL—Left leg.

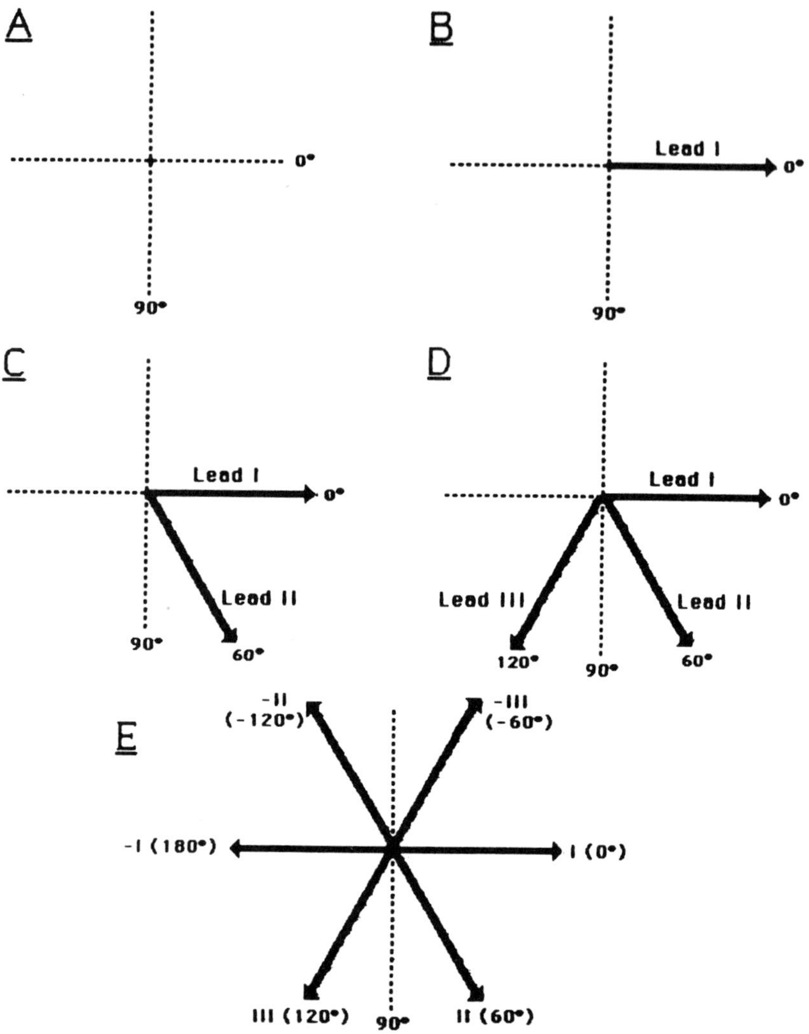

Figure 3-3. Reconstruction of the triaxial lead system.

Unipolar extremity leads (aVR, aVL, and aVF) were not added to the standard ECG until a number of years after the triaxial lead system had been established. When first described by Wilson, these leads were known as VR, VL, and VF. They were obtained by recording the electrical difference between an exploring electrode on each respective extremity and a null central terminal with an electric potential of zero formed by connecting the right arm, left arm, and left leg electrodes. Initially the QRS deflections obtained in this manner were of very small amplitude, and consequently were difficult to interpret on the ECG. By modifying the way in which the unipolar lead system was set up internally within the ECG machine itself (disconnecting the extremity lead of the exploring electrode from the central terminal), Goldberger showed that recorded voltages from unipolar leads could be *augmented* by 50%. Thus an "a" (for augmented) has been added to the original notations.

Fig. 3-4A illustrates the unipolar lead system. This is most easily remembered by noting that the three leads form a "Mercedes Benz triangle." Lead aVL views the heart from the left shoulder, and represents an axis of −30°. Lead aVF views the heart from the feet, and represents an axis of

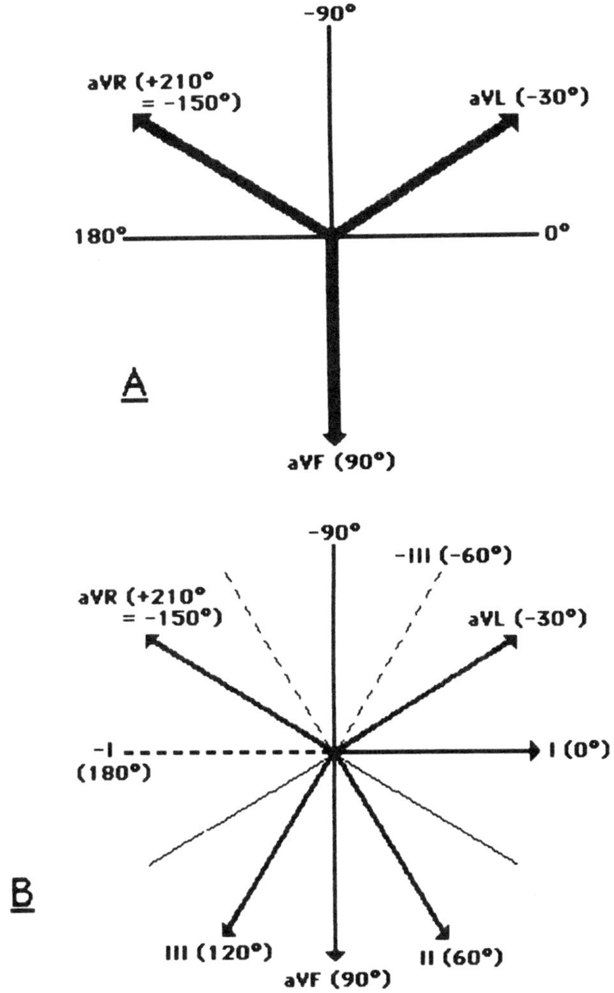

Figure 3-4. **A.** The unipolar lead system, consisting of leads aVR, aVL, and aVF. **B.** Superposition of the unipolar leads on the triaxial system to make the hexaxial lead system.

+90°. Lead aVR, representing an axis of +210°(= − 150°), has been termed an "extracavitary" lead, because it views the heart from the farthest distance away (from the right shoulder). This lead is usually the *least* helpful to us in our calculation of axis. Fig. 3-4B shows how we can construct the hexaxial lead system by superposition of the unipolar leads on the triaxial system.

Reconstruction of the hexaxial lead system can be accomplished easily if one follows the steps described above for construction of the triaxial lead system (Fig. 3-3A to 3-3E). To this, lead aVF looking directly up from the feet is added at 90°. Lead aVL at −30° bisects leads I and −III. The Mercedes triangle is then completed with lead aVR.

The Three Basic Laws of Electrocardiography

The final principle to understand in calculating QRS axis is derived from the three basic laws of electrocardiography:

- A wave of depolarization that approaches a monitoring electrode writes an upward (positive) deflection on the ECG.
- A wave of depolarization that recedes from a monitoring electrode writes a downward (negative) deflection on the ECG.
- A wave of depolarization that is perpendicular to a monitoring electrode writes an equiphasic (equally positive and negative) QRS complex.

These basic laws are illustrated in Fig. 3-5. Thus, the mean QRS axis will be most oriented *toward* (almost parallel to) the monitoring lead recording the greatest net QRS deflection. It will be *farthest* away from the monitoring lead recording the largest negative net deflection, and *perpendicular* to a monitoring lead with a net deflection of zero.

PROBLEM: Apply these laws to estimate the mean QRS axis of the representation shown in Fig. 3-6, in which monitoring leads are recording from a source of electrical activity located at the center of the circle.

ANSWER: Because the largest positive net deflection is recorded in lead I at 0°, the mean QRS axis will be most oriented toward this lead. The two standard limb leads closest to lead I are leads II (at +60°) and lead − III (at −60°). The amplitude of the QRS deflection in each of these leads is equal—the QRS complex is 4 little boxes (or 4 mm) tall. Thus, the mean QRS axis of the electrical activity in this representation must be located exactly between these two leads, or precisely at 0°.

Note that the deflection in leads aVF (at + 90°) and −aVF (at − 90°) is equiphasic or isoelectric (equal positive and negative components of the QRS complex with a net deflection of zero). These leads are perpendicular to the mean QRS axis. Monitoring leads that are less than 90° away from the mean QRS axis (leads II, aVL, and − III) record a net positive deflection.

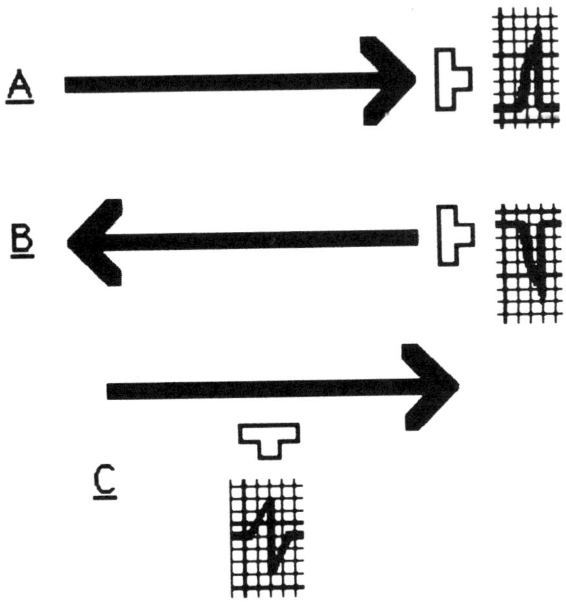

Figure 3-5. The three basic laws of electrocardiography.

Monitoring leads greater than 90° away (leads III, −I, and aVR) record a net negative deflection. The more negative the deflection, the farther away the monitoring lead must be from the mean QRS axis. Thus the largest negative deflection is seen in lead −I, which is expected because this is the lead directly opposite the wave of depolarization.

Two-Lead Method for Axis Determination

There are a number of ways to calculate the mean QRS axis. Perhaps the simplest is to inspect leads I and aVF. If the net QRS deflection in both of these leads is positive, then the mean QRS axis must lie between 0° and +90° (See Fig. 3-7). Although controversy still surrounds the issue of what constitutes a "normal" mean QRS axis, we find it easiest to use quadrants in our definition (see Fig. 3-8). Thus, if the net deflection in *both* leads I and aVF is positive, the mean QRS axis must be normal. Right axis deviation (RAD) will be present if the net QRS deflection is positive in lead aVF but negative in lead I, while left axis deviation (LAD) is present if the net QRS deflection is positive in lead I but negative in lead aVF (Table 3-1). If the net QRS deflection is negative in *both* leads I and aVF, then the mean QRS axis will be in "no man's land," which is located in the upper-right quadrant of our circle (between +180° and +270°). We define this axis as "indeterminate," since it is often impossible to determine if such an axis represents marked right or left axis deviation.

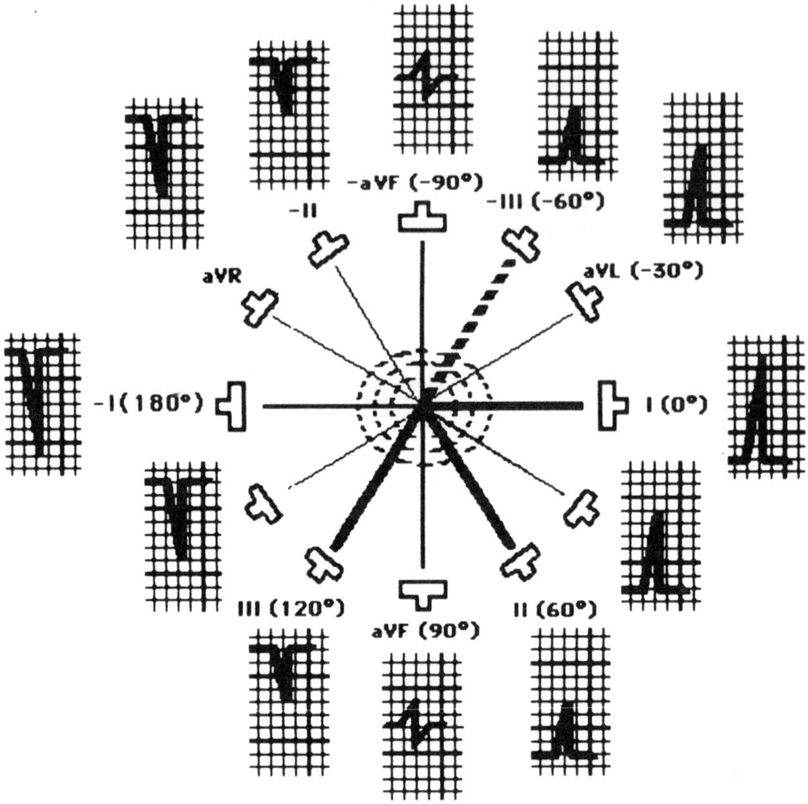

Figure 3-6

After localizing the mean QRS axis to one of the four quadrants by this method, one can then look to see if there is any lead in which the net QRS deflection is almost zero. The mean axis will be approximately 90° away from (perpendicular to) this lead. If the net deflection is slightly positive, the mean axis will be just less than 90° away. Similarly, if the net deflection is slightly negative, the mean axis will be just over 90° away.

PROBLEM: Estimate the mean QRS axis from the six limb leads of the ECG shown in Fig. 3-9 by this method.

ANSWER: One can tell at a glance that the mean QRS axis is normal in Fig. 3-9 since the net QRS deflection in both leads I and aVF is positive (see Table 3-1). The QRS complex is almost equiphasic in lead aVL, which lies at −30°. If it were exactly equiphasic, then the mean QRS axis would be perpendicular to this lead and lie at +60°. However, the net deflection in lead aVL is slightly positive, so the mean QRS axis must lie *less* than 90° away from lead aVL, or at about +50°.

Three-Lead Method for Axis Determination

This two-lead method is probably the easiest for the beginning electrocardiographer to master. A relative disadvantage, however, is that unless one of the leads is nearly isoelectric, only a rough estimation of axis is usually possible. A more precise method of axis calculation is the *three-lead* method, which uses inspection of the three standard limb leads (I, II, and III) to estimate axis. We have already seen how this works in Fig. 3-6. In that example, the mean QRS axis was seen to be oriented most toward lead I at 0°, as this was the lead with the greatest net positive deflection. Since the net deflection in leads II and −III was equal, the mean QRS axis was seen to lie exactly between these leads at 0°.

PROBLEM: Calculate the mean QRS axis from the three standard limb leads shown in Fig. 3-10. What would you expect lead aVF to look like?

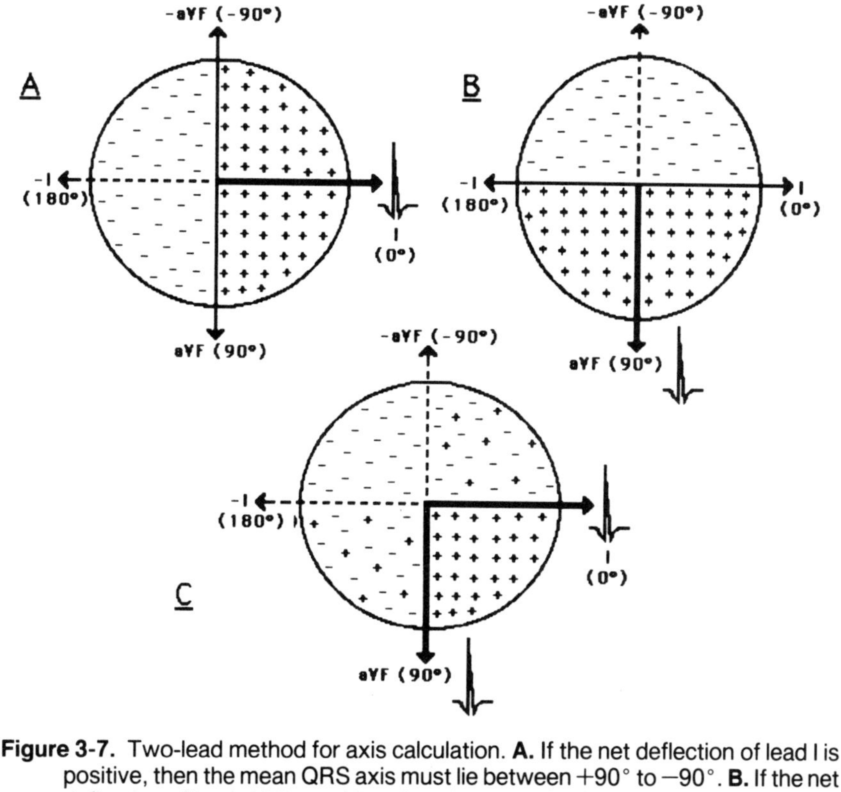

Figure 3-7. Two-lead method for axis calculation. **A.** If the net deflection of lead I is positive, then the mean QRS axis must lie between +90° to −90°. **B.** If the net deflection of lead aVF is positive, then the mean QRS axis must lie between 0° to +180°. **C.** If the net deflection in both leads I and aVF is positive, then the mean QRS axis must lie between 0° to +90°.

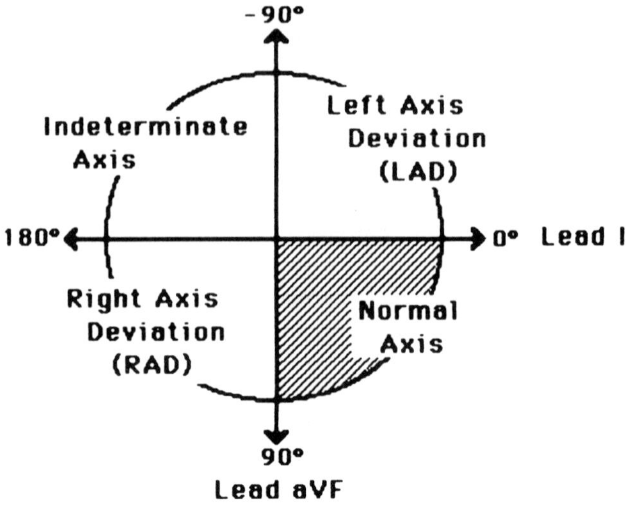

Figure 3-8. Suggested criteria for categorization of axis deviations according to quadrants.

Figure 3-9

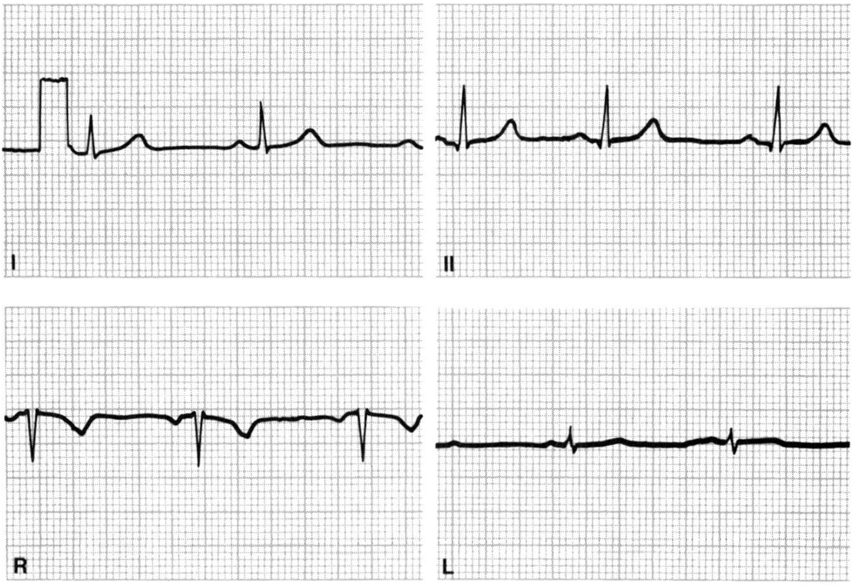

TABLE 3-1

Two-lead method for determining axis

	Normal Axis	RAD	LAD	Indeterminate Axis
Lead I	+	−	+	−
Lead aVF	+	+	−	−

ANSWER: Fig. 3-11 illustrates the rationale for determining the mean QRS axis of the three standard limb leads shown in Fig. 3-10. The axis is oriented most toward lead I at 0°, since this lead manifests the greatest net positive deflection. The net deflection of lead I = −2(Q wave) + 13(R wave) −2(S wave) = 9 mm. The two standard limb leads adjoining lead I are leads II and −III. If the net deflection of these two leads were exactly equal, then the mean QRS axis would lie exactly between them at 0°. However, since the net deflection in lead II (5 mm) is slightly greater than that in lead −III (3

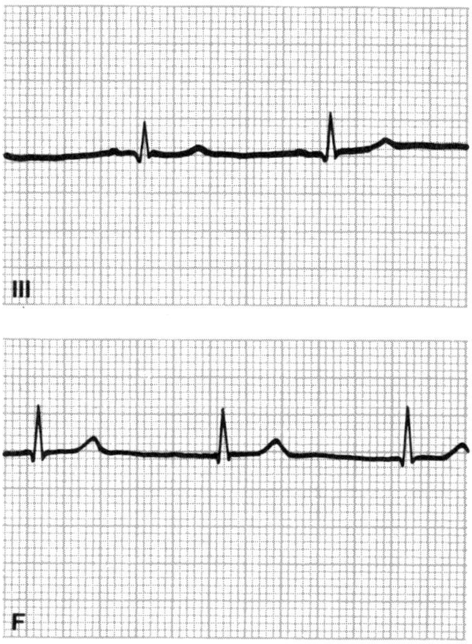

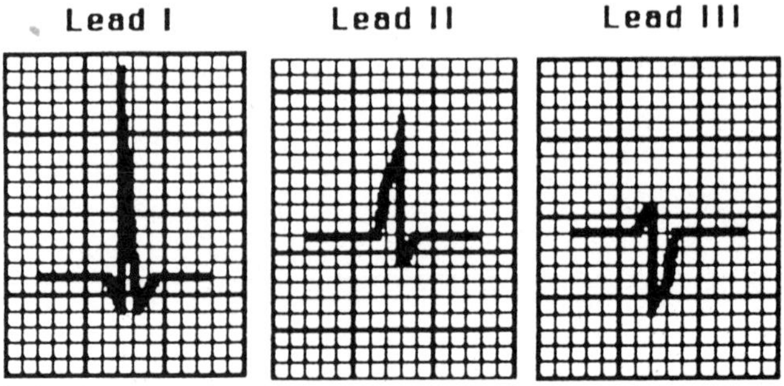

Figure 3-10

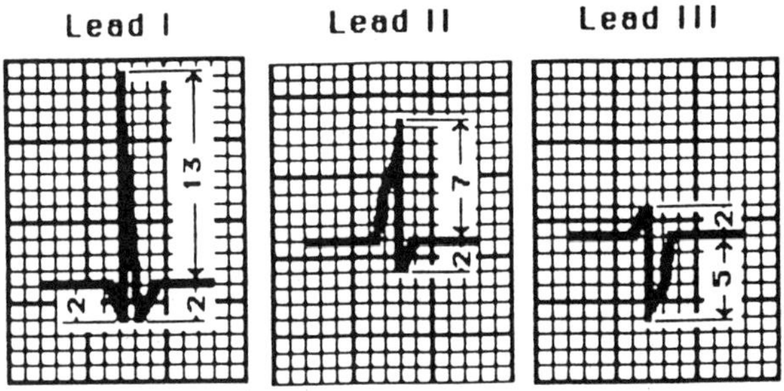

Deflection (in mm)

	Lead I	Lead II	Lead -III
Q Wave	-2	0	0
R Wave	+13	+7	+2
S Wave	-2	-2	-5
Net Deflection	+9	+5	+3

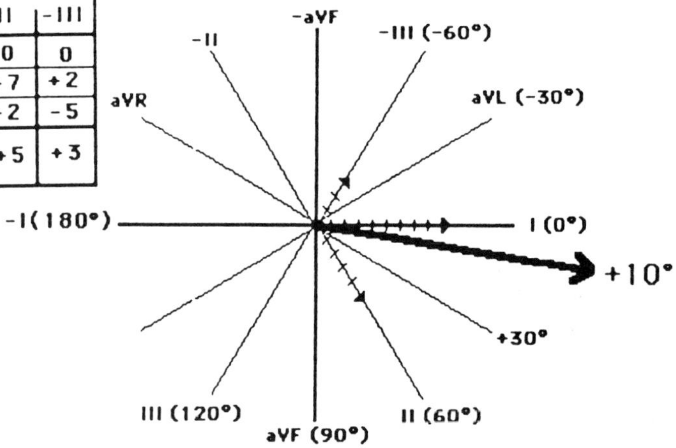

Figure 3-11. Explanation of axis calculation for Fig. 3-10.

mm), the axis must be slightly more oriented toward the former. We estimate it to be at about +10°.

Fig. 3-12 illustrates the expected appearance of lead aVF. If the mean QRS axis were exactly 0°, then one would expect lead aVF, which is perpendicular to 0°, to be equiphasic, However, since the axis was estimated to be slightly positive at +10°, lead aVF lies a little less than 90° away. Therefore, it should manifest a slightly positive net deflection. Inspection of Fig. 3-12 shows that it does.

Much greater precision can be achieved with this method because three rather than two leads are used to calculate the axis. With a little practice, axis calculation may be accomplished as rapidly as with the two-lead method. Inspection of a fourth lead (in this case lead aVF) may then be used, if desired, to further refine your estimation or to serve as a final check. (We prefer to use either lead aVL or aVF rather than the extracavitary lead aVR as the final check.)

We also prefer choosing the three standard limb leads (I, II, and III) when using this method of axis calculation, rather than the three augmented limb leads (aVR, aVL, and aVF), or interchanging among the two systems. Each standard limb lead is equidistant from its neighbor (60° away, by Einthoven's Law). Thus, if the net deflection of two of the limb leads is equal, the axis must lie *exactly* between the two. The same *cannot* be said if the amplitude of a standard limb lead and that of an augmented lead is equal, because the displayed QRS voltage of the *augmented* leads has been increased by 50% over the actual voltage recorded from that respective extremity.

A final consideration is the dynamic nature of the mean QRS axis. The inferior portion of the heart sits on the diaphragm. Consequently, leads III and aVF that view this aspect of the heart may be significantly affected by the phasic diaphragmatic movement of normal respiration. Similarly, changes in body position such as turning or standing may also at times have a dramatic affect on the mean QRS axis.

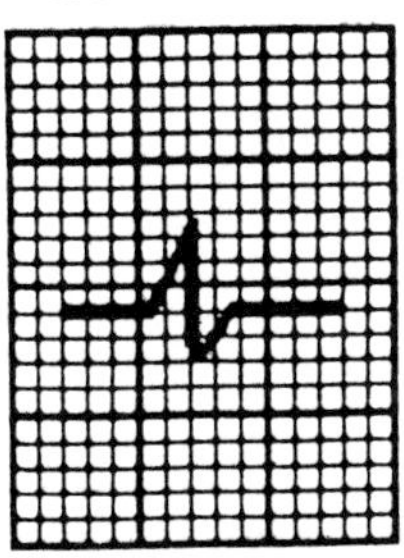

Figure 3-12. Expected appearance of lead aVF for the three standard limb leads shown in Fig. 3-9. Since the mean QRS axis is +10°, lead aVF should manifest a slightly positive net deflection.

In the past, all ECGs were obtained from single-channel machines, which recorded one lead at a time. Currently, most hospitals and many office practices have switched to simultaneous three-channel ECG machines, which save time by recording three leads at the same time. Usual groupings are as follows: leads I, II and III; leads aVR, aVL, and aVF; leads V_1, V_2, and V_3; and leads V_4, V_5, and V_6. Thus, when a simultaneous three-channel ECG machine is used, an additional reason for not interchanging standard limb leads with augmented leads for axis calculation is the security of knowing that QRS deflections of leads I, II, and III will all be recorded at the same instant in time, whereas those of leads I and aVF will not be.

With this as a background, let us now apply these methods for axis calculation to the examples in the rest of this chapter. Our rationale for the axis determinations of the first two examples will be illustrated on the hexaxial lead system in a similar manner as was done in Fig. 3-11. After this, you're on your own!

NOTE: You may find it helpful at first to draw out the hexaxial lead system (Fig. 3-13) to assist in your calculation. Visualization of axis determination is often much easier when plotted out. With practice, you will probably find yourself performing these calculations in your head.

PROBLEM: Estimate the mean QRS axis from the leads shown in Fig. 3-14.

ANSWER to Fig. 3-14: The largest net positive deflection in the standard limb leads is in lead II at 60°. The mean QRS axis is most oriented toward this lead (Fig. 3-15A). If lead I (at 0°) and lead III (at 120°) were exactly equal, the mean QRS axis would be precisely at 60°. Since the net deflection of lead

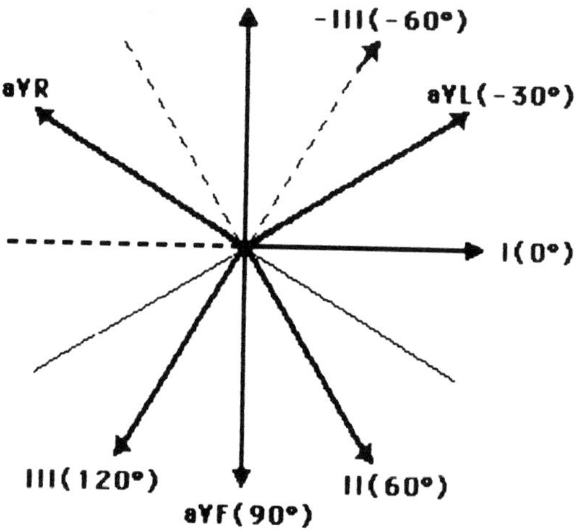

Figure 3-13. The hexaxial lead system.

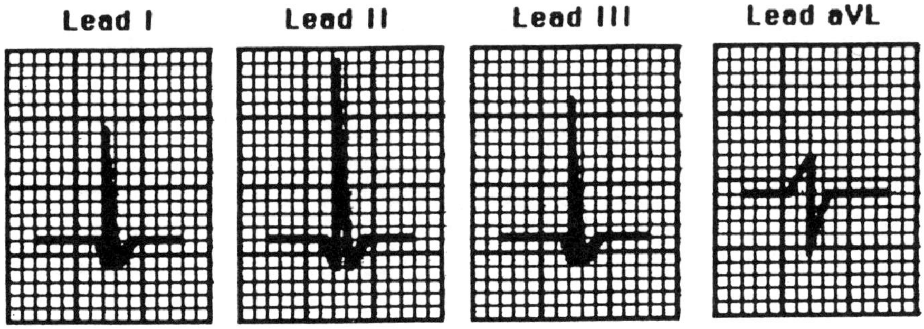

Figure 3-14

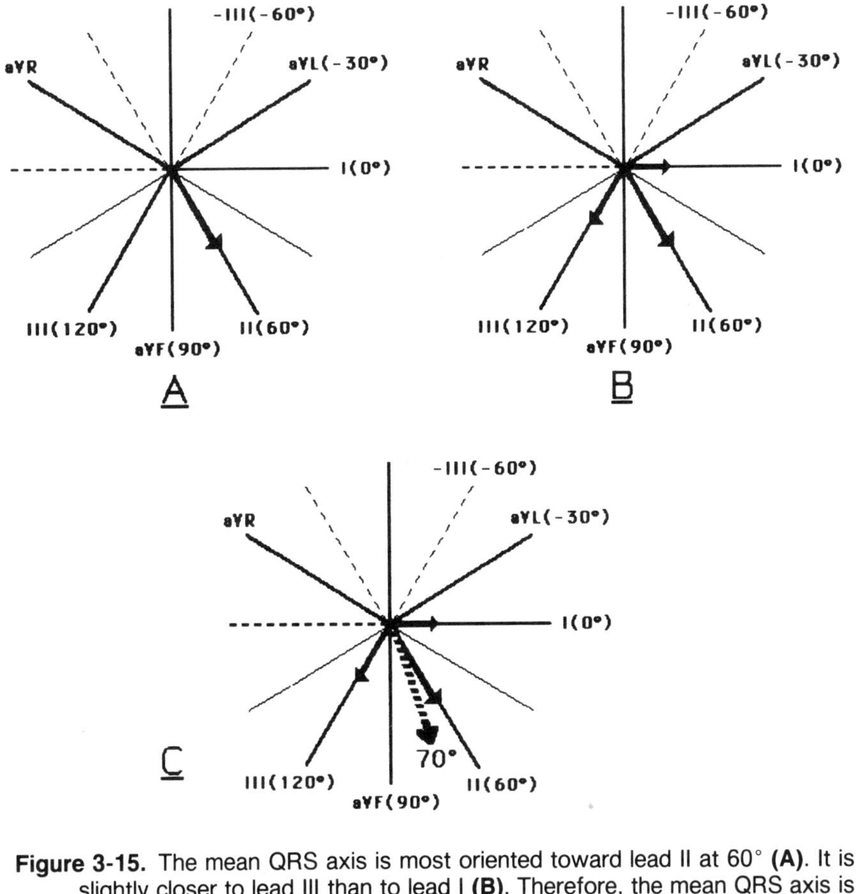

Figure 3-15. The mean QRS axis is most oriented toward lead II at 60° **(A)**. It is slightly closer to lead III than to lead I **(B)**. Therefore, the mean QRS axis is about +70° **(C)**. As a check of this calculation, note that lead aVL is slightly negative in Fig. 3-14 as it should be for an axis of +70°.

III is greater than that of lead I, however, the axis will be closer to lead III, or at about 70° (Fig. 3-15B and C).

Lead aVL confirms this estimation. If lead aVL (at −30°) were equiphasic, the mean QRS axis would be 90° away, or at +60°. Since the net deflection of lead aVL is slightly negative, the axis must be just over 90° away, or at about +70° as estimated above.

PROBLEM: Estimate the mean QRS axis from the leads shown in Fig. 3-16.

ANSWER to Fig. 3-16: The largest net deflection in the standard limb leads is in lead I (Fig. 3-17A). Since the net deflection of lead III [+2(R wave) −7(S wave) = −5, or 5 mm net deflection in the direction of lead −III] is slightly greater than the net deflection in lead II [+4(R wave) −2(S wave) = +2, or 2 mm net deflection], the mean QRS axis will be most oriented toward lead I (at 0°), but closer to lead −III (at −60°) than to lead II (at +60°) (Fig. 3-17B). Thus the mean QRS axis is about −15° (Fig. 3-17C). Lead aVF at 90° is consistent with this estimation, because it is slightly negative.

PROBLEM: Estimate the mean QRS axis from the leads shown in Fig. 3-18.

ANSWER to Fig. 3-18: There is no one dominant deflection in this example. Instead, the net deflections of leads II (at +60°) and III (at +120°) are identical. One would expect the mean QRS axis to lie midway between at +90°. Lead I confirms this in that it is equiphasic.

Right Axis Deviation

We have previously defined right axis deviation (RAD) as a mean QRS axis of greater than 90°. This holds true mainly for adults; slight RAD may be normal in children. Fig. 3-18 then would manifest borderline RAD in an adult.

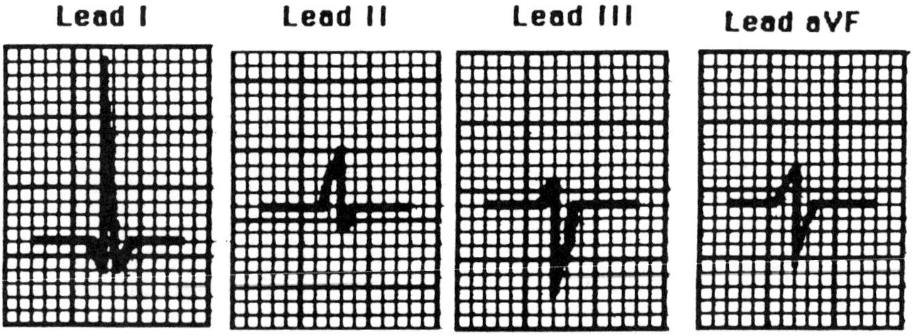

Figure 3-16

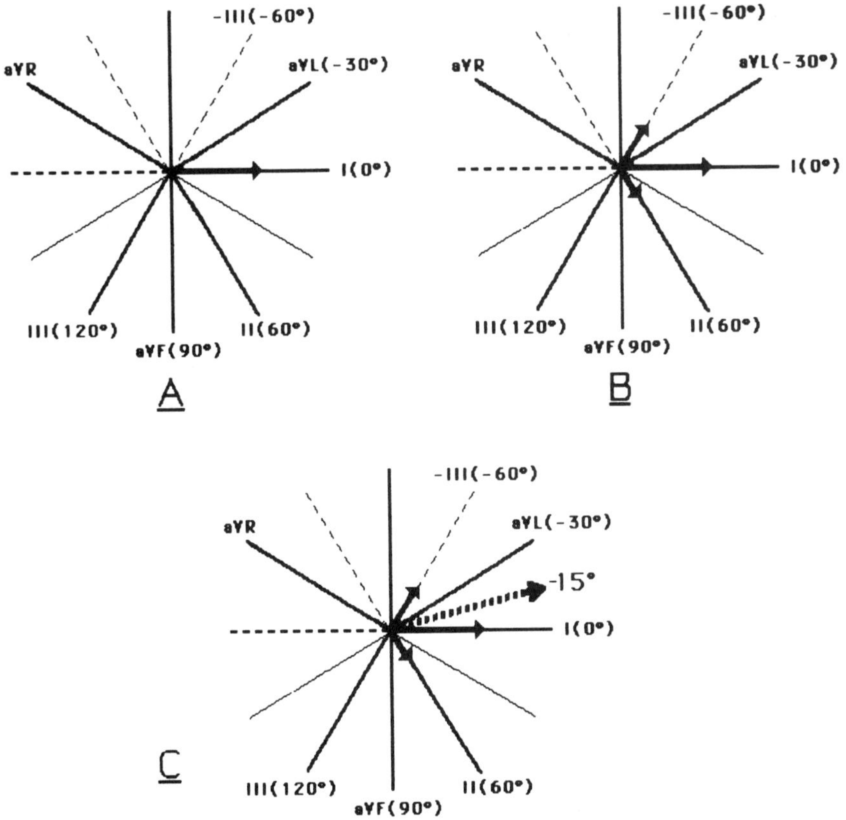

Figure 3-17. The mean QRS axis is most oriented toward lead I at 0° **(A)**. It is slightly closer to lead −III than to lead II **(B)**. Therefore, the mean QRS axis is about −15° **(C)**. As a check of this calculation, note that lead aVF is slightly negative in Fig. 3-16 as it should be for an axis of −15°.

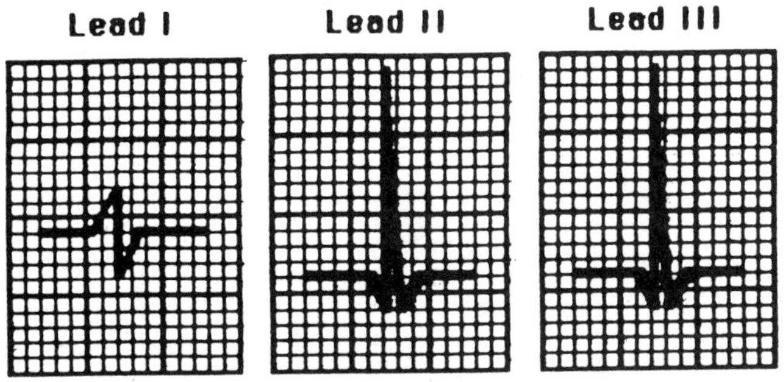

Figure 3-18

PROBLEM: How can one tell at a glance if there is definite RAD? Examine Fig. 3-19. Is RAD present in either A or B in this figure?

ANSWER to Fig. 3-19: One can tell at a glance if RAD is present simply by looking at lead I. If lead I (at 0°) has a net negative deflection, the mean QRS axis must be more than 90° away from this lead, and RAD must be present. This condition is satisfied in Fig. 3-19A. The axis is about +100°. Since lead I is positive in Fig. 3-19B, RAD is not present. The axis here is about +80°

Up to now we have determined the net deflection of a particular QRS complex by counting the number of millimeters of positive deflection and subtracting the number of millimeters of negative deflection. While in most instances we can arrive at an extremely accurate estimate of mean QRS axis by this method, this may *not* be true if the QRS complex is widened. Actually, it is *not* the number of millimeters in a deflection that counts, but rather the *area* enclosed by that deflection that is most important. As one might imagine, calculation of axis often poses a problem in bundle branch block.

PROBLEM: Consider Fig. 3-20. What is the mean QRS axis?

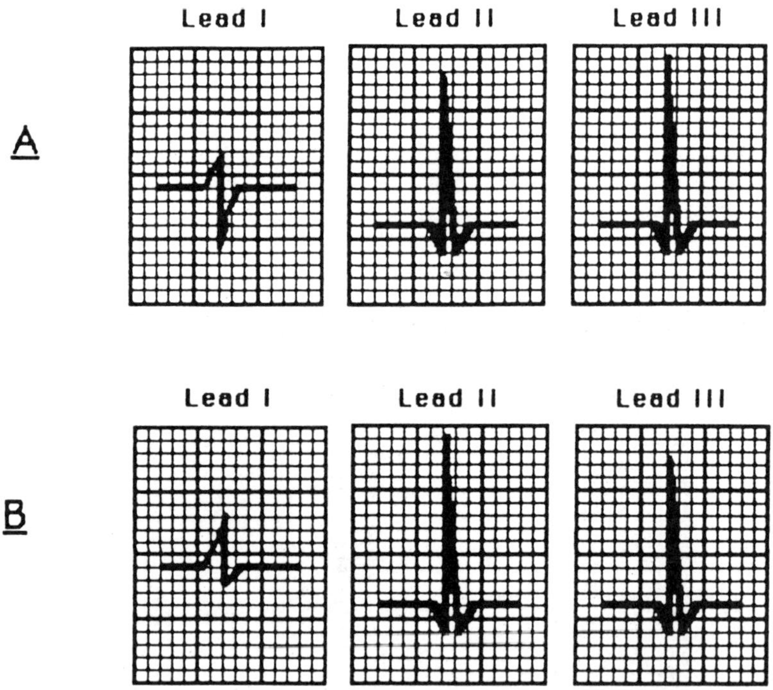

Figure 3-19

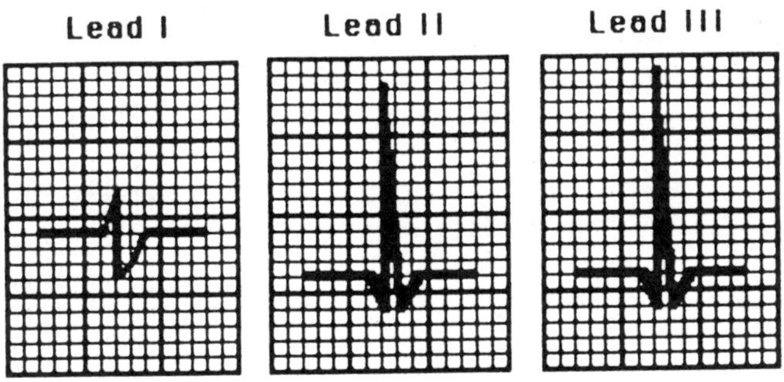

Figure 3-20

ANSWER to Fig. 3-20: Once again, there are two dominant net deflections in leads II and III. The mean QRS axis is thus oriented between them at about +90°. Inspection of lead I reveals the R wave in this lead to be equal in amplitude to the S wave (3 mm). However, the area encompassed by the negative deflection is clearly greater than that contained within the R wave. Thus, the net deflection of lead I is somewhat negative, and the mean QRS axis in this example must be greater than +90°.

PROBLEM: Estimate the mean QRS axis from the leads shown in Fig. 3-21.

ANSWER to Fig. 3-21: There are two dominant deflections in leads I (at 0°) and II (at +60°). Since the latter net deflection is slightly greater, the mean QRS axis is also closer to the latter, or at about +40°. This is confirmed by the slight positivity of lead III that puts the axis at less than 90° away from this lead.

PROBLEM: Estimate the mean QRS axis from the leads shown in Fig. 3-22.

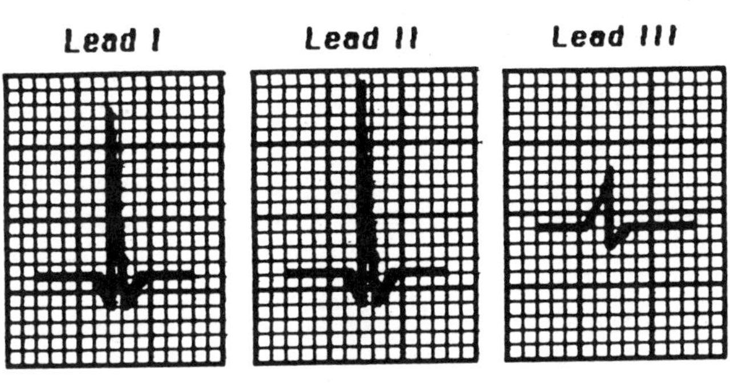

Figure 3-21

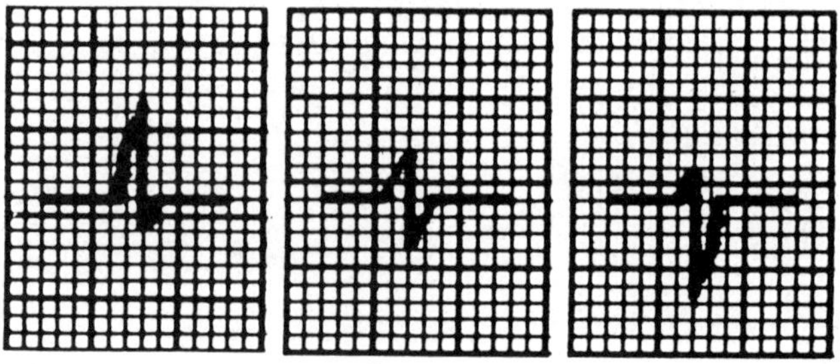

Figure 3-22

ANSWER to Fig. 3-22: There is no dominant QRS deflection in this example. Instead, the net deflection of lead I (+6 −2 = +4) appears to be about as positive as the net deflection in lead III is negative (+2 −6 = −4). Thus, the mean QRS axis should be oriented about midway between lead I (at 0°) and lead −III (at −60°), or at about −30°. This is confirmed by the equiphasic complex in lead II.

Left Axis Deviation

We have previously defined left axis deviation (LAD) as a mean QRS axis that is more negative than 0°. However, many elderly individuals develop various degrees of LAD as part of the aging process, without necessarily developing a discrete abnormality in their conduction system. Thus, we usually do not define a leftward axis as *pathologic* until the mean QRS axis becomes more negative than −30°.

PROBLEM: How can one tell at a glance if pathologic LAD is present? Examine Fig. 3-23. Is a pathologic LAD present in either tracing?

ANSWER to Fig. 3-23: If lead II (at +60°) is isoelectric, the mean QRS axis will be 90° away, or at −30°. To determine if pathologic LAD is present, one need therefore *only* look at lead II. If the net deflection in this lead is negative, the mean QRS axis must be greater than 90° away, and there is pathologic LAD.

Thus, pathologic LAD is present in Fig. 3-23A, but not in Fig. 3-23B. (The actual mean QRS axis is about −45° in the former and −15° in the latter.)

PROBLEM: Estimate the mean QRS axis from the leads shown in Fig. 3-24.

ANSWER to Fig. 3-24: All of the QRS complexes in this example are approximately equiphasic. Because it is inconceivable for the mean QRS

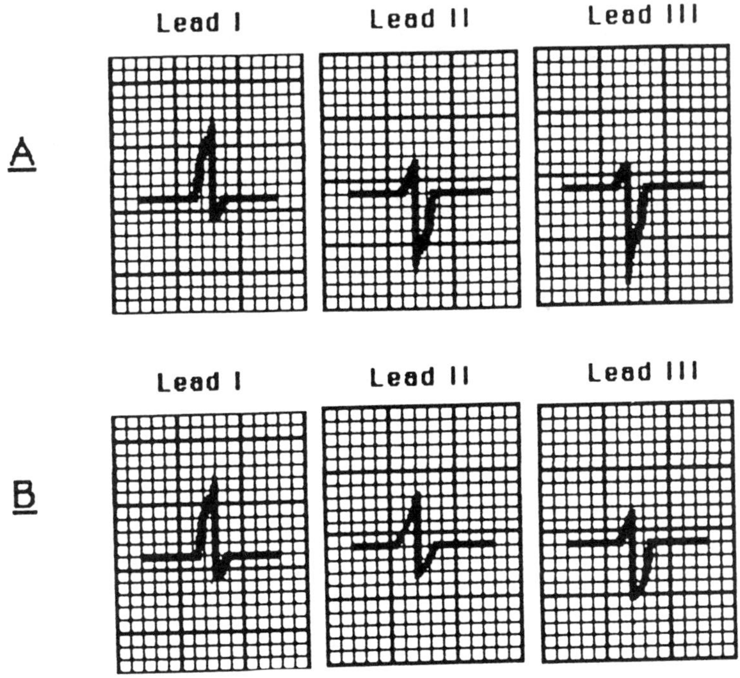

Figure 3-23

axis to be perpendicular to each of the standard limb leads, calculation of axis becomes a virtually impossible task.

Indeterminate Axis

When one cannot determine a mean QRS axis because no predominant deflection exists in the standard limb leads, we say the axis is "indeterminate." This is the case in Fig. 3-24. Almost by default, we place the axis in

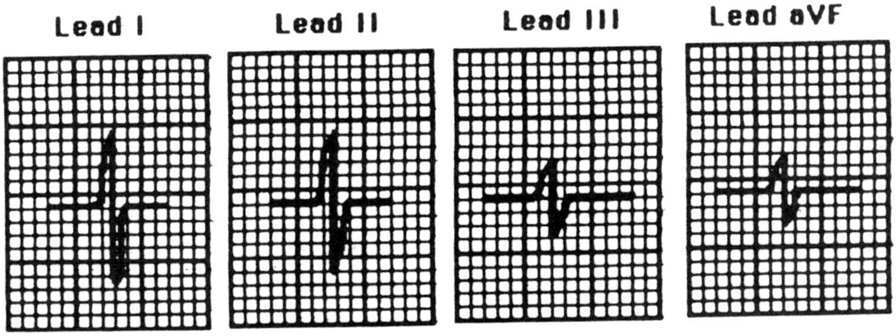

Figure 3-24

the right upper quadrant (180° to 270°) of our axis categorization circle (Fig. 3-8). Clinically, indeterminate axis is most often seen in patients with right ventricular hypertrophy or chronic obstructive pulmonary disease. It may also occur as a normal variant.

Clinical Significance of Axis Determination

Now that you're able to determine mean QRS axis rapidly and accurately, you might be asking what the clinical significance of this calculation is. Does one ever really need to say more than whether an axis is normal or not?

To answer this question it might be helpful to consider the following scenario. A baseline ECG obtained on a patient reveals a mean QRS axis of +15°. Sometime later the patient returns complaining of the acute onset of dyspnea and pleuritic chest pain. Repeat ECG now shows the mean QRS axis to be +85°. Whereas the axis in both tracings is "normal" (within 0° to +90°), the 70° shift of the axis to the right in the above-described setting would increase one's suspicion of pulmonary embolism as a possible cause of the patient's symptoms.

Determination of axis is important in the diagnosis of conditions such as bundle branch block, left anterior and posterior hemiblock, right ventricular hypertrophy, and congenital heart disease (see Tables 3-2 and 3-3). LAD and RAD may occur as normal variants, in chronic obstructive pulmonary disease, with pericardial effusion, or with pneumothorax. In pregnancy, obesity, or in the elderly, LAD is common, whereas an acute right axis shift as described in the above scenario may alert the clinician to the possibility of pulmonary embolism. Thus, calculation of the mean QRS axis to within 15° becomes more than an academic exercise, and one should never be content with merely describing the axis as "normal."

PROBLEM: As a final exercise, determine the mean QRS axis of the ECG shown in Fig. 3-25. Which of the causes of RAD listed in Table 3-3 would you suspect?

ANSWER to Fig. 3-25: There is marked RAD, with the mean QRS axis

TABLE 3-2

Causes of left axis deviation (LAD)

Normal variant
Left anterior hemiblock (LAHB)
Left bundle branch block (LBBB)
Left ventricular hypertrophy (LVH)
Elevated diaphragm (pregnancy, ascites)
Obesity
Inferior infarction

TABLE 3-3

Causes of right axis deviation (RAD)

Normal variant
Left posterior hemiblock (LPHB)*
Right ventricular hypertrophy (RVH)*
Acute cor pulmonale (pulmonary embolism)
Lateral infarction
Limb-lead reversal
Dextrocardia
Childhood

**Note: Right bundle branch block per se usually does* not *cause RAD unless there is associated LPHB or RVH.*

oriented between negative lead I (at +180°) and positive lead III (at +120°), or at about +150°.

PROBLEM: Is there anything unusual in Fig. 3-25 about the appearance of the P wave, QRS complex and T wave in lead I?

ANSWER: They are all negative! Global negativity of the P wave, QRS complex, and T wave should *never* normally be seen in lead I. Its presence implies that all electrical activity must be moving *away* from the left (where the heart normally lies within the chest) toward the right. This ECG pattern can occur under only two circumstances:

- Dextrocardia, in which the cardiac apex is located on the right side of the chest
- Limb-lead reversal

Statistically, limb-lead reversal is *far* more likely than dextrocardia.

Limb-Lead Reversal

Commission of technical errors during the recording of an ECG occurs more often than is generally appreciated. It is most frequently seen when persons who do not usually obtain ECGs are called on to perform this function—for instance, when the regular ECG technician is unavailable, or at night on the hospital ward after the ECG team has gone home. Even among the best of technicians, however, limb-lead reversal is bound to occur at some time simply because people are human and subject to error.

Surprisingly, physicians and other health-care professionals often have more difficulty recognizing technical errors such as limb-lead reversal than they do in interpreting standard ECG findings. This may have major clinical implications, because limb-lead reversal can closely simulate the picture of acute myocardial infarction. Patients have been admitted to the hospital with this diagnosis, only to have their Q-wave and ST-T wave changes "disappear" the next day when a follow-up ECG, performed with the leads applied correctly, is normal.

Figure 3-25

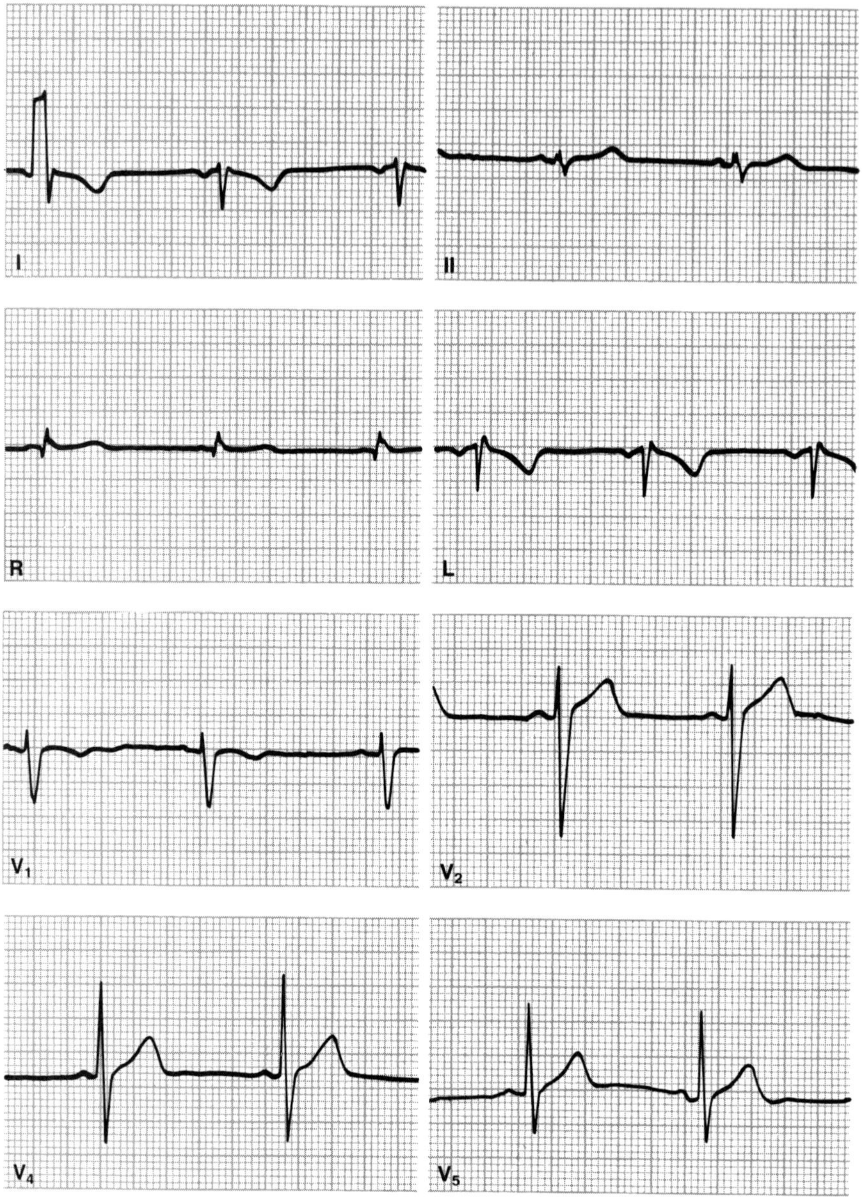

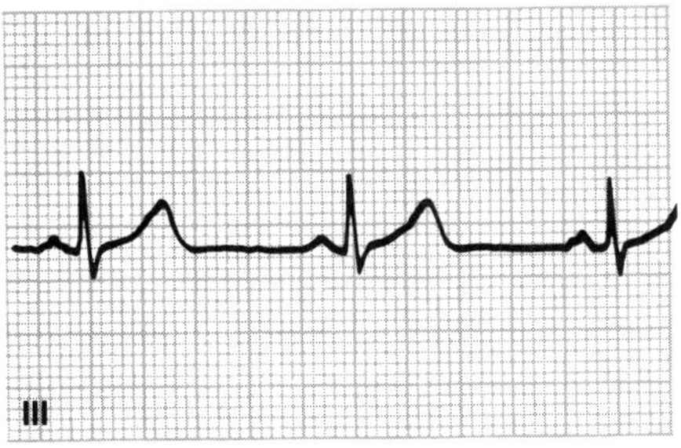
III

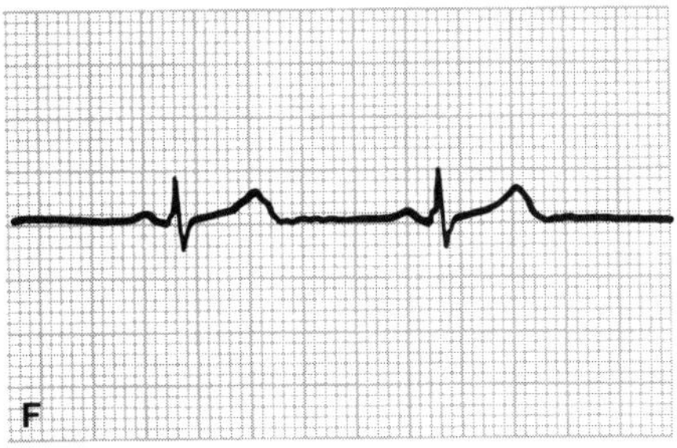
F

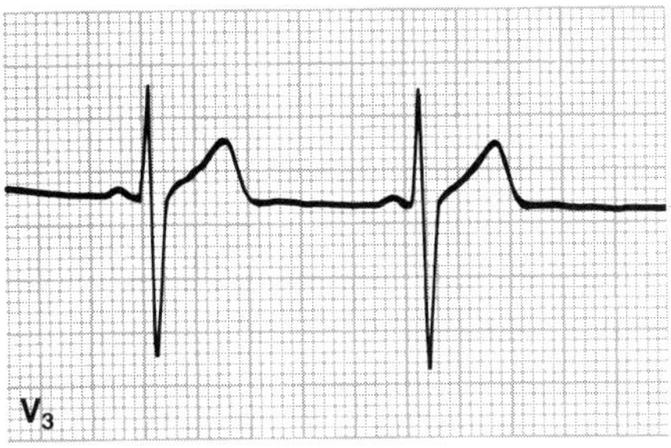
V_3

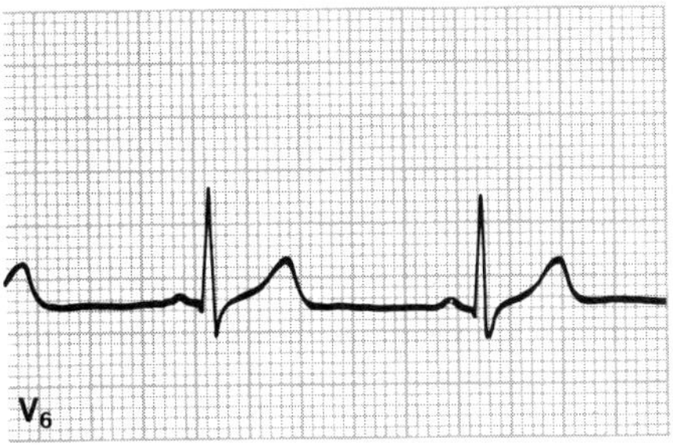
V_6

Figure 3-26

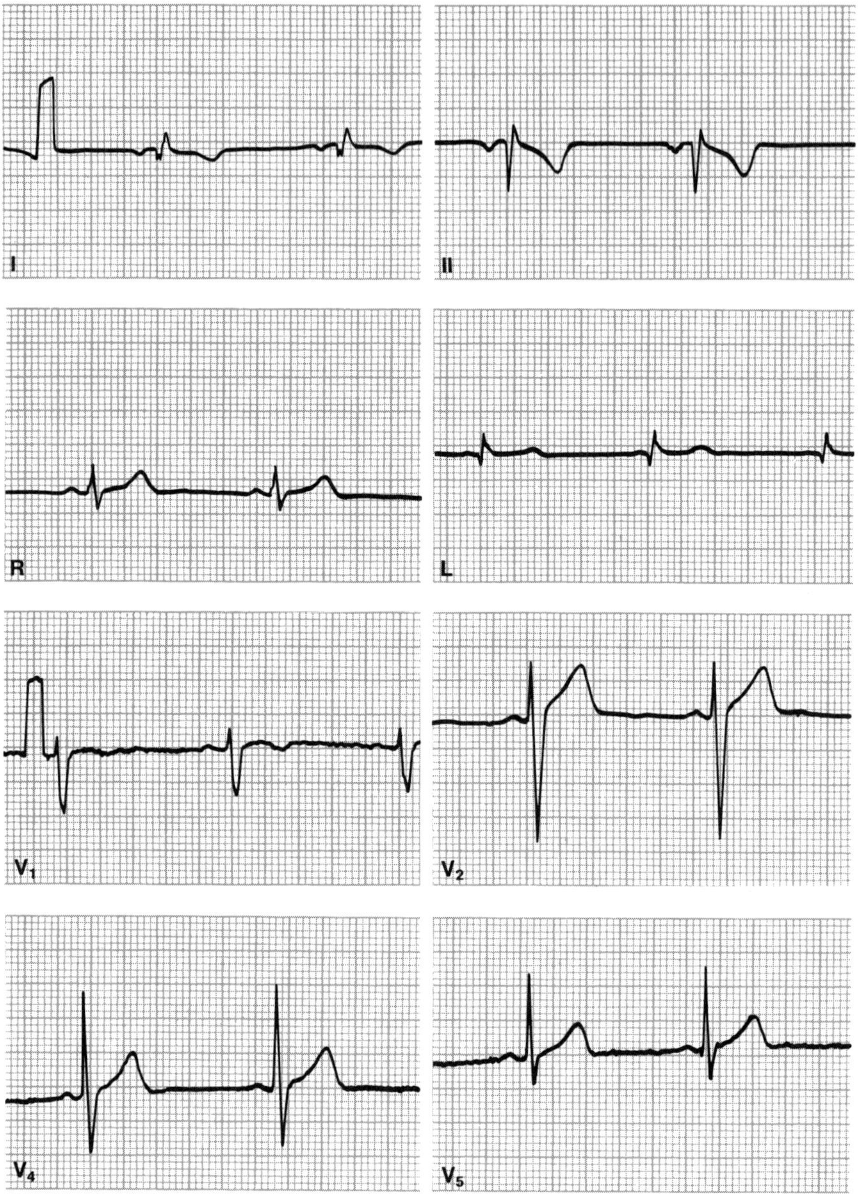

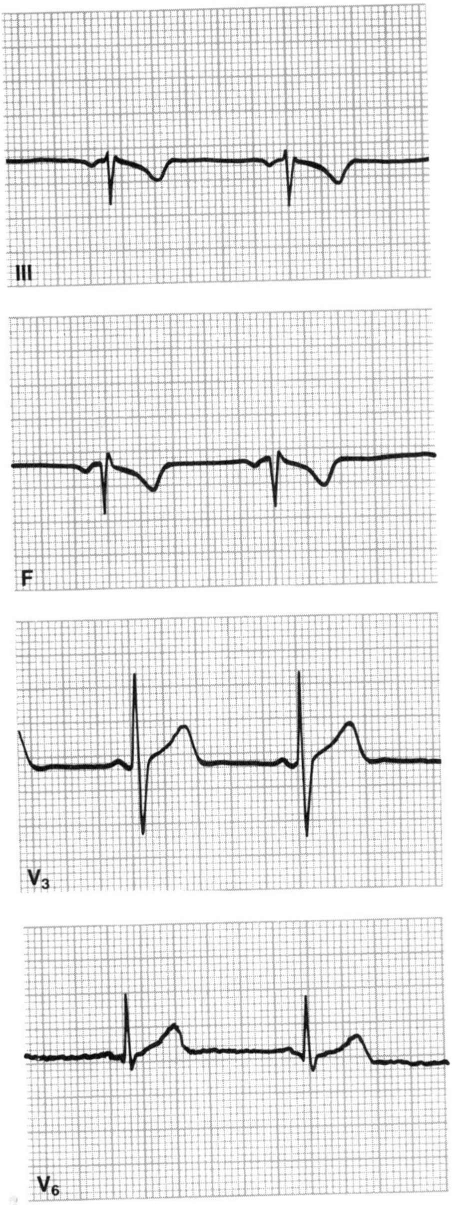
III
F
V_3
V_6

Figure 3-27. ECG from the same patient who demonstrated lead reversal due to interchange of the left and right arm electrodes (Fig. 3-25), and of the right arm and left leg electrodes (Fig. 3-26). In this figure, the recording electrodes are correctly applied.

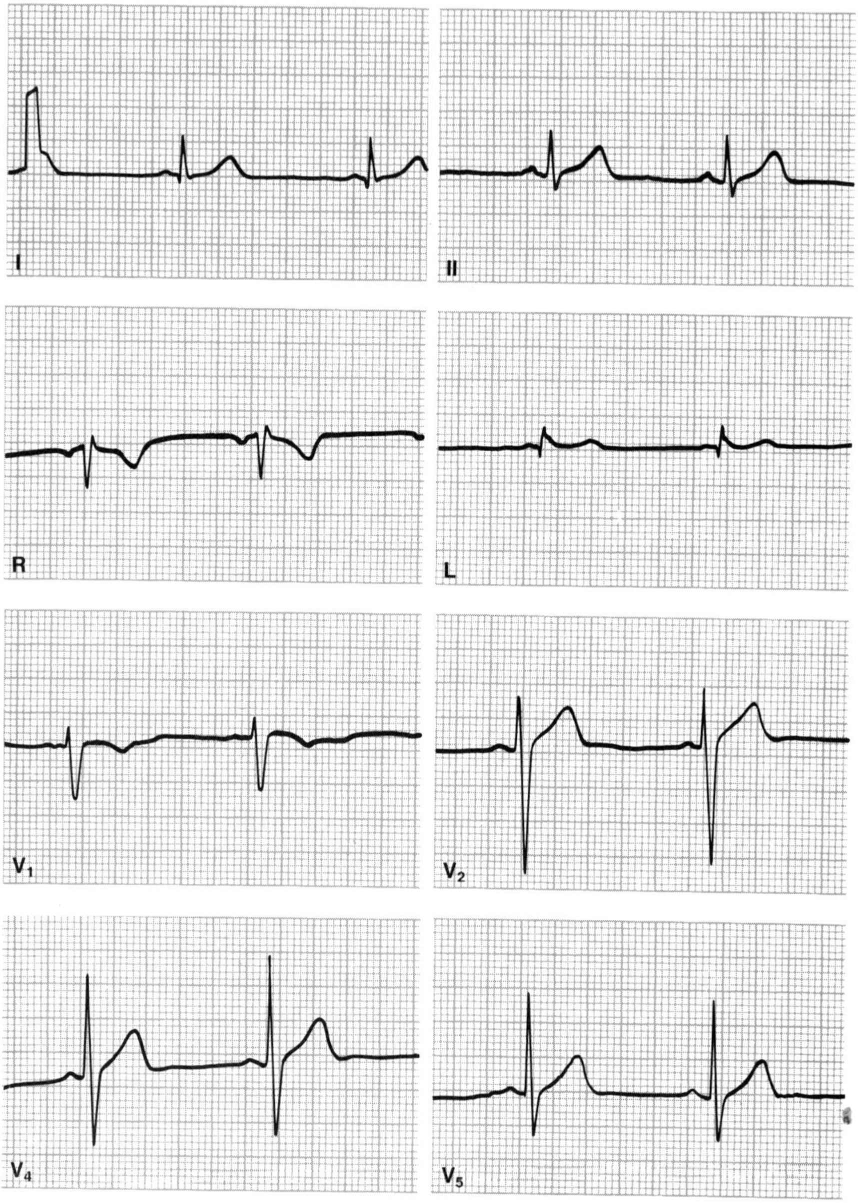

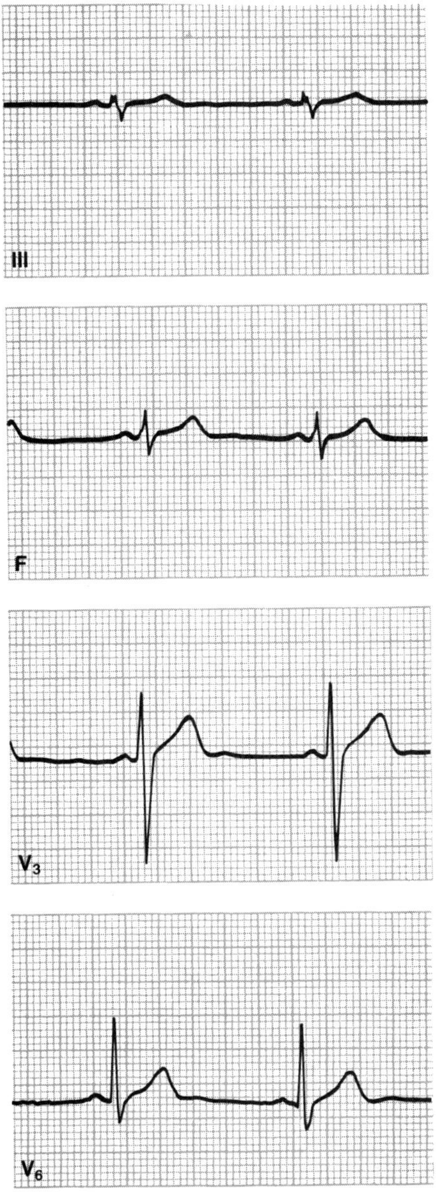
III
F
V_3
V_6

One of the main reasons limb-lead reversal is so commonly missed is that it occurs infrequently, so the novice electrocardiographer may have had little prior experience in recognizing it. In reality, identification of limb-lead reversal is usually *not* difficult at all.

The most common error that produces limb-lead reversal is interchanging the left-arm electrode with the right-arm electrode. When this is done, the expected recording for lead aVR will appear in lead I, and the expected recording for lead I will appear in lead aVR. This is the case in Fig. 3-25. *Limb-lead reversal in this tracing should be suspected because the P wave, QRS complex, and T wave are all predominantly negative in lead I.* In addition, the QRS complex in lead aVR is predominantly *positive.* Lead aVR looks at the heart's electrical activity from the right shoulder. It will almost always be predominantly *negative,* because the depolarization wavefront normally spreads to the left (—*away* from lead aVR.)

PROBLEM: The ECG in Fig. 3-26 is an example of a different type of limb-lead reversal in the same patient. Is there anything unusual in leads II and aVR that might make you suspect something is awry?

ANSWER: The P wave is inverted in lead II of this tracing. This should never occur under usual circumstances with normal sinus rhythm. In addition, the QRS complex is again predominantly positive in lead aVR, whereas with normal lead positioning it is almost always predominantly negative. The right-arm and left-leg recording electrodes were interchanged in this case.

Confirming the diagnosis of limb-lead reversal is easy to do if the patient is still present. Simply repeat the ECG, verifying lead placement. This is done in Fig. 3-27. Note that when the leads are correctly placed:

- The P wave, QRS complex, and T wave are predominantly *positive* in lead I.
- The P wave, QRS complex, and T wave are predominantly *negative* in lead aVR.
- The P wave is *upright* in lead II (as it is supposed to be under usual circumstances with normal sinus rhythm).

Dextrocardia

Dextrocardia may be distinguished electrocardiographically from limb lead reversal by the type of R-wave progression observed in the precordial leads. Normally, the R wave becomes progressively taller as one moves across the precordium. Since reversal of limb-lead electrodes will not interfere with precordial lead placement, one would expect R-wave progression to be normal in limb-lead reversal. This is the case in Figs. 3-25 and 3-26. In contrast, when the heart is situated in the right side of the chest, the height of R waves should *decrease* as one moves from lead V_1 toward lead V_6.

CHAPTER 4

THEORETICAL CONSIDERATIONS

This chapter will discuss theoretical considerations one must keep in mind when interpreting any ECG. Understanding this material will be crucial to understanding the practical examples to follow in the remainder of the book, and constant reference will be made to this chapter. Some of the material *will* be advanced for those without a sound prior background in electrocardiography. Do *not* be concerned if you find it hard to digest during this initial reading. Skim through the more difficult material now and return to it later. Rest assured that the theory presented here will become much clearer when reexamined in the clinical context of ECGs discussed in succeeding chapters.

Normal Ventricular Depolarization

Having discussed rate, rhythm, and axis, let us now trace the development of the QRS configuration in the various leads of the normal ECG. To do this, a firm appreciation of the usual sequence of ventricular activation is needed. Later, we'll apply these principles to understanding the ECG alterations that accompany myocardial infarction, chamber enlargement, and bundle branch blocks.

Let us review the schematic diagram of the atrioventricular conduction system that was introduced in Chapter 1. As seen in Fig. 4-1A, after the impulse originates in the SA node (1), it is conducted through the interatrial and internodal tracts (2), the AV node (3), and the bundle of His (4). It next enters the left and right bundle branches that course down each side of the septum (5). Because arborizations from the left bundle branch activate the septum at a higher level than do arborizations from the right bundle branch, *the impulse will normally depolarize the left side of the septum first* (6). Appreciation of this fact is crucial to understanding the sequence of normal depolarization. As a result, the middle-left side of the septum is activated first, and septal depolarization proceeds from left to right. In reality, the process of ventricular depolarization takes place in *three* dimensions, so that in addition to a rightward direction, the mean vector of septal depolarization is usually oriented downward and anteriorly.

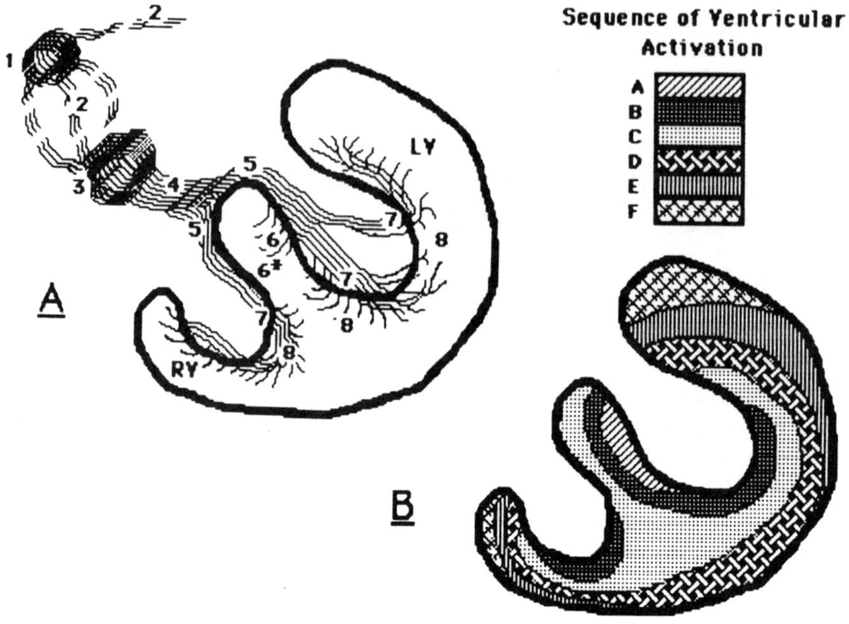

Figure 4-1. A. Atrioventricular conduction system. **B.** Sequence of ventricular activation. LV—Left ventricle; RV—Right ventricle; 1—SA node; 2—Interatrial and internodal tracts; 3—AV node; 4—Bundle of His; 5—Division of His into left and right bundle branches; 6—First activation of the septum by arborizations from the left bundle branch; 6*—Spread of electrical impulse through the septum; 7—Travel through distal bundle branch system; 8—Exit from terminal ramifications of Purkinje system.

As the septum is being activated (6*), the depolarization wavefront continues to spread extremely rapidly throughout the remainder of the bundle branch system and the specialized Purkinje network (7). This activates the endocardial surface of the left and right ventricular cavities.

Conduction velocities of the depolarization impulse are slowest through the AV node (≈ 50 mm/sec). They are significantly faster in the atria (≈900 mm/sec), and fastest of all in the bundle branches and specialized Purkinje system (≈2000 mm/sec). As the impulse arrives at the terminal ramifications of the Purkinje system (8 in Fig. 4-1A), conduction velocity again slows down (≈400 mm/sec) as the impulse begins its journey through the ventricular myocardium.

As can be seen, the process of ventricular depolarization is complex. In Chapter 3 we saw that at any given moment during this process, the heart's electrical activity could be represented by numerous small instantaneous vectors, each with its own magnitude and direction (Fig. 3-1 in Chapter 3). These vectors are constantly changing with time as the depolarization wavefront spreads through the ventricles. Fig. 4-1B illustrates the approximate time sequence of this electrical wavefront as it spreads through the ventricles to activate the heart. Note that the first area to be activated is the middle left portion of the septum (Panel A in Fig. 4-1B). As described above, the depolarization wavefront is then transmitted via specialized conduction fibers to the endocardial surface of the left and right ventricular cavities at the same time the septum is being activated (Panel B). This is followed in sequence by activation of the ventricular apex, and then the bulk of the left and right ventricular free walls (Panels C and D). The last portions of the heart to be activated are the posterobasal wall of the left ventricle and the right ventricular outflow tract (Panels E and F). Activation is delayed in these areas because they generally lack a well-developed Purkinje fiber network.

In summary, the ventricular depolarization wavefront begins in the middle-left third of the septum, then spreads rightward as it moves toward the endocardial surfaces of the ventricular cavities, following which it penetrates and travels through the myocardium until arriving at the outer epicardial border. The whole process (Panels A to F in Fig. 4-1B) in the normal heart takes less than 0.10 second.

Ventricular repolarization takes place in the opposite direction. Instead of proceding from endocardium to epicardium, the process of ventricular repolarization in the normal human heart proceeds from epicardium to endocardium (Fig. 4-2)! This is because the first portion of the heart to be depolarized (the endocardium) has the longest refractory period and is thus the last to be repolarized. This sequence of activation resembles the events illustrated in Fig. 1-3E of Chapter 1 for the theoretical myocardial cell, and explains why the T wave will usually be oriented in a similar direction as the QRS complex in most leads of a normal ECG.

Several important anatomic points should be emphasized. The left ventricular wall in a normal adult is approximately three times as thick as the right ventricular wall. The electrical potential it generates may be up to ten times greater than that generated by the right ventricular myocardium.

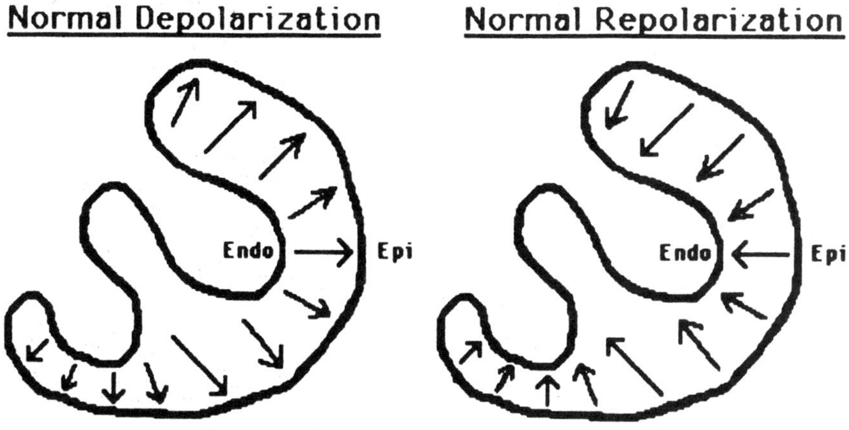

Figure 4-2. Direction of normal ventricular depolarization and repolarization. Endo — Endocardium; Epi — Epicardium.

Thus, left ventricular events totally predominate during the process of ventricular depolarization! Furthermore, the ventricular septum that divides the left and right ventricular cavity is really part of the left ventricle. As such, it is *not* the slender fragile structure we sometimes think, but rather has the same thickness as the left ventricular free wall. Consequently, a similar amount of time is needed for the activation wavefront to pass through the septum as for it to be conducted through the left ventricular free wall. The final point to emphasize is that events are always occurring in *three* dimensions. Thus, septal activation is accomplished in a rightward, downward, and anterior direction. Right and left ventricular activation occur not only in the direction that their name implies, but also in an anterior and posterior sense, respectively, since the ventricles are really anterior and posterior structures. This becomes important later in this chapter when we discuss chamber enlargement and fascicular blocks.

Although the above stated explanation of events comprising ventricular depolarization may appear somewhat complicated, it fortunately can be greatly simplified. Instead of the multitude of instantaneous vectors depicted in Fig. 3-1 of Chapter 3, the process of ventricular depolarization can be accurately represented by the two principal forces shown in Fig. 4-3. The reason we are able to ignore the overwhelming majority of electrical forces generated during ventricular activation is that most of them are spatially oriented in opposing directions. As a result, many of these forces cancel each other out; only a minority of them are left to generate the QRS deflections that we see on the ECG.

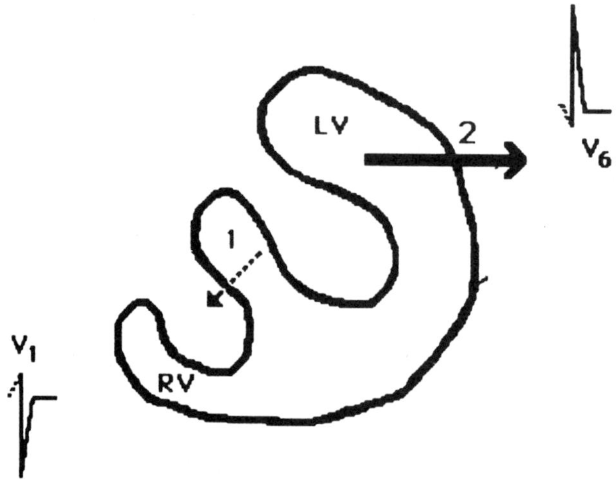

Figure 4-3. Normal ventricular depolarization. The process can be accurately represented by two principal forces: a small vector of septal depolarization (1), and a larger vector of left ventricular depolarization (2). The small r wave in V_1 and the narrow q wave in V_6 (dotted lines) are important normal findings that reflect septal depolarization.

As illustrated by vector 1 in Fig. 4-3, ventricular depolarization begins in the middle-left third of the septum, and travels in a downward and left-to-right direction. This initial vector of electrical activity will be seen by a right-sided lead such as V_1 as coming directly toward it. As a result, a small r wave (positive deflection) is written on the ECG in lead V_1. Similarly, septal depolarization will be seen by a left-sided lead such as V_6 as moving directly away, and a small q wave (negative deflection) forms the first portion of the QRS complex that is written in lead V_6. These events of septal depolarization are depicted in Fig. 4-3 as dotted lines.

Two points deserve special mention. The presence of a small r wave in lead V_1 implies that septal activation is intact. With septal infarction, this r wave is lost, and a QS complex will be seen in lead V_1. Similarly, the small q wave seen in lead V_6 also reflects normal septal depolarization. Such small and narrow q waves are commonly seen in the lateral leads (I, aVL, V_5, and V_6), and do not necessarily imply infarction.

When the heart is oriented in a more vertical position, "normal septal q waves" may also be seen in the inferior leads (Fig. 4-4). Here vector 1 is again directed to the right, but this time points superiorly. Initial septal forces will therefore be oriented away from an inferior lead such as aVF, and a small q wave may normally be seen in this lead. Differentiation of normal inferior septal q waves from infarction q waves can usually be made by the fact that the former are often smaller in size and tend to occur in otherwise young and healthy individuals who have a relatively vertical heart. At times as we will see later, this differentiation may become extremely difficult.

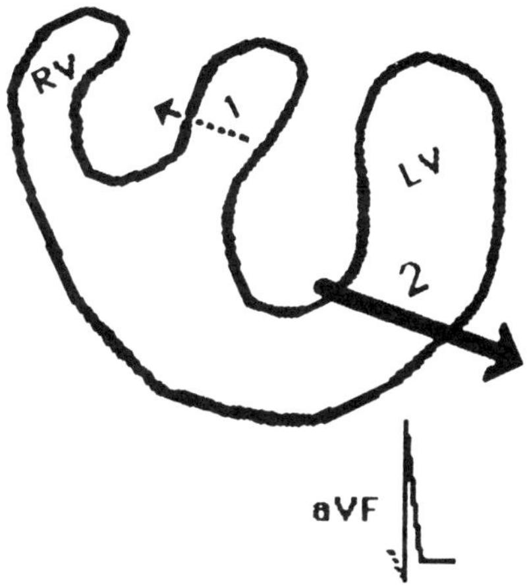

Figure 4-4. Occurrence of normal inferior septal q waves in the presence of a vertical mean QRS axis. Although vector 1 (dotted vector) is still directed from left to right, it now points superiorly. Thus, initial forces are oriented away from an inferior lead such as aVF, and a normal septal q wave (dotted line) may be inscribed.

Let's return to Fig. 4-3. Following activation of the septum, left ventricular depolarization dominates the remainder of the depolarization process. This is represented in the diagram by the solidly drawn vector 2, which is much larger than the initial vector of septal depolarization. Although right ventricular depolarization is occurring simultaneously, right ventricular forces will be dwarfed by left ventricular events in the normal adult heart. Consequently, we can omit them from our schematic representation of the depolarization process. Vector 2 will be seen by the left-sided lead V_6 as coming directly toward it. It writes a tall R wave (positive deflection) in lead V_6. On the other hand, vector 2 will be seen by the right-sided lead V_1 as moving directly away. Consequently it will write a deep S wave (negative deflection) in lead V_1.

Left Ventricular Hypertrophy

PROBLEM: Can you predict the morphology of the QRS complex in leads V_1 and V_6 for a patient with left ventricular hypertrophy (LVH)?

ANSWER: The answer is illustrated in Fig. 4-5. With the increase in left ventricular mass that occurs in LVH, vector 2 becomes correspondingly larger. Left-sided leads reflect these increased forces by writing taller R waves in some or all of the lateral leads (I, aVL, V_5, and V_6). On the other hand, right-sided leads now see more activity directed away from them. As a result, the S wave in leads such as V_1 and V_2 becomes deeper. Although the septum also becomes thicker with LVH (since it is part of the left ventricle), its increase in size is usually not reflected on the ECG.

Criteria for diagnosing LVH will be reviewed in detail later. For the moment, consider the possibility of LVH when any of the *voltage* criteria shown in Table 4-1 are present in an adult *35 years of age* or older.

R-Wave Progression

Up to this point we have almost exclusively discussed events as if they occurred only in the frontal plane. Let us now examine spread of the activation wavefront as it is seen by the precordial leads in the transverse (or horizontal) plane (Fig. 4-6).

Orientation of the spread of ventricular depolarization as it varies with time during a single cardiac cycle is represented by the irregularly shaped ellipse in this figure. This is known as a *vector loop.* Normally the loop is inscribed in a counterclockwise (ccw) direction in the horizontal plane. Initial forces of septal activation travel anteriorly, and from left to right. The vector loop continues in its counterclockwise direction as the major portion of the left ventricle is activated. Forces are now directed posteriorly and to the left where the left ventricle lies in the thorax. Completion of the cycle occurs with return of the loop to its point of origin.

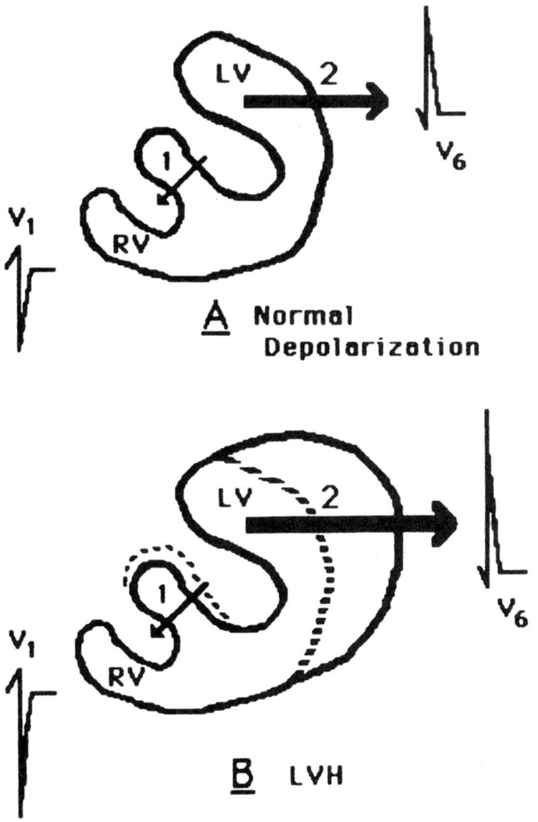

Figure 4-5. Ventricular depolarization with left ventricular hypertrophy (LVH).

As described in Fig. 4-3, forces of ventricular depolarization can be simplified into two basic components: one vector representing septal depolarization and another representing depolarization of the major portion of the left ventricle. These are indicated by vectors 1 and 2 in Fig. 4-6.

Typical ECG recordings from the precordial leads are also shown in the figure. Note that R-wave amplitude becomes progressively greater as one moves from lead V_1 (which primarily sees the left ventricular activation

TABLE 4-1

Voltage criteria for LVH (adults ≥ 35 years old)

- R wave in lead aVL ≥12 mm
- R wave in lead V_5 ≥25 mm
- Sum of S wave in lead V_1 or V_2 + R wave in lead V_5 or V_6 ≥35 mm

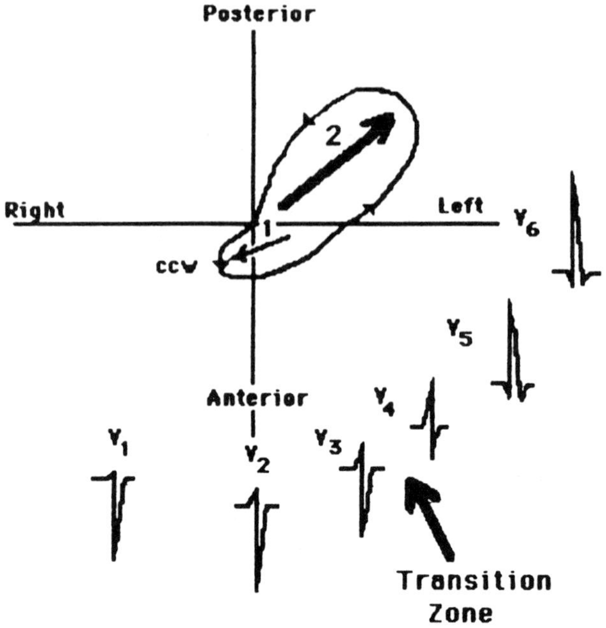

Figure 4-6. Horizontal (transverse) vector loop of normal depolarization. Note counterclockwise (ccw) orientation. There is normal R-wave progression with transition between leads V_{3-4}.

wavefront as moving away from it), toward lead V_6 (which sees the majority of forces from vector 2 as directly approaching). Thus, one can say that "R-wave progression" is *normal.* Note also that a point is reached where the QRS complex changes from predominantly negative to predominantly positive. This is known as the *transition zone,* and it is usually situated between leads V_3 and V_4 as shown here.

At times, transition may be *delayed,* so that the change from predominant negativity to positivity of the QRS complex in the tranverse plane doesn't occur until lead V_4 to V_5 or later. If the height of the r waves in leads V_1 to V_4 remains extremely small, we say that there is "poor R-wave progression." This condition is frequently seen in patients with chronic obstructive pulmonary disease (COPD), in whom a marked rightward and posterior shift ("posterior-axis deviation") may occur in the orientation of the horizontal vector loop (Fig. 4-7). The principal forces of ventricular activation (vector 2 in Fig. 4-7), are now directed *away* from all of the precordial leads, and the zone of transition never occurs (r waves in the precordial leads of Fig. 4-7 never become larger than their corresponding S waves). Such *persistence of S waves* throughout the precordial leads is a useful ECG clue to the presence of COPD.

Poor R-wave progression is an important ECG finding that may be

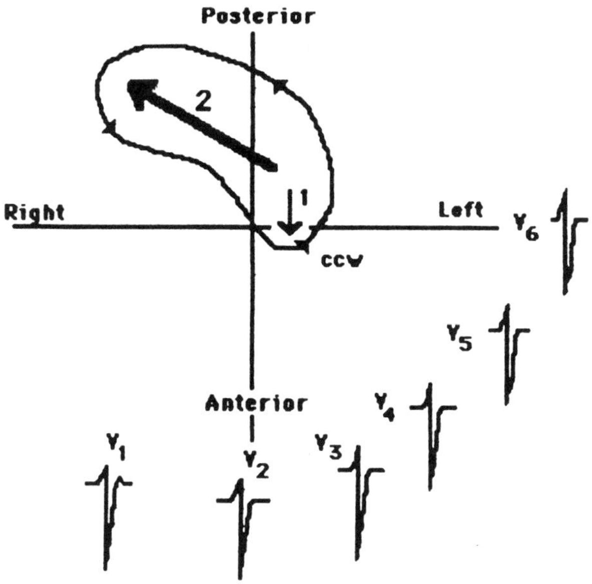

Figure 4-7. Chronic obstructive pulmonary disease. Due to the posterior and rightward shift in orientation of forces in the horizontal plane vector loop, there is poor R-wave progression in the precordial leads with delayed transition.

associated with a number of other conditions (Table 4-2). Consider Fig. 4-8, which illustrates the horizontal vector loop of a patient with an anteroseptal infarction. Because of the infarction, there is a loss of septal forces. Consequently, initial forces will no longer be oriented rightward and anteriorly, but are directed immediately posteriorly (dotted vector loop in Fig. 4-8). Electrocardiographically, QS complexes will be seen in the anterior leads since initial forces move away from leads V_1 to V_4.

TABLE 4-2

Common causes of poor R-Wave progression

Anteroseptal infarction
Left ventricular hypertrophy
Right ventricular hypertrophy (type C)
Chronic obstructive pulmonary disease
Left bundle branch block
Left anterior hemiblock
Cardiomyopathy
Lead misplacement
Normal variant

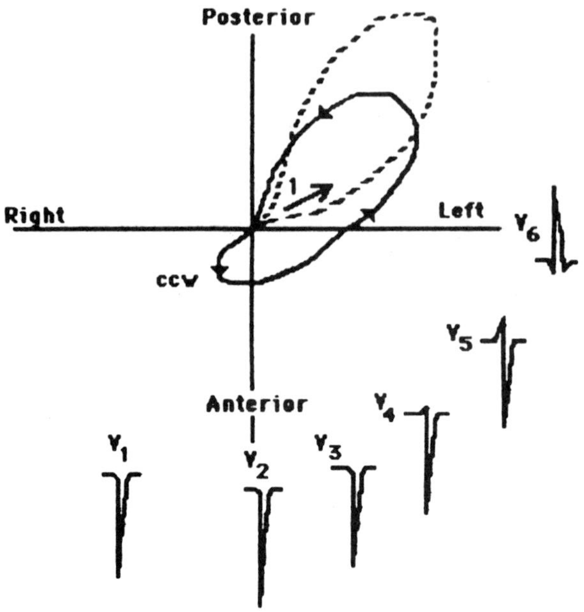

Figure 4-8. Anteroseptal infarction. Vector 1 is oriented posteriorly due to the loss of anterior and rightward initial forces. Precordial leads show poor R-wave progression with QS complexes in leads V_{1-3}.

PROBLEM: Compare the QRS morphology of leads V_1 to V_6 in Fig. 4-7 and 4-8. Is there any way electrocardiographically to distinguish the poor R-wave progression of a patient with COPD from one who has an anteroseptal infarction?

ANSWER: Although there is poor R-wave progression in the schematic representation of COPD (Fig. 4-7), small r waves *are* present in all of the precordial leads. R waves are completely lacking, however, in leads V_1 to V_3 of the schematic representation of anteroseptal infarction (Fig. 4-8). In addition, note that "transition" never occurs in Fig. 4-7. Instead, deep S waves persist across the entire precordium, as is commonly seen in patients with COPD. While still delayed, transition *does* finally occur (between leads V_5 and V_6) in Fig. 4-8. Once past the area of infarction, the horizontal vector loop resumes its normal progression leftward and posteriorly, and a relatively normal-appearing QRS complex appears in lead V_6.

Clinically, as you may imagine, it is sometimes extremely difficult to distinguish between COPD and anterior infarction. At times, small precordial r waves may be completely absent in the former or present in the latter. To complicate matters further, technical errors, such as placing the precordial leads an interspace too high, or over too far, may also produce a picture of poor R-wave progression that simulates anterior infarction. The scope of this problem may be more fully appreciated when one considers the usual course of events for a patient admitted to rule out infarction: *serial* ECGs are obtained on *successive* days by *different* ECG technicians. Unless meticulous care is taken to place the precordial leads in their precise position (or a mark is made on the patient's chest to guarantee identical lead placement for serial tracings), minor variations in initial or serial lead placement may occur that have a profound effect on interpretation of the ECG.

PROBLEM: As a final illustration of this problem, consider Fig. 4-9, which shows how the normal transverse plane vector loop (solid vector loop in figure) is altered by LVH (dotted vector loop). Can you explain why LVH might also produce poor R-wave progression in the precordial leads?

ANSWER: Because of the increase in left ventricular forces that occurs with LVH, vector 2 in the figure becomes larger and more *posteriorly* oriented. With this comes a corresponding reduction in rightward and anterior forces. Thus, R waves increase their amplitude in the lateral leads, while in the anterior leads, the r wave diminishes in height and the S wave deepens.

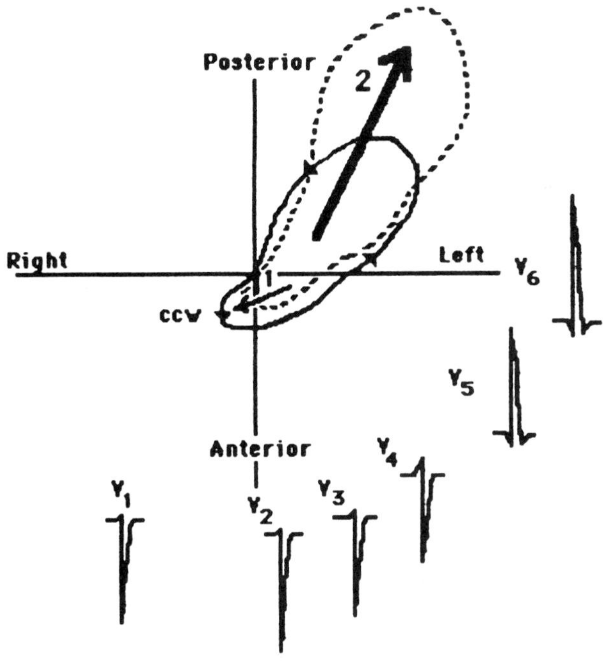

Figure 4-9. Left ventricular hypertrophy. The transverse plane vector loop is oriented more posteriorly due to the increase in left ventricular forces. There is poor R-wave progression in the precordial leads which may stimulate anterior infarction.

PROBLEM: Should you suspect anterior infarction in addition to LVH from the precordial lead sequence shown in Fig. 4-9?

ANSWER: Although septal infarction is unlikely in Fig. 4-9 (since the presence of small but definite r waves in leads V_1 to V_2 implies that septal depolarization is intact), overall anterior forces are reduced. Even though actual Q waves are not present, the poor R-wave progression seen in leads V_1 to V_4 is consistent with possible anterior infarction. The dilemma lies in determining whether such poor R-wave progression is purely the reflection of an increase in left ventricular forces (from LVH), a decrease in anterior forces (from anterior infarction), or a combination of the two (from concomitant LVH and anterior infarction). While consideration of the clinical setting, comparison with previous tracings, and examination of the rest of the ECG for other clues may be helpful, at times it is impossible clinically to resolve the issue from inspection of the 12-lead ECG alone.

Genesis of Q Waves

As a natural extension of the discussion on R-wave progression, we can explain the genesis of Q waves that occur with myocardial infarction. Fig. 4-10A illustrates a cross-sectional view of the left ventricle. The arrows in the figure indicate the initial outward direction of left ventricular depolarization that proceeds from endocardium to epicardium.

With necrosis (myocardial infarction), there will be loss of these initial outward forces over the electrically inert infarcted area. For example, with infarction of a portion of the anterior wall of the left ventricle (shaded area in Fig. 4-10B), anterior forces will be lost. A monitoring electrode directly overlying this area of necrosis would now see unopposed posterior forces during the initial portion of ventricular depolarization. Consequently, a Q wave (negative deflection) will be inscribed on an ECG recording taken from this lead. Thus, Q waves that develop with myocardial infarction result from the *loss* of forces over the infarcted area that leaves forces from the opposite wall of the heart unopposed.

Q waves are not always pathologic. We have already seen how small, narrow q waves reflecting septal depolarization may *normally* be seen in either lateral or inferior leads (Figs. 4-3 and 4-4). Such q waves are said to be insignificant, because of themselves, they are not suggestive of myocardial infarction.

Q waves become *significant* (suggestive of myocardial infarction) when they are abnormally wide ($\geq$0.04 second or one little box in duration) or abnormally deep ($\geq$25% the height of the R wave in a given lead). In general, the wider and deeper the Q wave, and the greater the number of neighboring leads in which Q waves are recorded, the more extensive the infarction. Unfortunately, numerous exceptions to this general rule exist.

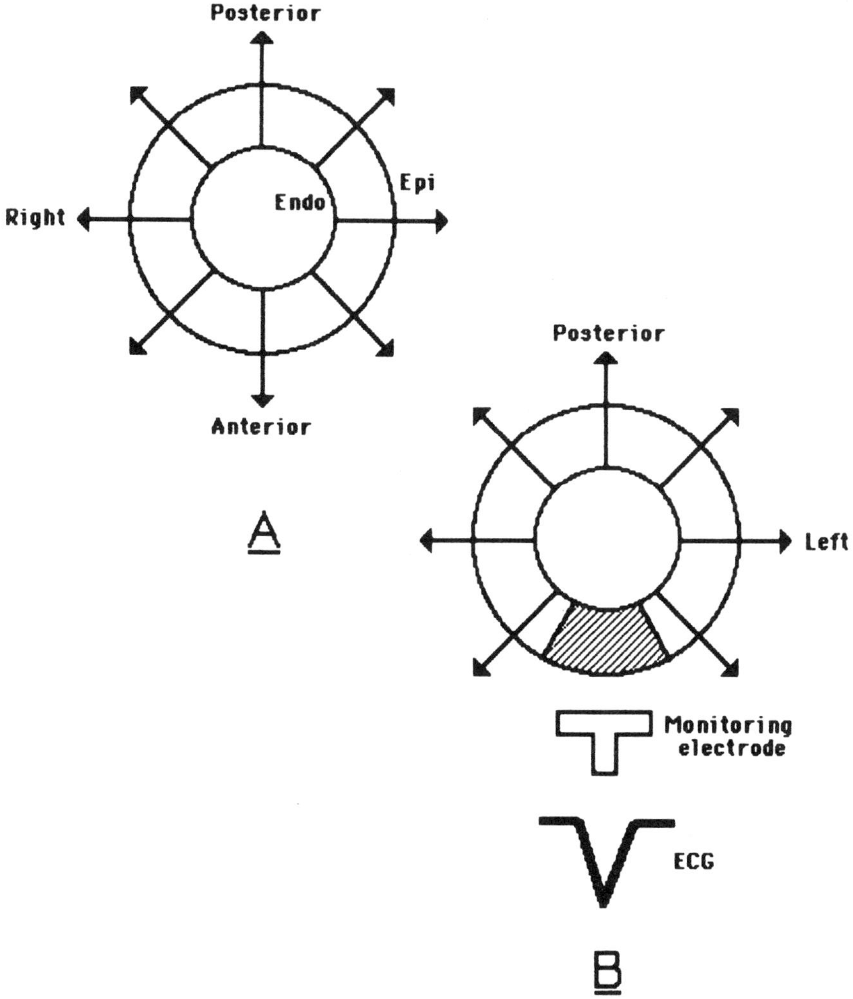

Figure 4-10. Genesis of infarction Q waves. Cross-sectional view of the left ventricle. Panel **A** indicates the initial outward direction of normal left ventricular depolarization. With infarction of a portion of the anterior wall of the left ventricle (shaded area in Panel **B**), there is loss of anterior forces. Posterior forces are now unopposed, and a Q wave is recorded in a monitoring electrode overlying the electrically inert anterior area. Endo—Endocardium; Epi—Epicardium.

Although Q waves usually persist following myocardial infarction, this is not always the case. Q waves sometimes decrease in amplitude following infarction. Occasionally, they may even disappear entirely. Thus, although the q waves in the three inferior leads (II, III, and aVF) of Fig. 4-11 appear benign (and certainly do not meet the above stated criteria for "signifi-

Figure 4-11. Although the q waves in leads II, III, and aVF in this ECG do not meet the criteria for "significance" in that they are neither 25% the height of their respective R wave, nor are they 0.04 sec in duration, one cannot absolutely rule out a prior inferior infarction on the basis of this tracing alone.

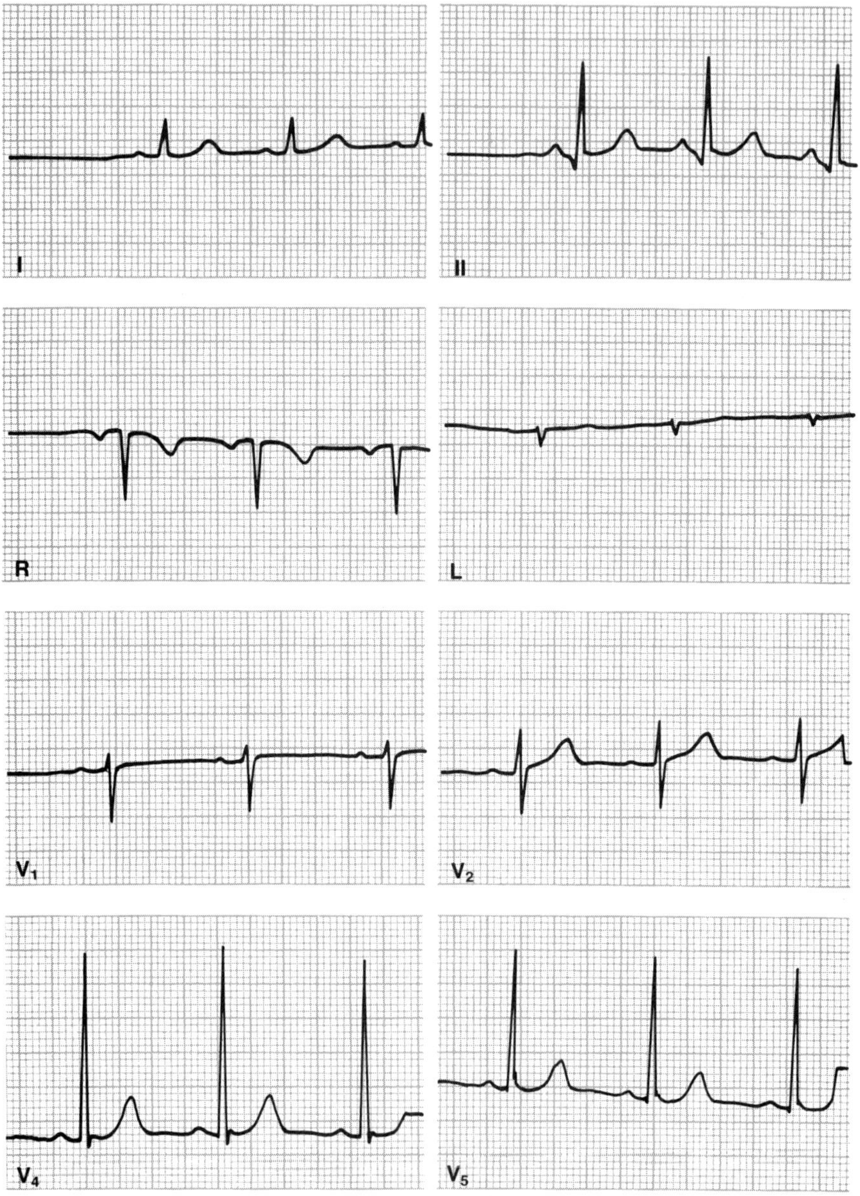

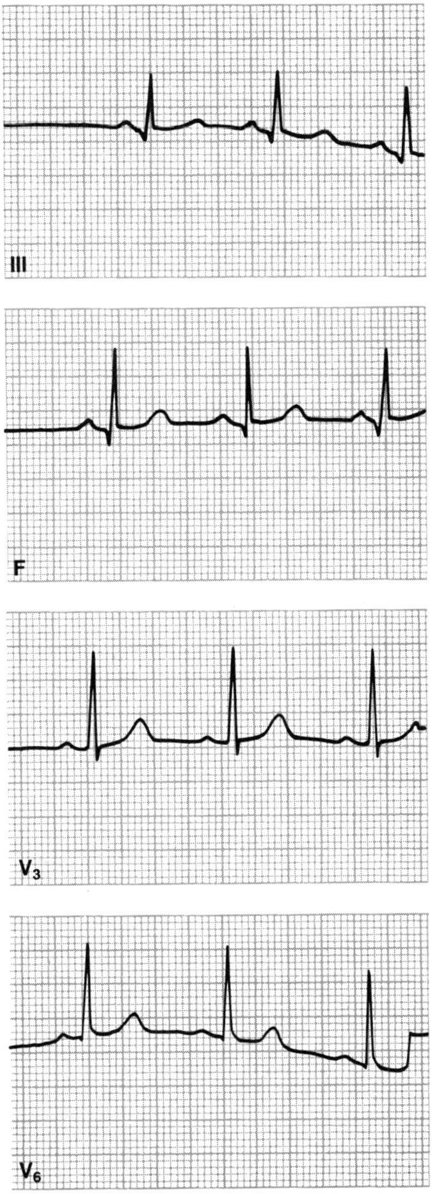
III
F
V_3
V_6

cance"), one could *not* be absolutely sure from this ECG alone that this 60-year-old patient had not had a prior inferior myocardial infarction.

To complicate matters further, up to 10% of the *normal* population have abnormally wide or deep Q waves in either lead III or aVL. The clinical importance of Q waves often *cannot* be judged on their appearance alone.

Right Ventricular Hypertrophy

Let us return to the derivation of ventricular hypertrophy. The situation with right ventricular hypertrophy (RVH) is more complex than with LVH. As illustrated in Fig. 4-12A, the left ventricle in the normal adult is approximately three times as thick and generates up to *ten* times as much electrical potential as the right ventricle. Consequently, left ventricular forces predominate during normal ventricular depolarization (solid lined scale in Fig. 4-12A). Even with a *threefold* increase in right ventricular forces, there may be little appreciable alteration of this left ventricular dominance (dotted scale in Fig. 4-12A). *Thus, it is often only after marked degrees of right ventricular enlargement has occured in adults that it becomes detectable electrocardiographically.*

Electrocardiographic evidence of RVH is much easier to see in children. This is because the relative predominance of the right ventricle during fetal development and early childhood affords this chamber with a comparable (if not larger) electrical potential compared to the left ventricle. Thus, since the right and left ventricles start out at approximately equal electrical potentials in Fig. 4-12B (solid lined scale), even lesser degrees of RVH are able to produce a significant alteration in the balance of ventricular forces (dotted scale).

Electrocardiographic manifestations of various degrees of RVH are illustrated in Fig. 4-13. Even though the right ventricle has approximately doubled in size in Fig. 4-13A ("mild RVH"), only minimal changes are seen on the electrocardiogram. These consist of a slight increase in height of the r wave in lead V_1 and perhaps some deepening of the S wave in the lateral leads. With more moderate degrees of RVH (Fig. 4-13B), R-wave amplitude progressively increases and S-wave depth diminishes in right-sided chest leads. Finally, with massive right ventricular enlargement (Fig. 4-13C), an R wave predominates as the S wave eventually disappears in lead V_1. Note that as R-wave amplitude has increased in the right-sided leads, the S wave has become progressively deeper in the lateral leads. This reflects the chamber enlargement taking place away from the left (in the right ventricle). If you now compare the QRS morphology of leads V_1 and V_6 in Figs. 4-5B and 4-13C, it becomes clear that the relative relationship between the left and right ventricle has reversed.

Three types of RVH (types A, B, and C) have been described, depend-

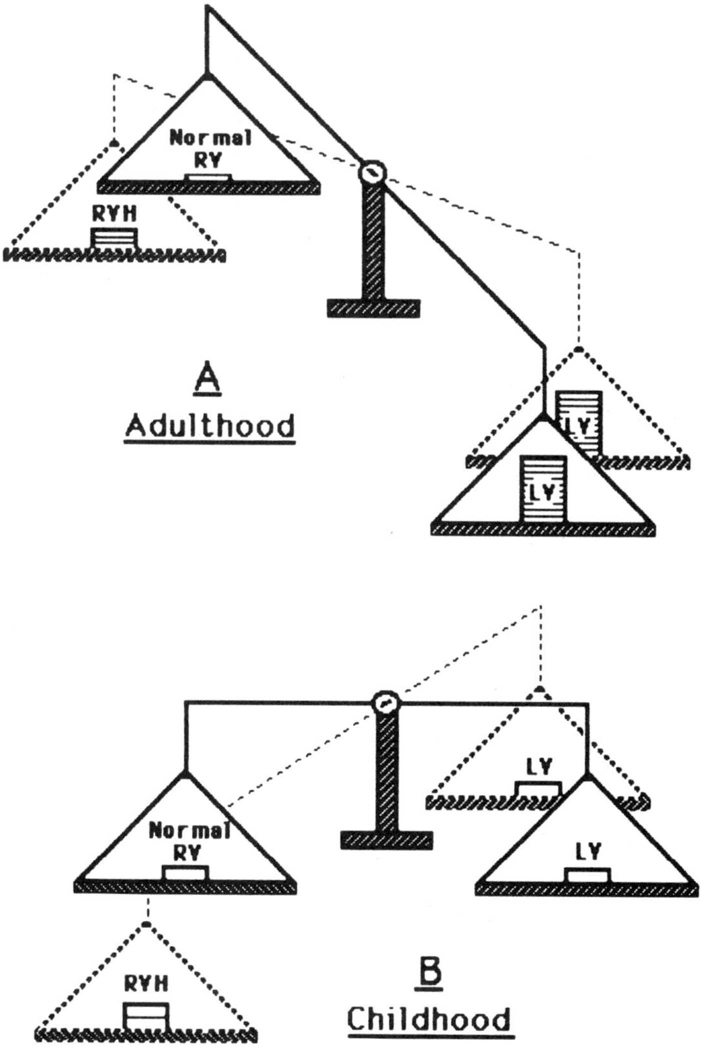

Figure 4-12. Relative electrical forces of the right and left ventricles in childhood and adulthood.

ing on the alteration of forces in the transverse plane (Fig. 4-14). Comparison with the horizontal vector loop of normal ventricular depolarization (dotted lines) is shown in the figure.

In *type A RVH,* the direction of activation for the horizontal vector loop becomes clockwise and is accompanied by a tremendous increase in anterior forces (Fig. 4-14A). This type of RVH primarily occurs in congenital heart disease (pulmonary stenosis, tetralogy of Fallot, Eisenmenger's syn-

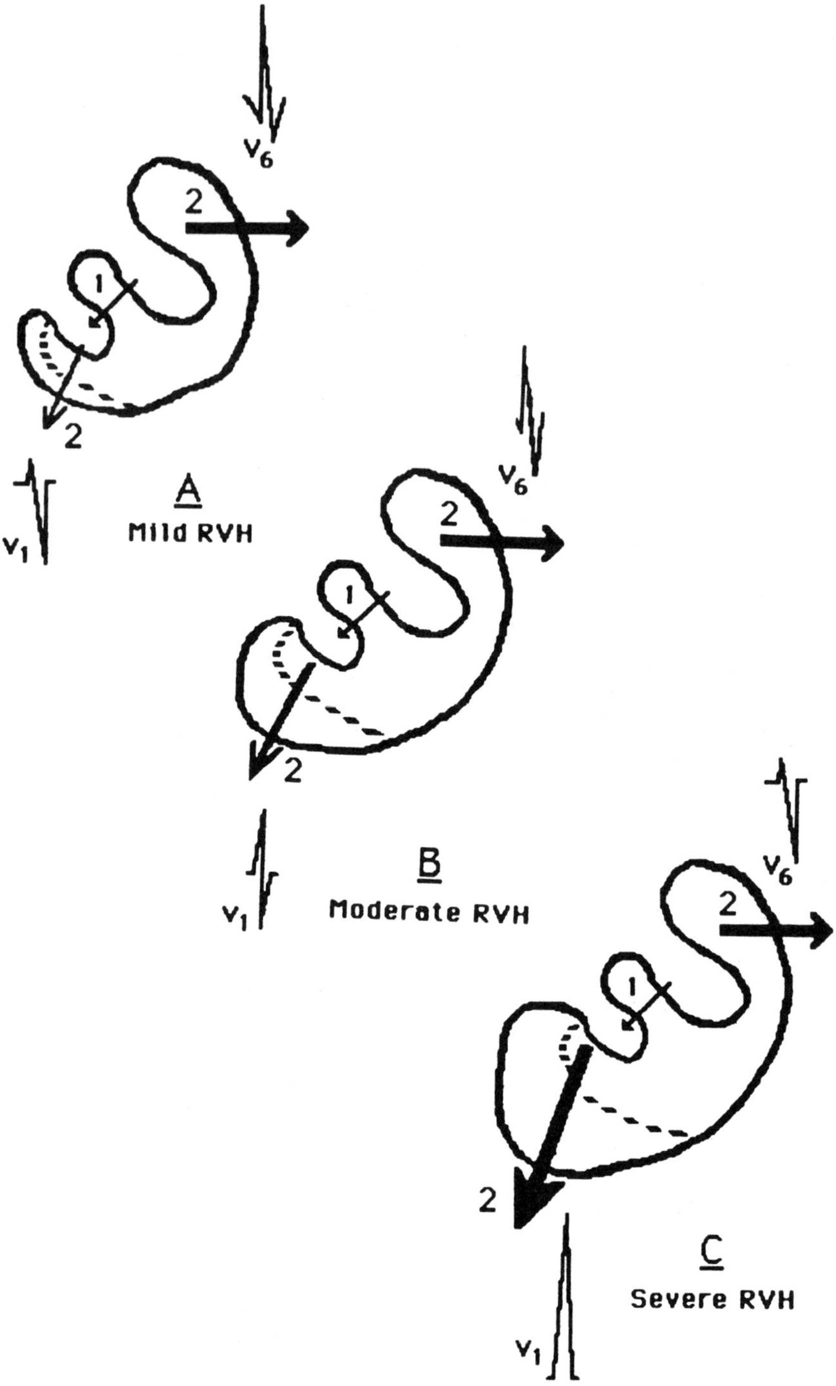

Figure 4-13. Ventricular depolarization with right ventricular hypertrophy (RVH).

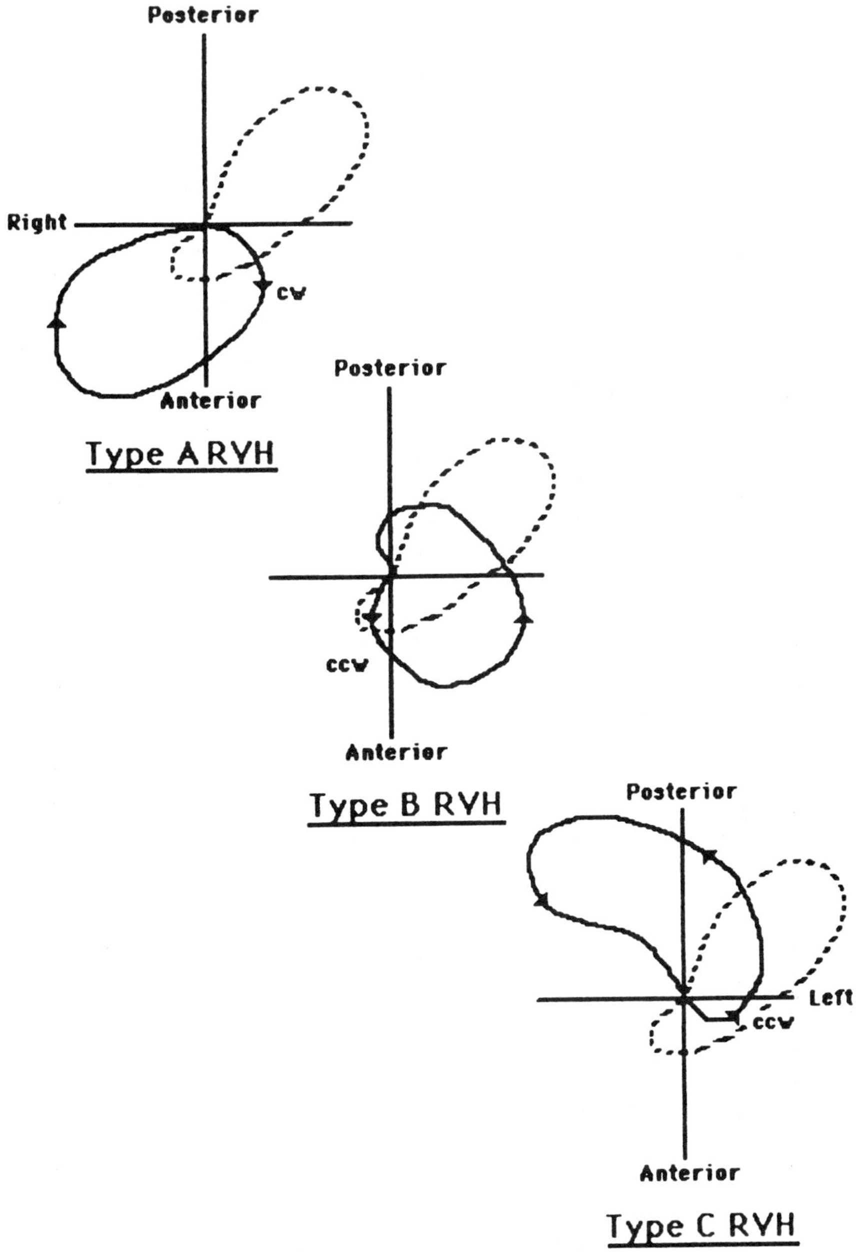

Figure 4-14. Horizontal plane vector loop representations (solid lined loops) of types A, B, and C right ventricular hypertrophy (RVH). Type A RVH is oriented in a clockwise (cw) direction, while types B and C retain the counterclockwise (ccw) orientation of normal depolarization. (The horizontal vector loop of normal depolarization is superimposed on each figure in dotted lines for comparison.)

drome), and reflects severe pressure overload states. It is rare in adults. The ECG picture produced often resembles that shown in Fig. 4-13C.

Type B RVH is less severe than type A RVH. Right ventricular forces are inscribed in a normal counterclockwise direction, but with significant anterior displacement (Fig. 4-14B). This pattern of RVH may be seen with some of the same conditions that produce type A RVH, or with severe mitral stenosis, pulmonary hypertension, or cor pulmonale. A similar horizontal vector loop may also occur in normal children in whom right ventricular forces are still relatively dominant.

Type C RVH is the kind most commonly seen in adults. As was discussed earlier in this chapter (with the explanation for Fig. 4-7), ventricular forces of the horizontal plane vector loop for this type of RVH are inscribed with normal counterclockwise rotation, but with significant posterior and rightward displacement (Fig. 4-14C). Development of this pattern is often seen in patients with *pulmonary disease.* Associated findings include poor R-wave progression and persistence of S waves across the precordium. S waves may also be seen in all three standard limb leads (I, II, and III). In addition, *low voltage* in the limb leads (QRS amplitude not exceeding 5 mm in any of the six limb leads) is common. This has been attributed to the increase in distance between the chest wall and heart of patients with emphysematous lungs. Superposition of right ventricular enlargement on this picture (development of cor pulmonale) may be signaled by the appearance of right atrial enlargement (RAE), incomplete right bundle branch block (IRBBB), and right axis deviation (RAD). The combination of these findings constitutes the fully developed picture of type C RVH.

The degree of RVH shown in Fig. 4-13C almost *never* develops in adults. Increase in R-wave amplitude even to the extent depicted in Fig.4-13B (R wave $>$S wave in lead V_1), usually does not develop until a far advanced stage of COPD has been reached and/or significant pulmonary hypertension supervenes. In contrast, more than half of all newborns have a horizontal vector loop resembling the pattern of type A RVH shown in Fig. 4-14A. Normal newborns frequently manifest an ECG picture similar to that shown in Fig. 4-13B or even Fig. 4-13C (R-wave amplitude in V_1 may be much greater than S-wave amplitude in this lead). Although left ventricular forces rapidly increase after birth, an R/S ratio >1 in lead V_1 often persists for the first few years of life. By age 5, most children will show an R/S ratio <1 in lead V_1.

Appreciation of the vectorcardiographic derivation for the different types of RVH is important in understanding the ECG appearance of this often-elusive entity. Practically speaking, one can simplify recognition of RVH by listing ECG manifestations of the two most common types: types A and C (Table 4-3). The former is usually associated with congenital heart disease and can be easily identified by the predominant R wave it produces in lead V_1. Recognition of type C RVH is much more subtle and must be based on the constellation of findings listed in the table.

TABLE 4-3

Criteria for right ventricular hypertrophy

Type A RVH:*	Type C RVH:*
Predominant R wave in lead V_1 Right axis deviation Right atrial enlargement Deep S waves in leads V_{5-6} Strain pattern in the anterior precordial leads	Right axis deviation or indeterminate axis Right atrial enlargement Persistence of S waves across the precordium S waves in leads I, II, and III Incomplete right bundle branch block Low voltage in the limb leads.

**Type B RVH is a less common intermediate form.*

Atrial Enlargement

To complete the ECG derivations for chamber enlargement, let us discuss the changes one might expect in P-wave morphology with enlargement of the right and left atria (Fig. 4-15). Both individual contributions of left and right atrial depolarization, as well as the results of combined atrial activity in leads II and V_1, are shown in the figure.

Consider first the development of the normal P wave. Since atrial activation begins in the sinus node of the right atrium, the wave of atrial depolarization will first begin spreading through this chamber before activating the left atrium. Consequently, a "right-sided" lead (lead V_1) will view the initial portion of atrial depolarization as approaching it, and an initial positive deflection will be inscribed in lead V_1 (solid lines in Fig. 4-15A). With left atrial depolarization, right-sided monitoring leads now see the wave of atrial depolarization as moving away, and a terminal negative deflection will be inscribed in lead V_1 (dotted lines in Fig. 4-15A). Thus a *biphasic* P wave may *normally* be seen in lead V_1, in which the initial positive component reflects right atrial activation, and the terminal negative component, left atrial activation.

In contrast, depolarization of both the left and right atria is seen as a positive deflection in lead II. Combined atrial activity should therefore *always* result in a positive P wave in lead II when there is normal sinus rhythm.

Now consider what happens with pure right atrial enlargement (RAE). In this case, the first component of atrial activation becomes more prominent, and resultant P waves (the combined atrial activity) become tall and **p**eaked in the inferior (right-sided or **p**ulmonary leads). To satisfy criteria for RAE, P-wave amplitude must at least equal or exceed 2.5 mm in one of the three inferior leads (II, III, or aVF). P-wave duration is usually not pro-

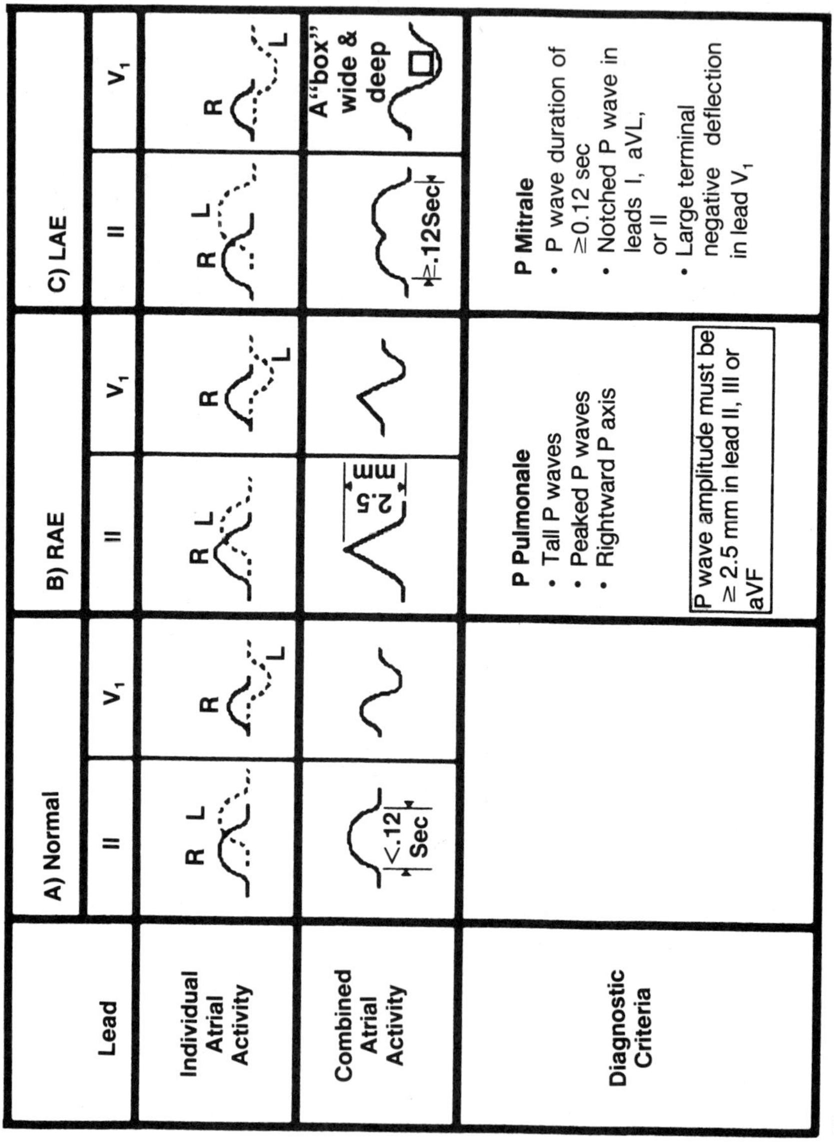

Figure 4-15. Atrial Enlargement

longed. RAE is most commonly associated with disorders such as **pul**monary stenosis in congenital heart disease or chronic obstructive **pul**monary disease in adults. The term "P **pul**monale" may help recall its ECG features (Fig. 4-15B).

Although the initial (right) atrial component of the P wave in lead V_1 may also become peaked and more prominent with RAE, this criterion is not nearly as helpful clinically as is development of tall peaked P waves in the inferior leads.

In contrast, with pure *left atrial enlargement (LAE),* it is the second component of atrial depolarization that becomes larger (Fig. 4-15C). Duration of atrial depolarization may become prolonged, and P waves often take on a *notched* appearance. Because of its frequent association with mitral stenosis and/or regurgitation, LAE has been referred to as "P **m**itrale," where the shape of the letter **"m"** may help recall the notch that is seen in the left-sided (mitral) leads.

An even better criterion for evaluating LAE than P-wave prolongation and notching in leads I, II, and aVL is enlargement of the terminal negative component of the P wave in lead V_1. The diagnosis of LAE is suggested when this terminal negative deflection becomes 1 box deep and 1 box wide. Fig. 4-15C reviews these criteria.

Conditions other than atrial enlargement may affect P-wave morphology. Rapid changes in intra-atrial pressure, certain electrolyte disorders, and intra-atrial conduction defects may all produce P-wave changes that simulate RAE or LAE. In addition, abnormal P waves can sometimes be seen as a normal variant in otherwise healthy individuals without evidence of underlying heart disease. To acknowledge the fact that P-wave changes may be due to many factors other than actual chamber enlargement, we prefer the terms right atrial abnormality (RAA) and left atrial abnormality (LAA) to RAE and LAE, except in those cases in which true atrial enlargement is known clinically to exist. Both terms are used in the literature.

Right Bundle Branch Block

Let us now look at the sequence of ventricular depolarization with the bundle branch blocks. In *right bundle branch block (RBBB),* the direction of the initial wave of ventricular activation (septal depolarization), remains the same. This is because the electrical wavefront is still able to be conducted down the left side of the septum by the intact left bundle branch. Thus, with RBBB, septal depolarization proceeds normally from left to right (vector 1 Fig. 4-16A).

Following septal activation, the mass of the left ventricle is depolarized (vector 2 in Fig. 4-16A). However, simultaneous activation of the right ventricle is unable to occur because of the conduction block in the right bundle branch. It is only toward the end of left ventricular depolarization that the depolarization wavefront is able to complete its spread back through

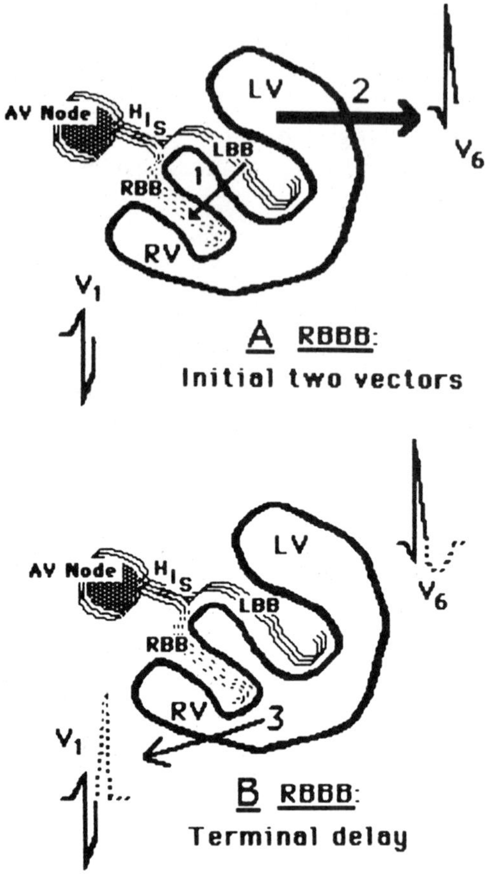

Figure 4-16. Derivation of right bundle branch block (RBBB). **A.** The initial sequence of ventricular activation (vectors 1 and 2) with RBBB is identical to that for normal depolarization. **B.** Terminal delay (vector 3) produced by RBBB.

ventricular myocardium to activate the right ventricle (vector 3 in Fig. 4-16B). Thus, the fundamental defect with RBBB is one of *terminal conduction delay,* with the final phase of ventricular activation oriented anteriorly and to the right (in the direction of the right ventricle). Compare Fig. 4-16A with Fig. 4-3 to verify again that the initial two vectors of depolarization in RBBB are virtually identical to those that occur with normal depolarization.

RBBB is recognized electrocardiographically by prolongation of the QRS complex to at least 0.11 second, the presence of an rSR′ in lead V_1, and the appearance of wide S waves in leads I and V_6. The terminal R′ in lead V_1 (drawn in dotted lines in Fig. 4-16B) results from the return of electrical activity toward the right as represented by vector 3 in this figure. Similarly, lateral leads such as V_6 will see this terminal electrical activity as moving away, and inscribe an S wave (drawn in dotted lines in Fig. 4-16B). This terminal negative deflection (the S wave) is *wide* in the lateral leads, because it represents terminal conduction *delay*. The depolarization wavefront on its return (vector 3) must now activate the right ventricle by traveling through individual myocardial fibers, since the right bundle branch is blocked. This takes more time.

Left Bundle Branch Block

In contrast to RBBB, with *left bundle branch block (LBBB),* the initial phase of septal activation can no longer originate from the left, because the conduction block prevents propagation of electrical activity down this side of the septum. Consequently, the wave of depolarization must travel down the intact right bundle branch, where it initiates septal activation from the right side. *Thus, septal activation, proceeds from right to left with LBBB* (vector 1 in Fig. 4-17B).

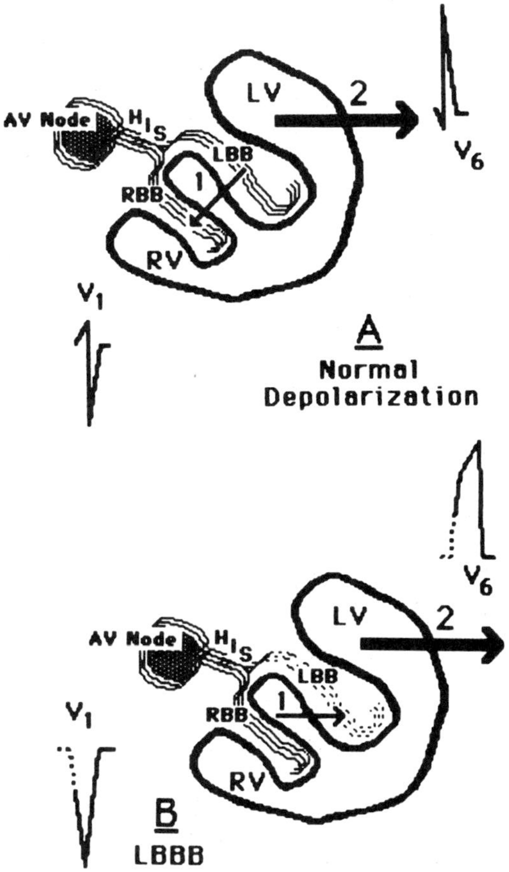

Figure 4-17. Derivation of left bundle branch block (LBBB). **A.** Sequence of normal depolarization. **B.** Illustration of how LBBB alters the initial vector of ventricular activation.

Following septal activation, the mass of the left ventricle must be stimulated through ordinary ventricular myocardium rather than the specialized conduction system of the left bundle branch. This produces significant delay in left ventricular activation. Even though right ventricular depolarization is occurring simultaneously (in a normal fashion through the intact right bundle branch), it is overshadowed by dominant left ventricular forces. Thus, the remaining vector of ventricular depolarization can be represented by a single large force oriented to the left and posteriorly (vector 2 in Fig. 4-17B).

Dotted lines at the origin of the QRS complexes in leads V_1 and V_6 of Fig. 4-17B illustrate the effect that the altered direction of septal activation has on the ECG appearance of LBBB. The septal q wave that is usually seen with normal ventricular depolarization in lead V_6 (Fig. 4-17A) is *absent,* since septal activation is oriented *toward* this left-sided lead in the presence of this conduction defect (vector 1 in Fig. 4-17B). Similarly, the small initial r wave that is usually seen in lead V_1, with normal ventricular depolarization may be lost with LBBB.

About a third of the time, a small initial r wave may still be seen in lead V_1 *despite* the presence of LBBB. This is because the right bundle branch occasionally activates the free wall of the right ventricle before it activates the septum. When this is the case, initial depolarization still travels toward lead V_1, and a small initial positive deflection may be seen in this lead. *However, septal Q waves should never be seen in lateral leads with pure LBBB!*

In summary, LBBB is recognized electrocardiographically by prolongation of the QRS complex to at least 0.12 second, loss of initial septal q waves in leads I, aVL, V_5, and V_6, and development of a monophasic upright (and occasionally notched) QRS complex in these lateral leads. The QRS complex in lead V_1 is predominantly negative, reflecting the fact that ventricular activation is taking place *away* from this lead (toward the left ventricle). It may or may not manifest a small initial r wave.

Detection of Myocardial Infarction with Bundle Branch Block

PROBLEM: Would you expect any difficulty in detecting the Q wave of myocardial infarction in patients with left or right bundle branch block?

ANSWER: By definition, Q waves form the first portion of the QRS complex. Since the first portion of ventricular depolarization (septal activation) is *not* altered in RBBB (Fig. 4-16), genesis of Q waves is unaffected, and one can usually still recognize myocardial infarction. However, the sequence of septal activation (initial depolarization) with LBBB is reversed. As a result, detection of Q waves is for the most part unreliable in the presence of this conduction defect, and recognition of myocardial infarction is often masked.

An easy way to remember these concepts is to recall that myocardial infarction is essentially a *left* ventricular event. Even though some involvement of the right ventricle may occur in up to 25 percent of inferior infarctions, most of the time such involvement is not clinically significant. Since LBBB alters the sequence of left ventricular activation, it is logical that this conduction defect would make detection of a left-sided event such as myocardial infarction difficult. On the other hand since left ventricular activation is unaffected by RBBB, detection of left-sided events such as myocardial infarction is often unimpaired.

Detection of Ventricular Hypertrophy with Bundle Branch Block

PROBLEM: Would you expect any difficulty in detection of left or right ventricular hypertrophy in patients with bundle branch block?

ANSWER: Once again, since LBBB alters the sequence of left ventricular activation, one would expect ECG detection of LVH to be much more difficult in the presence of this conduction disorder. This feeling had been the prevalent view by most authorities in the field, who until recently recommended that no attempt be made to diagnose LVH with LBBB. Recent evidence to the contrary (Kafka, Burggraf, Milliken, 1985; Noble, Humphrey, Monaghan, 1984) suggests that if voltage is extremely prominent (if, for example the S wave in lead V_2 is *deeper* than 30 mm), or if there is associated LAA, ECG diagnosis of LVH can probably be made with accuracy *despite the presence of LBBB.*

Clinically, it is well to note that most hospitalized patients who have LBBB will also have LVH, as the disease processes associated with both these entities are similar (hypertension, ischemic heart disease, cardiomyopathy, congestive heart failure, and aortic valvular disease).

On the other hand, ECG detection of RVH is virtually impossible when LBBB is present. This is because right ventricular activation is overshadowed by simultaneous left ventricular activation.

What about ECG detection of ventricular hypertrophy when RBBB is present? RBBB does not affect the normal process of left ventricular activation. Consequently, ECG detection of LVH is possible despite the presence of RBBB. Although criteria employing depth of the S wave in lead V_1 or V_2 cannot be used (since there is now a terminal R′ in these leads), LVH is probably present when there is a marked increase in amplitude of the R wave in the lateral leads of patients with RBBB.

Electrocardiographic detection of RVH in the presence of RBBB is also occasionally possible, though more difficult than detection of LVH. Whereas lesser degrees of RVH in adults are often masked by the simultaneous occurrence of dominant left ventricular forces (Fig. 4-12A), activation of the right ventricle in RBBB (vector 3 in Fig. 4-16B) occurs alone *after* activation of the left ventricle is complete. Although alteration in the sequence of right ventricular activation does make recognition of right-sided events more difficult, RVH is probably present in addition to RBBB when the terminal rightward deflection (the R′) of the QRS complex in lead V_1 is extremely tall (greater than 15 mm).

Table 4-4 summarizes the pertinent points from this discussion on bundle branch blocks.

Hemiblocks

Let us complete the section on bundle branch blocks with discussion of the hemiblocks. A schematic representation of the major divisions of the ventricular conduction system is illustrated in Fig. 4-18. As can be seen, the bundle of His (HIS in the figure) divides into the right and common left bundle branches (RBB and LBB, respectively). The *right bundle branch* courses along the right side of the interventricular septum as a slender non-

TABLE 4-4

Characteristics of bundle branch blocks

	RBBB	LBBB
Typical appearance in lead V_1	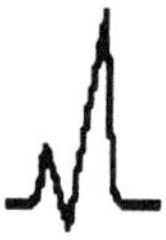	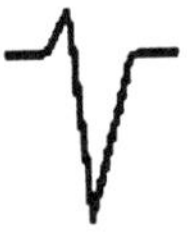 or 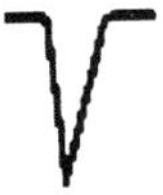
Typical appearance in lead I or V_6*	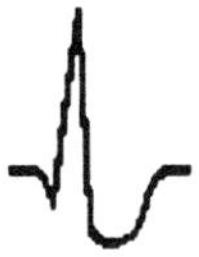	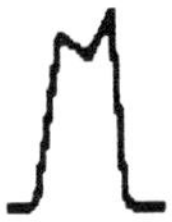 or 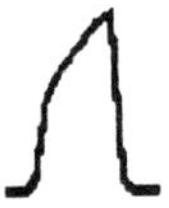
Effect on normal ventricular depolarization	Terminal conduction delay	Reversal of initial (septal) depolarization

Ability to diagnose associated conditions in the presence of this conduction defect:

Associated condition	RBBB	LBBB
Myocardial infarction	Good	Poor
LVH	Fair	Poor (?)**
RVH	Poor	Extremely poor

**The morphology of the QRS complex in lead I has a similar appearance to that of lead V_6 with typical bundle branch blocks.*

***Up until recently it was felt that electrocardiographic diagnosis of LVH in the presence of LBBB was unreliable. Recent evidence to the contrary suggests the LVH can probably be diagnosed with accuracy despite LBBB if there is very prominent voltage, associated LAA, or both.*

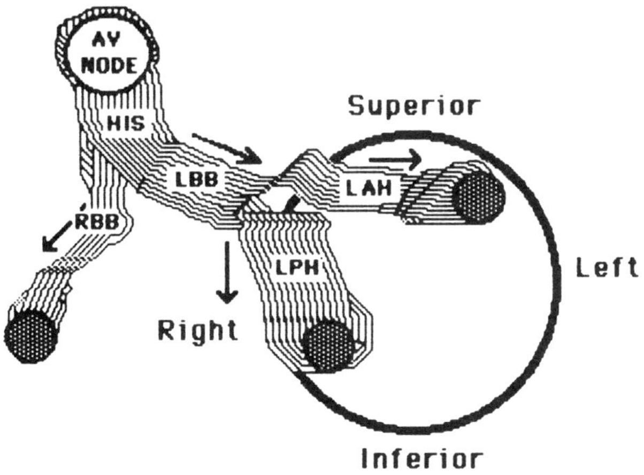

Figure 4-18. Schematic representation of the major fascicles of the ventricular conduction system. HIS—bundle of His. RBB—Right bundle branch (the most slender fascicle). LBB—Common left bundle branch. LAH—Left anterior hemidivision of LBB. LPH—Left posterior hemidivision of LBB (thickest fascicle). Solid circle depicts cross-sectional view of the left ventricular cavity showing leftward and superior orientation of LAH and rightward and inferior orientation of LPH.

branching fascicle almost until it reaches the apex of the right ventricle. There it finally branches into its terminal ramifications that activate all areas of the right ventricle.

The *common left bundle branch* continues intact for only a short distance before dividing into *left anterior* and *left posterior* hemidivisions (LAH and LPH, respectively). Left anterior and posterior hemiblocks are felt to result from a block in conduction at the level of these hemidivisions. In reality, the major fascicles of the ventricular conduction system are *not* discrete structures, but rather ill-defined groupings of fibers having a general orientation, with numerous interconnections between them. A third division of the common left bundle branch (a septal fascicle) is thought to exist in many individuals. It is infinitely simpler (and fortunately equally accurate from an electrocardiographic point of view) to think of the common left bundle branch as dividing into two major fascicles for conduction of the depolarization impulse through the left ventricle.

Though commonly used, the anatomic terms that describe these two major fascicles are misleading. As depicted in the cross-sectional circle of the left ventricular cavity in Fig. 4-18, the LAH is really *not* an anterior structure. Rather, it is directed in a leftward and superior orientation. Similarly, the LPH is *not* a posterior structure, but instead is directed rightward and inferiorly. Appreciation of these anatomical relationships is crucial to understanding the ECG derivation of the hemiblocks.

Left Anterior Hemiblock

By definition, with *left anterior hemiblock (LAHB)* the impulse is prevented ("blocked") from traveling along the left anterior hemidivision. After emerging from the common left bundle branch, it begins activation of the left ventricle via the intact left posterior hemidivision (Fig. 4-19). As stated above, orientation of the LPH is rightward and inferior. Consequently, standard lead III (which is also oriented rightward and inferiorly) will see initial activation of the left ventricle as approaching it, and will thus inscribe a small initial positive deflection (r wave). Standard lead I, oriented to the left and superiorly, will see initial activation of the left ventricle as moving away, and thus writes an initial negative deflection (q wave).

The last portion of the left ventricle to be activated will be the area supplied by the blocked fascicle. Consequently, *terminal* activation forces will be oriented leftward and superiorly (where the anterior hemidivision lies). Since lead I views these terminal forces as approaching, a large positive deflection (R wave—drawn as a dotted line in the figure) is inscribed in this lead. Similarly, lead III views these terminal forces as moving away and writes a terminal negative deflection (a deep S wave—drawn as a dotted line in Fig. 4-19).

Although activation of the left ventricle is necessarily slower in the presence of LAHB, the delay is usually minimal (generally less than 0.03 second) due to the presence of the multiple interconnections between the major fascicles. Thus, the overall duration of the QRS complex with isolated LAHB is either normal or minimally prolonged (≤0.10 second).

Finally, because the terminal forces with LAHB are oriented to the left and superiorly, left axis deviation (LAD) is a characteristic feature of this

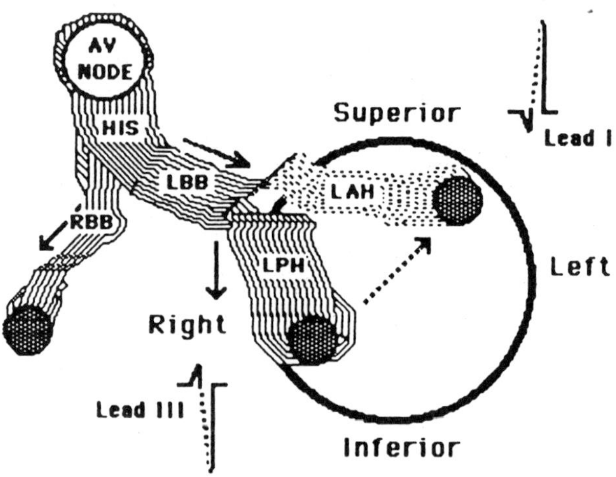

Figure 4-19. Derivation of left anterior hemiblock (LAHB).

hemiblock. But the degree of LAD needed to make this diagnosis confidently is still the subject of controversy. While some authorities accept an axis of $-30°$ as consistent with this condition, others insist on at least $-60°$. For simplicity, we favor a *pathologic degree of LAD* (a mean QRS axis that is more negative than $-30°$) as our standard.

PROBLEM: Using the criterion that a mean QRS axis more negative than $-30°$ is indicative of LAHB, how can this diagnosis be made at a glance?

ANSWER: As discussed in Chapter 3, lead II (at $+60°$) is the key lead to focus on in deciding whether pathologic LAD exists. If lead II is equiphasic, then the mean QRS axis must be perpendicular to ($90°$ away from) lead II and lie at $-30°$. LAHB will thus be present if the net QRS deflection in standard lead II is negative (if the mean QRS axis is more negative than $-30°$).

Left Posterior Hemiblock

With *left posterior hemiblock (LPHB),* activation of the left ventricle begins through the intact left anterior hemidivision (Fig. 4-20). Since this conduction fascicle is oriented to the left and superiorly, a small initial upright deflection (the r wave) is initially inscribed in lead I, at the same time as a negative initial deflection (the q wave) is inscribed in lead III. Terminal forces with LPHB are oriented to the right and inferiorly (in the direction of the blocked posterior hemidivision). Thus, the QRS complex in lead III manifests a large positive deflection (the tall R wave—drawn in dotted lines

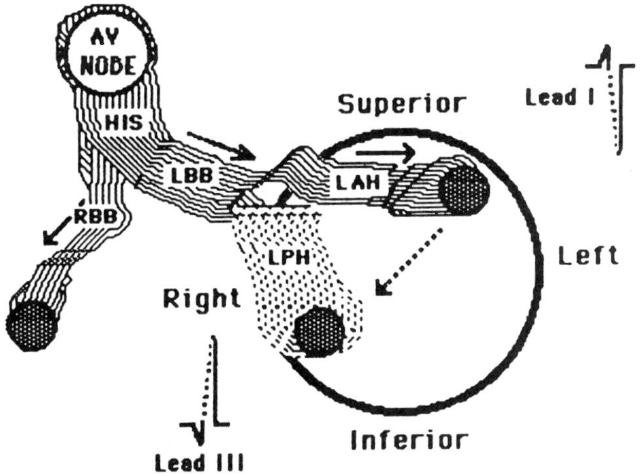

Figure 4-20. Derivation of left posterior hemiblock (LPHB).

in Fig. 4-20); lead I shows a deep negative deflection (the deep S wave—drawn with dotted lines).

Because the terminal forces with LPHB are oriented to the right and inferiorly (and a deep S wave is produced in lead I), there will be *right axis deviation (RAD).* Although also subject to controversy, the degree of RAD needed to make this diagnosis is felt by most authorities to be *at least* +105° (if not, +120°).

LPHB occurs far less commonly than LAHB. It rarely is seen as an isolated conduction defect, but rather tends to occur in association with RBBB (as bifascicular block). Anatomically, the LPH is a much thicker fascicle than the LAH. It also has a dual blood supply (from the right coronary artery and left anterior descending branch of the left coronary artery), as compared to the thinner LAH, which is only supplied by the left coronary artery. Thus, the LPH is much less susceptible to injury than the LAH. Development of LPHB consequently portends a poorer prognosis, as it implies a greater degree of myocardial damage than does LAHB.

Table 4-5 summarizes the pertinent points from this discussion on the hemiblocks.

A last point to consider regards the theoretical derivation of LBBB. In Fig. 4-17, the block in conduction for LBBB was illustrated as occurring at the level of the common left bundle branch *before* its bifurcation into the LAH and LPH. LBBB may also occur from a more *distal* block in the left ventricular conduction system, provided that *both* the LAH and LPH were blocked. As one might imagine, because of the diffuse ramifications of the ventricular conduction system, a more distally occurring LBBB would imply a far greater extent of myocardial damage than the more frequent proximal lesion that occurs where the common left bundle branch is still a fairly discrete structure. Electrocardiographically, if left axis deviation (and, rarely, right axis deviation) is seen in association with LBBB, it is probably the result of a more distal and diffuse type of LBBB in which a relatively greater degree of block has occurred in the left anterior (or posterior) hemidivision.

The Coronary Circulation

As a conclusion to this chapter on theoretical considerations, let us briefly review the coronary circulation and its impact on ECG findings, such as myocardial infarction and intraventricular conduction disturbances.

The coronary circulation is illustrated in Fig. 4-21. The two main coronary arteries originate from the aorta. The right coronary artery (RCA) travels down the right side of the heart and supplies the right atria and ventricle. In about 90 percent of subjects it then continues along the undersurface of the heart as the posterior descending branch (3 in Fig. 4-21) to vascularize the lower portion of the interventricular septum.

TABLE 4-5

Characteristics of hemiblocks

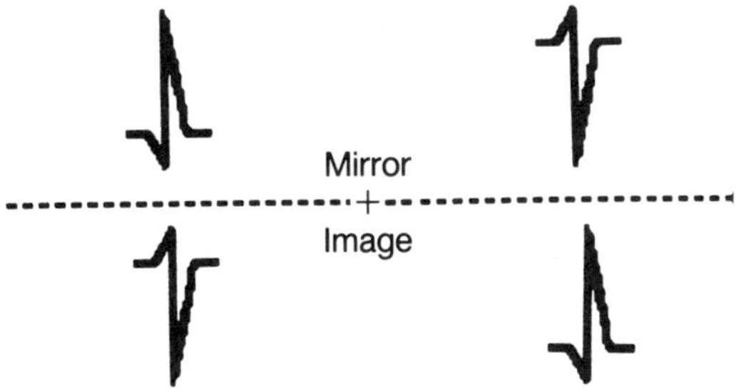

	LAHB	LPHB
Typical appearance in lead I		
Typical appearance in lead III (or II)		
Mean QRS axis	More negative than −30°	At least + 105°
Clinical clue to its presence	If lead II has a net negative deflection	If in the presence of RBBB, lead I is markedly negative (*both* deep & wide)
Relative frequency of occurrence	Much more common	Uncommon
Reason for this frequency	Thinner fascicle; blood supply from only left coronary artery	Thicker fascicle; dual blood supply (from both left and right coronary artery)
Occurrence as an isolated defect in conduction	Common	Uncommon
Occurrence in association with RBBB	Common	Common

Note: Facility for recall of the QRS morphology of the hemiblocks may be prompted by realization that the lead III appearance of LAHB is the mirror-image of its lead I appearance. The morphology for LPHB can then be easily reconstructed by simply reversing the lead I and lead III appearance of LAHB.

Acute occlusion of the right coronary artery usually results in *inferior* and/or *posterior* myocardial infarction. It may also cause *right* ventricular infarction. As previously mentioned, even though involvement of the right ventricle may occur in up to 25 percent of inferior infarctions, most of the time such involvement is not clinically significant. Acute inferior infarction may occasionally result in complete RBBB since the proximal portion of the right bundle branch is supplied by branches from the right coronary artery.

The left coronary artery begins as a short left main branch. It rapidly divides into the circumflex artery (4), which wraps around the lateral portion

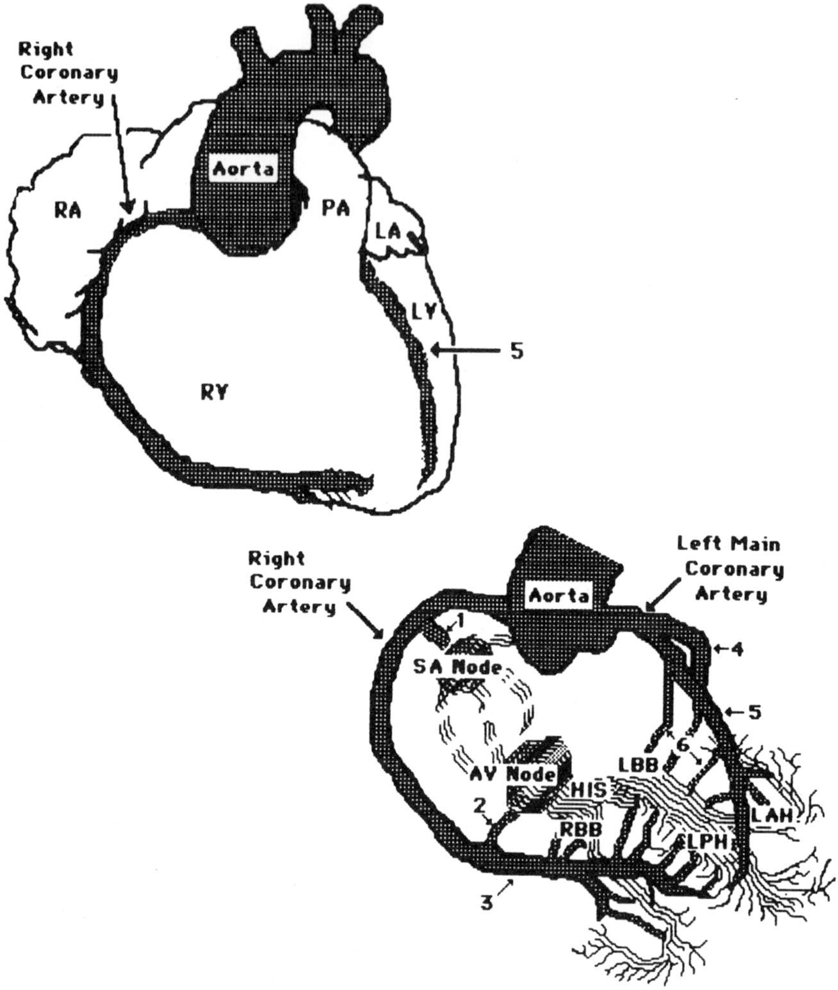

Figure 4-21. The heart and the coronary circulation. RA—Right atrium. LA—Left atrium. RV—Right ventricle. LV—Left ventricle. PA—Pulmonary artery. 1—SA nodal artery. 2—AV nodal artery. 3—Posterior descending artery. 4—Circumflex artery. 5—Left anterior descending artery. 6—Septal perforating arteries.

of the left ventricle, and the left anterior descending artery (LAD—5), which runs along the anterior portion of the heart.

Acute occlusion of the left main coronary artery is usually rapidly fatal, as this cuts off the blood supply for the major portion of the left ventricle. These patients often die within minutes of an acute myocardial infarction from irreversible cardiogenic shock.

Acute occlusion of the circumflex artery usually results in *lateral* myocardial infarction. In about 10% of subjects, the circumflex artery (rather than the right coronary artery) continues to run along the undersurface of the heart to form the posterior descending artery. In such cases, acute occlusion of the circumflex artery may also give rise to a *posterior* infarction.

Acute occlusion of the LAD results in *anterior* myocardial infarction. As shown in the figure, a number of septal perforator branches (6) arise from the LAD. These penetrating branches are important in supplying the conduction tissue that lies within the interventricular septum (the main trunk of the right bundle branch and both fascicles of the left bundle branch). Clinically, therefore, anterior infarction is much more likely than inferior infarction to result in either LAHB or complete LBBB. Should acute occlusion of the LAD occur *proximal* to the first septal perforator, development of a significant interventricular conduction disturbance becomes even more likely.

As discussed in the section on hemiblocks, LPHB occurs much less commonly than LAHB. Anatomically, the thicker LPH has a dual blood supply (from the RCA and LAD branch of the left coronary artery), whereas the thinner LAH is only supplied by the left coronary artery. In ischemic heart disease, LPHB often occurs in association with complete RBBB. Its presence implies extensive myocardial damage with involvement of both the right and left coronary circulation.

There is considerable variation in vascularization of the SA node. About 60 percent of the time, the SA nodal artery (1) arises from the right coronary artery. In most remaining cases this artery arises from the left circumflex artery, although in rare instances both coronary arteries may each give off a branch to the SA node.

On the other hand, the AV nodal artery (2) is almost always (90% of the time) supplied by the right coronary artery. Clinically, this explains the reason that inferior myocardial infarction is much more likely than anterior infarction to result in 2°, Mobitz type I (Wenckebach) AV block.

The final point to consider regarding the extent of injury that occurs from acute coronary occlusion deals with the degree of development of the collateral circulation. Although we have divided the coronary circulation into branches that arise from either the right or left coronary arteries, one must remember that numerous interconnections (collaterals) exist between these two principal vessels. For example, septal perforator branches (6), which arise from the LAD and supply the uppermost portion of the interventricular septum, freely anastomose with septal perforators arising from the posterior descending artery (3), which supply the lower portion of the septum.

With progressive narrowing of a coronary artery, widening of collateral channels may occur with time in an attempt to assist in vascularization of an underserved area. Thus, the 30-year-old man with acute onset of ischemic heart disease who has not had time to develop his collateral circulation may be at much higher risk of infarcting a large area of the heart than an older individual with a more gradual onset of disease. Unfortunately, severity of symptoms is of *no* assistance in judging either the extent of coronary narrowing or the degree of development of the collateral circulation, and coronary angiography is often needed to define the anatomy.

Enough theory! On to application of the principles that have been covered up to now.

References

Kafka H, Burggraf GW, Milliken JA: Electrocardiographic diagnosis of left ventricular hypertrophy in the presence of left bundle branch block: An echocardiographic study. *Am J Cardiol* 1985; 55:103–106.

Noble LM, Humphrey SB, Monaghan GB: Left ventricular hypertrophy in left bundle branch block. *J Electrocardiol* 1984; 17:157–160.

PART TWO

Clinical Applications

CHAPTER 5

THE ST SEGMENT IN HEALTH AND DISEASE

In this chapter we'll discuss the appearance of the ST segment in health and disease. Special emphasis will be devoted to recognition of the normal ECG, because only by having a good appreciation of what we mean by "normal" can one define the abnormal. For the most part, ECGs in this and the remaining chapters will be analyzed according to the systematic approach presented in Chapter 1 and summarized in Table 1-6. Greatest benefit will be derived if you take a moment to develop your own interpretation of each ECG *before* looking at our answers!

Normalcy and Its Variations

PROBLEM: Start by interpreting the ECG shown in Fig. 5-1. Do you feel that the ST-segment changes represent health or disease?

INTERPRETATION of Fig. 5-1

Rate and rhythm: The rhythm is fairly *regular* and *sinus-initiated,* as normal (albeit rather small) upright P waves are seen before each QRS complex in lead II. The R-R interval is between 4 and 5 large boxes long. If it were exactly 4 large boxes, the rate would be 75 beats/min. If it were 5 large boxes, it would be 60 beats/min. The heart rate is about 65 beats/min since it is closer to the latter.

Intervals

PR interval: Normal (less than 0.20 second), and measuring about 0.14 second in lead II.

QRS interval: Normal (and measuring about 0.08 second).

QT interval: Normal (clearly less than one-half of the R-R interval). (Determination of QT-interval prolongation was discussed in Chapter 1.)

Axis: Definitely normal, since the QRS complex is upright in both leads I and aVF. (See Table 3-1 for 2-lead method for axis determination.)

Figure 5-1

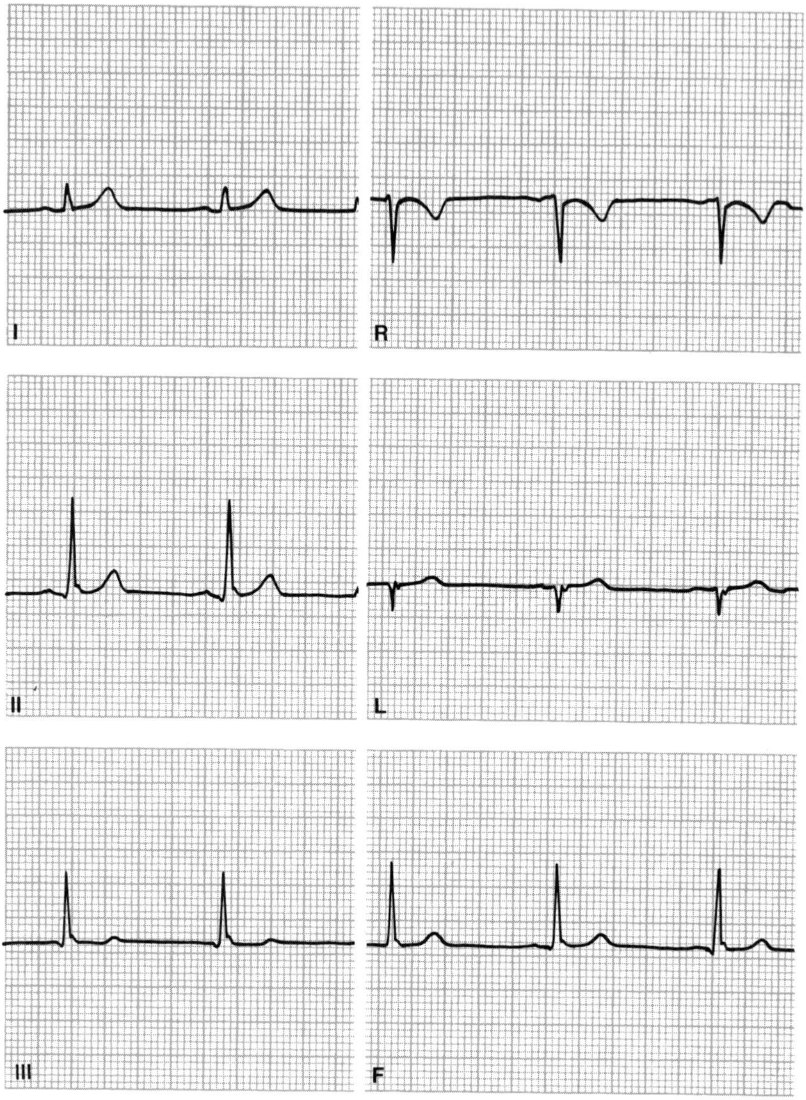

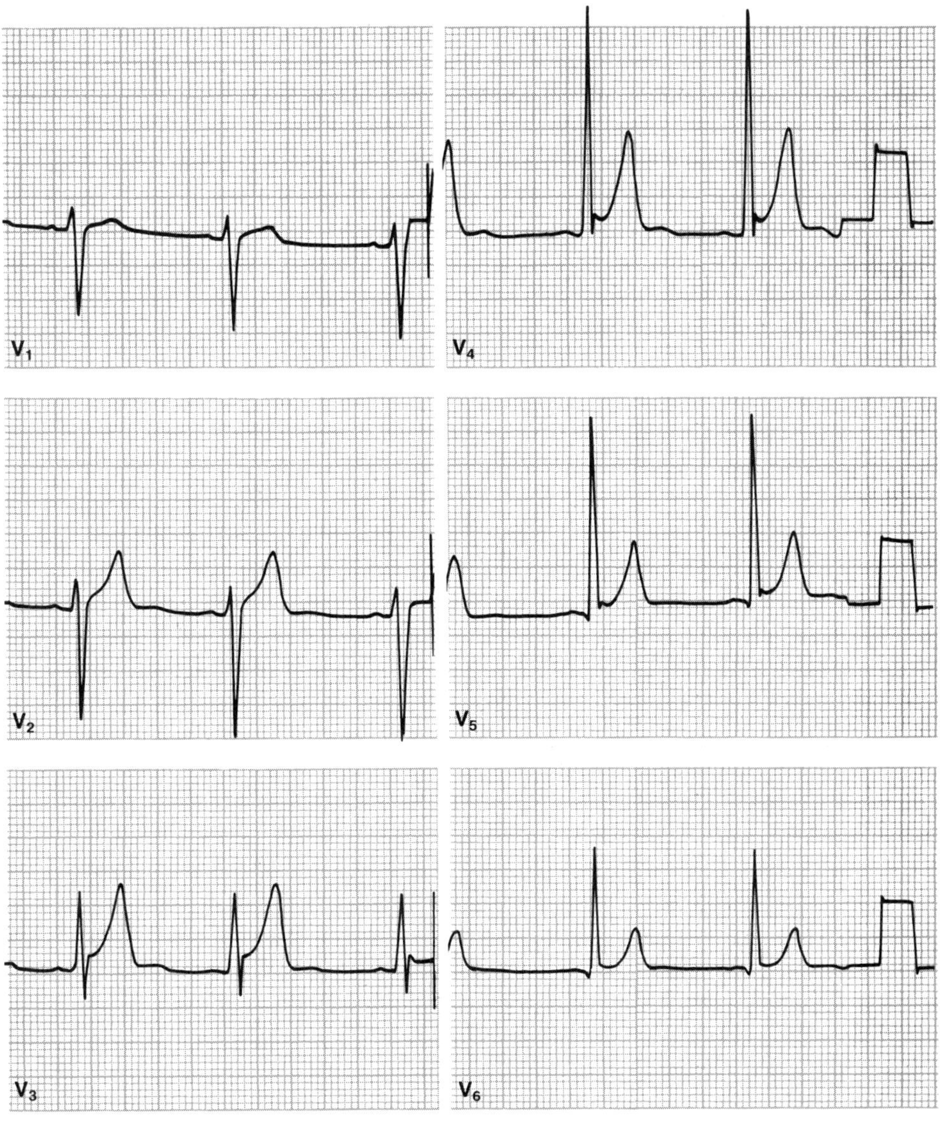
V1
V2
V3
V4
V5
V6

Should one desire to more accurately determine the mean QRS axis, the 3-lead method (see Chapter 3) may be used. Among the three standard limb leads, the predominant QRS deflection is seen in lead II (at +60°). Therefore, the mean QRS axis is most closely oriented toward this lead (Fig. 5-2A). Since lead III (at +120°) is definitely more positive than lead I (at 0°), the mean QRS axis will be much closer to the latter, or at about +80° (Fig. 5-2B and C).

One can check this estimation by examining lead aVL (at −30°). If this lead were exactly isoelectric, the mean QRS axis would be 90° away (or at +60°). The net deflection of lead aVL is negative, so the axis has to be farther to the right than +60°.)

Chamber enlargement: Theoretical considerations in the diagnosis of chamber enlargement were introduced in Chapter 4. There is no suggestion in Fig. 5-1 for either RVH or atrial enlargement. However,

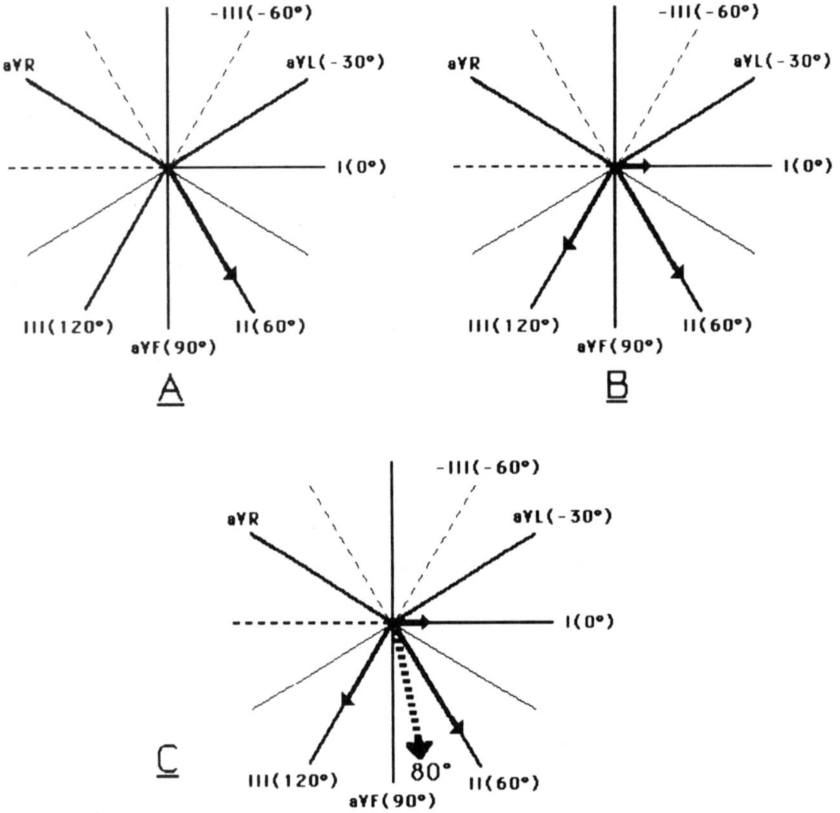

Figure 5-2. The mean QRS axis is most oriented toward lead II at 60° **(A).** It is much closer to lead III than to lead I **(B).** Therefore, the mean QRS axis is about +80° **(C).** As a check of this calculation, note that lead aVL is negative as it should be for an axis of +80°.

impressive QRS voltage is present, suggesting the possibility of LVH. Amplitude of the R wave in lead V_5 alone equals 28 mm. In addition, the sum of the deepest S wave in V_1 or V_2 and the tallest R wave in V_5 or V_6 far exceeds the 35 mm needed to satisfy the *voltage criteria* for LVH given in Chapter 4.

QRST changes:

Q waves: Very small q waves are present in the inferior leads (II, III and aVF) and in V_5 and V_6.

R-wave progression: Normal. (The R wave becomes progressively taller as one moves across the right precordial leads. R-wave amplitude in leads V_4 or V_5 will often be greater than in V_6, as it is here.) *Transition* does occur a little early (R-wave amplitude exceeds S wave amplitude between leads V_2 and V_3), but this is a common, perfectly normal findings. (R-wave progression was discussed in Chapter 4.)

ST-segment elevation or depression: The ST segment is clearly elevated in leads V_2 to V_5, and to a lesser extent probably also in leads II and aVF

T-wave inversion: None.

If the history for this patient were that of an adult presenting for the first time with the acute onset of chest pain, the ST-segment elevation seen in most of the precordial leads would certainly be cause for concern. If no prior ECG were available for comparison, one would have to consider an acute event such as myocardial infarction or pericarditis. In addition, the marked increase in amplitude of QRS complexes in the precordial leads easily satisfies voltage criteria for LVH.

If, on the other hand, this patient were an otherwise healthy, totally asymptomatic, athletic 22-year-old man who had this ECG performed as part of his routine employment physical examination, the electrocardiographer would most probably arrive at an entirely different interpretation. The point to emphasize is that ECGs *MUST always be interpreted in light of the clinical setting!* Failure to do so will consistently result in over- or under-interpretation.

Unfortunately, in practice, one is frequently called on to interpret ECGs without the benefit of desired clinical information. When this occurs, should there by any question at all about a tracing, it becomes the electrocardiographer's *responsibility* to correlate ECG findings to history before rendering a final interpretation. In a less than ideal world, the bare minimum information that should accompany every ECG would be the age of the patient and the reason for admission to the hospital and/or why the ECG was performed. Prior tracings for comparison, when available, are invaluable.

In fact, the ECG shown in Fig. 5-1 was obtained from a healthy, asymptomatic 22-year-old man. Given this clinical setting, the tracing is entirely normal. QRS voltage is not increased considering the patient's age (QRS voltage is often increased in individuals under 35 years of age who do not have LVH), the small and narrow q waves in the inferior and lateral leads are "normal septal q waves" (previously discussed and illustrated in Figs. 4-3 and 4-4), and the ST-segment elevation represents a normal variant known as *early repolarization.*

In evaluating ST-segment elevation, the *shape* of the ST segment is often a more important parameter to consider than the actual number of millimeters that the ST segment is elevated above the baseline. Although the ST segments in leads V_2 to V_6 of Fig. 5-1 *are* elevated, they demonstrate an *upward concavity.* As previously illustrated (by the "smiley" figure at the bottom of Fig. 1-5), this type of ST-segment elevation *usually* has benign clinical implications. In addition, a prominent *J point* is present. The J point (illustrated in Fig. 1-5C) marks the ***junction*** of the end of the QRS complex and the beginning of the ST segment. It is most prominent and appears as a notch in leads V_4 and V_5 of Fig. 5-1. With the acute injury pattern of acute myocardial infarction, it is extremely unusual for the QRS complex to descend to the baseline in an S wave, rise back to a J point, and then descend again to form a gradually up-sloping ST segment. Thus in Fig. 5-1, the combination of upward-sloping ST segments with J-point elevation and lack of *significant* Q waves in the setting of an asymptomatic 22-year-old person overwhelmingly favor early repolarization as the etiology of the ST-segment elevation.

Finally, one might remark that the T waves in Fig. 5-1 are rather tall and peaked in most of the precordial leads. As will be discussed later in this chapter, these T waves do not represent hyperkalemia, but instead are more consistent with a repolarization variant in an otherwise healthy, asymptomatic 22-year-old subject.

PROBLEM: Apply this information in evaluating the likely significance of the ST-segment elevation seen in Figs. 5-3 and 5-4. Would you hospitalize one or both of these patients?

Note: *We will continue to explain each ECG according to the systematic approach presented in Table 1-5, although not in nearly as much detail as for Fig. 5-1. Greatest benefit to the reader may be derived from resisting the temptation to jump ahead with answers to the problems posed before having systematically analyzed each tracing either mentally or in writing.*

INTERPRETATION of Fig. 5-3

Rate and Rhythm: Regular sinus rhythm is present at a rate of about 95 beats/min.

Intervals

PR interval: Normal (and measuring about 0.19 second).

QRS interval: Normal (and measuring about 0.08 second).

QT interval: Prolonged. This is best seen in leads V_2, V_3 and V_4 in which the interval from the onset of the Q wave until the end of the inverted T wave is clearly greater than half the R-R interval.

Axis: About 0°. (The predominant QRS deflection is seen in lead I at 0°, so the mean QRS axis is most closely oriented toward this lead. Since the QRS complex is essentially isoelectric in lead aVF at 90°, the mean QRS axis should be perpendicular to this lead, or at about 0°.)

Chamber enlargement: None. The P wave in lead II appears somewhat prominent, but it is not peaked and does not fulfil the 2-1/2 mm voltage requirement needed to diagnose RAA. Although there is a terminal negative component to the P wave in lead V_1, it is not deep enough to contain one little box from the ECG grid, and therefore does not satisfy the criteria for LAA.

QRST changes: Amplitude of the QRS complexes in this tracing is decreased, although strict criteria for *low voltage* in the limb leads (that all QRS complexes in the limb leads are ≤ 5 mm tall) are not quite met because the R wave in lead I is 6 mm tall. Decreased voltage in the limb and/or precordial leads is commonly seen in patients with chronic obstructive pulmonary disease. However, it is probably of no clinical significance when it occurs without other associated findings of this disorder (as it does here).

Q waves: An isolated Q wave of unknown significance is present in lead III. QS complexes suggestive of anterior infarction are seen in leads V_1 to V_3, with small q waves persisting out to leads V_4 and V_5.

R-waved progression: Poor, due to the QS complexes in leads V_1 to V_3. Transition occurs between leads V_4 and V_5.

ST-T wave changes: The ST segments are *coved* ("convex up") in virtually all of the precordial leads. Although the ST segments themselves are only elevated by a few millimeters, their shape (the "frowny" configuration), the associated symmetric (ischemic-looking) T-wave inversion, the absence of a prior ECG for comparison, and the history of a 59-year-old woman having chest pain, would make one assume that the anterior infarction was acute until proven otherwise. Hospitalization in an intensive care unit would be strongly advised.

INTERPRETATION of Fig. 5-4

Rate and rhythm: Each impulse is *sinus-initiated,* as normal upright P waves are again seen in lead II. However, there is slight but definite variation in the R-R interval between leads, with the heart rate ranging from 60 to 70 beats/min. Thus, the rhythm is *sinus arrhythmia.* (Diagnosis of sinus arrhythmia was discussed in Chapter 1.)

Intervals

PR interval: 0.18 second.

QRS interval: 0.08 second.

QT interval: Normal.

Axis: About +10°. (Again the predominant QRS deflection among the three standard limb leads is seen in lead I at 0°, so the mean QRS axis is oriented most toward this lead (Fig. 5-5A). The net QRS deflection of

Figure 5-3. ECG from a 59-year-old woman complaining of chest pain. No prior ECG available.

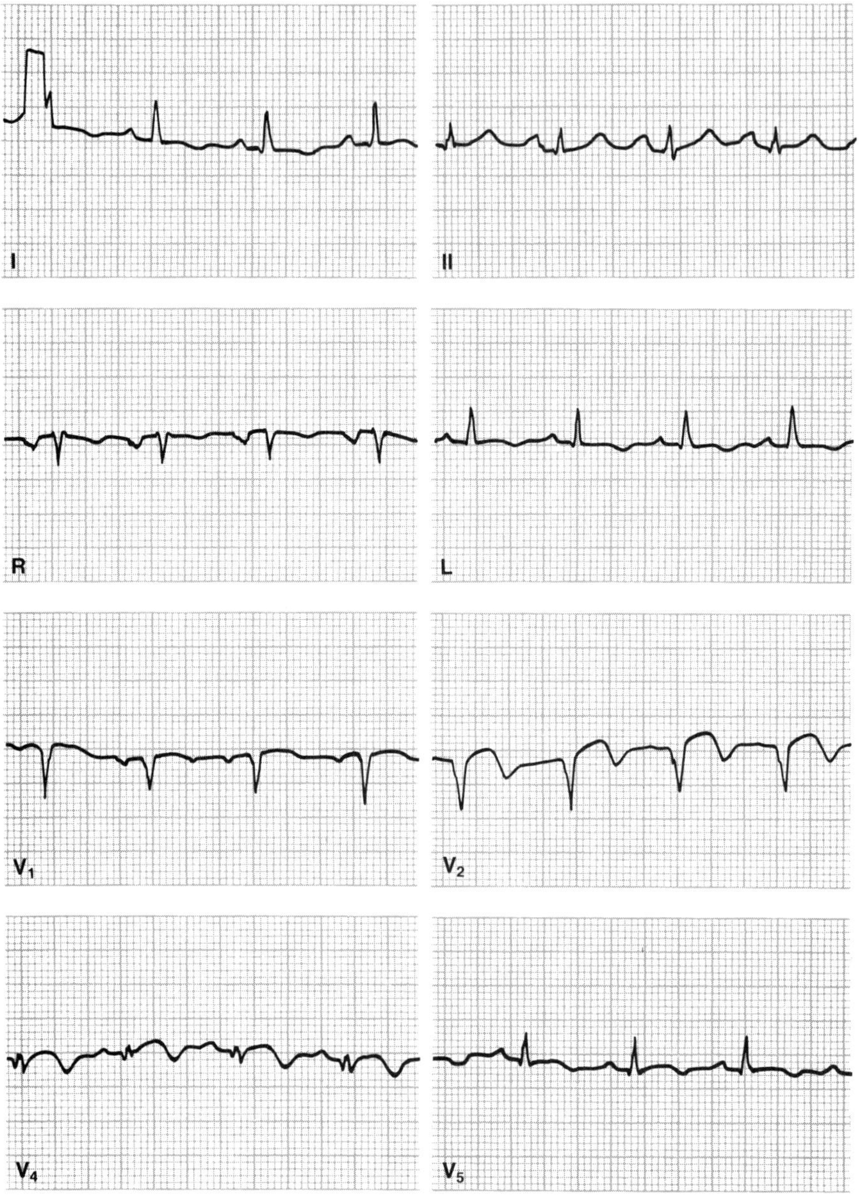

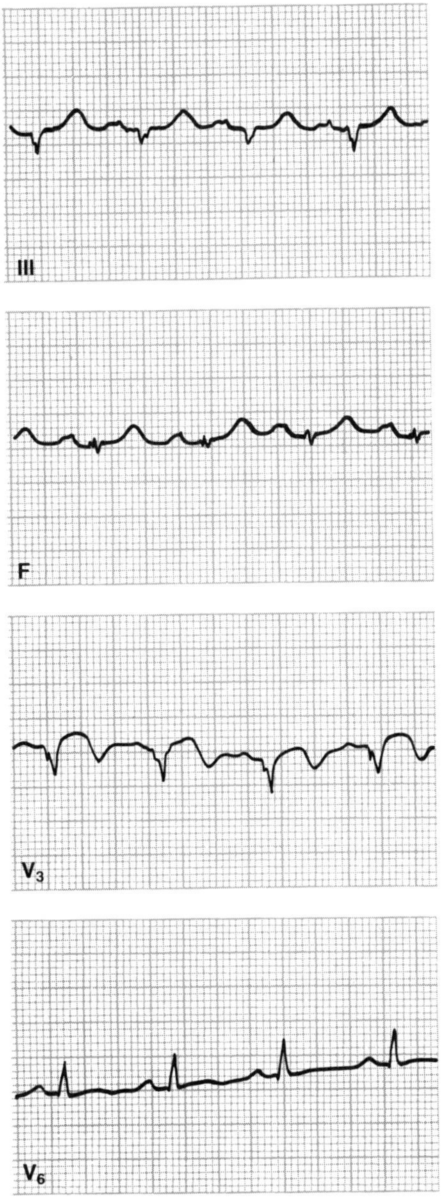
III
F
V3
V6

Figure 5-4. ECG performed as part of a routine physical examination on an asymptomatic 39-year-old man. No prior ECG available.

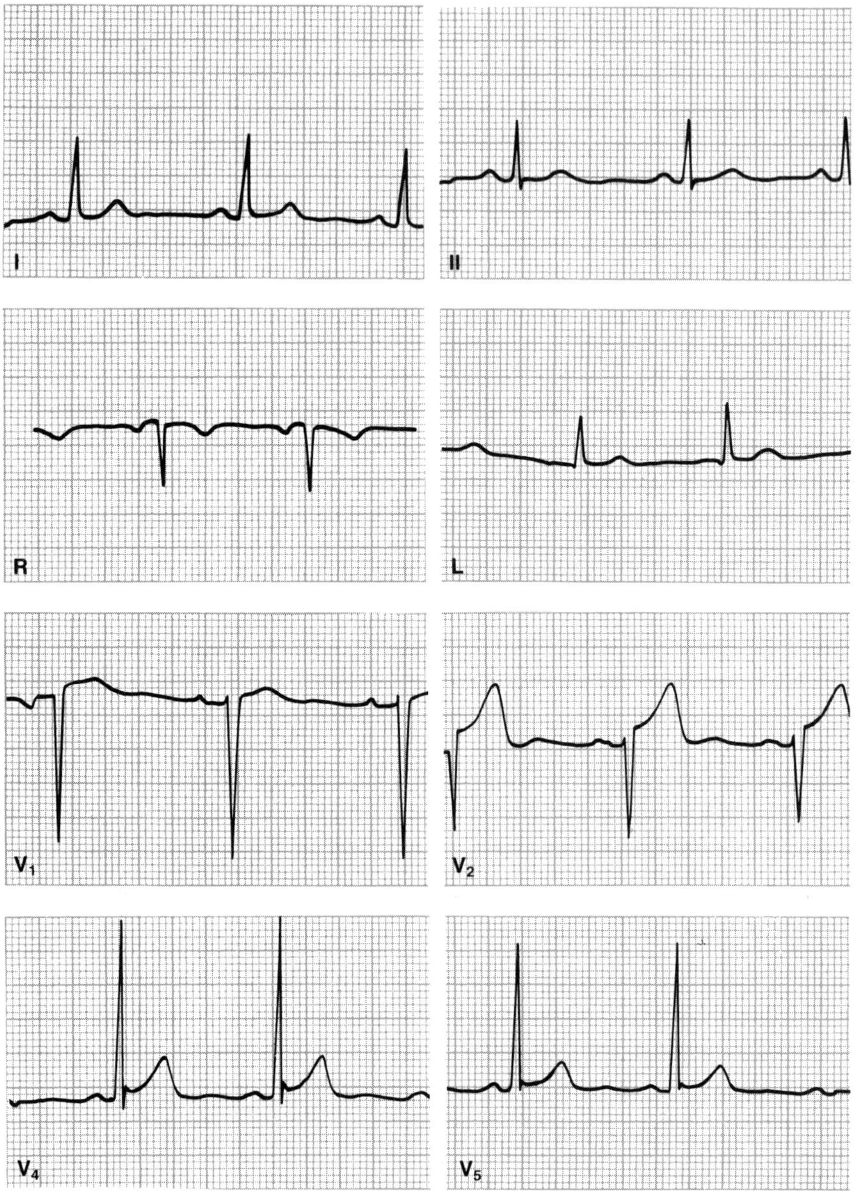

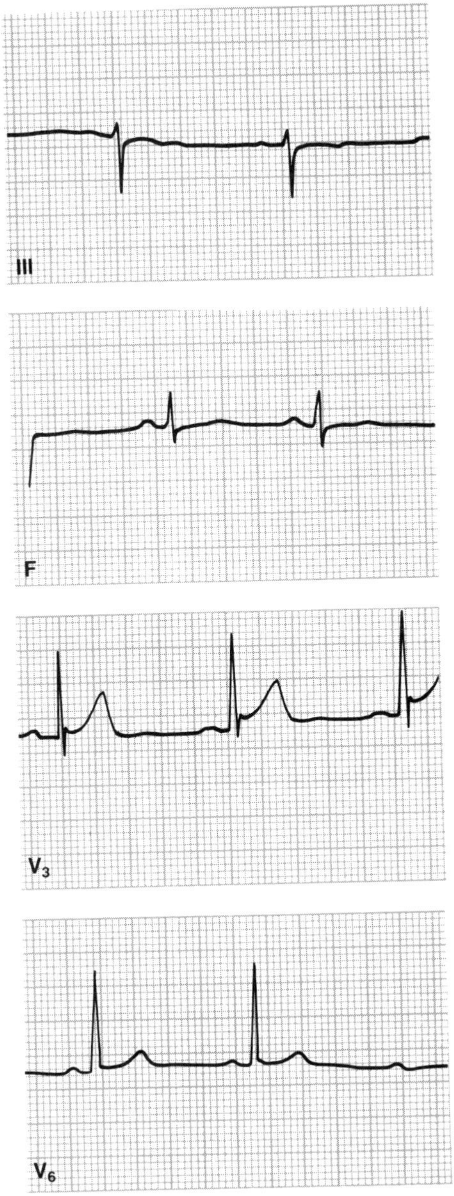
III
F
V3
V6

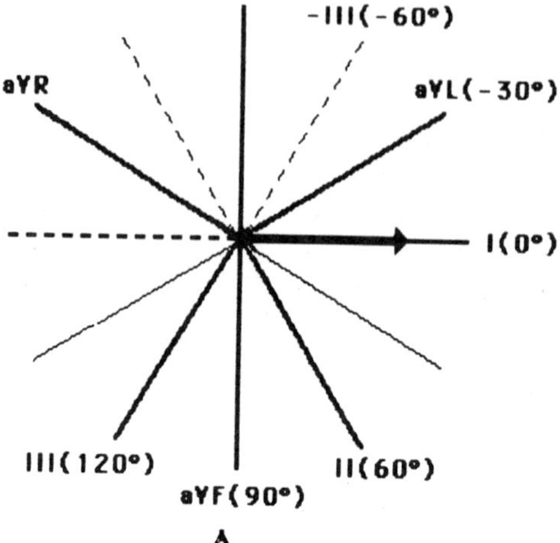

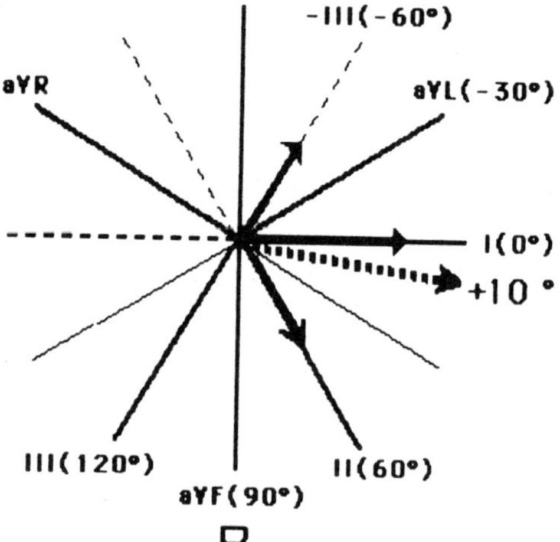

Figure 5-5. The mean QRS axis is most oriented toward lead I at 0° **(A).** The net deflection of lead II at +60° is about equal to that of lead −III at −60°, putting the QRS axis approximately midway between these two leads. Since the net deflection of the QRS complex in lead aVF is positive, however, the mean QRS axis must lie slightly less than 90° away from this lead, or at about +10° **(B).**

lead II at +60° is about as positive as lead III at −60° is negative, putting the mean QRS axis approximately midway in between (or at about 0°). However, since the net QRS deflection in lead aVF of Fig. 5-4 is positive, the mean QRS axis must lie slightly less than 90° away from this lead, or at about + 10° (Fig. 5-5B).

Chamber enlargement: There is voltage for LVH ($SV_1 + RV_5 > 35$ mm).

QRST changes

Q waves: Q waves or QS complexes are commonly seen in lead aVR and can virtually always be *ignored.* A small, narrow "normal septal q wave" is present in lead aVL of this tracing.

R-wave progressiion: Normal. Transition occurs between V_2 and V_3.

ST-T wave changes: Nonspecific ST-segment flattening is present in leads III and aVF. Although several millimeters of ST-segment elevation is seen in leads V_2 to V_4, the upward concavity of the ST segment (the "smiley" configuration), the prominent J point, and the absence of significant Q waves, in the setting of an ECG performed on an otherwise healthy, asymptomatic 39-year-old man strongly suggest early repolarization as the reason for the ST-segment elevation. No further workup is indicated, and this individual definitely would not need hospitalization.

It is important to emphasize that were this 39-year-old man having chest pain at the time the ECG shown in Fig. 5-4 was taken, one would be hard pressed to exclude the possibility of acute injury, particularly if no prior ECG were available for comparison. In this case, admission at least to an observation unit in the hospital might be strongly considered.

PROBLEM: Let us return to our discussion of the normal ECG. Examine the ECG shown in Fig. 5-6, taken from a 29-year-old woman who was seen in the office for a syncopal episode. Should you be concerned about the T-wave inversion seen in leads III and V_1?

INTERPRETATION of Fig. 5-6

Rate and rhythm: There is slight variation in the R-R interval between beats with the heart rate ranging between 52 and 65 beats/min. However, normal upright P waves are seen in lead II with a constant PR interval. Thus, the rhythm is *sinus arrhythmia* and *bradycardia.*

Intervals

PR interval: 0.18 second.

QRS interval: 0.08 second.

QT interval: Normal (clearly less than half the R-R interval).

Axis: About +20°. The mean QRS axis is oriented between lead I (at 0°) and lead II (at 60°) (Fig. 5-7A). It is closer to the former because the net deflection of the QRS complex in lead I is greater than that for lead II (Fig. 5-7B). Confirmation that the mean QRS axis is less than +30° is forthcoming from the inspection of lead III (at +120°). If the net deflection of this lead were isoelectric, then the mean axis would be 90° away at exactly +30°. Since it is negative, the mean QRS axis must be more than 90° away, or at about +20°.

Figure 5-6. ECG from a 29-year-old woman with a syncopal episode. Note the T-wave inversion in leads III and V_1.

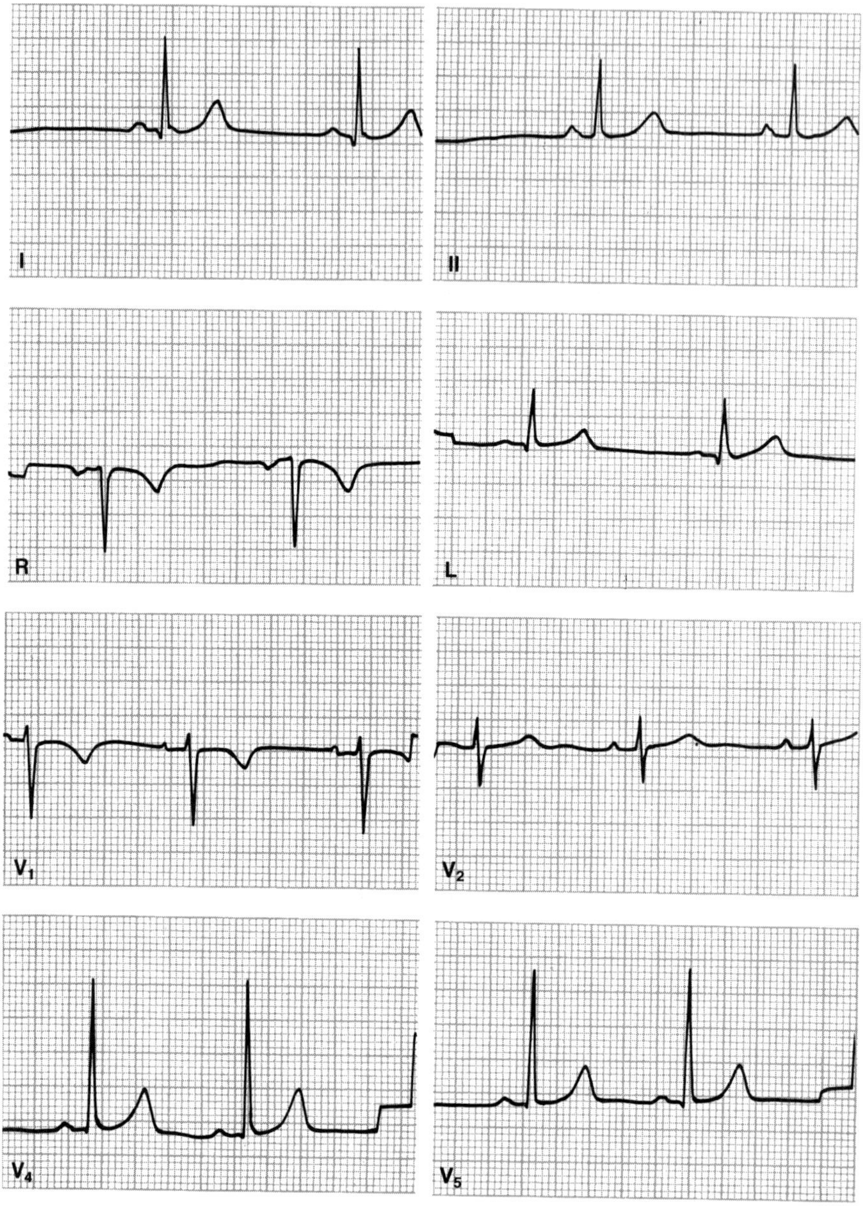

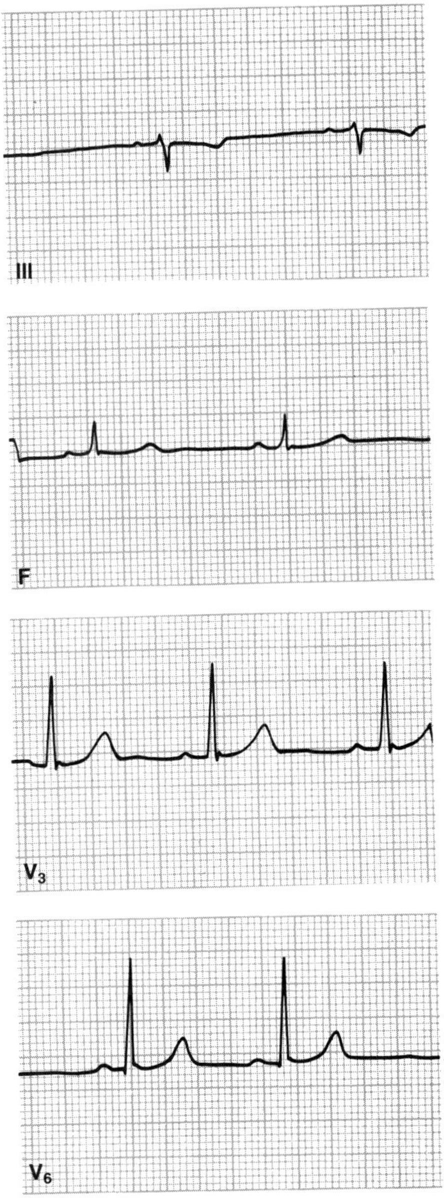
III
F
V3
V6

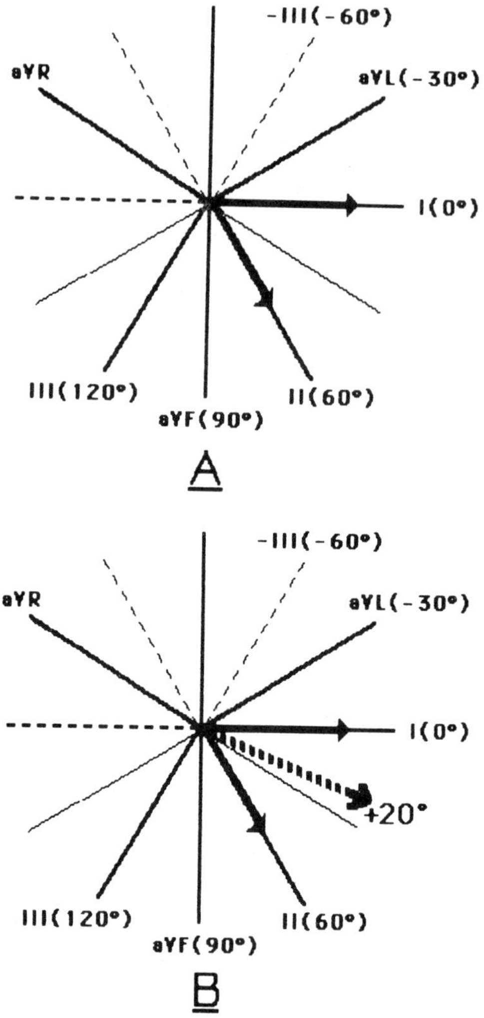

Figure 5-7. The mean QRS axis is oriented between lead I at 0° and lead II at 60° (A). It is slightly closer to the former, and lies at about +20° (B). As a check of this calculation, note that lead III at 120° is negative as it should be for an axis of +20°.

Chamber enlargement: None.

QRST changes

Q waves: Normal septal q waves are seen in the lateral leads (I, aVL, V_5, and V_6).

R-wave progression: Normal. Transition occurs between leads V_2 and V_3.

ST-T wave changes: The ST segments are normal. As stated above, T-waves are symmetrically inverted in leads III and V_1.

Fig. 5-6 is a perfectly normal ECG! In adults, T waves may *normally* be inverted in a number of leads, including leads III, aVF, aVL, and V_1 (see Table 1-2 in Chapter 1). The reason for this is that, in general, the mean T-wave vector (the mean axis of ventricular repolarization) is oriented almost parallel to the mean QRS vector (the mean vector of ventricular depolarization, or the mean QRS axis). Thus, when the QRS deflection is predominantly negative in inferior leads III (as it is in Fig. 5-6) or aVF, the T wave tends to "follow" closely behind and also be negative. In patients with a vertical axis in whom the QRS complex in lead aVL is predominantly negative, T-wave inversion normally may be seen in that lead for the same reason. Finally, in lead V_1, the T wave normally may be upright, flat, or inverted in adults. It usually becomes upright by lead V_2 in *adults,* and remains so over the rest of the precordial leads.

Examine the morphology of the ST segments in Fig. 5-6 carefully. Note that there is a smooth and gradual transition in most leads from the end of the QRS complex to where it merges into the ST segment. The ST segment itself gently curves upward until it blends in with the T wave.

PROBLEM: Compare the shape of the ST segments in Fig. 5-6 with those of the ECG shown in Fig. 5-8. The latter tracing was obtained from a 69-year-old mentally retarded patient who was complaining of some chest discomfort. Are the ST segments in Fig. 5-8 normal?

INTERPRETATION of Fig. 5-8

Rate and rhythm: Sinus rhythm at 65 beats/min.

Intervals: All intervals are normal.

Axis: About $+60°$. (The greatest absolute QRS deflection is in lead II at 60°. Almost equal *net* QRS deflections are seen in leads I and III, putting the mean QRS axis right in between these leads at 60°. Lead aVL at $-30°$ serves as a final check of this estimate. Since the QRS complex in this lead is isoelectric, the mean QRS axis *must* be perpendicular to lead aVL, or at about 60°.)

Chamber enlargement: None.

QRST changes: Although in most leads the T wave is upright and ST segments do not appear to be displaced from the baseline, something is unusual about the appearance of these ST segments. Close inspection reveals a loss of the smooth and gradual up-sloping that was characteristic of the previous normal tracing. The most important point to derive from this example is that the ST segments in Fig. 5-8 are *not* normal! The abnormality *(nonspecific ST-segment flattening)* is highlighted in Fig. 5-9.

Figure 5-8. ECG from a 69-year-old mentally retarded patient with chest discomfort.

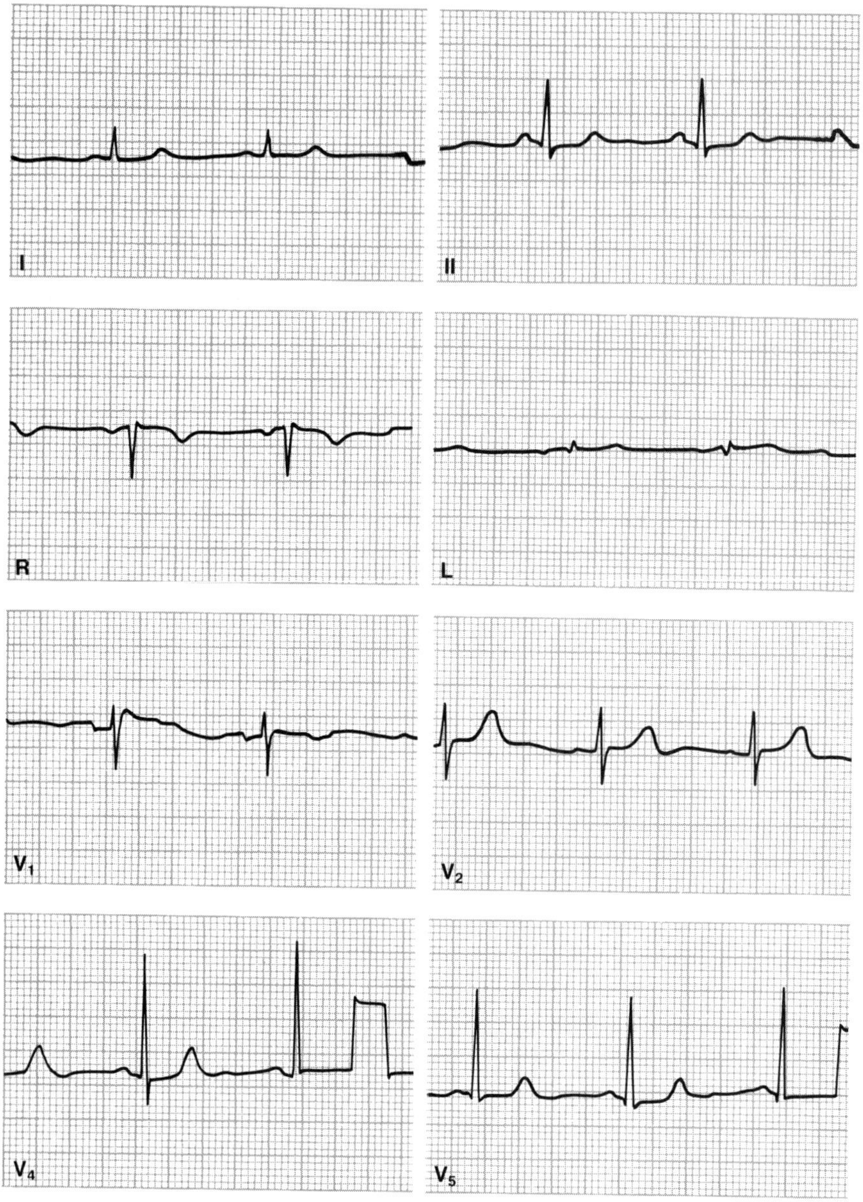

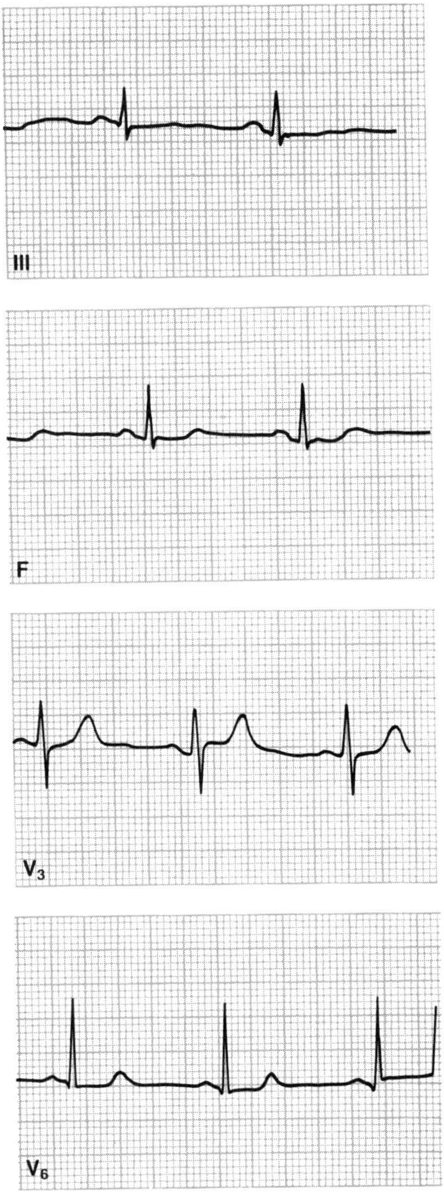
III
F
V_3
V_6

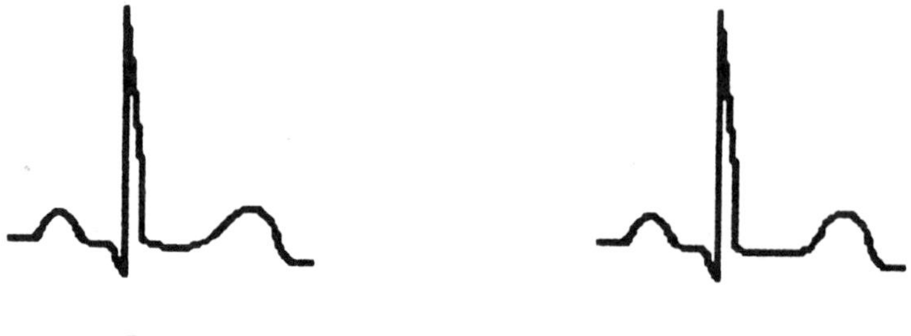

Figure 5-9. **A.** Normal ST segment. There is a smooth and gradual upsloping of the ST segment as it melts into the T wave. **B.** Nonspecific ST-segment flattening. There has been a loss of the gradual up-sloping contour of the ST segment. This change is often subtle.

Nonspecific ST-T Wave Abnormalities

Occasionally, ST-segment flattening of the type seen in Fig. 5-8 may be a subtle sign of underlying coronary artery disease. One might suspect this to be the case in this example, considering the patient's age and presenting complaint. Most of the time, however, ST-segment flattening is a very *non-specific* change without definable etiology.

PROBLEM: Examine the ST segments and T waves of the ECG shown in Fig. 5-10, taken from a 31-year-old man who presented to the emergency department with an acute anxiety attack.

INTERPRETATION of Fig. 5-10

Rate and rhythm: Sinus tachycardia at 115 beats/min. The PR and QRS intervals are normal. The only lead in which one can clearly measure the QT interval is lead V_2. Although appearing to be greater than half the R-R interval in this lead, QT-interval prolongation is much more difficult to evaluate at heart rates over 100 beats/min.

Axis: $+70°$.

Chamber enlargement: None, considering the age of the patient.

QRST changes: Small (probably normal septal) q waves are present in the inferior and lateral precordial leads. Transition occurs between lead V_3 to V_4, and R-wave progression is normal. Diffuse ST-segment and T-wave flattening are seen in virtually all leads except for V_2 and V_3.

The written interpretation for this ECG might read as follows:

"Sinus tachycardia at 115 beats/min. *Nonspecific ST-T wave abnormalities (NS ST-T Abns).*

This is *not* a normal ECG. The ST segments and T waves are altered in almost every lead. Yet there is not much else that can be said about this tracing. Any of a number of causes might be responsible for these abnormalities including ischemia, drug effects, electrolyte disturbances, and ventricular hypertrophy. In fact, this patient's abnormalities were probably the result of hyperventilation from his acute anxiety attack, since a follow-up ECG done soon after he had calmed down was entirely normal!

In recognition of the fact that the tracing shown in Fig. 5-10 is not normal, while still acknowledging that there may be no indication as to what the ST-T wave abnormalities are caused by, changes such as these are called *nonspecific*. In practice, such changes may range from minimal flattening of the ST segment and/or T wave, to the diffuse flattening seen here. Nonspecific ST-T wave changes are probably the most common abnormality seen in electrocardiography.

Ischemia and Strain

In Chapter 1 we discussed the numerous factors that can affect T waves. Many of these were listed in Table 1-3. Although it is often impossible to determine the exact cause of ST-segment and T-wave abnormalities by simple inspection, a number of conditions are known to produce characteristic changes in the ECG. Included among these are the ST-segment and T-wave abnormalities that occur with ischemia and left ventricular strain.

As discussed in Chapter 1, ischemia typically produces a *primary* T-wave change. Since ischemia is usually fairly well localized to a particular portion of the myocardium, the overall sequence of left ventricular activation will not be greatly altered. *Symmetric* T-wave inversion is characteristically seen on the electrocardiogram (Fig. 5-11A). On the other hand, repolarization changes that accompany LVH ("strain") are the result of a *secondary* T-wave change in which the process of left ventricular activation *is* significantly altered by the increase in left ventricular mass. Electrocardiographically, secondary T-wave changes are usually represented by ST-segment depression and *asymmetric* T-wave inversion (Fig. 5-11B).

PROBLEM: Examine the precordial lead sequences shown in Figs. 5-12A and 5-12B. Are the ST segments and T waves more suggestive of ischemia or strain?

ANSWER to Fig. 5-12A: Coving of the ST segments and *symmetric* T-wave inversion in leads V_2 to V_6 of this example are suggestive of anterolateral ischemia.

ANSWER to Fig. 5-12B: The ST segments in leads V_4 to V_6 of this figure are sagging and slightly depressed. As opposed to Fig. 5-12A, T-wave inversion is *asymmetric*. The initial portion of the T wave gradually slopes down-

Figure 5-10. ECG from a 31-year-old man presenting with an acute anxiety attack.

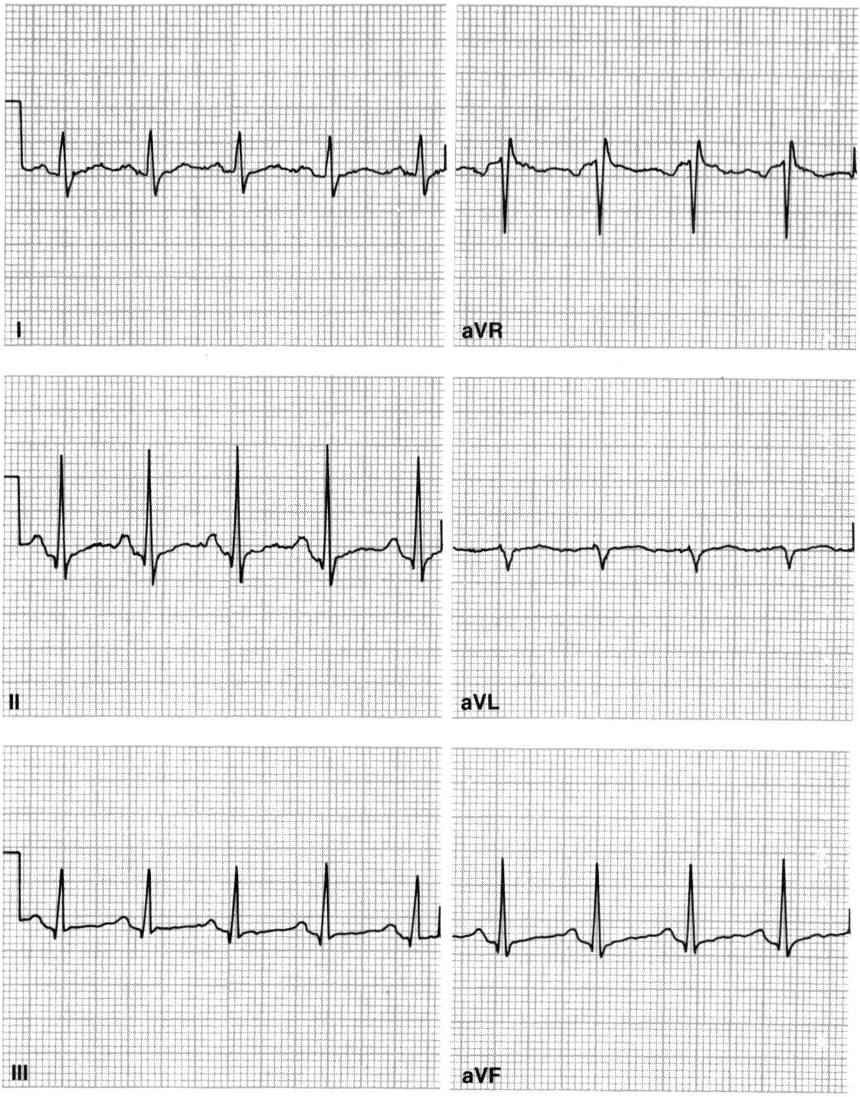

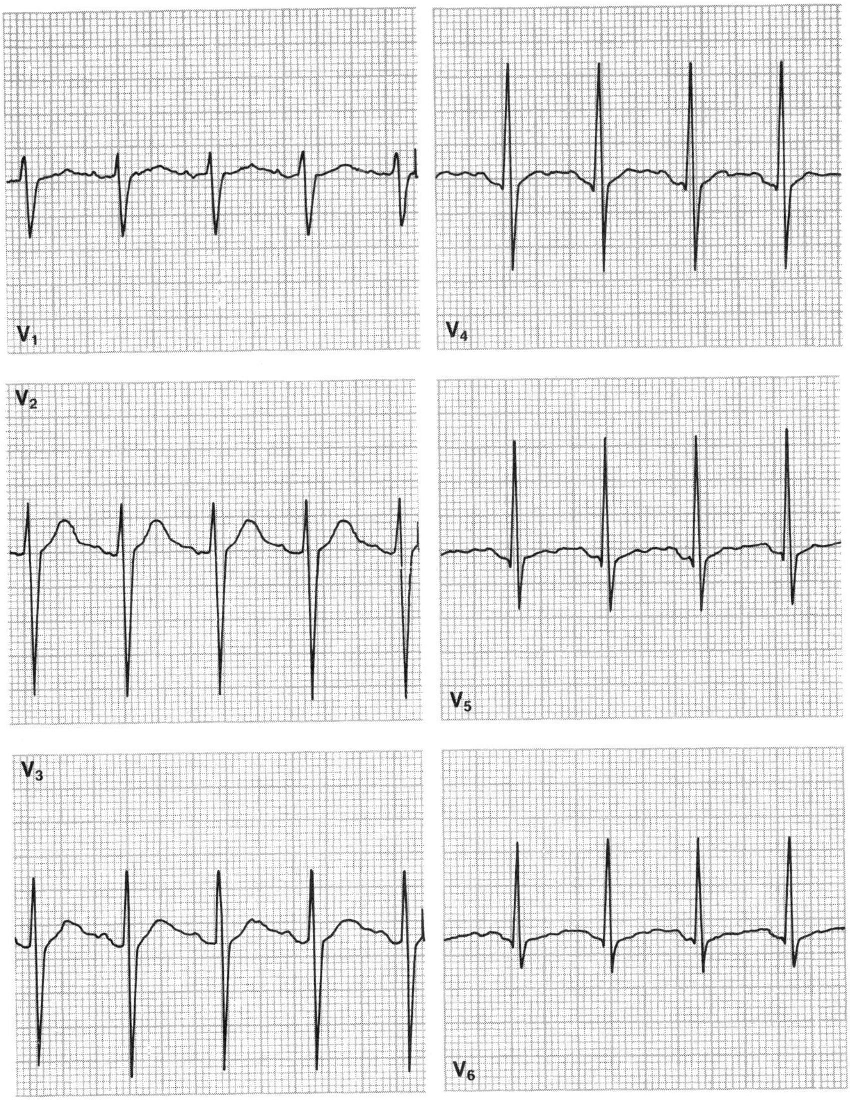
V1
V4
V2
V5
V3
V6

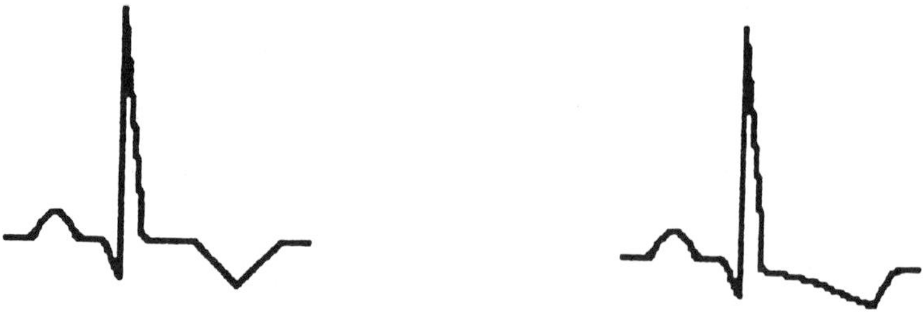

Figure 5-11. **A.** Primary T-wave change. Symmetric T-wave inversion is characteristic of ischemia. **B.** Secondary T-wave change. Sagging ST-segment depression with asymmetric T-wave inversion is characteristic of the repolarization change that is seen with LVH ("strain").

ward, blending imperceptibly with the sagging ST segment. The final portion of the T wave has a more rapid up-slope as it returns to the baseline. Voltage requirements for LVH are easily met, as the sum of the deepest S wave in V_1 to V_2 plus the tallest R wave in V_5 to V_6 exceeds the required 35 mm. The picture is typical of LVH with strain.

Up to now we have suggested that symmetric T-wave inversion was the principal ECG manifestation of ischemia. While this is true, it should be remembered that ST-segment depression may also be a manifestation of ischemia. As we will see in the next section, ST-segment depression may result from a number of other conditions, and is much less specific for ischemia than the pattern of symmetric T-wave inversion.

PROBLEM: Interpret the ECG shown in Fig. 5-13. Decide whether the ST segments and T waves are more suggestive of ischemia or strain.

INTERPRETATION of Fig. 5-13

Rate and rhythm: Sinus rhythm at a rate of 95 beats/min. The PR and QRS intervals are normal (0.17 second and 0.10 second, respectively). The QT interval is borderline prolonged (the QT interval is about half the R-R interval).

Axis: About $-10°$. (Left axis deviation must be present, since the net QRS deflection of lead aVF is negative. However, since the net deflection of lead II is definitely positive, the mean QRS axis is clearly less than $-30°$.)

Chamber enlargement: QRS amplitude is markedly increased in all of the lateral leads, easily satisfying voltage criteria for LVH.

QRST changes: A QS complex is present in lead V_1. This is probably of no clinical significance. Transition occurs early between leads V_1 and V_2.

Nonspecific ST-segment flattening and biphasic T waves are seen in leads III, aVF, and V_2 to V_4. The ST segments are depressed in leads II, V_5, and V_6, but an even more prominent finding in these leads is the fairly deep, symmetric T-wave inversion. This suggests ischemia. However, the tremendous QRS voltage in the lateral leads, together with the more typical appearance of "strain" of the ST segments in leads I and aVL, strongly suggests that LVH is *also* present.

This ECG offers a good example of how the primary T-wave changes of ischemia may partially or totally mask the secondary T-wave changes of strain. Perhaps the best way to interpret this ECG would be:

"Sinus rhythm at 95 beats/min. LAD (left axis deviation). Early transition in the precordial leads. LVH *with* strain *and/or* ischemia."

Clinical correlation and/or comparison with prior tracings would be needed to determine whether the ST-segment depression and symmetric T-wave inversion represented an acute process.

Causes of ST-Segment Depression

There are only a handful of conditions in electrocardiography that require instant recollection by the interpreter of a list of differential diagnostic possibilities. The first such list that we will discuss deals with the most common causes of ST-segment depression.

PROBLEM: Examine the ECG shown in Fig. 5-14, taken from a 60-year-old woman with a history of congestive heart failure. The patient was being treated with digoxin and a diuretic. Can you list five possible reasons for the diffuse ST-segment depression that is present?

INTERPRETATION of Fig. 5-14

Rate and rhythm: A narrow-complex supraventricular tachycardia is present at a rate of approximately 200 beats/min. No P waves are evident.

Axis: About +55°. (The largest absolute deflection among the three standard limb leads is in lead II at +60°. Since the net deflection of lead aVL at −30° is slightly positive, the mean QRS axis is just less than 90° away from this lead, or at about +55°.)

Chamber enlargement: There is voltage for LVH ($SV_1 + RV_5 \geq 35$ mm).

QRST changes: Diffuse ST-segment depression is seen in multiple leads. This may result from one or more of the following: (1) strain (the patient has LVH); (2) ischemia; (3) rate-related ST-T wave changes induced by the tachycardia; (4) digitalis effect; or (5) hypokalemia (Table 5-1).

Figure 5-12

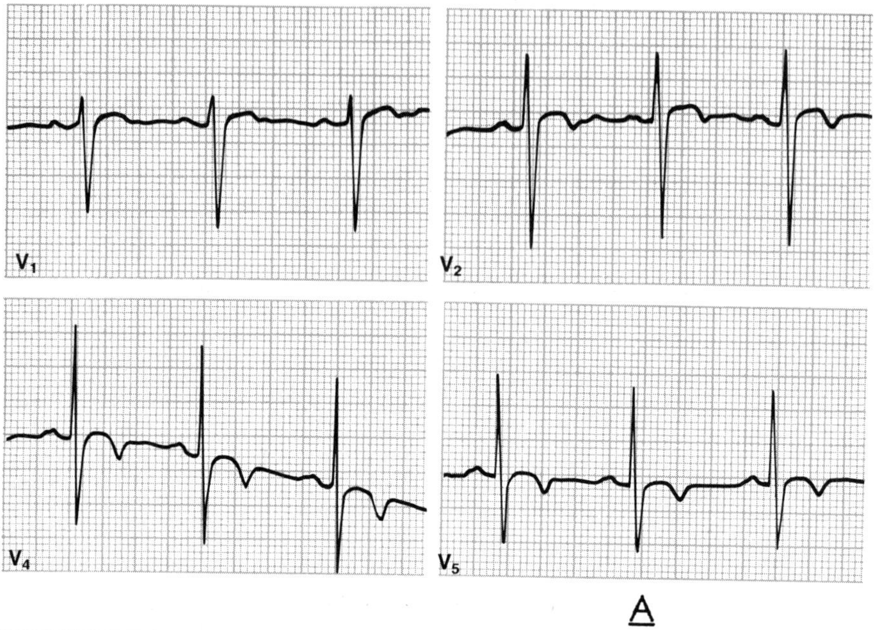

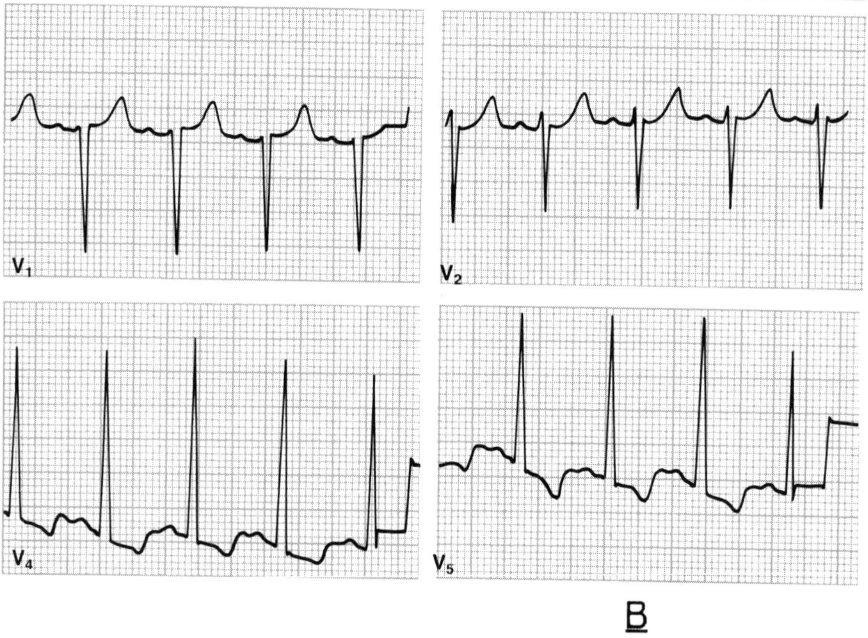

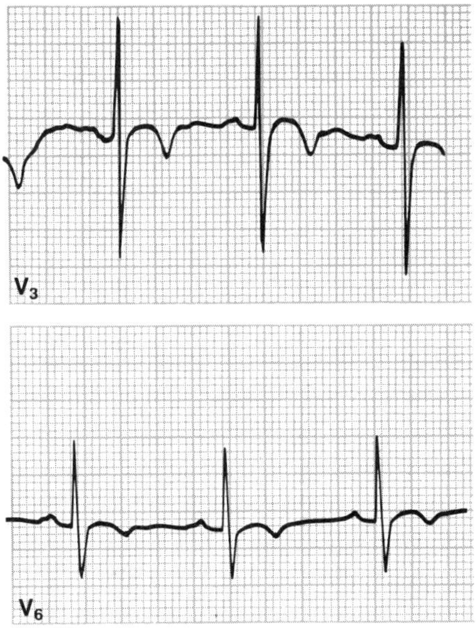
V3
V6

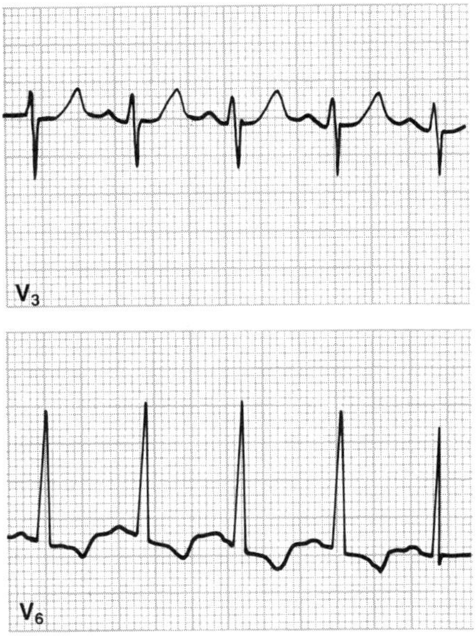
V3
V6

Figure 5-13

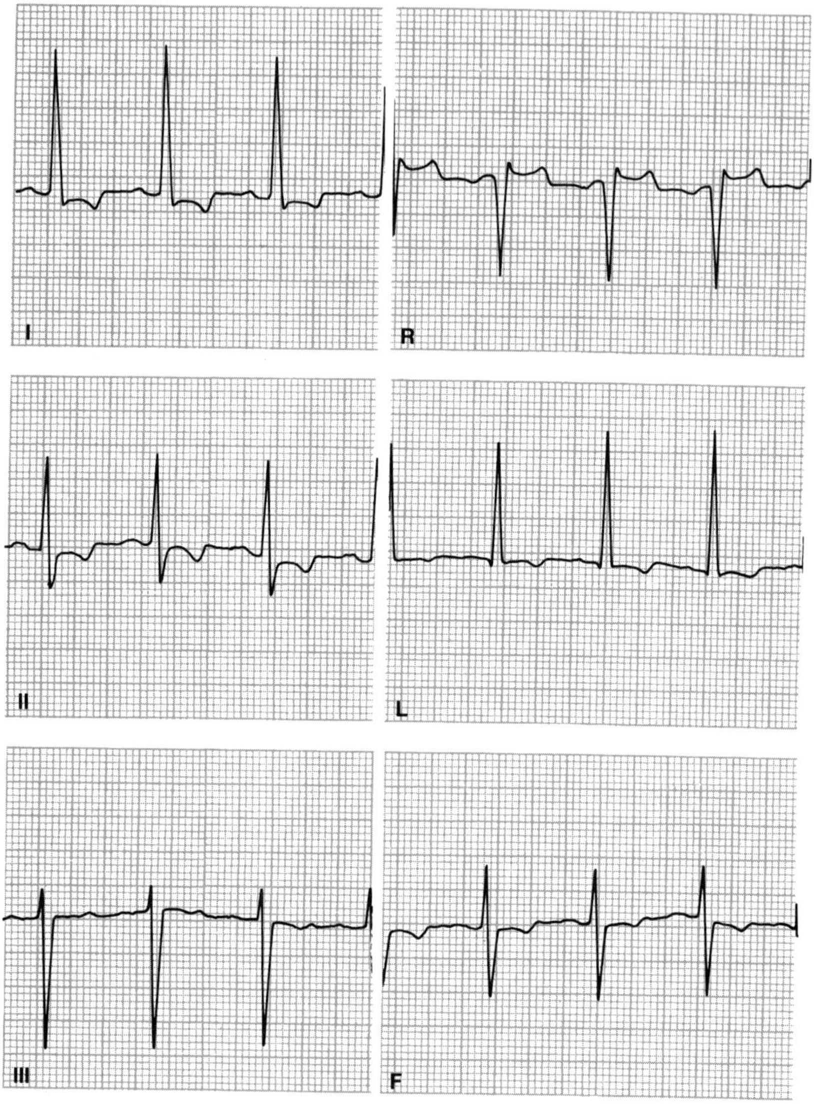

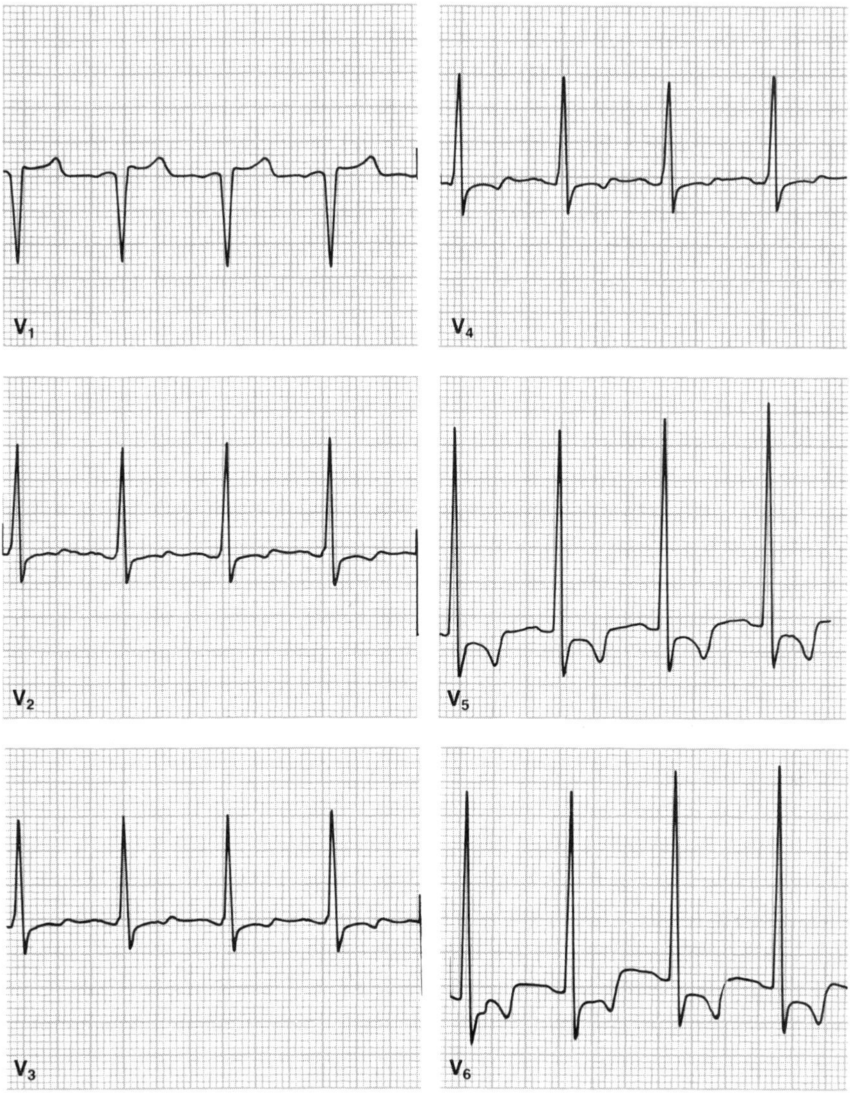
V1
V2
V3
V4
V5
V6

TABLE 5-1

Causes of ST-segment depression

"Strain" (from LVH)
Ischemia
Rate-related ST-segment depression
Digitalis effect
Hypokalemia

Fig. 5-15 illustrates this patient's ECG following conversion to normal sinus rhythm. Note that much of the ST-segment depression has resolved. This implies that *ischemia* and *rate-related* ST-T wave changes that were associated with the tachycardia accounted for at least some of the ST-segment depression seen in Fig. 5-14. However, since the ST segments are still depressed in most leads of the post-conversion tracing, and the patient is *hypokalemic,* takes *digoxin,* and demonstrates ECG voltage criteria for *LVH*, one or more of these factors may also have contributed to the ST-segment depression seen in Fig. 5-14.

Figure 5-14. Supraventricular tachycardia at a rate of about 200 beats/min with diffuse ST-segment depression.

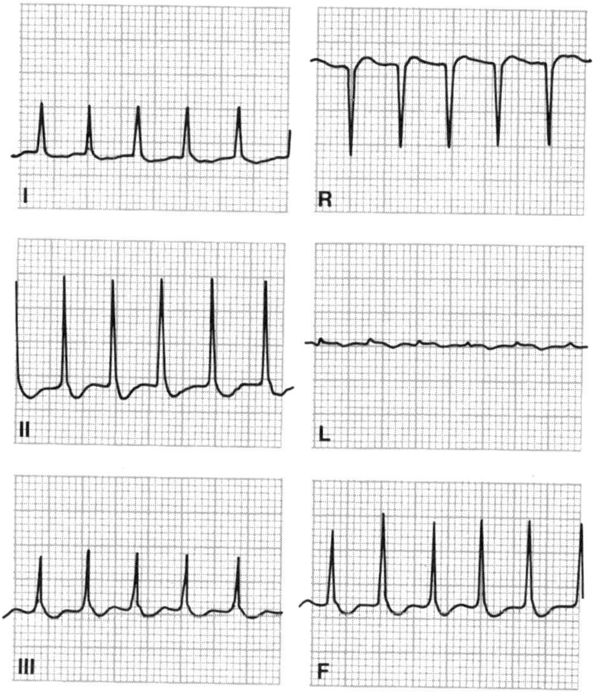

In summary, whenever one encounters ST-segment depression in an ECG, each of the five factors listed in Table 5-1 should be considered as a possible contributing cause. Let us now consider in greater detail how some of these factors affect the ECG.

Digitalis Effect

Digitalis has been employed in the treatment of patients with cardiac disorders since the drug was first described by William Withering in the late eighteenth century. It remains one of the most commonly used agents in the treatment of congestive heart failure and supraventricular tachydysrhythmias today.

Digitalis exerts two principal actions on the heart. The first is to increase the force of cardiac contraction (positive inotropic effect). This is felt to increase stroke volume and improve cardiac output in patients with congestive heart failure. The second is to prolong the refractory period of the AV node and to slow the conduction velocity of the cardiac impulse through this structure. As a result, the ventricular response of supraventricular ta-

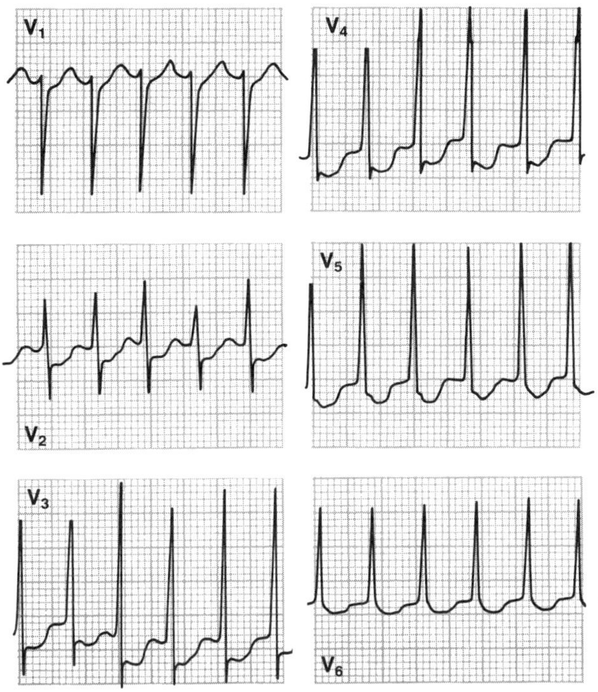

chydysrhythmias is slowed, and the PR interval in normal sinus rhythm may be prolonged.

Digitalis characteristically produces one of two effects ("digitalis effect") on the ECG. In some patients, a scooping or "hockey stick" deformity of the ST segment is seen (Fig. 5-16A). A way to remember this is to think of the "little white pill" (digoxin) rolling back and forth along the curved surface of the ST segment (inset of Fig. 5-16A). Associated with the increased force of contraction, the period of electrical systole may shorten. Thus, the QT interval in digitalized patients may become *shortened,* although this effect is often not noticeable on the ECG.

The other characteristic effect that digitalis may have on the ECG is to produce ST-segment depression and asymmetric T-wave inversion that may be indistinguishable from left ventricular strain (Fig. 5-16B).

When taken in excess, digitalis can produce virtually any cardiac dysrhythmia. Dysrhythmias that are especially suggestive of digitalis toxicity include atrial tachycardia with AV block, accelerated junctional rhythms, atrial fibrillation with either a slow or regularized ventricular response, Mo-

Figure 5-15. After conversion to sinus rhythm, much of the ST-segment depression has resolved. Changes consistent with LVH with "strain," digitalis effect, or both remain.

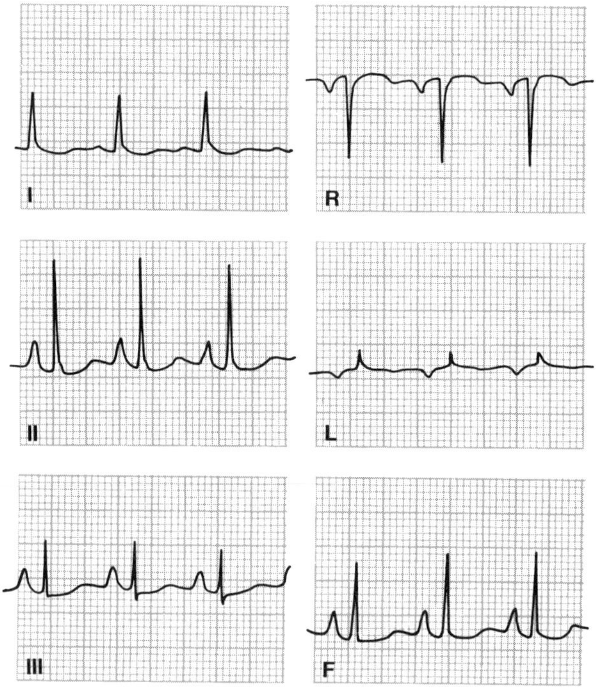

bitz I (Wenckebach) 2° AV block, and complex ventricular dysrhythmias. The point to emphasize is that the arrhythmogenic effect of excess digitalis is totally independent of the effect the drug has on the ST segment and T wave. *Not* all patients on digitalis manifest digitalis effect. Furthermore, the presence or absence of digitalis effect does *not* necessarily correlate with serum levels of the drug. Thus a patient with a markedly toxic serum digoxin level may have a totally normal ECG!

Hypokalemia

Potassium is the principal intracellular cation. Over 98 percent of the body's potassium is contained within the cells. Normal serum potassium concentration is 3.5 to 5.5 mEq/L. It is important to emphasize that *only* potassium in the extracellular fluid (ECF) compartment is reflected by the serum concentration. Yet despite the fact that ECF potassium makes up less than 2 percent of total body potassium, it has a profound effect on cardiac and neuromuscular function.

A number of factors other than total body potassium content affect the

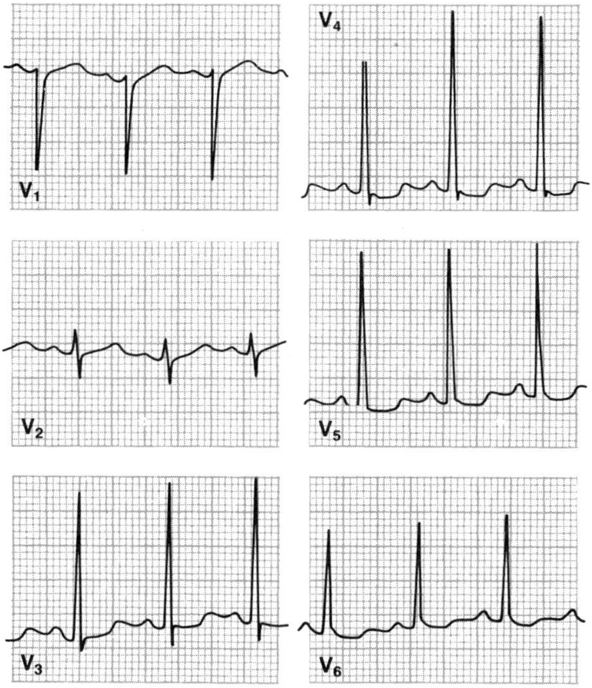

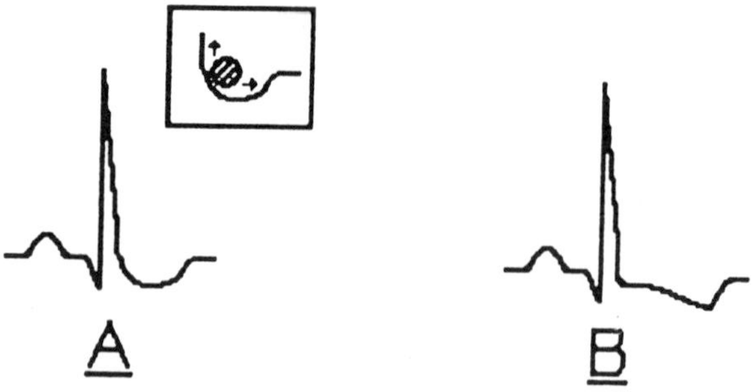

Figure 5-16. Digitalis effect. **A.** ST-segment "scooping" deformity (or "pill-rolling" effect—insert) with shortening of the QT interval. **B.** ST-segment depression with asymmetric T-wave inversion. Although patients on digoxin may manifest either of these ECG effects, there is a poor correlation between serum digoxin levels and the ECG.

serum concentration of potassium. Especially important is acid–base balance. Acidosis tends to shift potassium out of cells into the ECF, while alkalosis usually results in movement of potassium from the ECF back into the cells. Thus a patient with severe total body potassium depletion may have a normal or even increased serum potassium concentration if acidosis is present.

Hypokalemia is said to exist when serum potassium is less than 3.5 mEq/L. Patients most at risk of developing this electrolyte abnormality include those with poor dietary intake, excessive vomiting or diarrhea, or use of potassium-wasting diuretics (furosemide or thiazides).

The ECG may be affected in a number of ways by hypokalemia (Fig. 5-17). Early changes may be subtle and amount to little more than a decrease in amplitude of T waves. With greater degrees of hypokalemia, T waves flatten, U waves become evident and increase in amplitude, and nonspecific ST-segment depression develops in a number of leads. With marked hypokalemia (serum $K^+ < 2.0$ mEq/L), ST-segment depression may become quite pronounced.

U waves are usually best seen in leads V_2 to V_4. Although their presence is a nonspecific finding that may be associated with bradycardia, use of certain drugs (quinidine, procainamide, phenothiazines), central nervous system disorders, and left ventricular hypertrophy, identification of U waves that exceed T waves in amplitude strongly suggests hypokalemia. Differentiation between the T wave and U wave may become extremely difficult at this point (Fig. 5-17F).

For unexplained reasons, P waves may get taller and more peaked in the inferior leads with hypokalemia. This pattern may be indistinguishable from that which occurs with right atrial abnormality (RAA). The term "pseudo P-pulmonale" has been used to describe these changes in P-wave morphology, where "pseudo" acknowledges that peaking and increased am-

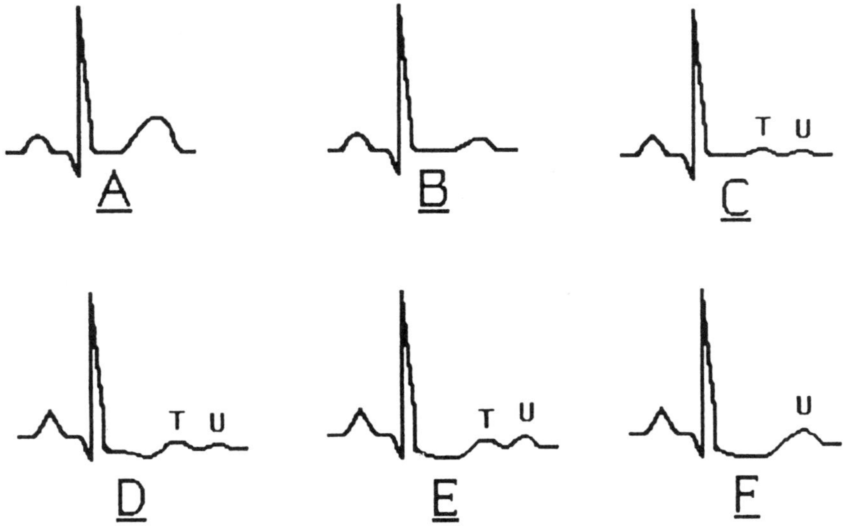

Figure 5-17. ECG changes of hypokalemia. **A.** Normal. Earliest changes are flattening of the T wave **(B)**, with development of U waves **(C)**.Diffuse ST-segment depression and a "pseudo P-pulmonale" pattern **(D)** may follow. ST-segment depression may become fairly marked with progressive increase in U wave amplitude **(E)**. Although overall, ECG changes with hypokalemia are nonspecific, the diagnosis should be strongly considered if U-wave amplitude ever exceeds T-wave amplitude. Differentiation between the T wave and U wave may become extremely difficult at this point **(F)**.

plitude of P waves may have nothing to do with the dimensions of the right atrium.

It is important to remember that the ECG is neither a sensitive nor a specific indicator of hypokalemia. Many patients manifest nonspecific ST-T wave abnormalities but have totally normal serum potassium concentrations. Conversely, many patients with mild to moderate hypokalemia (serum $K^+ \approx 2.5$ to 3.5 mEq/L) do not manifest any ECG abnormalities at all.

PROBLEM: Examine the ECG shown in Fig. 5-18. Comment on QT-interval duration and ST-T wave morphology.

INTERPRETATION of Fig. 5-18

Rate and rhythm: Sinus bradycardia at about 55 to 60 beats/min. 1° AV block is present. The QT interval appears to be greatly prolonged.

Axis: About 0°.

Chamber enlargement: None.

QRST changes: Q waves of uncertain significance are present in the inferior

Figure 5-18

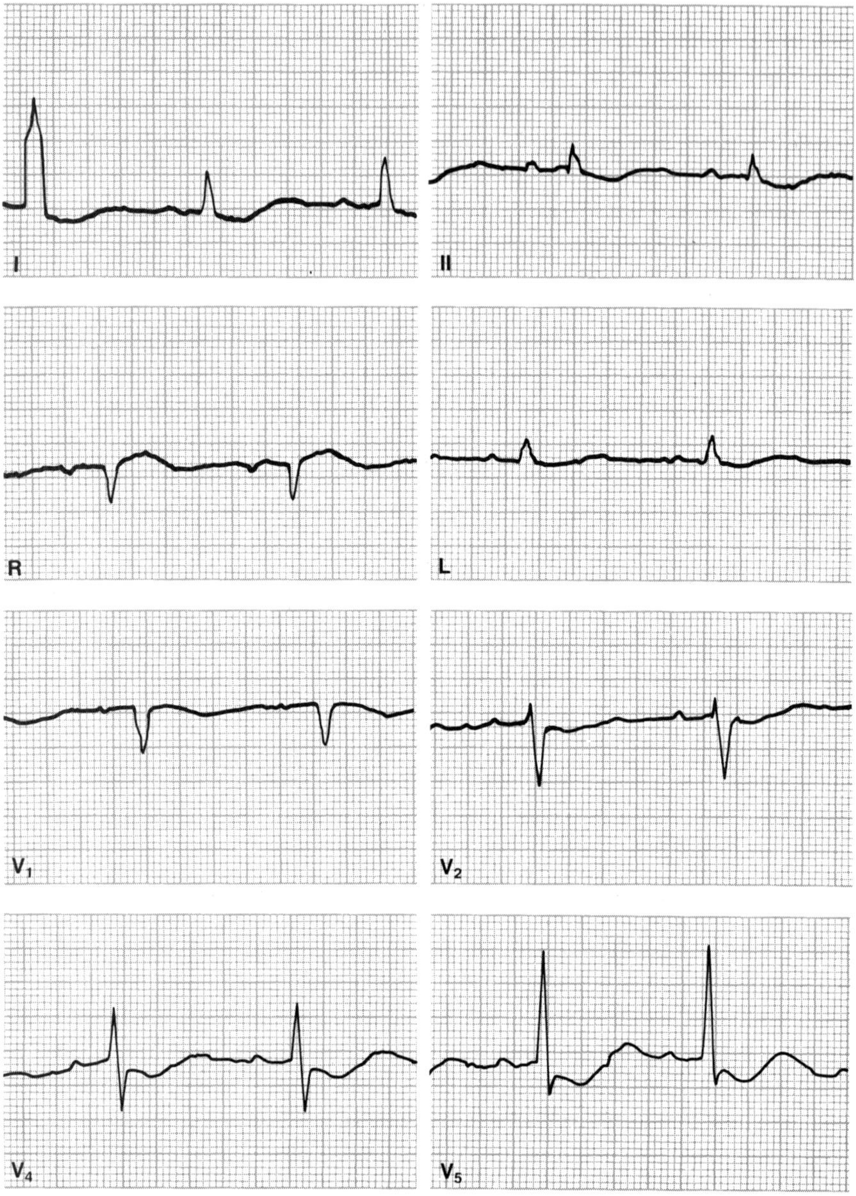

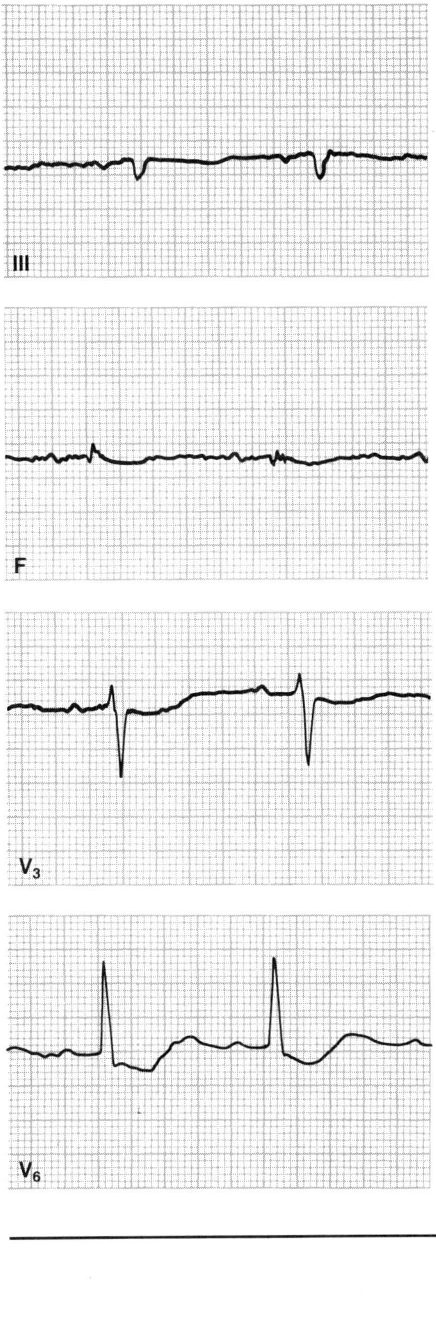
III
F
V3
V6

leads. R-wave progression is normal. ST segments are "scooped" and markedly depressed in multiple leads.

The most striking findings of this ECG are diffuse ST-segment depression and marked QT-interval prolongation. The latter should suggest one or more of the entities listed in Table 1-4 as the reason for QT prolongation.

Serum potassium concentration of the patient whose ECG is shown in Fig. 5-18 was <2.0 mEq/L at the time this tracing was recorded. Large U waves have fused with the terminal portion of flattened T waves to give the appearance of a greatly prolonged QT interval, when in fact the QU interval is what is being measured. With correction of the serum potassium, all ECG abnormalities reverted to normal.

Hyperkalemia

As opposed to the situation with hypokalemia, the ECG is a much more sensitive indicator of increased ECF concentrations of potassium. Yet once again, serum potassium concentration does *not* necessarily reflect total body stores of this cation. This is especially true for the patient with severe acidosis in whom rapid shifts between intracellular and extracellular potassium commonly occur. Acidosis may result in transient hyperkalemia with flooding of potassium from the cells into ECF despite normal or even decreased total body stores of potassium. With correction of acidosis, potassium reenters the cells and serum potassium concentration may drop precipitously.

The usual sequence of ECG alterations that takes place with hyperkalemia is illustrated in Fig. 5-19. The earliest change is peaking of the T wave (Fig. 5-19B and C). This usually occurs when serum potassium is in the range of 6 to 7 mEq/L. With progressively increasing degrees of hyperkalemia, T waves continue to become taller and more peaked, P waves decrease in amplitude, the PR interval lengthens, and the QRS complex widens (Fig. 5-19D). P waves then disappear. Although the ECG may simulate a ventricular rhythm at this stage (absent P waves, wide QRS complexes), intracardiac electrophysiologic studies have shown origination of the impulse from the SA node and transmission to the AV node are usually both still intact. Thus there is *sinoventricular conduction.* However, since atrial depolarization is unable to occur in the presence of such severe hyperkalemia, P waves are not inscribed on the ECG.

With preterminal hyperkalemia (serum $K^+ \approx$ 10mEq/L), the QRS complex becomes sinusoid (Fig. 5-19E). Ventricular fibrillation and/or asystole follow shortly thereafter.

Although the finding of tall, peaked T waves in multiple leads of an ECG is strongly suggestive of hyperkalemia, several caveats should be borne

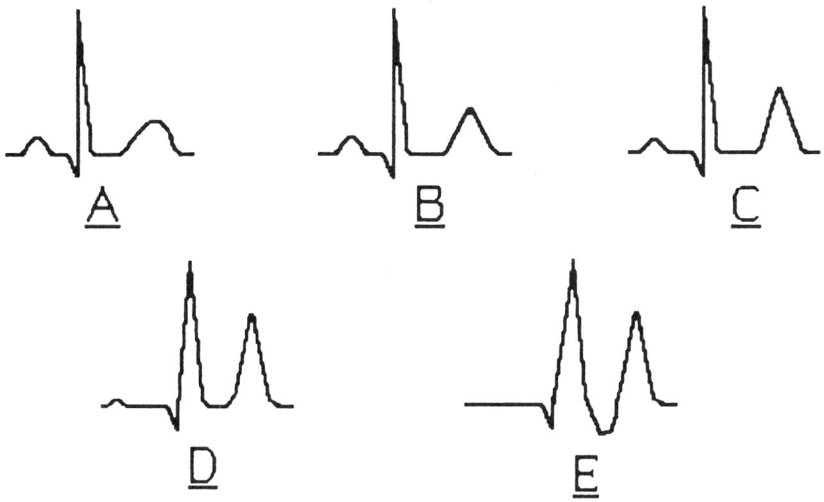

Figure 5-19. ECG changes of hyperkalemia. **A.** Normal. **B.** Earliest change is peaking of T wave ($K^+ \approx 6-7$ mEq/L). **C.** T wave amplitude becomes taller and more peaked ($K^+ \approx 7-8$ mEq/L). **D.** P-wave amplitude becomes less, the PR interval lengthens, and the QRS complex widens ($K^+ > 8$mEq/L). **E.** P waves disappear (sinoventricular rhythm) and the QRS complex becomes sinusoid ($K^+ > 10$ mEq/L). Ventricular fibrillation and/or ultimately asystole follow.

in mind. Clinically, hyperkalemia is much less common than hypokalemia. When it does occur, hyperkalemia is almost always associated with renal insufficiency, acidosis, or the use of potassium-sparing diuretics (spironolactone, dyrenium, etc.). Absence of precipitating factors should raise the question of whether another condition that mimics hyperkalemia might be present instead.

The most common condition to do this is a type of *repolarization variant.* Differentiation between the tall, peaked T waves produced by hyperkalemia and those produced by this repolarization variant is illustrated in Fig. 5-20. The shape of the T wave with hyperkalemia may be remembered by thinking of the Empire State Building (Fig. 5-20A and accompanying inset). That is, the sides of the T wave are symmetric and its base is *narrow.* While the T wave may be equally tall with the repolarization variant, its sides tend to be less symmetric, its summit less peaked, and its base wider (Fig. 5-20B).

PROBLEM: Examine the ECGs shown in Figs. 5-21 and 5-22. Is one or both of the ECGs suggestive of hyperkalemia?

INTERPRETATION of Fig. 5-21

Rate and rhythm: Sinus rhythm at about 70 beats/min. All intervals are normal.

Axis: $-30°$(LAD).

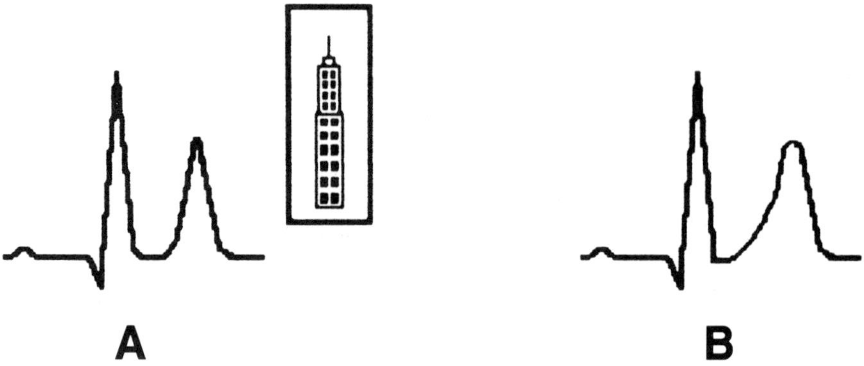

Figure 5-20. Tall T waves. **A.** Hyperkalemia. T waves are tall and peaked. Like the skyscraper in the insert, the base of the T wave is narrow. **B.** Repolarization variant. The T wave may be equally tall, but its sides tend to be more asymmetric, its summit is not as peaked, and the base of the T wave is wider.

Chamber enlargement: There is borderline voltage for LVH ($SV_2 + RV_5 \approx$ 35 mm).

QRST changes: QS complexes and ST-segment elevation of uncertain significance are present in leads V_1 and V_2. R-wave progression is normal. Striking T waves that are both tall and peaked are seen inferiorly and across the precordium. The base of these T waves is especially narrow in leads V_3 to V_5 where the T waves are tallest. In a patient with renal failure, this tracing should strongly suggest hyperkalemia. Serum potassium concentration was 8.4 mEq/L.

INTERPRETATION of Fig. 5-22

Rate and rhythm: Sinus bradycardia and arrhythmia at about 55 to 65 beats/min. All intervals are normal.

Axis: 60°.

Chamber enlargement: None.

QRST changes: There are no Q waves, and R-wave progression is normal. Although T waves are tall and peaked in the precordial leads, the ascending limb of the T wave rises slower than the descending limb comes down (the sides of the T wave are *asymmetric*), the summit of the T wave is not pointed, and its base is wide. The picture much more resembles Fig. 5-20B (the repolarization variant) than 5-20A (hyperkalemia). In addition, it would be highly unlikely for an otherwise healthy 45-year-old man on no medications to develop hyperkalemia.

Return now to Fig. 5-1, which we discussed at the beginning of this chapter, and carefully reexamine the morphology of T waves in the precordial leads. Although tall and peaked, the sides of these T waves are asymmetric (particularly in leads V_2 and V_3), and their base is wide. Considering that this tracing was taken from an otherwise healthy asymptomatic 22-year-old man who was not on a potassium-sparing diuretic, it would be safe to assume that the ECG represented a normal repolarization variant.

A final point to make regarding the diagnosis of hyperkalemia is that while a fairly good correlation exists between the development of tall, peaked T waves on the ECG, and the occurrence of mild-to-moderate elevations of serum potassium ($K^+ \approx 5.5$ to 7.0 mEq/L), the correlation is *not* perfect. Some patients do not develop ECG abnormalities until after the serum potassium has exceeded 7.0 mEq/L. Others develop them much sooner. Consequently, *both* the ECG *and* the serum level of potassium should be obtained in making the diagnosis of hyperkalemia, and *both* should be followed in treating such patients until serum potassium has returned to normal.

Hyper- and Hypocalcemia

The other cation that is known to affect the ECG is calcium. Disturbances of calcium ion concentrations occur much less commonly than do those of potassium ion concentrations.

Normal serum calcium ranges between 8.8 and 10.4 mg/dL. *Hypercalcemia* ($Ca^{++} > 10.4$ mg/dL) may be caused by numerous conditions including malignancy, hyperparathyroidism, vitamin D intoxication, milk alkali syndrome, sarcoidosis, myeloma, Paget's disease, and hyperthyroidism. Symptoms include anorexia, nausea, abdominal pain, constipation, polyuria, and headache. The principal ECG manifestation of hypercalcemia is *shortening* of the QT interval. This effect will usually *not* be seen until serum calcium levels have risen above 12 mg/dL.

Severe hypercalcemia ($Ca^{++} \geq 14$ mg/dL) is a medical emergency that can lead to psychosis, coma, and death. Most of the time, it will be known long before an ECG is obtained that a patient has hypercalcemia. However, on rare occasions, recognition of a short QT interval may provide that invaluable first clue to the diagnosis in an unconscious patient.

Hypocalcemia ($Ca^{++} < 8.8$ mg/dL) most commonly occurs with chronic renal insufficiency. As a result, it is frequently associated with hyperkalemia. Electrocardiographically, hypocalcemia produces the opposite effect of hypercalcemia—namely, *lengthening* of the QT interval. A normal-appearing T wave may occur at the end of a long isoelectric ST segment. Electrocardiographic characteristics of hyper- and hypocalcemia are illustrated in Fig. 5-23.

PROBLEM: Examine the ECG shown in Fig. 5-24, taken from an acutely ill 38-year-old woman with severe metabolic acidosis and renal failure. What electrolyte abnormalities are suggested?

INTERPRETATION of Fig. 5-24

Rate and rhythm: The rhythm is regular at about 115 beats/min; however, *no atrial activity is seen.*

Figure 5-21. ECG from an elderly adult with renal insufficiency.

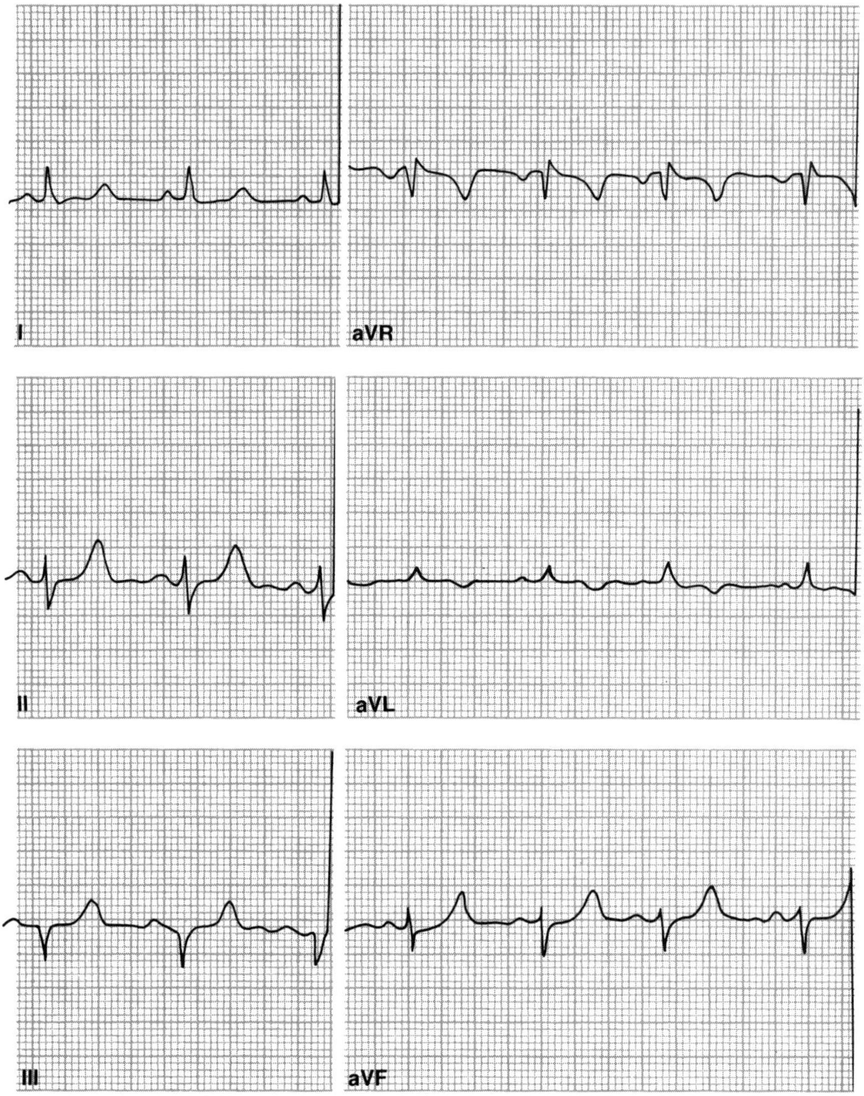

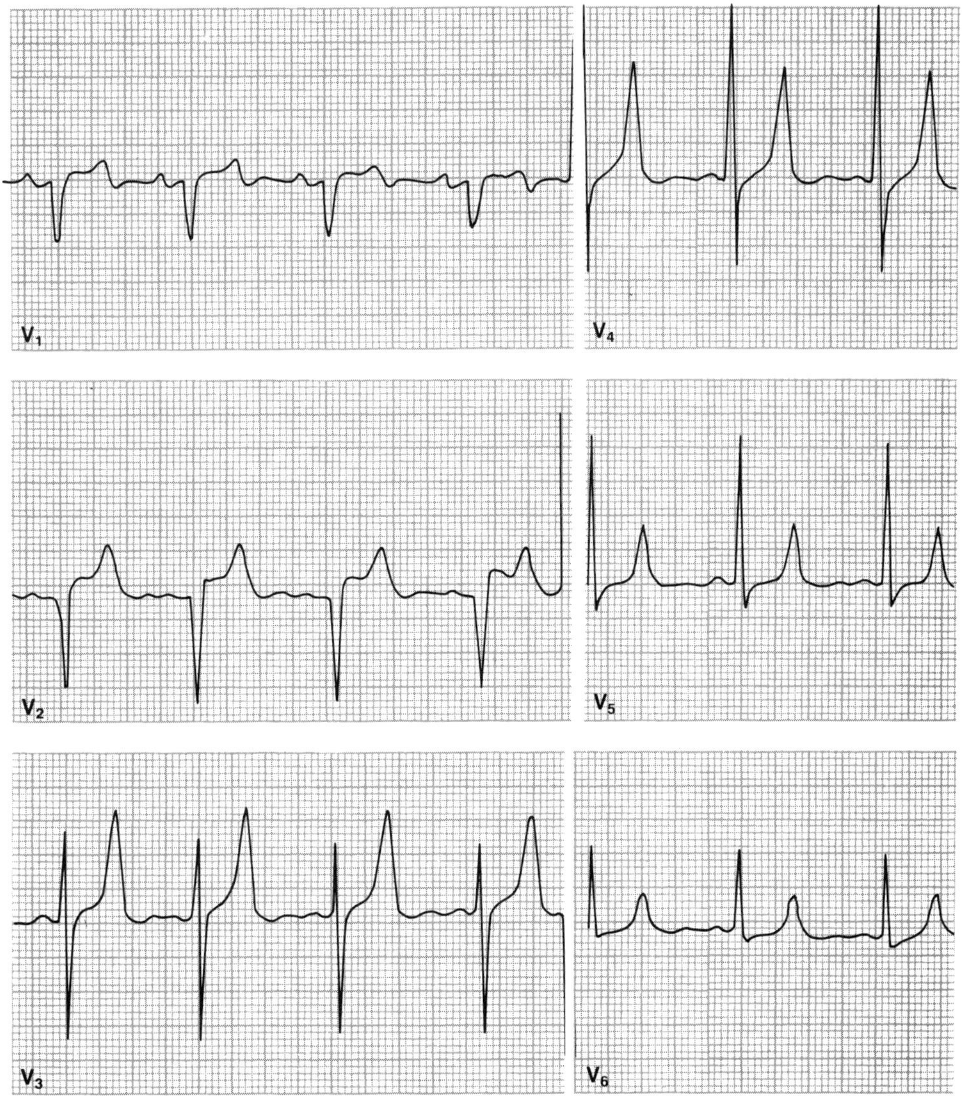
V1
V4
V2
V5
V3
V6

Figure 5-22. ECG from a healthy, asymptomatic 45-year-old man who is on no medications.

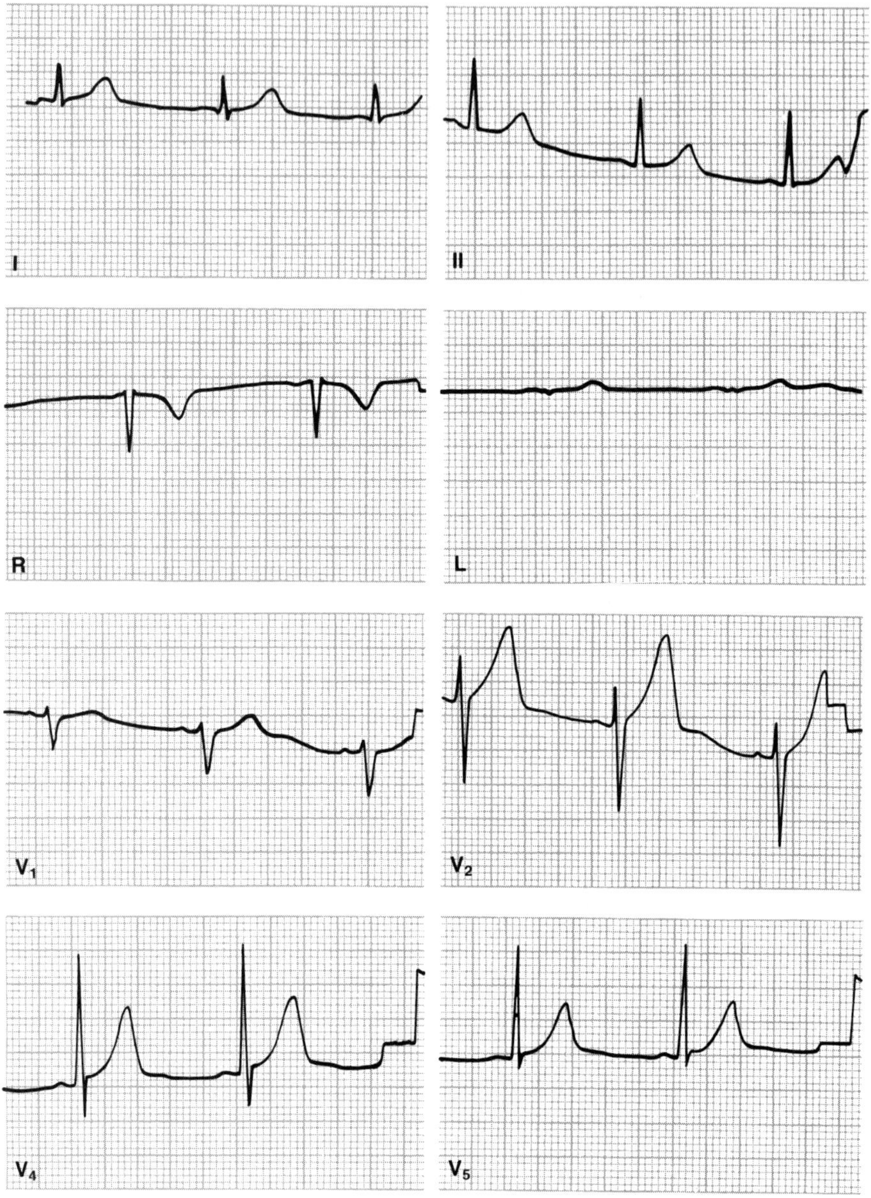

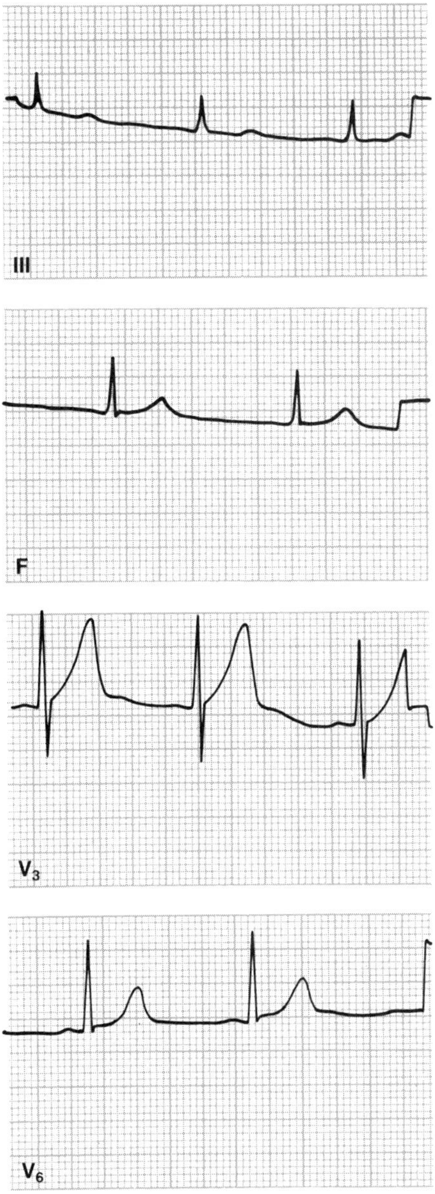
III
F
V3
V6

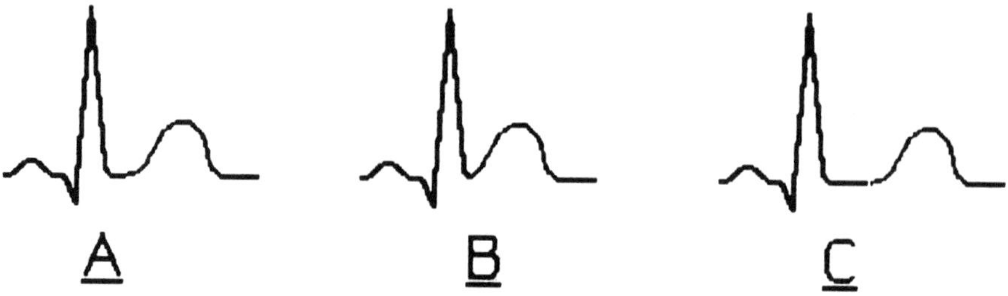

Figure 5-23. ECG changes of hyper- and hypocalcemia. **A.** Normal. **B.** Hypercalcemia. There is shortening of the QT interval. **C.** Hypocalcemia. There is lengthening of the QT interval. A relatively normal-appearing T wave occurs at the end of a long isoelectric ST segment.

Intervals

QRS interval: Borderline prolonged (about 0.10 second).

QT interval: Markedly prolonged. Our rule of thumb for determining QT-interval prolongation (that the QT interval should be less than one-half the R-R interval) is not as accurate with heart rates over 100 beats/min; nevertheless, the QT interval in this example takes up such a large portion of the R-R interval that it almost certainly is prolonged, regardless of the tachycardia.

Axis: About 20°, although hard to determine because of *low voltage* of the QRS complexes in the limb leads.

Chamber enlargement: None.

QRST changes: T waves are tall and peaked, and have a narrow base, particularly in leads V_2 and V_3. In an acutely ill acidotic patient with renal failure, one should strongly suspect hyperkalemia. In addition, prolongation of the QT interval in this setting suggests associated hypocalcemia.

A moderate-to-severe degree of *hyperkalemia* ($K^+ > 7.0$ mEq/L) might be suspected in this example, since the QRS is beginning to widen and there is no atrial activity (*Sinoventricular conduction* as explained in this chapter is probably present, although one could not rule out an accelerated junctional and/or ventricular rhythm.)

Central Nervous System Disorders

The final cause of ST-segment and T-wave abnormalities that we will discuss in this chapter is central nervous system (CNS) disorders. Although much of the time the ECG will be normal or show only minimal nonspecific ST-T wave abnormalities, CNS disorders such as stroke, subarachnoid or intracerebral hemorrhage, head trauma, and brain tumor occasionally produce striking changes. ST segments may be markedly elevated or profoundly depressed, presenting a picture that strongly resembles acute myocardial infarction or ischemia. T waves may be upright or deeply inverted. They are often extremely *broad,* and consequently may greatly prolong the QT interval.

PROBLEM: As an example, examine the ECG shown in Fig. 5-25, obtained from a 15-year-old boy who had just shot himself in the head.

INTERPRETATION of Fig. 5-25

Rate and rhythm: Sinus tachycardia at 145 beats/min.

Axis: About 75°.

Chamber enlargement: RAA is suggested by the tall, peaked P waves in the inferior leads. (The P waves exceed 2-1/2 mm in amplitude in lead II.) QRS voltage is normal in the precordial leads considering the patient's age.

QRST changes: Dramatic and diffuse ST-segment depression is seen in virtually all leads, except in aVR and aVL where there is ST-segment elevation. If one did not know the history in this case, myocardial infarction and/or ischemia would have to be strongly suspected.

Surprisingly, the ECG of this patient had almost reverted to normal when it was repeated several hours later. The boy died shortly thereafter.

PROBLEM: Let us conclude this chapter by examining the ECGs shown in Figs. 5-26, 5-27, and 5-28. A brief history is given in the legend of each tracing. Do you feel that the ST and T wave changes represent health or disease?

INTERPRETATION of Fig. 5-26

Rate and rhythm: Sinus rhythm at 80 beats/min. The PR and QRS intervals are normal. The QT interval is borderline prolonged.

Axis: About 20°.

Chamber enlargement: P waves are somewhat prominent and peaked in the inferior leads, but do not meet the 2-1/2 mm amplitude requirement for RAA. There is no ventricular enlargement.

QRST changes: ST segments are flattened and depressed in multiple leads. U waves are evident as a small, round upright deflection that follows the T wave in leads II, III, aVF and V_2 to V_5.

The triad of nonspecific ST-segment depression, U waves, and "pseudo P-pulmonale" is highly suggestive of *hypokalemia.* The patient was being treated with a diuretic for his hypertension, and had a serum potassium of 3.2 mEq/L at the time of this tracing.

INTERPRETATION of Fig. 5-27

Rate and rhythm: Sinus arrhythmia. All intervals are normal.

Axis: +100°. This degree of RAD in a child may be normal.

Figure 5-24. ECG from an acutely ill 38-year-old woman with severe metabolic acidosis and renal failure.

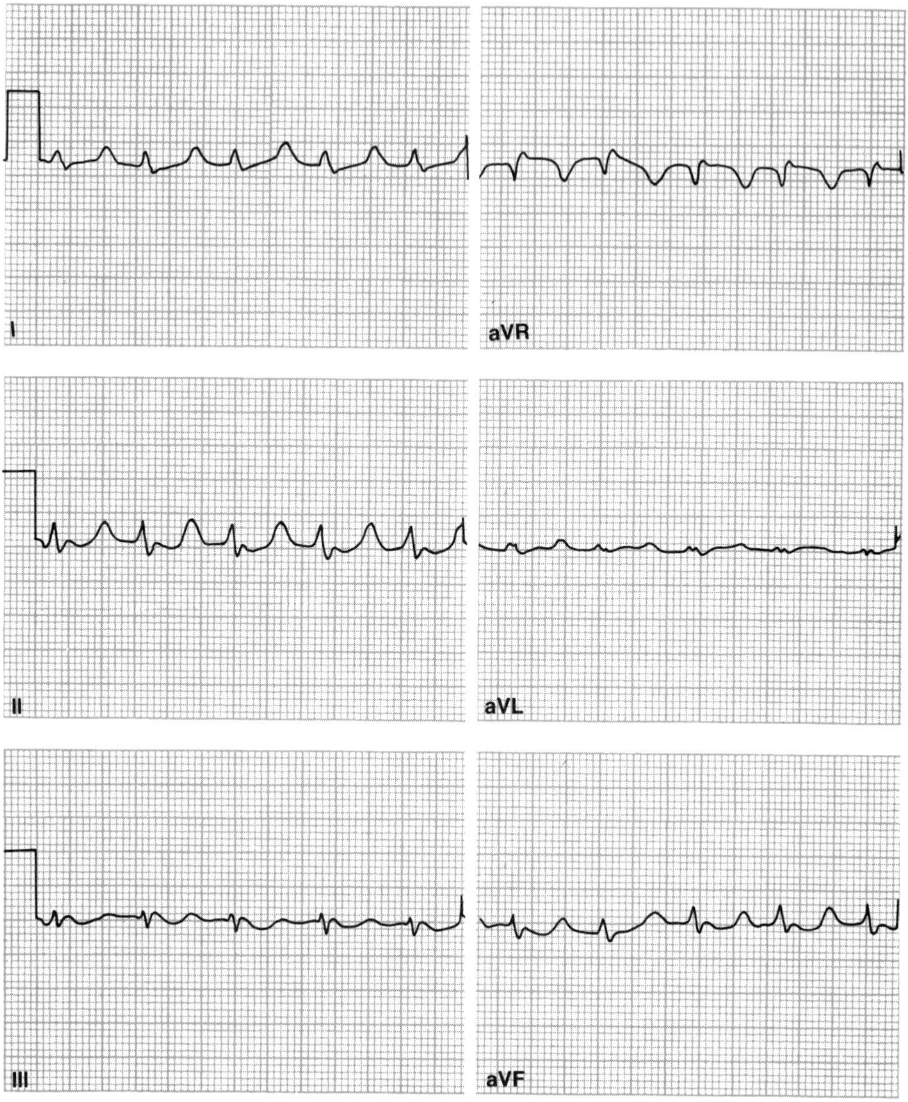

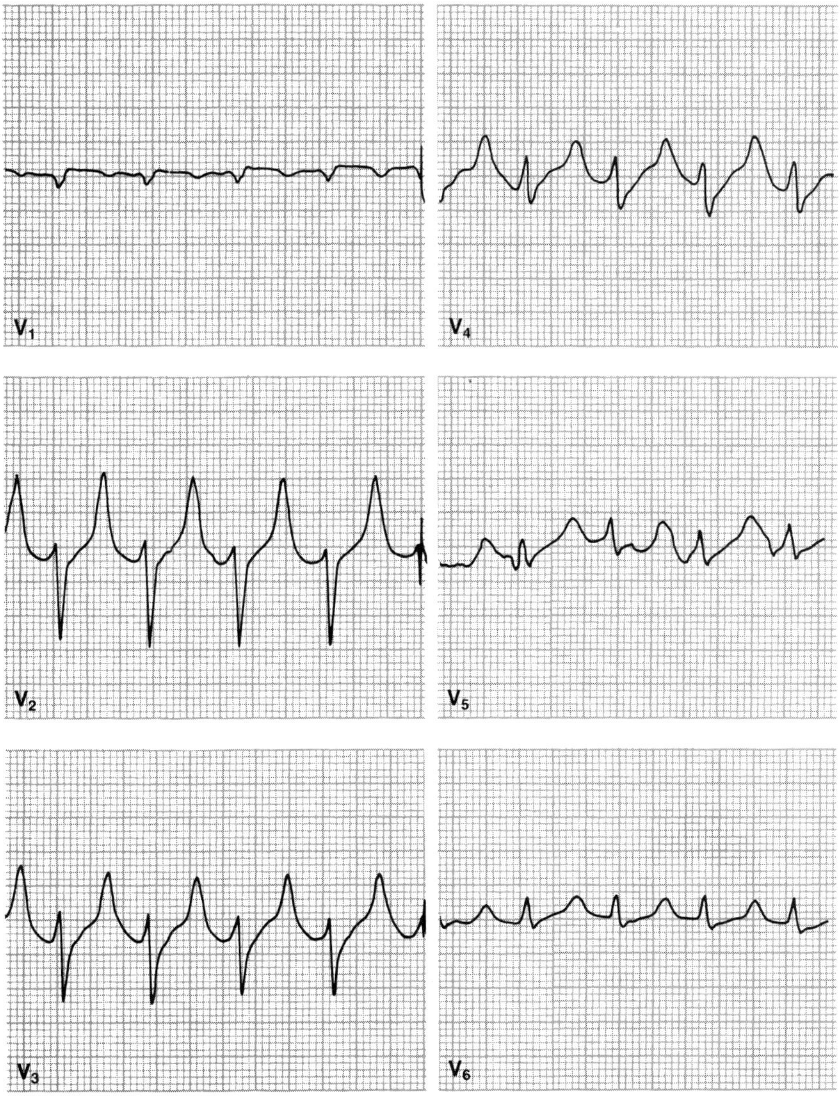
V1
V4
V2
V5
V3
V6

Figure 5-25. ECG from a 15-year-old boy with a gunshot wound to the head.

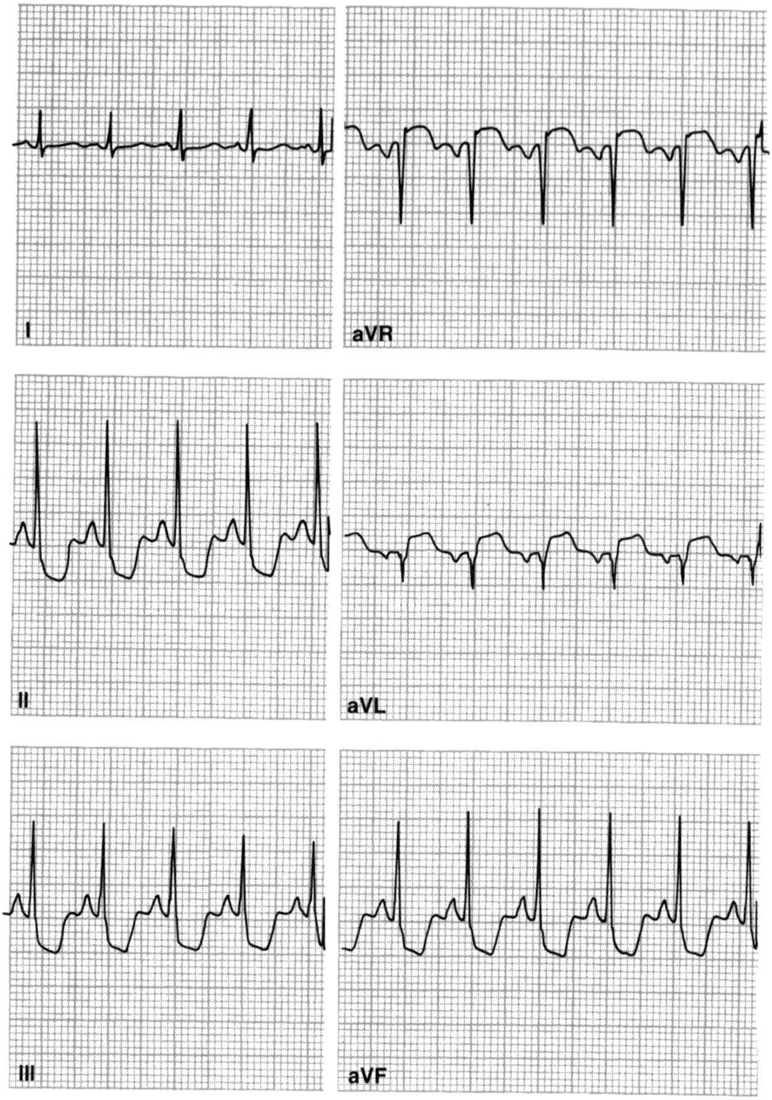

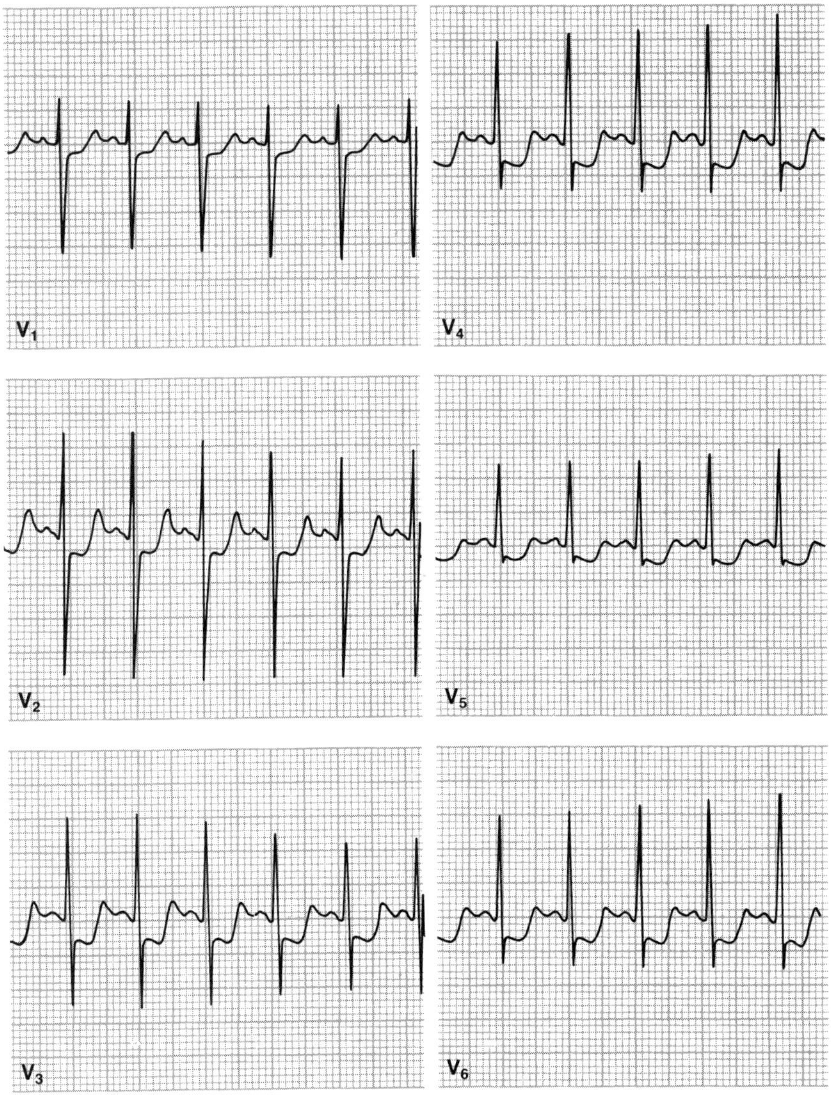
V1
V4
V2
V5
V3
V6

Figure 5-26. ECG from a 60-year-old man with hypertension.

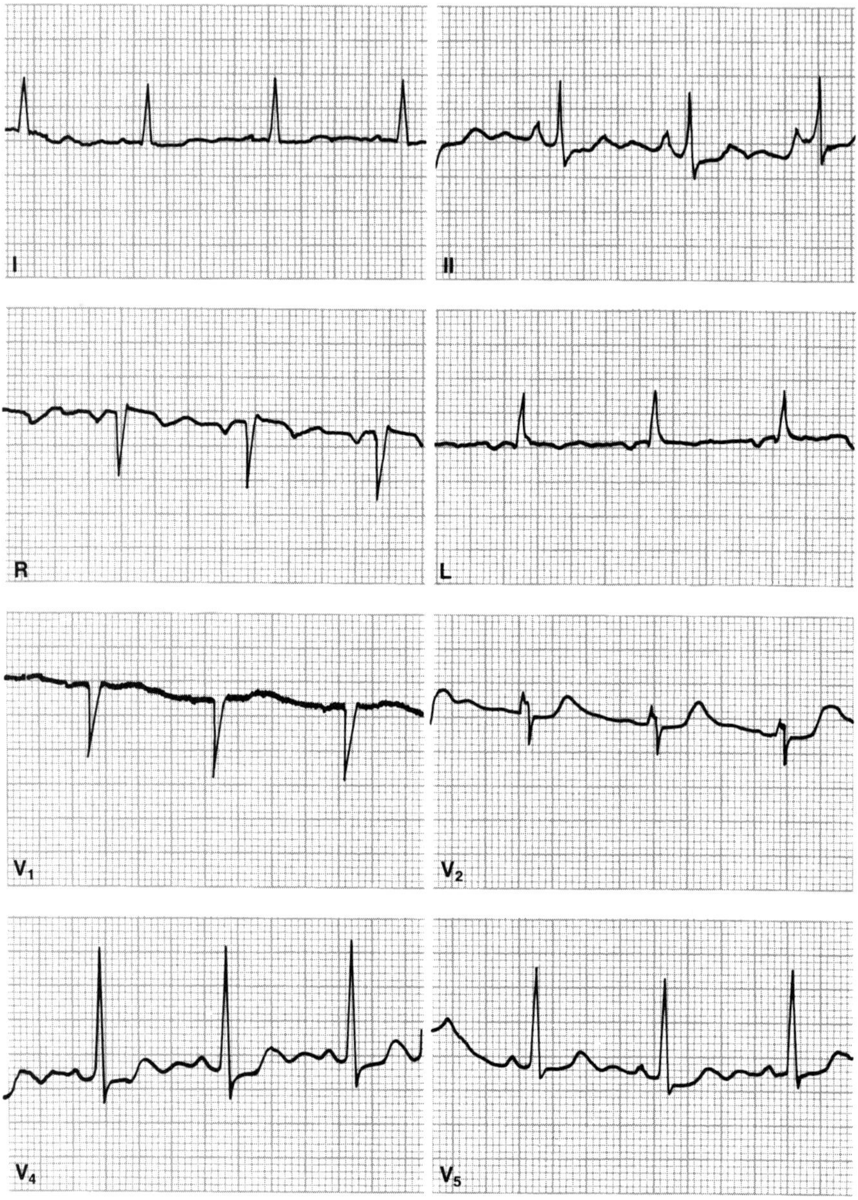

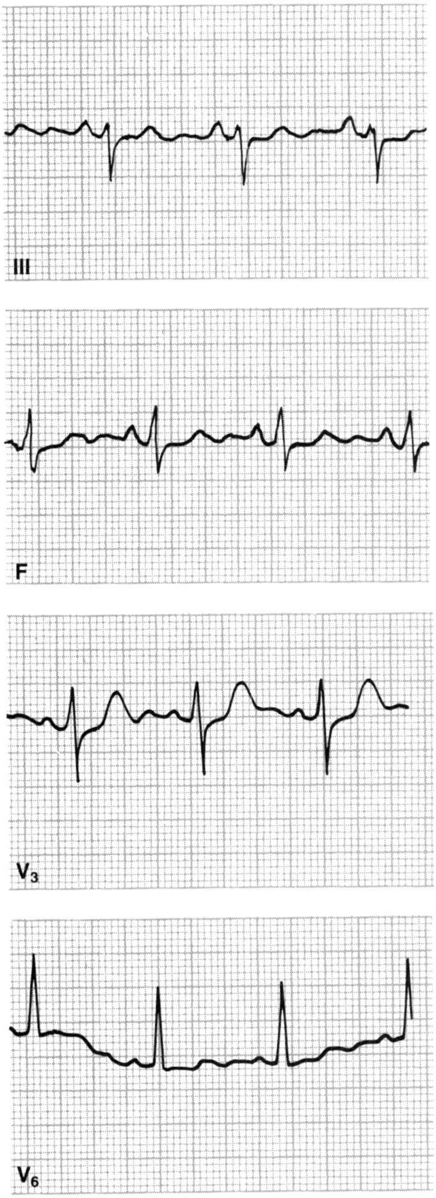
III
F
V3
V6

Figure 5-27. ECG from a playful 7-year-old child.

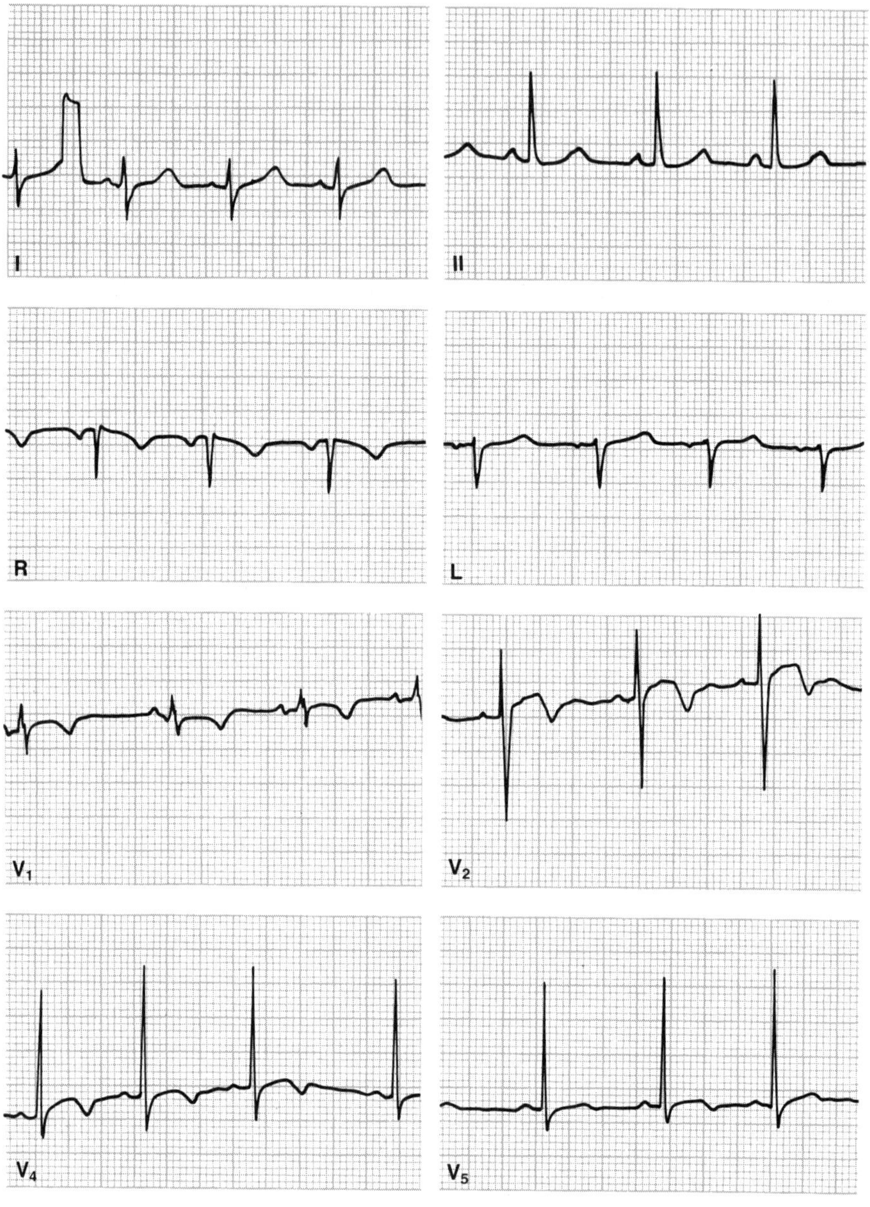

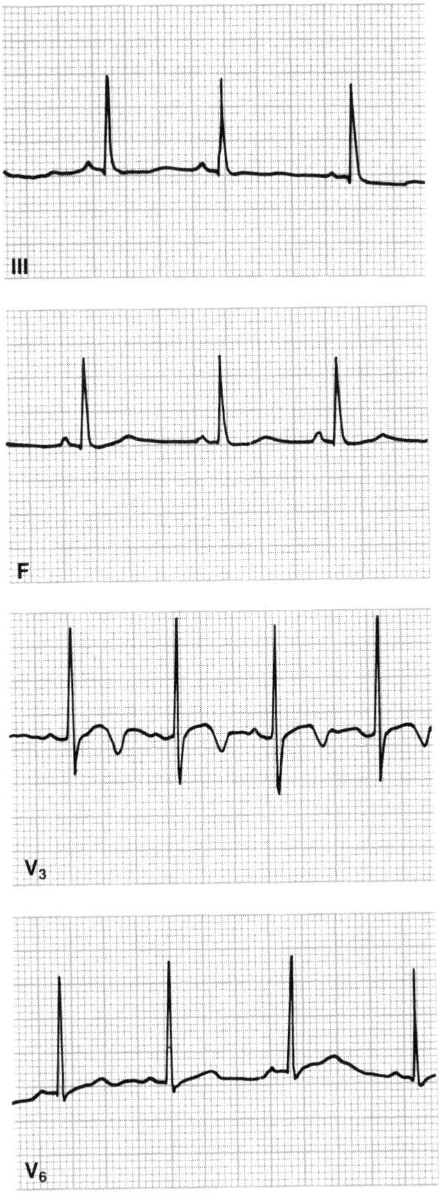
III
F
V_3
V_6

Figure 5-28. ECG from a 73-year-old man with a history of cardiac dysrhythmias.

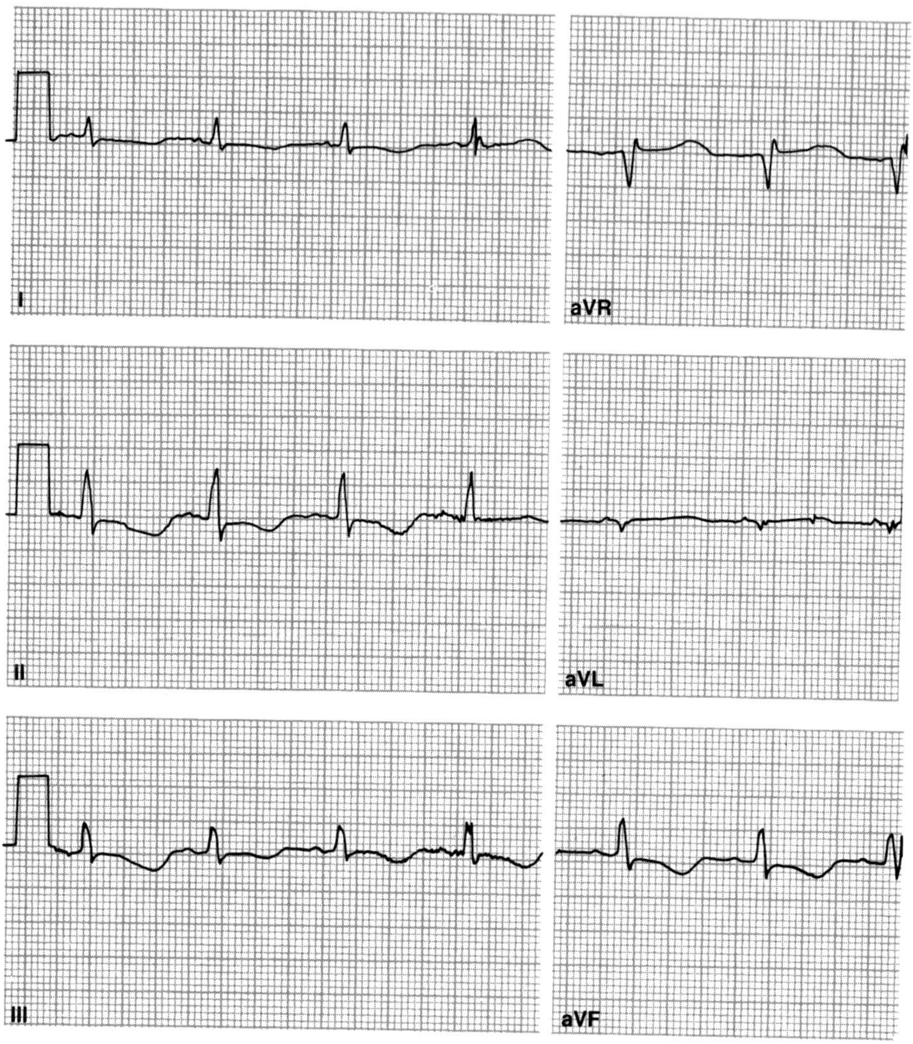

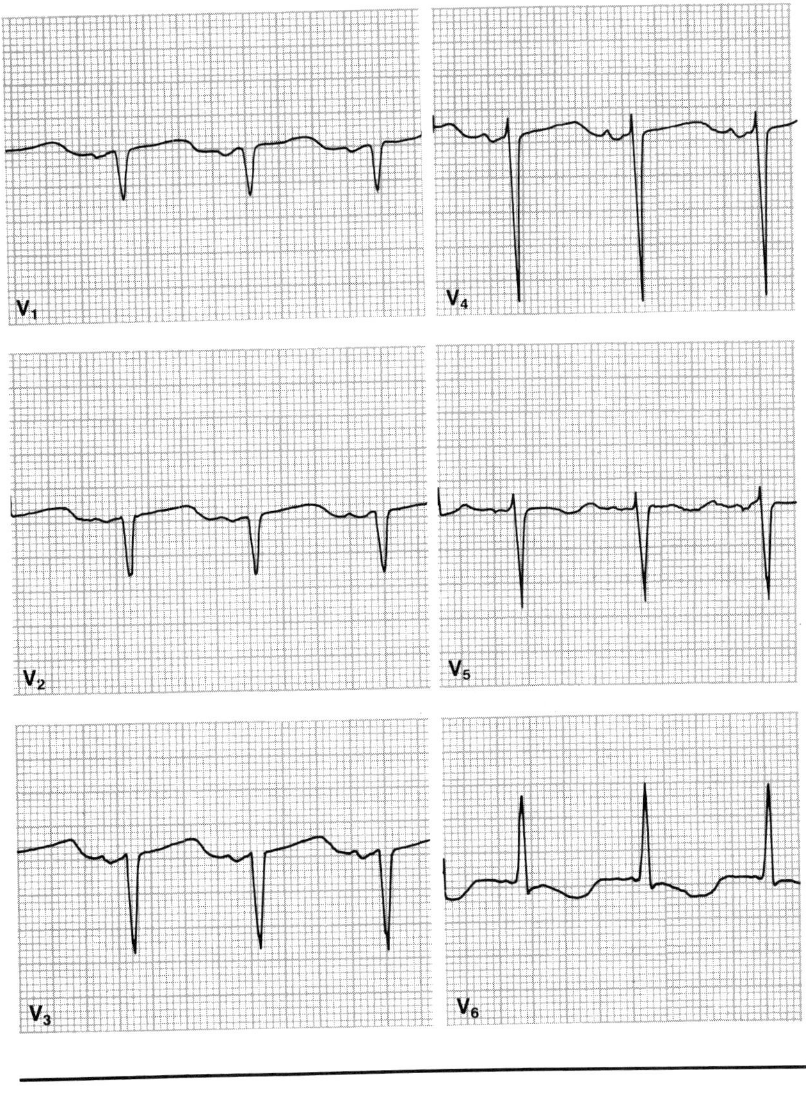
V_1
V_4
V_2
V_5
V_3
V_6

Chamber enlargement: Although increased anterior forces are present (the amplitude of the R wave equals that of the S wave in lead V_1, and transition occurs early between leads V_2 and V_3), they are not of sufficient magnitude to satisfy the criteria for RVH in this age group. In addition, the absence of RAE and the lack of a prominent S wave in the lateral precordial leads argue against RVH.
QRST changes: ST segments are coved, and T waves are symmetrically inverted in leads V_1 to V_4.

The Juvenile T-Wave Pattern

If this tracing had been taken from a middle-aged adult complaining about chest pain, one would strongly suspect anterior ischemia as the cause of symptoms. Instead, the child in question was playful and totally unaware of the concern her ECG was causing her physician.

As discussed in Chapter 1, the T wave in the adult ECG may normally be negative in lead V_1. In adults, T waves usually become positive by lead V_2, and remain so for the other precordial leads. In children, however, T waves may normally be inverted in a number of anterior precordial leads. Persistence of T-wave inversion in lead V_1 up to and including lead V_4 is a common normal ECG variant of childhood, and is termed the *juvenile T-wave pattern.* Occasionally this pattern may last into adulthood. Should such a patient then present to an emergency department complaining of chest pain, it might be extremely difficult to determine whether the anterior precordial T-wave inversion was due to a persistent juvenile pattern or ischemia.

INTERPRETATION of Fig. 5-28
Rate and rhythm: Sinus rhythm at about 75 beats/min. The PR and QRS intervals are normal. The QT interval is markedly prolonged!
Axis: About 65°.
Chamber enlargement: None.
QRST changes: QS complexes are seen in leads V_1 and V_2. R-wave progression is poor, and transition does not occur until leads V_5 to V_6. The patient may have had a prior anterior infarction. In addition, T waves are broad and inverted in the inferolateral leads.

The most striking finding about this tracing is the dramatic QT interval prolongation. As previously discussed in Chapter 1 (and summarized in Table 1-4), *three conditions should be considered in the presence of definite QT interval prolongation*—drugs, electrolyte disturbance, and CNS disorders. The patient in question was being treated with quinidine for his cardiac dysrhythmias, and had developed QT-interval prolongation as a toxic response to this drug.

CHAPTER 6

INTRAVENTRICULAR CONDUCTION DELAYS

An intraventricular conduction delay is a disturbance in conduction of the electrical impulse that originates *below* where the bundle of His bifurcates into the right and left main bundle branches. As a result, ventricular activation is delayed and the QRS complex is widened.

Intraventricular conduction delay should be distinguished from atrioventricular (AV) block. With AV block, *transmission* of the impulse from the atria to the ventricles is delayed or blocked. In contrast with intraventricular conduction delay, transmission of the impulse from the atria to the ventricles proceeds normally, but the *sequence* of ventricular activation is altered.

Morphologic Characteristics of the Bundle Branch Blocks

There are three principal types of intraventricular conduction delays. Electrocardiographic derivation of two of these, right and left bundle branch block, was discussed in Chapter 4. Table 6-1 reviews characteristic morphologic features in the identification of these conduction defects.

Right bundle branch block (RBBB) is recognized by the presence of a RBBB pattern (an rSR′) in lead V_1, and a wide terminal negative deflection (a wide S wave) in the lateral leads. The QRS complex is prolonged to at least 0.11 second.

Left bundle branch block (LBBB) is recognized by the presence of a monophasic upright QRS complex (which may or may not be notched) in the lateral leads, and a predominantly negative QRS complex in the anterior precordial leads. A narrow r wave may sometimes precede the negative QRS deflection in the anterior leads. However, septal q waves should *never* be seen in any of the lateral leads with pure LBBB. The QRS interval tends to be prolonged to a greater extent with LBBB than with RBBB (since the left ventricle is much thicker than the right ventricle), and a duration of at least 0.12 second is required before the diagnosis of LBBB can be made.

TABLE 6-1

Morphologic characteristics of right bundle branch block (RBBB) and left bundle branch block (LBBB)

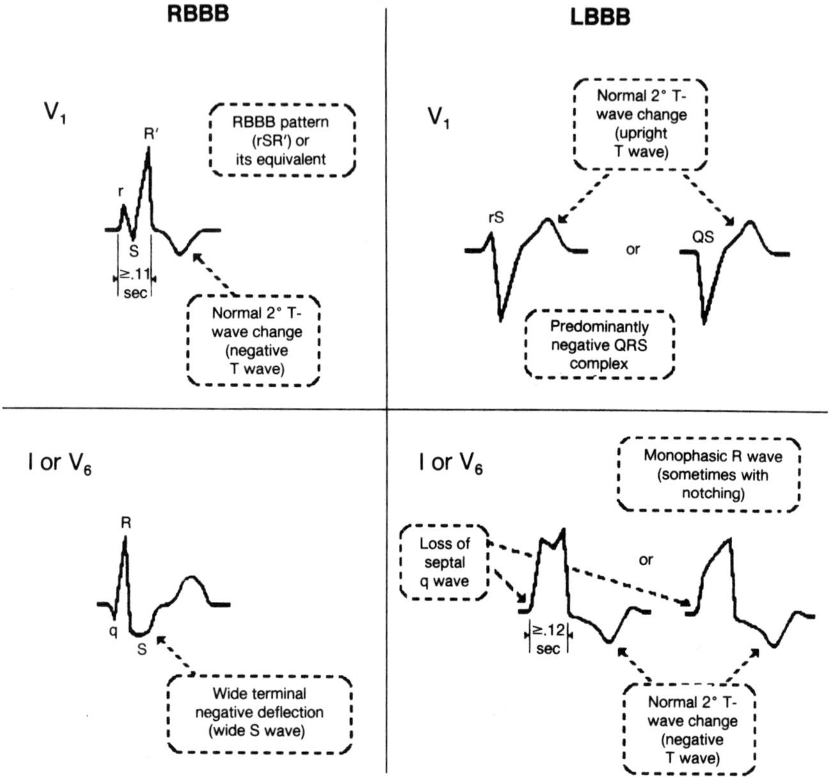

Although the typical appearance of RBBB and LBBB is described according to morphologic changes that occur in "lateral" and "anterior" precordial leads, accurate identification of bundle branch blocks can be readily accomplished by concentrating one's attention on only a few select leads. This is because a similar ECG picture is usually evident in *all* lateral leads with both LBBB and RBBB. One should therefore not have to look at *each* lateral lead (leads I, aVL, V_5, and V_6) to make the diagnosis. Inspection of one limb lead (preferably lead I) and one precordial lead (preferably lead V_6) generally suffices.

With LBBB, a similar ECG picture (predominantly negative QRS complexes) is usually seen in each of the *anterior* precordial leads (leads V_1 to V_3). However, with RBBB, leads V_2 and V_3 may differ appreciably in appearance from lead V_1. Not infrequently, lead V_1 will be the only precordial lead to manifest a typical RBBB pattern. As a result, this is the key anterior precordial lead to focus on.

Thus, diagnosis of RBBB and LBBB may be made by inspection of the *three key leads* (leads I, V_1, and V_6) for the morphologic characteristics illustrated in Table 6-1.

Secondary T-Wave Changes with Bundle Branch Block

A final point to note when evaluating an ECG for the presence of bundle branch block is the direction of T waves. With pure RBBB or LBBB, the T wave is directed *opposite* to the terminal portion of the QRS complex. Thus, the T wave would be negative in lead V_1 with RBBB (since the terminal deflection—the R′—is positive), and positive in leads I or V_6 (since the terminal deflection—the S wave—is negative). For similar reasons, with LBBB the T wave should be upright in lead V_1 and inverted in leads I or V_6. These T-wave changes (known as *secondary T-wave changes*) reflect the fact that terminal depolarization forces of the heart and repolarization forces are oriented in opposing directions with a pure conduction disturbance. The T-wave change is the direct result of (it is *secondary* to) the altered sequence of ventricular activation.

If the T wave in one of the three key leads is not directed opposite to the terminal portion of its respective QRS complex, then a *primary T-wave change* is said to be present, and something other than a pure conduction disturbance (myocardial ischemia or infarction) may be going on. Because it is often difficult to detect ischemia and infarction electrocardiographically when they occur in association with bundle branch block, recognition of primary T-wave changes in this setting sometimes provides an important clue.

PROBLEM: Examine the ECGs shown in Figs. 6-1 and 6-2. The QRS complex is prolonged in both of these tracings. Is the pattern suggestive of LBBB or RBBB? Pay particular attention to the type of T-wave change that is present in each of the key leads.

INTERPRETATION of Fig. 6-1
Rate and rhythm: Sinus rhythm at 65 to 70 beats/min.
Intervals

PR interval: Normal.

QRS interval: Prolonged (to 0.14 second). The characteristic pattern of RBBB that was illustrated in Table 6-1 is seen—rSR′ in lead V_1, and terminal wide negative deflection (S wave) in leads I and V_6.

Figure 6-1

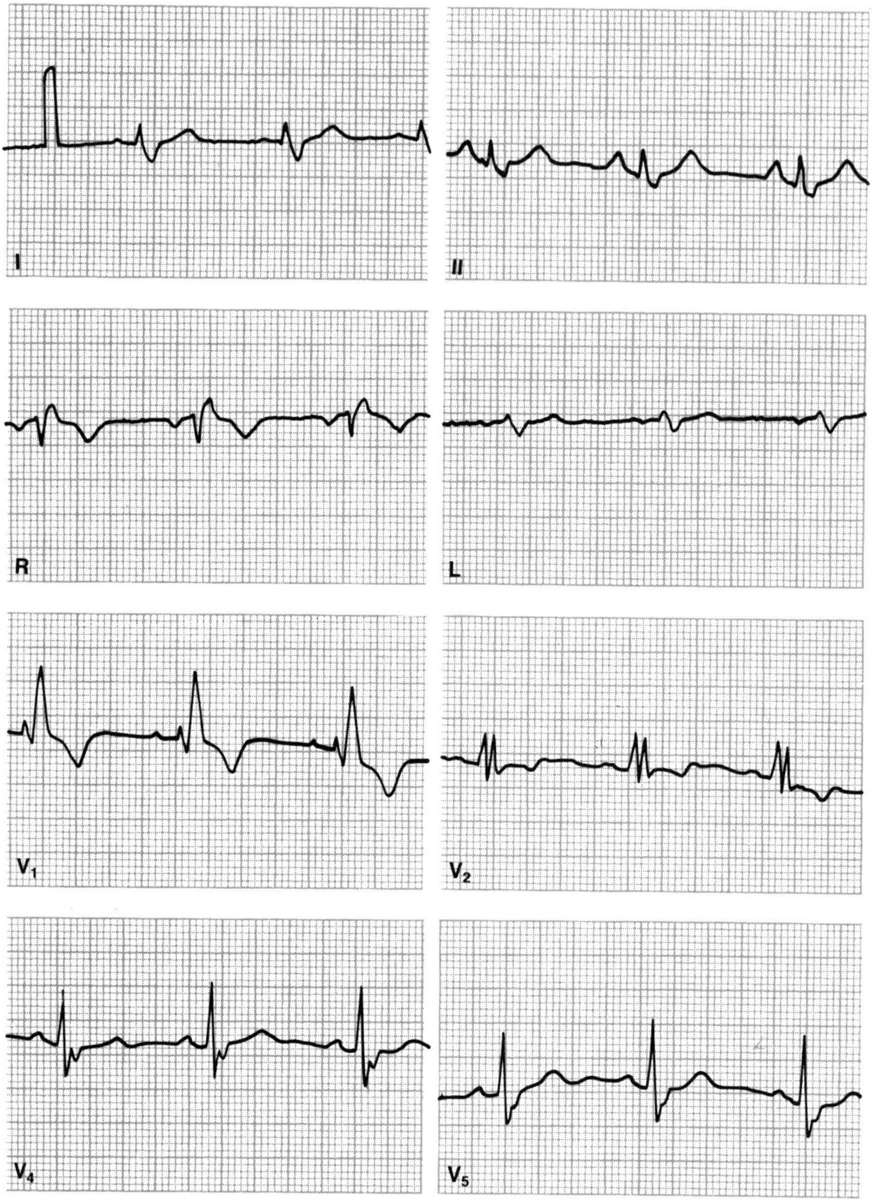

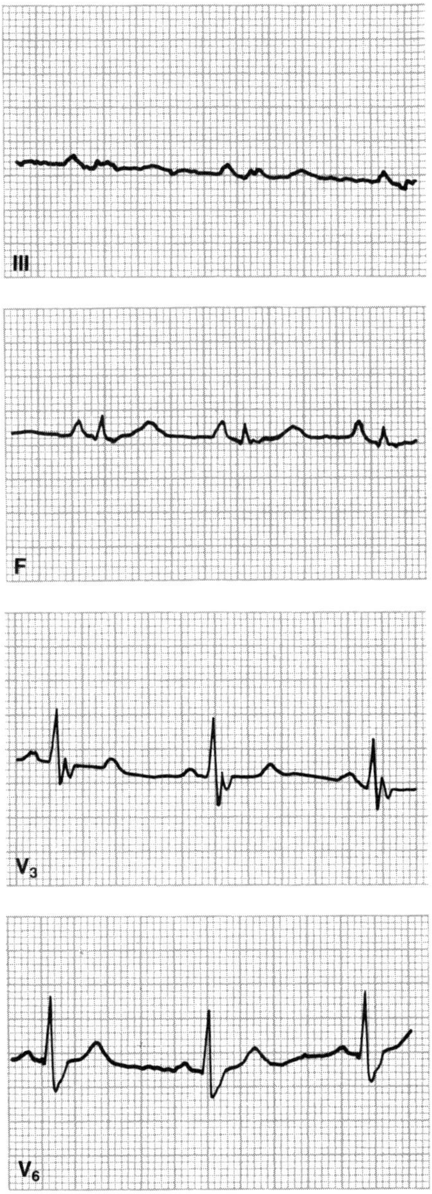
III
F
V3
V6

Figure 6-2

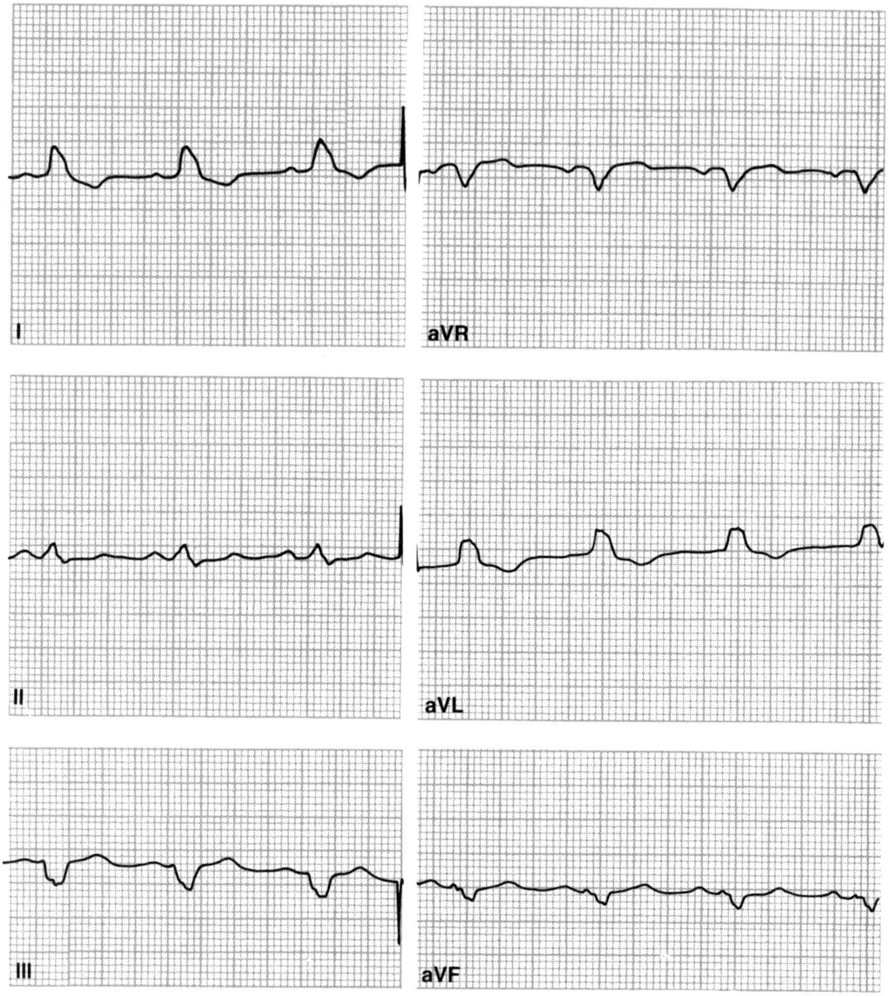

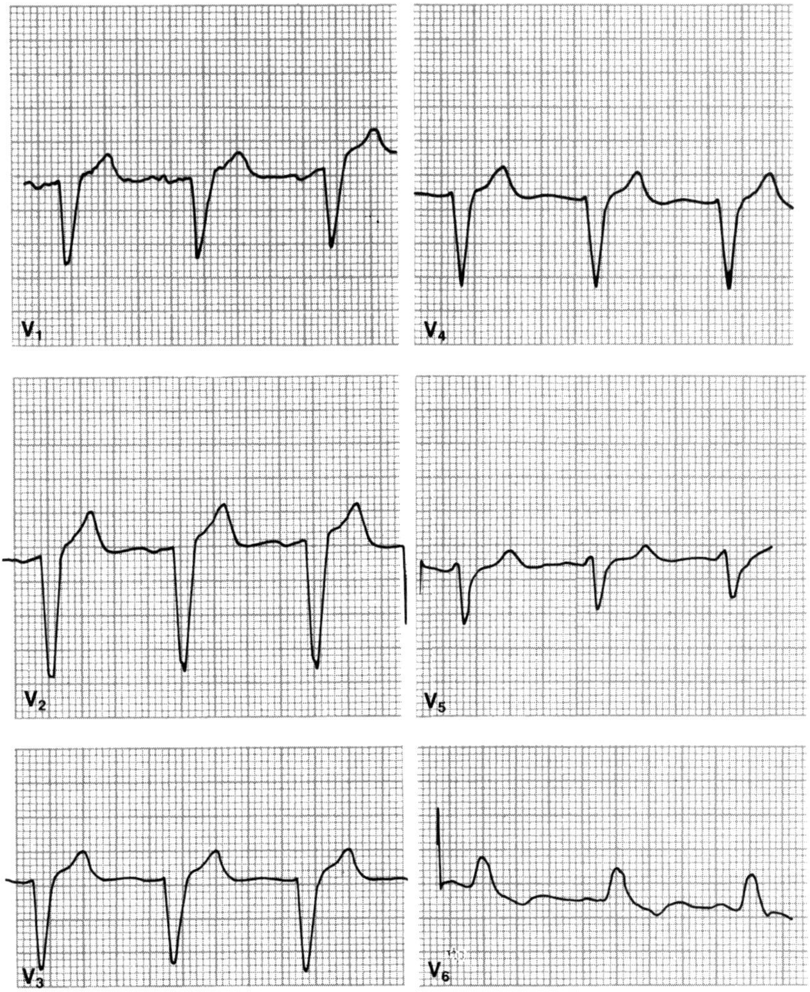
V1
V4
V2
V5
V3
V6

Chamber enlargement: RAA (tall, peaked P waves in the inferior leads that attain 2-1/2 mm in amplitude in lead II).

QRST changes: The expected secondary T-wave changes of RBBB are present in leads V_1 and V_2 (the T wave is inverted and opposite in direction to the terminal portion of the QRS complex in these leads). There are no acute changes.

INTERPRETATION of Fig. 6-2

Rate and rhythm: Sinus rhythm at 75 beats/min.

Intervals

PR interval: Normal.

QRS interval: Prolonged (to 0.13 second). The characteristic pattern of LBBB that was illustrated in Fig. 6-1 is evident—monophasic R wave with absence of a septal q wave in leads I and V_6, and predominantly negative QRS complexes in lead V_2 and the other anterior precordial leads. Transition in this example is delayed until V_5 to V_6, and QRS complex is still predominantly negative in the lateral lead V_5. Yet the pattern is typical of LBBB since the findings illustrated in Fig. 6-1 *are* present in the three *key* leads.

Chamber enlargement: None.

QRST changes: The expected secondary T-wave changes of LBBB are present (the T wave is inverted in leads I and V_6 and upright in lead V_1).

Clinical Significance of Complete Bundle Branch Block

Bundle branch block (RBBB or LBBB) is an ECG diagnosis that indicates a disordered sequence of intraventricular conduction. Mechanically, this results in dyssynchronous ventricular contraction. However, the dyssynchrony per se is rarely clinically significant, and cardiac function is almost always normal with both RBBB and LBBB.

A typical example of the ECG diagnosis of complete RBBB is illustrated in Fig. 6-1. The incidence of this common conduction disorder is about 1 percent in the general adult population, with its prevalence increasing among older individuals. Clinical implications of RBBB differ depending on the age of the patient. Although RBBB may occur with congenital heart disease (particularly with lesions that affect the right side of the heart, such as pulmonary stenosis and atrial septal defect), most younger adults with this conduction defect do not have any underlying cardiac disorder. Prognosis is excellent in this group.

Associated organic heart disease is much more common among older adults (over 50 years of age) who develop RBBB. Most have hypertension prior to the onset of the conduction defect. Other conditions commonly associated with development of RBBB are ischemic heart disease, congestive heart failure, cardiomyopathy, chronic obstructive pulmonary disease, and pulmonary hypertension. Abrupt development of RBBB is one of the most characteristic ECG manifestations of acute pulmonary embolism. Finally, pure degenerative disease of the conduction system (without evidence of other organic heart disease) may lead to RBBB, particularly among the elderly.

A typical example of the ECG diagnosis of complete LBBB is illustrated in Fig. 6-2. LBBB also has an incidence of approximately 1 percent in the general adult population, becoming more prevalent among the elderly. Unlike RBBB, which may occur as an isolated conduction disorder in otherwise healthy young adults, LBBB tends to occur in older individuals, and almost always in association with underlying heart disease. Most patients have hypertension prior to the onset of LBBB. Other common associated conditions include ischemic heart disease, congestive heart failure, cardiomyopathy, and valvular heart disease (especially aortic stenosis or aortic regurgitation). Pure degenerative disease of the conduction system (particularly among the elderly) may also lead to LBBB.

RBBB and LBBB share a number of clinical features. Although either may occasionally complicate acute myocardial infarction, these bundle branch blocks much more frequently develop as "clinically silent" events that are discovered only incidentally long after they occur. Progression of chronic bundle branch block to complete heart block can occur with either RBBB or LBBB, but is surprisingly uncommon—less than 1 percent per year. Consequently, patients with chronic bundle branch block who die suddenly usually do so from complications of their underlying cardiac disease rather than from development of complete heart block. On the other hand, when bundle branch block occurs as a complication of acute myocardial infarction, it has a much higher incidence of progression to complete heart block with a higher associated mortality. As will be discussed later, this increased mortality is primarily due to extensive necrosis from the infarction with resultant cardiogenic shock rather than progression to complete heart block.

In summary, overall prognosis of patients who develop RBBB or LBBB in either the acute or chronic setting is usually determined *not* by the presence of the conduction disorder, but instead by the severity of associated cardiovascular disease.

PROBLEM: The QRS complex is also prolonged in Fig. 6-3. Is the pattern suggestive of typical LBBB or typical RBBB?

INTERPRETATION of Fig. 6-3

Rate and rhythm: Sinus rhythm at about 60 beats/min.

Intervals

PR interval: Prolonged (to 0.23 second). First-degree AV block is present.

QRS interval: Prolonged (to 0.17 second). Although the pattern is

Figure 6-3

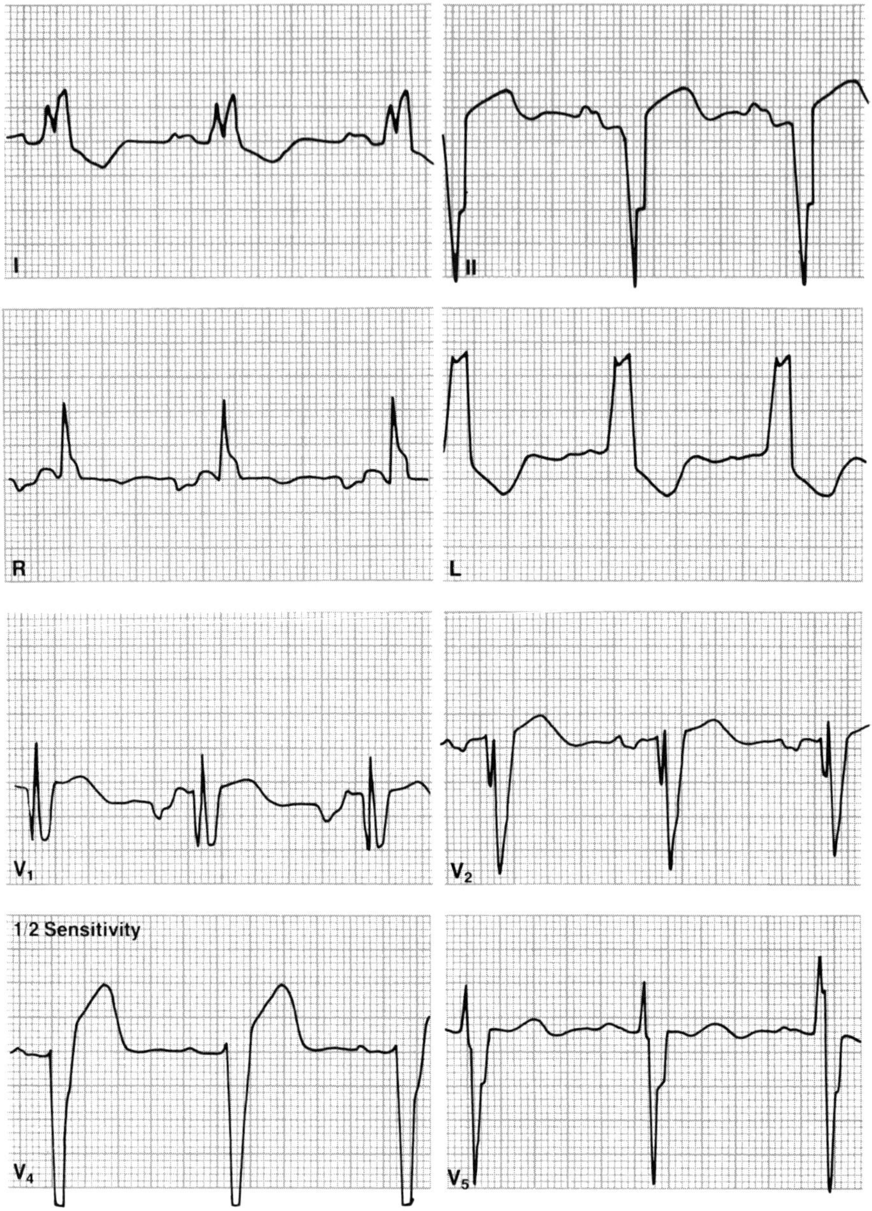

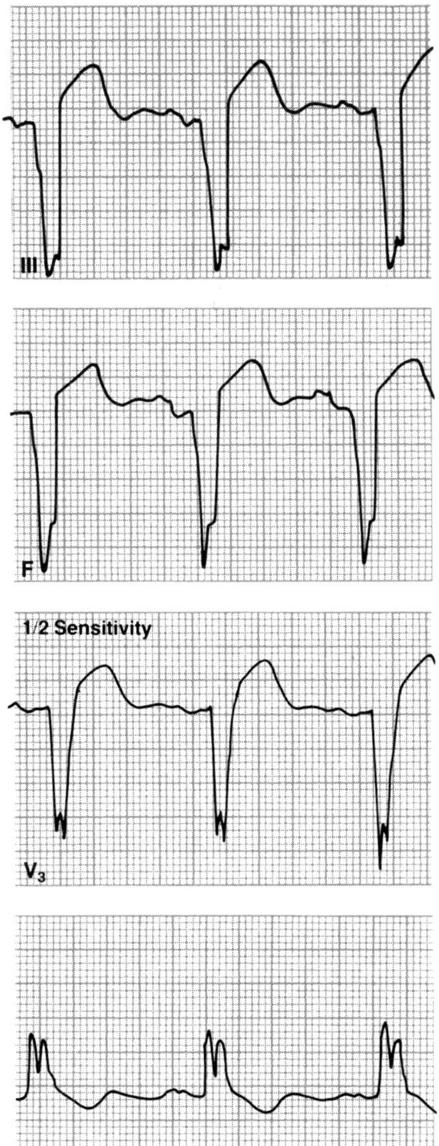
III
F
1/2 Sensitivity
V3
V6

suggestive of LBBB in lateral leads I and V_6 (monophasic R wave, absence of septal q waves, typical secondary T-wave change), the same *cannot* be said for the appearance of the QRS complex in lead V_1. The bizarre complex in this lead describes a Q-R-S morphology (deep Q wave, R wave, wide S wave), that suggests, if anything RBBB.

Chamber enlargement: LAA. The P wave is prolonged in duration, notched in leads I and II, and deeply negative in lead V_1.

Nonspecific Intraventricular Conduction Defect

The reason the QRS morphology is so unusual in Fig. 6-3 is that this ECG comes from a 17-year-old male with corrected transposition of the great vessels. In this disorder, the right ventricle acts as the physiologic left ventricle and pumps blood to the systemic circulation. The point to emphasize is that *a widened QRS complex may not always fit neatly into the category of left or right bundle branch block.* When it doesn't, the third type of intraventricular conduction delay is said to be present. Although a variety of terms have been used to describe this type of conduction defect (infarction or peri-infarction block, parietal ventricular block, peripheral block, etc.), we prefer the designation *nonspecific intraventricular conduction defect,* or simply *IVCD.*

Thus, when confronted with a 12-lead ECG that demonstrates sinus rhythm and a widened QRS complex, one might follow the line of reasoning outlined in Fig. 6-4 to arrive at the correct diagnosis of the type of conduction defect that is present.

QT-Interval Determination with Bundle Branch Block

Let us return for a moment to our interpretation of Figs. 6-1, 6-2, and 6-3. Note that we have not yet commented on QT-interval duration, mean QRS axis, ventricular enlargement, or the presence of infarction.

As discussed in Chapter 1, the QT interval represents the time period from the onset of ventricular depolarization (Q wave) until ventricular repolarization is complete (end of T wave). Recognition of QT-interval prolongation is clinically important, since it sometimes is the only sign of a metabolic problem, pharmacologic drug effect, or other ECG abnormality (Table 1-4). Intraventricular conduction disturbances by definition alter the sequence and prolong the duration of ventricular depolarization. Repolarization is similarly altered, and usually also prolonged. Therefore, the mere presence of a conduction defect will often result in QT-interval prolongation. However, since it is virtually impossible to separate the effect on the QT interval of a drug or electrolyte abnormality from the effect of a conduction

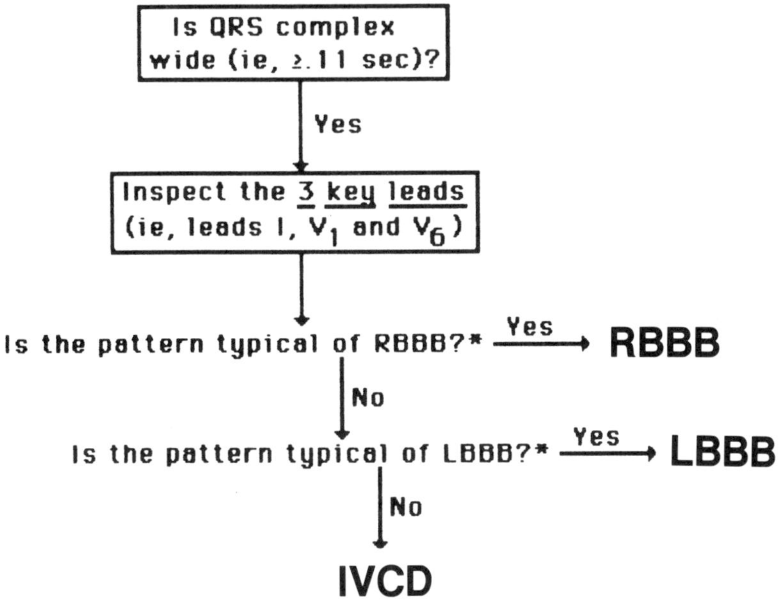

*Criteria for diagnosis of RBBB and LBBB are illustrated in Fig. 6-1.

Figure 6-4. Suggested flow sheet for evaluation of 12-lead ECG with sinus rhythm and QRS widening. RBBB—Right bundle branch block. LBBB—Left bundle branch block. IVCD—Nonspecific intraventricular conduction delay.

defect, the clinical utility of this measurement in the setting of bundle branch block is extremely limited.

Calculation of Mean QRS Axis with Bundle Branch Block

What about calculation of the mean QRS axis in the setting of an intraventricular conduction delay? For the most part, calculation of axis is accomplished in the same manner with LBBB or nonspecific IVCD as it is with QRS complexes of normal duration. Either of the methods for axis determination explained in Chapter 3 (the two-lead or the three-lead method) may be used, depending on the preference of the interpreter. The only difference is that rather than using amplitude (the *number* of little boxes) of a QRS deflection to assess relative magnitude of a vector in a particular lead, *area* enclosed by the QRS complex should be used. This concept was illustrated in the explanation of the axis determination for Fig. 3-20.

Thus, in Fig. 6-2 the axis is slightly leftward (about $-10°$ to $-20°$), since there is a negative net deflection in lead aVF. Marked LAD (of at least

$-75°$) is present in Fig. 6-3, since both leads II and III demonstrate overwhelmingly negative QRS complexes.

An exception to the rules for axis determination exists when complete RBBB is present. Calculation of axis in the setting of this conduction defect has been the source of much confusion. *When mean QRS axis with complete RBBB is normal or shows only slight left or right axis deviation, precise determination of axis is not clinically important.* However, superposition of marked left or right axis deviation on top of RBBB should be looked for because it may signal development of bifascicular block (RBBB and left anterior or posterior hemiblock).

Even if one wanted to calculate mean QRS axis with complete RBBB, controversy exists as to how this should be accomplished. Perhaps *two* mean QRS axes (an initial "unblocked" axis and subsequent "blocked" axis) should be determined to reflect the fact that the depolarization wavefront with RBBB undergoes a dramatic change in direction midway through its journey. First it travels toward the left (to activate the left ventricle) via the intact left bundle branch. The direction of this part of the journey (the "unblocked" axis) is reflected by the initial portion of the QRS complex, which is upright in lead I. The depolarization wavefront then returns to the right (by slow, myocardial cell-to-cell conduction) to activate the right ventricle. The direction of this final part of the journey (the final "blocked" axis) is best reflected by the terminal negative deflection in lead I (the wide S wave). Calculation of only *one* mean QRS axis in an attempt to determine an "average spatial orientation" for the heart's electrical activity with complete RBBB does *not* accurately reflect the true chain of events, because right and left ventricular depolarization take place *sequentially* rather than simultaneously with this conduction defect.

For practical purposes—our attempt to simplify this otherwise complicated issue—we will largely ignore calculation of mean QRS axis when complete RBBB is present, if the axis appears to be normal or only slightly leftward or rightward in orientation. Precise determination of mean QRS axis in this situation is of little (if any) clinical importance. If marked (a *pathologic* degree of) LAD is present—if the net deflection in lead II is negative—we will say that both RBBB *and* LAHB are present. If, on the other hand, a marked degree of RAD is present (if the r wave in lead I is small and the S wave is both very deep and wide), we will say that both RBBB *and* LPHB are present.

PROBLEM: Examine the ECG shown in Fig. 6-5. Is there RBBB?

INTERPRETATION of Fig. 6-5

Sinus rhythm at a rate of about 90 beats/min is present. The PR interval is at the upper range of normal (about 0.19 second). RBBB is present, as evidenced by QRS widening (to at least 0.13 second), a wide terminal negative deflection in lateral leads I and V_6, and an "RBBB-equivalent" pattern in lead V_1.

PROBLEM: A QR complex is present in lead V_1 of Fig. 6-5 rather than the more typical rSR′ that is usually seen with RBBB. Can you explain why no initial positive deflection precedes the Q wave in lead V_1 of this tracing?

ANSWER: The reason no r wave precedes the Q wave in lead V_1 of Fig. 6-5 is that there is anterior infarction. Wide Q waves are present in leads V_2 and V_3, small q waves persist in leads V_4 and V_5, and R-wave progression remains poor across the precordium. Coved ST-segment elevation in leads V_1 to V_3 suggests that the infarction is acute.

RBBB-Equivalent Patterns

Three important points should be made from this ECG. *First, diagnosis of RBBB does not absolutely require an rSR′ pattern to be present in lead V_1.* Coexistence of a complicating condition such as anterior infarction (as in Fig. 6-5), posterior infarction, or RVH may significantly alter morphology of the QRS complex in this lead. Provided that the QRS complex is sufficiently wide (≥0.11 second), and the typical morphology exists in lateral leads I and V_6 (a wide terminal negative deflection), diagnosis of RBBB can be made when any of the *"RBBB-equivalent patterns"* illustrated in Table 6-2B are present in lead V_1.

TABLE 6-2

Typical RBBB and RBBB-equivalent patterns.

A) Typical RBBB pattern (rSR′)

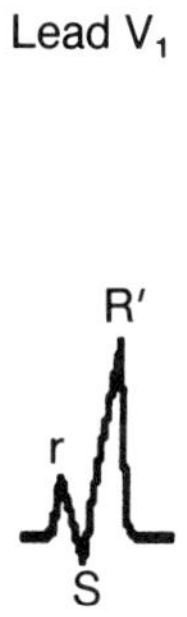

B) RBBB-equivalent patterns

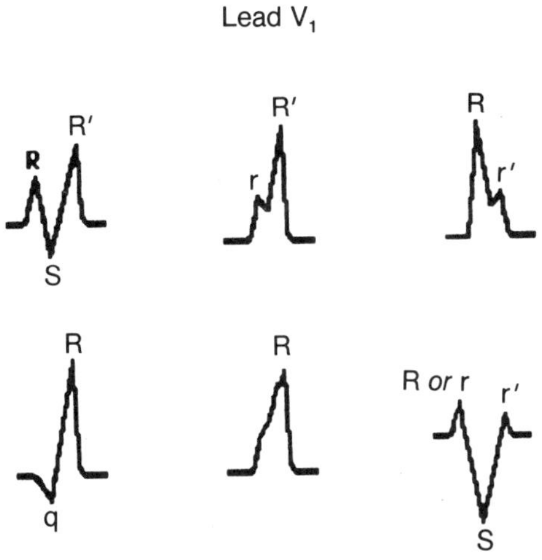

Figure 6-5

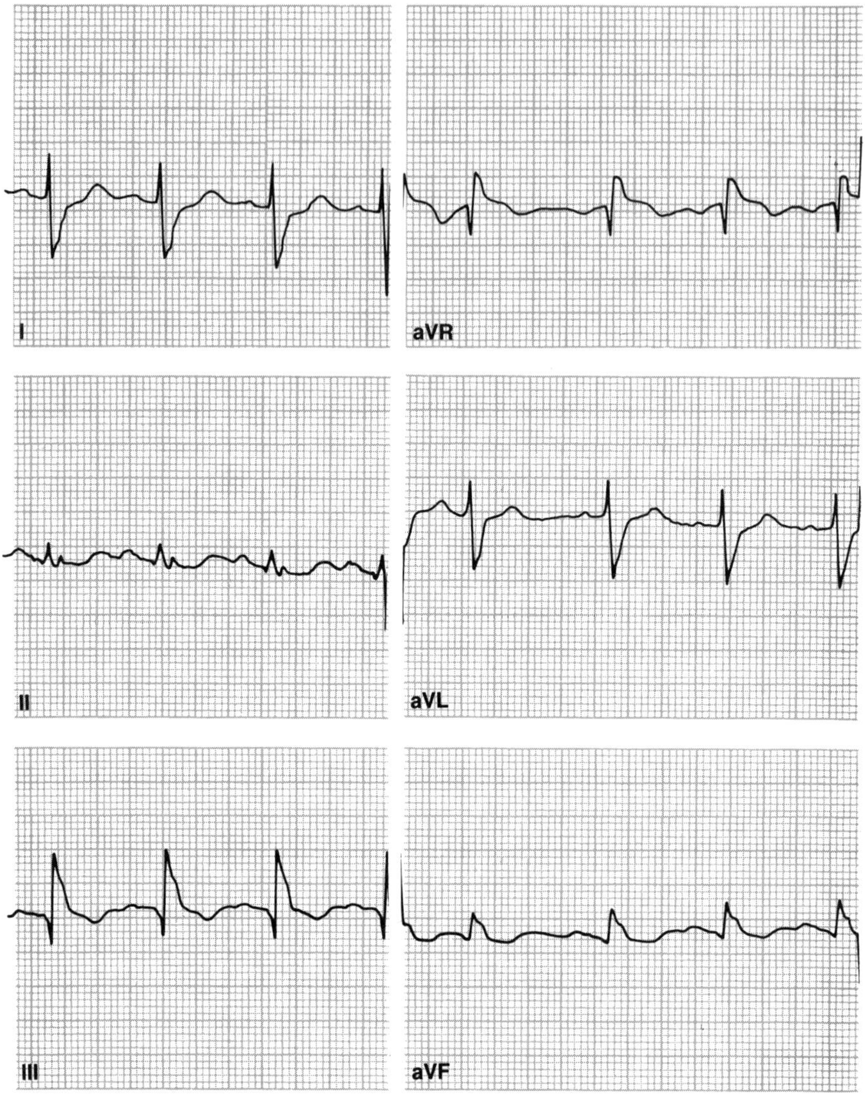

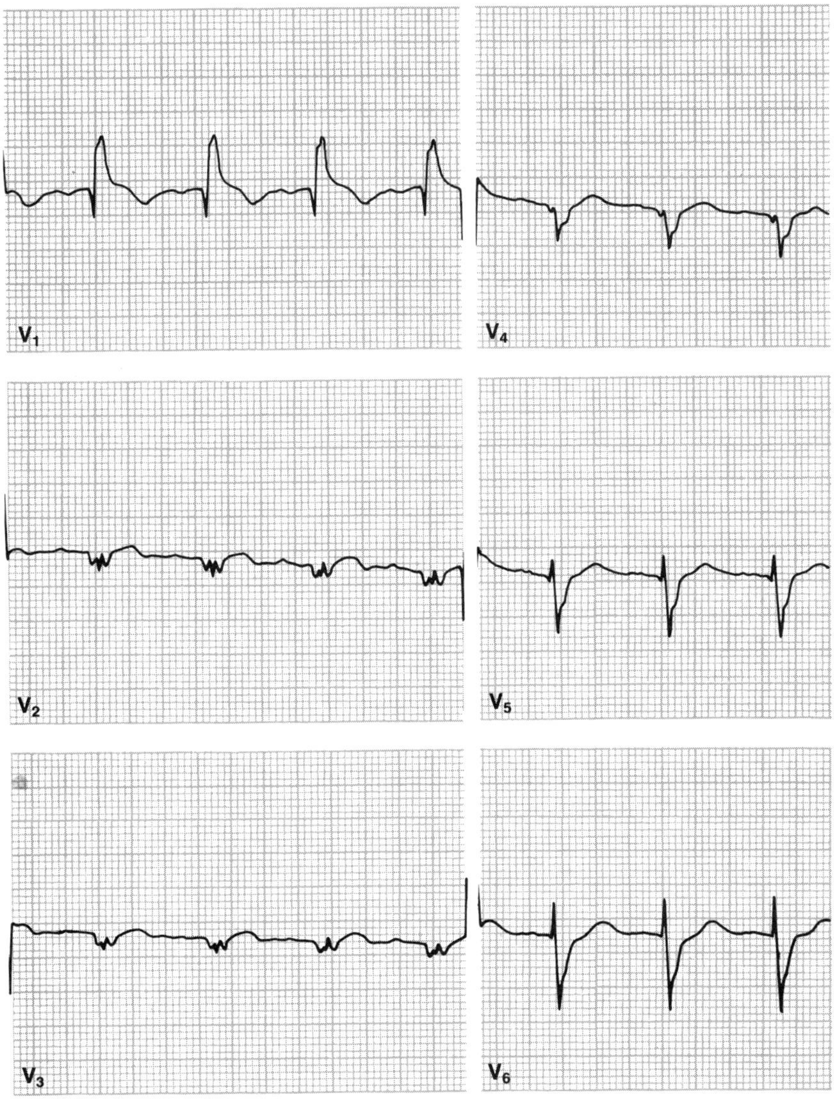
V1
V4
V2
V5
V3
V6

Diagnosis and Clinical Implications of Bundle Branch Block with Myocardial Infarction

The second point is that diagnosis of myocardial infarction can often be made despite the presence of RBBB. As discussed in Chapter 4, the initial vector of septal depolarization is undisturbed with RBBB. Consequently, Q waves (which are inscribed during the initial portion of ventricular activation) retain their diagnostic significance with this conduction defect. Note that in addition to the Q waves that are present in the anterior leads in Fig. 6-5, small q waves are also present in leads II and aVF, and a deep but narrow Q wave is seen in lead III. Previous inferior infarction may have also occurred in this patient.

The final point deals with clinical and prognostic implications of bundle branch block, and the need for prophylactic pacing. Although a certain percentage of patients with *chronic* RBBB or LBBB will go on to develop complete heart block, this percentage is quite low, and the asymptomatic patient does *not* need prophylactic insertion of a pacemaker. On the other hand, development of *new* bundle branch block in the setting of acute myocardial infarction (especially with anterior infarction) places the patient at much higher risk of developing complete heart block within the ensuing hours. These patients merit strong consideration for insertion of a prophylactic pacemaker. The risk of developing complete heartblock increases when the new bundle branch block is *bifascicular* (RBBB and LAHB, RBBB and LPHB, or complete LBBB), or if 1° AV block is associated with the bundle branch block.

A critical question that cannot be answered on the basis of a single ECG (such as the one in Fig. 6-5) is whether the bundle branch block is new or old. If a previous ECG from this patient also demonstrated the conduction disturbance, insertion of a prophylactic pacemaker would probably not be necessary, since progression to complete heart block would be much less likely.

Surprisingly, mortality in patients with acute anterior infarction associated with new bundle branch block is usually linked *not* to the development of complete heart block, but rather to development of cardiogenic shock. These patients have usually suffered extensive myocardial damage, which predisposes them to developing pump failure. Insertion of a prophylactic pacemaker may be advised in an attempt to protect these patients from the abrupt onset of complete heart block. Unfortunately, this intervention does little to improve the overall dismal prognosis.

PROBLEM: Reexamine Fig. 6-2. Is there evidence of prior inferior and/or anterior infarction?

ANSWER: Although one might be tempted to say that there is, remember that LBBB is present in this tracing. As discussed in Chapter 4, LBBB *does* alter the initial vector of septal depolarization. Consequently, detection of Q waves is for the most part unreliable with LBBB. *It is usually extremely difficult to diagnose infarction in the presence of LBBB.* Thus, interpretation of the ECG shown in Fig. 6-2 should read simply:

"Sinus rhythm at 75 beats/min. LBBB."

No more than this can be said about the tracing with certainty.

Imagine that the patient whose ECG was shown in Fig. 6-2 presented to the emergency department complaining of chest pain, and that no prior ECG was available. One would now be faced with the double dilemma of not being able to tell from the ECG whether the patient were infarcting (because of the LBBB), and also of not knowing if the LBBB were new.

Let us now return to the task of recognizing typical bundle branch block patterns.

PROBLEM: Examine Figs. 6-6 and 6-7. An RBBB or its equivalent pattern is present in the V_1 lead of each tracing. Do these ECGs represent typical RBBB?

INTERPRETATION of Fig. 6-6

Rate and rhythm: Sinus rhythm at 65 to 70 beats/min.

Intervals

PR interval: 0.15 second.

QRS interval: 0.09 second.

QT interval: Normal.

Axis: +40°.

Chamber enlargement: None.

QRST changes: Small q waves are seen in the inferior leads. These most likely are not significant.

Incomplete RBBB

Although an RBBB equivalent pattern (an rSr′) is present in lead V_1 and the T wave is inverted in this lead (typical secondary T-wave change for RBBB), the QRS interval is not prolonged. There are S waves in leads I and V_6, but these terminal negative deflections are *narrow* in both of these leads. Therefore, criteria for *complete* RBBB are not met. When morphologic characteristics of RBBB are evident but the QRS interval is not prolonged to at least 0.11 second, *incomplete RBBB (IRBBB)* is said to be present. Loosely applied, the designation of IRBBB is often given whenever an rSr′ pattern is seen in lead V_1 of an ECG regardless of whether there are S waves in the lateral leads.

IRBBB is a common ECG pattern that is estimated to occur in up to 5

Figure 6-6

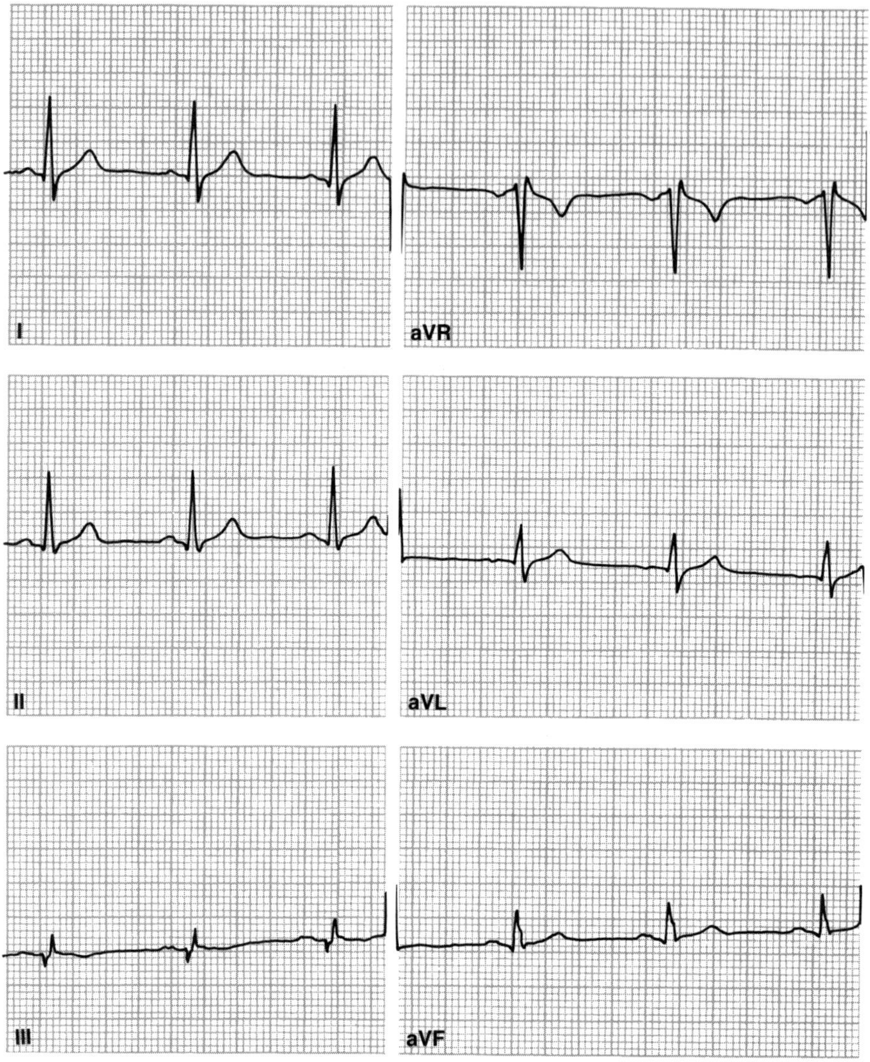

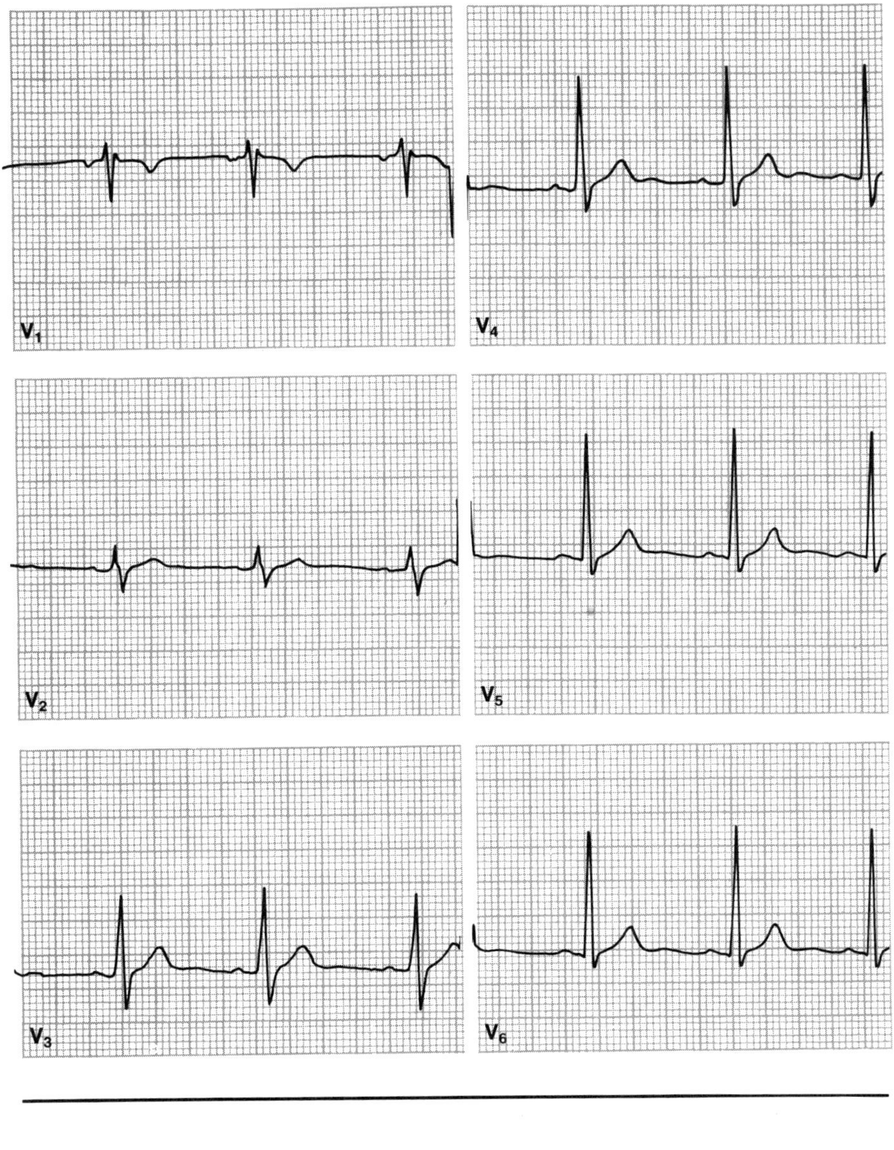
V1
V4
V2
V5
V3
V6

Figure 6-7

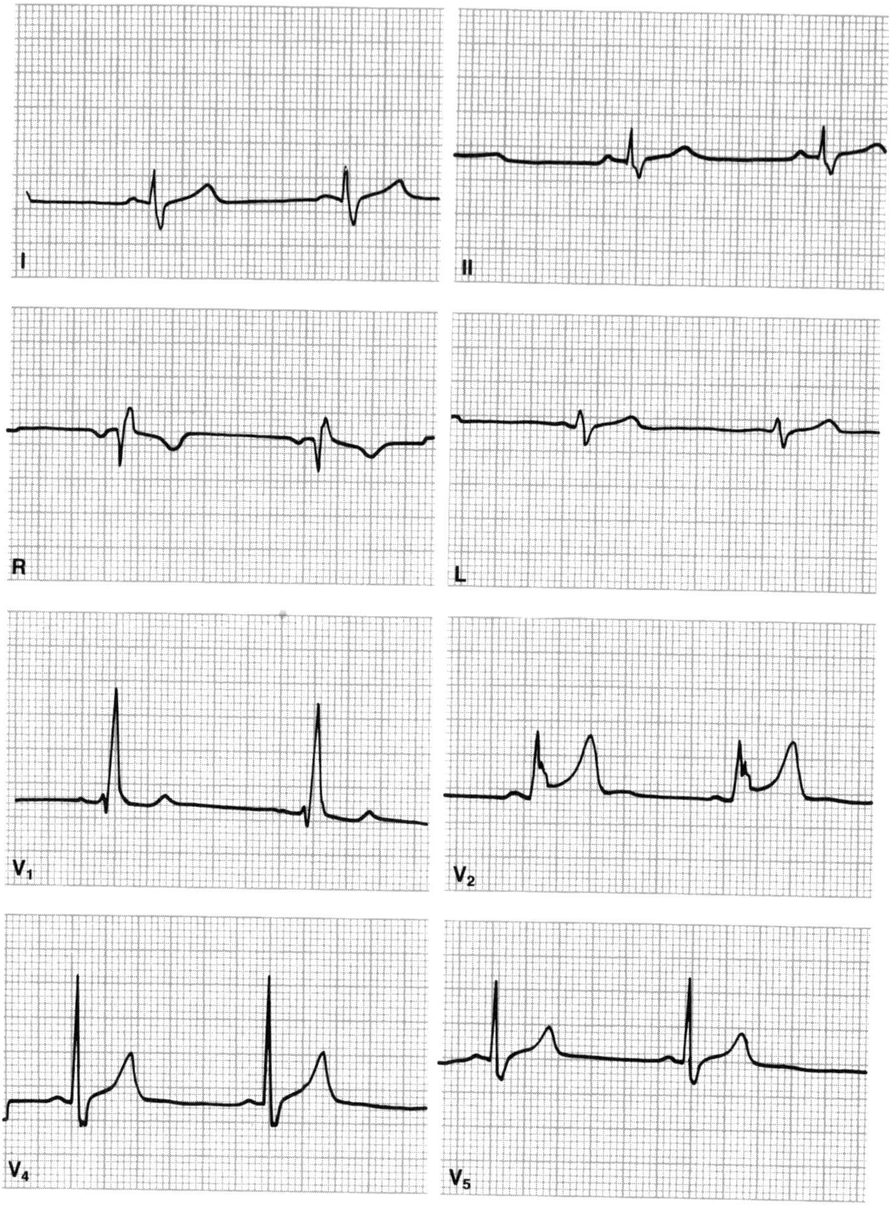

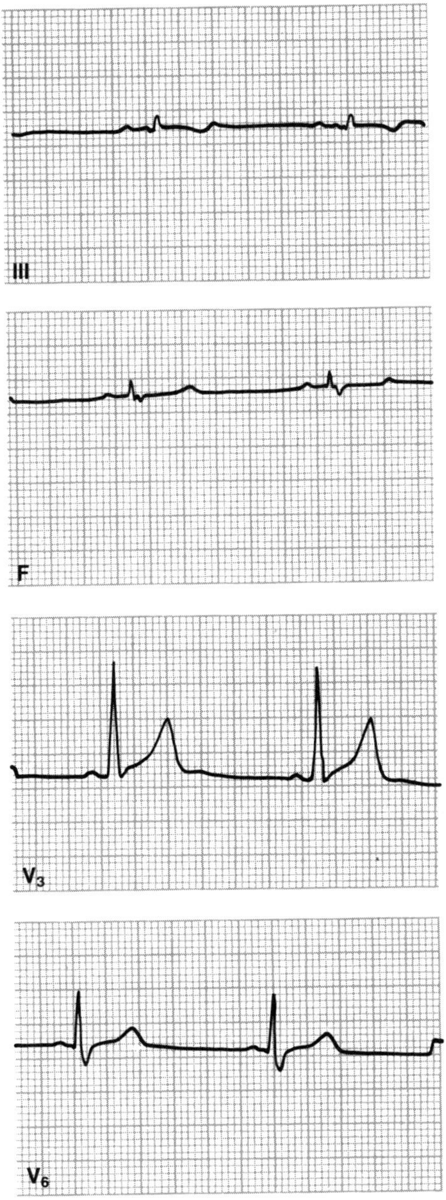
III
F
V3
V6

percent of the general population. Although it may be associated with any of the conditions that were listed for complete RBBB, IRBBB probably occurs most frequently as an isolated finding in otherwise healthy, asymptomatic individuals without underlying heart disease. In fact, many authorities feel that the rSr′ pattern in lead V_1 may not be a conduction disturbance at all. Instead, it may be a normal variant and reflect the fact that in some individuals, the last portion of the ventricles to be activated is the right ventricular outflow tract. (Note that mean QRS axis *can* accurately be determined with IRBBB.)

Incomplete LBBB

PROBLEM: Is there an incomplete form of LBBB?

ANSWER: If an incomplete pattern of RBBB has been described, one might logically assume that a corresponding pattern of incomplete LBBB also exists—and in fact it does, although the issue is not without controversy.

Incomplete LBBB presents similar morphologic characteristics as complete LBBB (a monophasic R wave in the lateral leads and predominantly negative QRS complexes in the anterior precordial leads), but with only a moderate degree of QRS-interval prolongation (to 0.10 or 0.11 second). The problem is the tremendous difficulty of differentiating incomplete LBBB from LVH. An essential feature of incomplete LBBB is the absence of septal q waves in the lateral leads, but septal q waves may also be missing from the lateral leads when there is marked LVH. QRS duration is not a failsafe distinguishing feature either, since LVH itself may produce some widening of the QRS complex because of the longer time required for activation of the hypertrophied left ventricle.

As a result of these limitations, diagnosis of incomplete LBBB may sometimes be possible only retrospectively by review of serial ECGs that demonstrate disappearance of septal q waves and progressive widening of the QRS complex over time with ultimate development of complete LBBB.

Clinically, one may be concerned that incomplete LBBB, like complete LBBB, could make LVH and myocardial infarction more difficult to detect. While this concern may be valid, practically speaking the overwhelming majority of patients who have incomplete LBBB will also have LVH. The reason is that similar underlying disease processes are associated with both of these disorders. Most of the time, therefore, ECG differentiation between incomplete LBBB and LVH is more of academic interest than of clinical importance.

A final issue to raise regarding the diagnosis of incomplete LBBB and its distinction from complete LBBB is at what point one should consider the block "complete." Although QRS prolongation to ≥ 0.12 second is generally accepted as the dividing point between these two entities, many patients with so-called "complete" LBBB continue to widen their QRS complex to as much as 0.16 second. Does this mean that their complete LBBB has now become "more complete"?

Theoretically, complete LBBB should be diagnosed only when the QRS complex has attained its maximal degree of prolongation. Clinically, there is no way to determine this in a prospective manner. For practical purposes (and in conformance with general practice), we will continue to use QRS prolongation to ≥0.12 second as our cutoff for diagnosing complete LBBB.

INTERPRETATION of Fig. 6-7

Rate and rhythm: Sinus bradycardia at 50 to 55 beats/min.

Intervals

PR interval: 0.17 second.

QRS interval: 0.12 second. Characteristic QRS morphology of RBBB is present—rsR′ in lead V_1, and a fairly wide terminal negative deflection in leads I and V_6.

QT interval: Normal (despite the presence of RBBB).

Chamber enlargement: Probably none.

QRST changes: Instead of the usual secondary T-wave change that one expects to see with uncomplicated RBBB, T waves are *upright* in leads V_1 and V_2. This represents a *primary T-wave change,* and suggests that something other than a pure conduction disturbance (such as ischemia or infarction) may be occurring. Although much of the time ischemia and infarction will not be detectable electrocardiographically in the setting of complete bundle branch block, keeping a keen eye out for subtle primary T-wave changes such as these will occasionally pay nice dividends.

PROBLEM: Examine the ECG shown in Fig. 6-8, taken from a 67-year-old woman complaining of chest pain. Does this tracing represent typical LBBB?

INTERPRETATION of Fig. 6-8

Rate and rhythm: Sinus arrhythmia with the rate varying between 70 and 95 beats/min.

Intervals

PR interval: 0.17 second.

QRS interval: 0.12 second. Characteristic QRS morphology of LBBB is present—absence of septal Q wave and monophasic R wave in leads I and V_6, and deep QS complex in lead V_1.

Axis: About +40°.

Chamber enlargement: Possibly LVH (very deep S wave >30 mm in lead V_2), although difficult to tell in the presence of LBBB.

Figure 6-8. ECG from a 67-year-old woman complaining of chest pain.

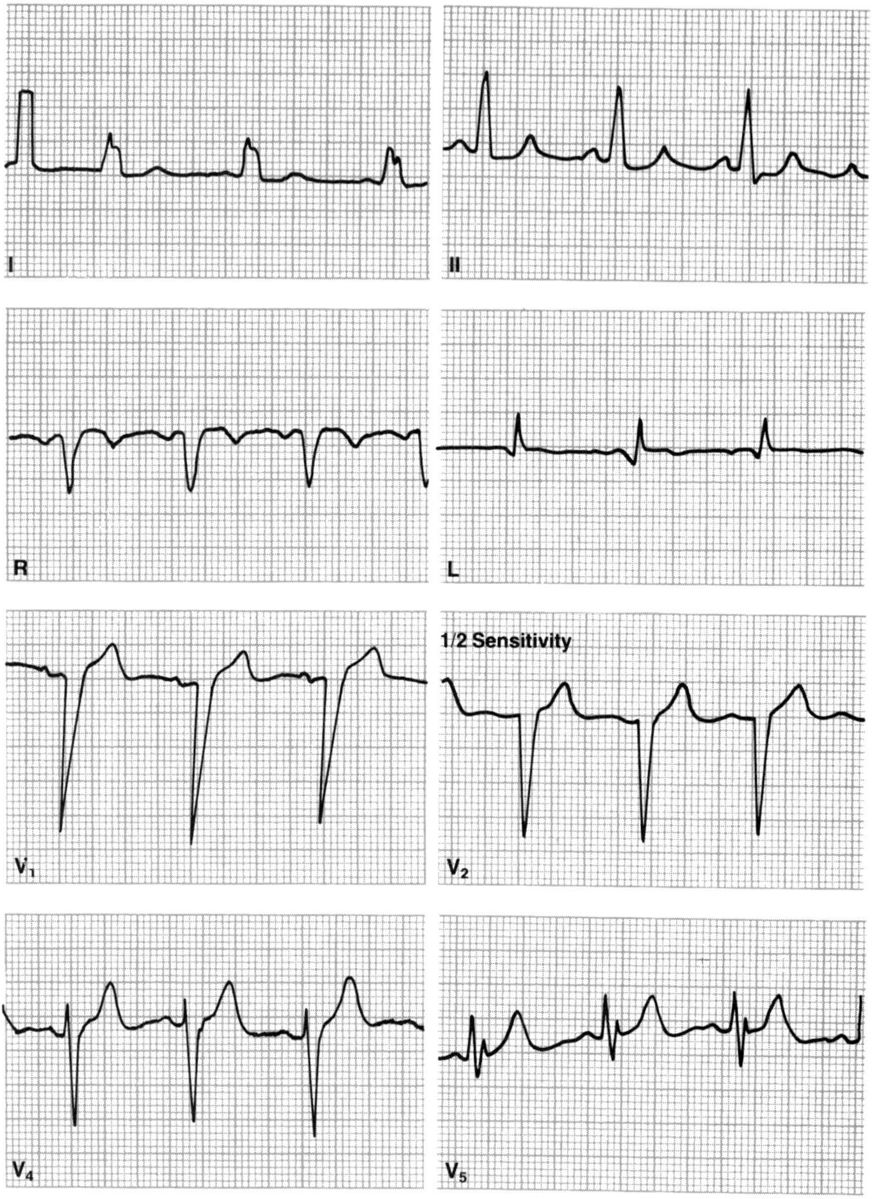

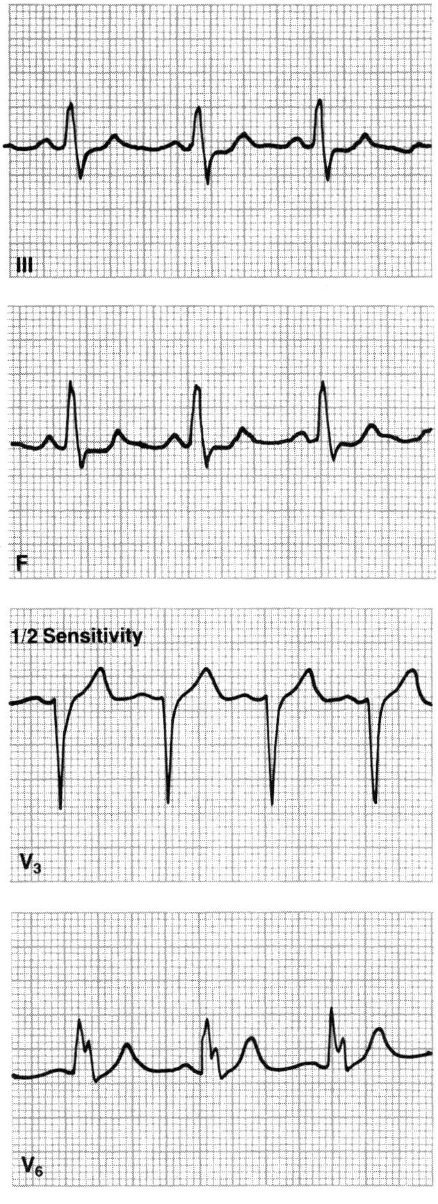
III
F
1/2 Sensitivity
V3
V6

QRST changes: A Q wave is present in lead aVL. R-wave progression is poor, and transition is delayed until leads V_4 and V_5, but this is commonly seen with LBBB. T waves are *upright* in leads I and especially V_6—primary T-wave change.

Although QRS morphology in leads I, V_1, and V_6 is typical for LBBB, the same cannot be said for the appearance of ST segments and T waves. Normally there is ST-segment depression and T-wave inversion in the lateral leads with LBBB. This is not the case in leads I and V_6 of this tracing. Thus, a primary T-wave change is present. In a 67-year old woman complaining of chest pain, this finding should suggest that ischemia or evolving infarction may be occurring in addition to the LBBB.

An additional finding of concern on this ECG is the Q wave that is seen in lead aVL. Normally Q waves should not be seen in *any* of the lateral leads with LBBB. Their presence suggests that possible anteroseptal infarction has occurred at some point in the past (or may be occurring at present).

Obtaining a comparison tracing (a previous ECG on this patient) would be extremely important in this case. Only in this way would one be able to determine whether the above two findings were likely to represent an acute process. Thus, the subtle findings present on this tracing (primary T wave change and presence of a septal q wave in a lateral lead) illustrate an exception to the general rule that infarction cannot be diagnosed in the setting of complete LBBB.

Chamber Enlargement with Bundle Branch Block

The subject of ECG diagnosis of chamber enlargement with bundle branch block was introduced in Chapter 4 (Detection of Ventricular Hypertrophy with Bundle Branch Block). Although LVH is more difficult to recognize when it occurs in the presence of LBBB, the diagnosis is suggested if voltage is extremely prominent (if the S wave in lead V_2 is *deeper* than 30 mm), or if there is associated LAA. Considering that leads V_2 and V_3 in Fig. 6-8 were recorded at *half-standardization,* the S wave in lead V_2 exceeds this voltage requirement.

Electrocardiographic detection of RVH is virtually impossible when LBBB is present. With RBBB, RVH is suggested if the terminal rightward deflection (the R′) of the QRS complex in lead V_1 is very tall (greater than 15 mm). Associated RAA provides supportive evidence. LVH is suggested with RBBB if the R wave in the lateral precordial leads (V_5 or V_6) is ≥ 25 mm, or if the R wave in lead aVL ≥ 12 mm.

Bundle branch block alters the sequence of ventricular activation, but has no effect on the sequence of atrial activation. Consequently, ECG diagnosis of atrial enlargement is not impeded in the presence of this conduction disturbance.

PROBLEM: Examine Figs. 6-9 and 6-10. Is *bifascicular* block present in either of these tracings?

INTERPRETATION of Fig. 6-9

Rate and rhythm: Sinus arrhythmia at 55 to 65 beats/min.

Intervals

PR interval: 0.19 second.

QRS interval: 0.12 second. Complete RBBB.

QT interval: Normal (despite the presence of RBBB).

Axis: Pathologic LAD is present (the net deflection of the QRS complex in lead II is negative), suggesting LAHB. The combination of complete RBBB and LAHB is a form of *bifascicular* block. (Conduction of the electrical impulse to the ventricles must be occurring down the remaining intact fascicle—the left posterior hemidivision of the left bundle branch.)

Chamber enlargement: RAA (tall peaked P waves in the inferior leads that exceed 2-1/2 mm in amplitude in lead II). Despite the presence of RBBB, *biventricular* hypertrophy is suggested in this tracing. Evidence favoring RVH is the very tall R′ (>15 mm) in lead V_1, and associated RAA. LVH is suggested by prominent voltage in lead aVL (R in aVL >12 mm) and in the lateral precordial leads.

QRST changes: The typical secondary T-wave change of RBBB is present in lead V_1.

INTERPRETATION of Fig. 6-10

Rate and rhythm: Sinus arrhythmia at 50 to 60 beats/min.

Intervals

PR interval: 0.20 second (or still within normal limits).

QRS interval: 0.12 second. Complete RBBB. (The qR complex in lead V_1 qualifies as an "RBBB-equivalent" pattern.)

QT interval: Normal (despite the presence of RBBB).

Axis: Marked RAD (of at least +105°) is present. This degree of RAD in the setting of RBBB suggests LPHB. (Note that the rS complex in lead I and the qR complex in lead III are consistent with the typical morphological characteristics of LPHB that were illustrated in Table 4-5.)

Chamber enlargement: None.

QRST changes: The T wave is upright in leads V_1 and V_2 (primary T-wave change). Clinical correlation and comparison with a prior tracing would be helpful in establishing the significance of this finding.

Bifascicular Block

The combination of complete RBBB and LPHB that is seen in Fig. 6-10 is another form of bifascicular block. (Conduction of the electrical impulse to the ventricles in this example of bifascicular block *must* be occur-

Figure 6-9

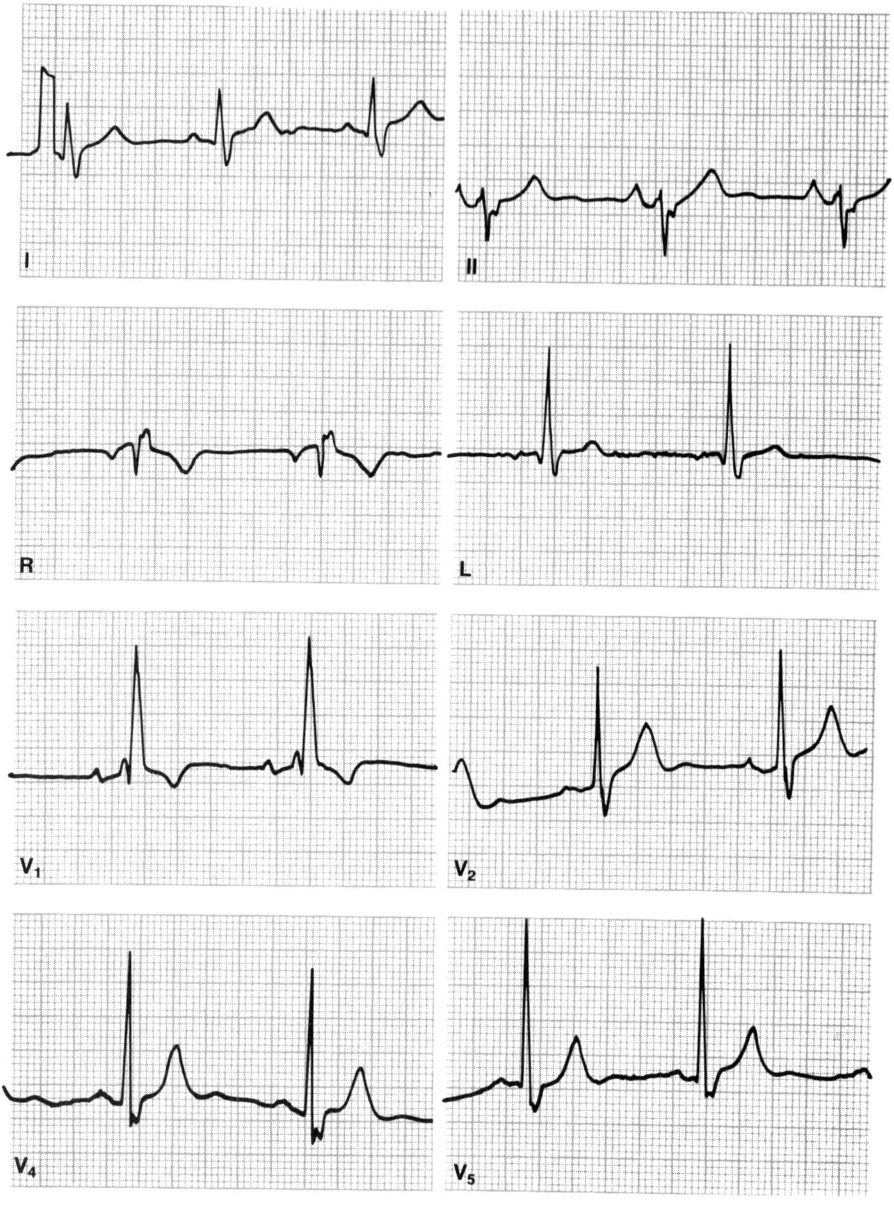

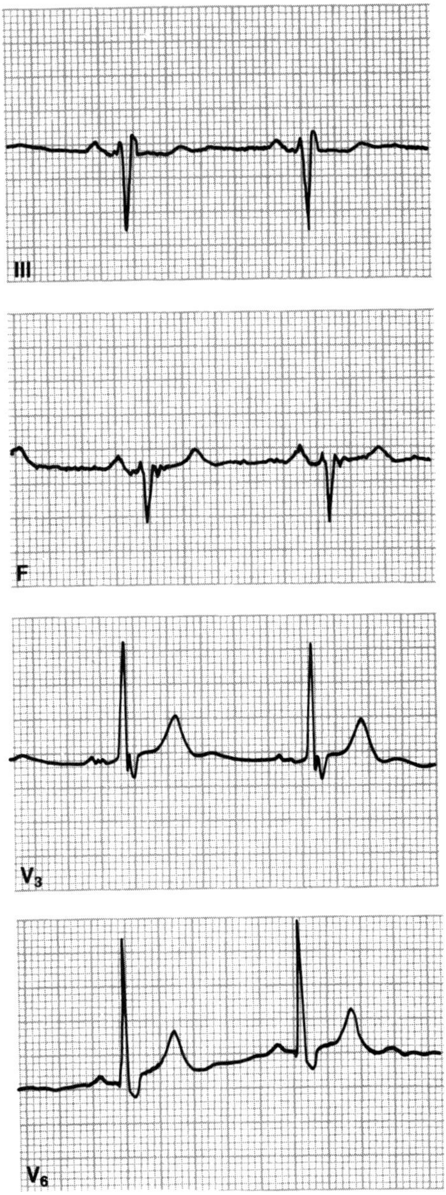
III
F
V3
V6

Figure 6-10

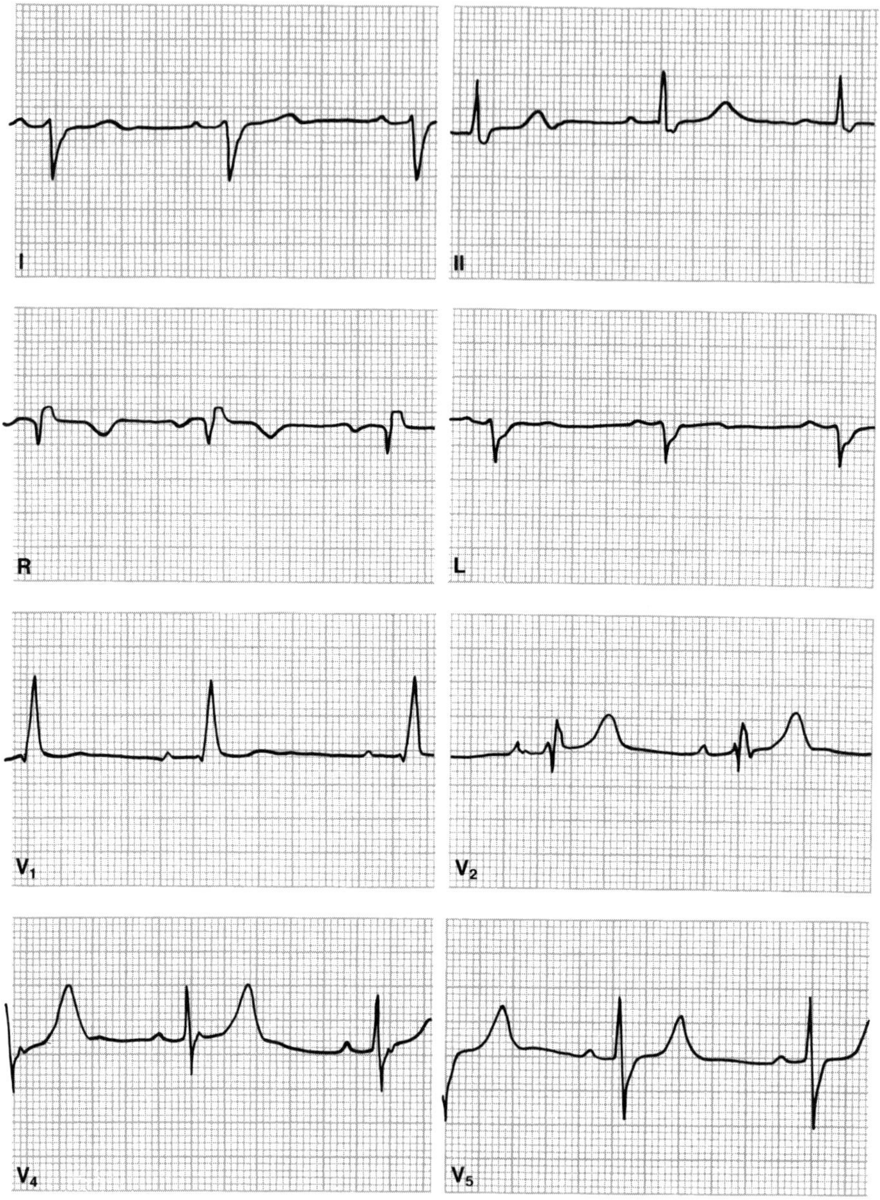

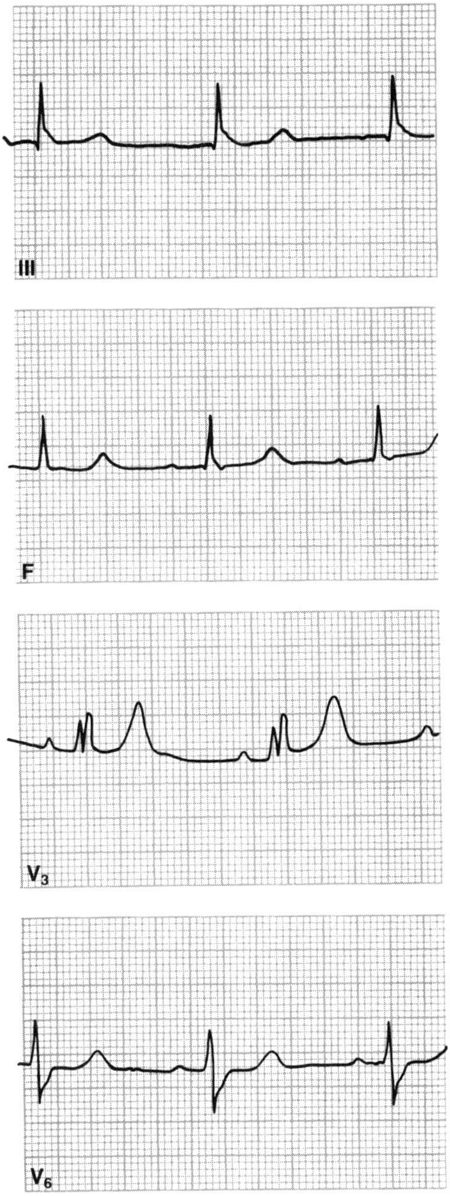
III
F
V_3
V_6

ring down the remaining intact fascicle—the anterior hemidivision of the left bundle branch). Reexamine the PR interval for a moment. Note that it is 0.20 second, or at the upper limits of normal. Precise measurement of the PR interval takes on added importance in the setting of bifascicular block, since if the PR interval is definitely prolonged (>0.21 second), it would imply that conduction of the impulse is also being *delayed* down the one remaining intact fascicle (that *trifascicular* block is present).

As discussed in Chapter 4 (Hemiblocks), the combination of RBBB and LPHB is a far less common form of bifascicular block than the combination of RBBB and LAHB, which was seen in Fig. 6-9. This is because of the dual blood supply of the left posterior hemidivision, and the fact that this fascicle is much thicker and consequently less susceptible to injury than is the anterior hemidivision. Consequently, when RBBB and LPHB are seen, it implies more extensive disease than when RBBB and LAHB are seen.

In a sense, one might consider complete LBBB a third form of bifascicular block; this conduction disorder by definition implies that conduction is impaired down *both* fascicles of the left bundle branch.

Differentiation Between Complete LBBB and IVCD

PROBLEM: Interpret the two ECGs shown in Figs. 6-11 and 6-12. Do one or both show LBBB?

INTERPRETATION of Fig. 6-11

Rate and rhythm: Sinus rhythm at 60 to 65 beats/min.

Intervals

PR interval: 0.19 second.

QRS interval: 0.15 second. Wide, notched monophasic R waves in leads I and aVL, and predominantly negative QRS complexes in the anterior precordial leads of this tracing suggest complete LBBB.

QT interval: Appears to be prolonged (greater than half the R-R interval) in leads such as III and aVL. However, determination of the QT interval is of little clinical utility in the setting of bundle branch block.

Axis: At least −40° (LAD).

Chamber enlargement: LAA. The P wave is notched and prolonged (>0.12 second in duration in lead II). LVH is more than likely present considering the greatly increased R-wave amplitude in aVL, the tremendous depth of S waves (all recorded at half standardization!) in the anterior precordial leads, and associated LAA.

QRST changes: The ST segments in leads I and aVL are depressed as one would expect with LBBB. However, the T wave is upright in these leads, albeit of greatly decreased amplitude. While the ST-T wave segments are not typical of what one usually sees in these lateral leads with uncomplicated LBBB (depressed ST segment and *inverted* T wave), probably they are not abnormal enough to qualify as a true primary T-wave change. In the anterior precordial leads, the ST segments are slightly elevated and the T waves are upright—consistent with typical secondary T-wave changes of LBBB.

Finally, ST-segment elevation and coving is also seen in leads III and aVF. Although this type of ST-segment change would be cause for concern under normal circumstances, in the setting of an intraventricular conduction delay it is of no diagnostic assistance.

Two interpretations might be given for this tracing—complete LBBB or IVCD. Both would be correct, depending on the criteria one chooses to define complete LBBB. Although QRS morphology is typical for LBBB in leads I, aVL, and the anterior precordial leads, the rSR′s′ configuration in lead V_6 is distinctly unusual for this conduction disorder. Since typical morphology for LBBB is not present in *each* of the key leads (I, V_1, *and* V_6), some electrocardiographers would classify this as a nonspecific IVCD. Others would ignore lead V_6 and accept the changes in the other leads as diagnostic of LBBB. Which answer *you* prefer is probably *not* important (either from a clinical or electrocardiographic point of view), as long as you understand the rationale followed for arriving at your conclusion.

Although we have been somewhat wordy in our description of the findings of this ECG, all that one need write for the ECG interpretation would be:

"Sinus rhythm at 60 to 65 beats/min.
LBBB (or IVCD, depending on your preference) with LAD.
LAA/Probable LVH."

In fact, the patient whose ECG is shown in Fig. 6-11 had congestive cardiomyopathy. The left atrial and ventricular chambers were grossly dilated, and the left ventricle was hypertrophied.

INTERPRETATION of Fig. 6-12
Rate and rhythm: Sinus rhythm at 90 beats/min.
Intervals

PR interval: 0.18 second.

QRS interval: 0.16 second.

QT interval: ——.

Axis: Pathologic LAD (of at least −60°).
Chamber enlargement: LAA (based on the significant terminal negative deflection of the P wave in lead V_1).
QRST changes: See below.

The QRS complex is definitely widened in this example, but it does not manifest the characteristic features of either RBBB or LBBB. According to

Figure 6-11

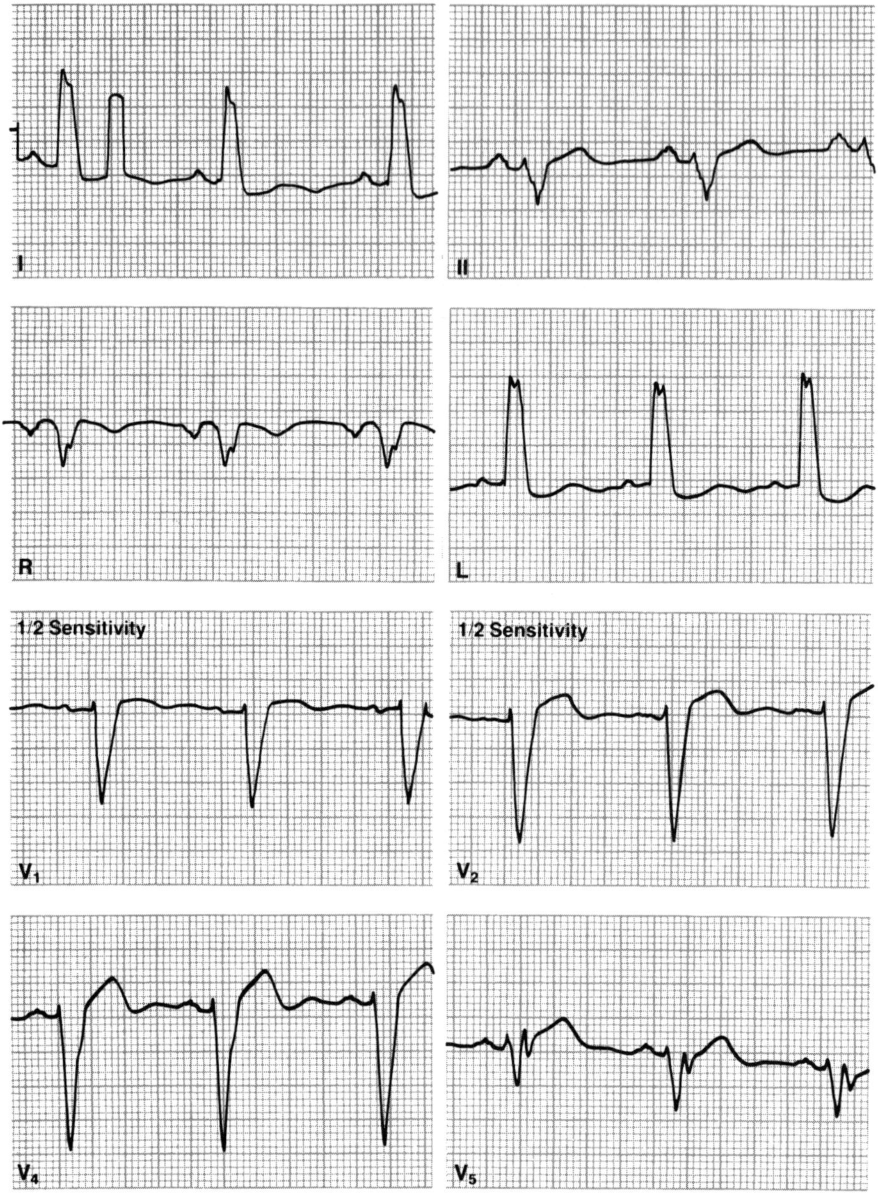

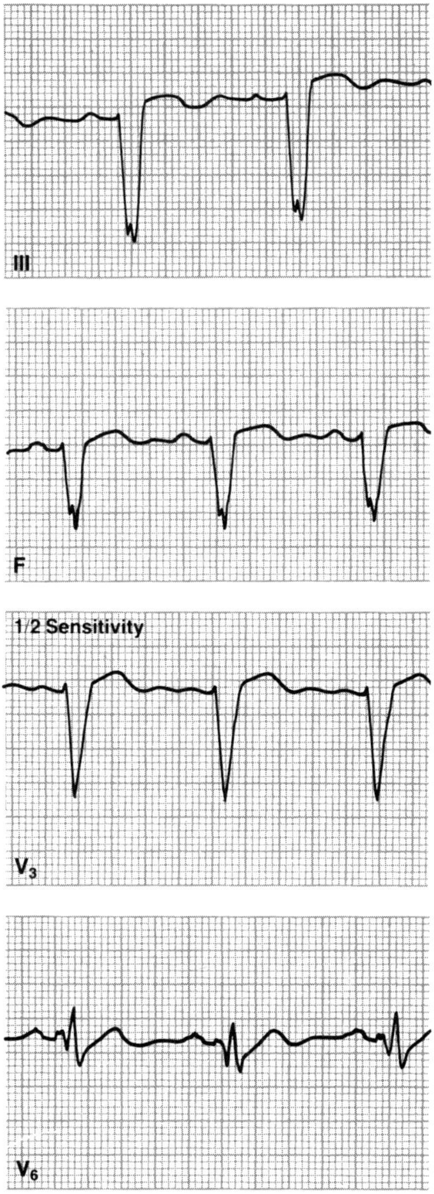
III
F
1/2 Sensitivity
V3
V6

Figure 6-12

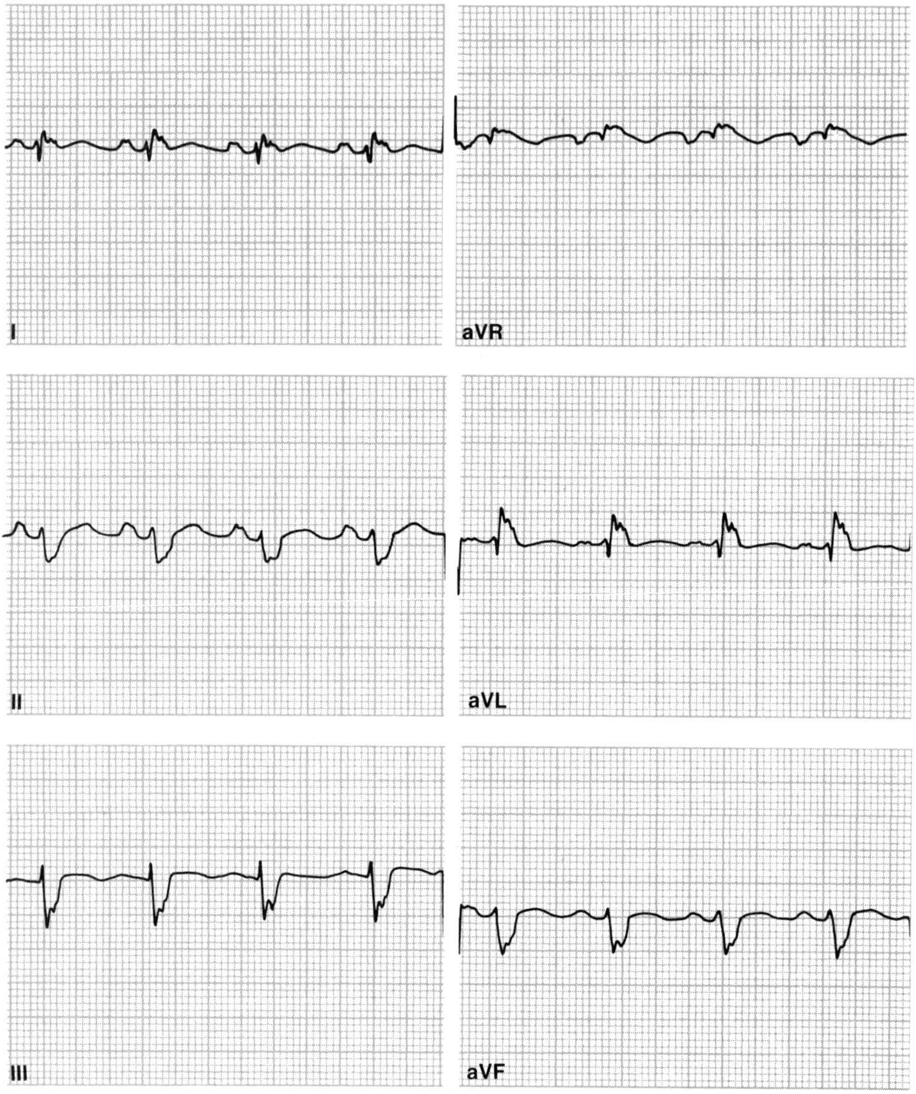

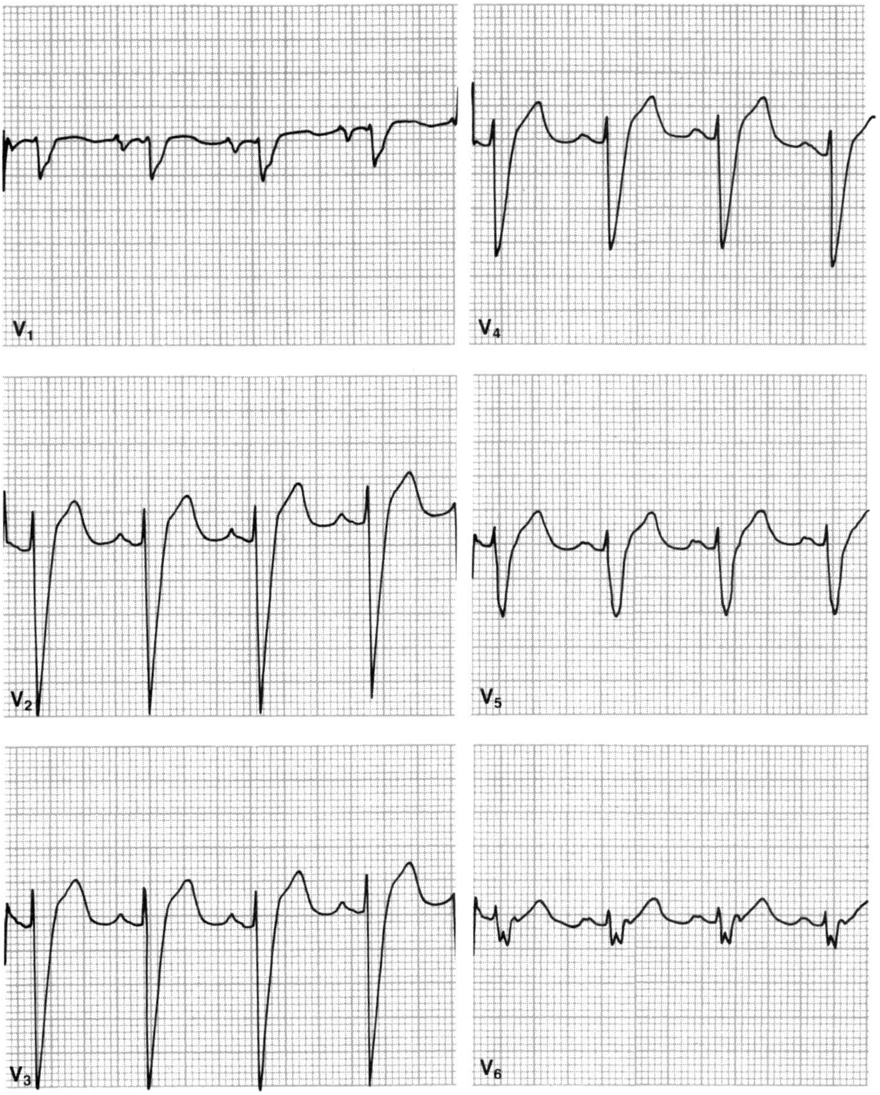
V1
V4
V2
V5
V3
V6

the flow sheet rationale of Fig. 6-4, this conduction defect should therefore be classified as IVCD. ST-T wave changes are consistent with secondary changes of the conduction disorder.

In fact, this patient also had congestive cardiomyopathy. A number of years before, a previous ECG had shown the typical pattern of complete LBBB. In the interim, she had a myocardial infarction (documented by enzymes). These clinical events *cannot* be deduced with certainty from inspection of this one single tracing. Without a prior tracing for comparison, all that one could (or should) write for the ECG interpretation of this tracing would be:

"Sinus rhythm at 90 beats/min. IVCD with LAD."

Patients with congestive cardiomyopathy may manifest any of a variety of electrocardiographic patterns, including LVH (and sometimes biventricular hypertrophy), RBBB, LBBB, or nonspecific IVCD. The type of pattern shown by this patient is typical.

PROBLEM: The ECG in Fig. 6-13 illustrates one more example of LBBB. Or does it?

ANSWER: The QRS complex is broad and slurred in the lateral leads and predominantly negative in the anterior precordial leads in a pattern that suggests complete LBBB. In addition, seemingly typical secondary ST-T wave changes are seen in the appropriate leads. However, this is *not* LBBB. Do you see why not?

Let's return to our format for systematic evaluation of ECGs.

Rate and rhythm: The rhythm is regular at 60 beats/min. Normal-appearing (upright) P waves are present, but the PR interval is short. It measures only 0.10 second before encountering the initial slurred portion of the QRS complex.

Accessory Pathways

The reason the PR interval is shortened in Fig. 6-13 is that the patient has Wolff-Parkinson-White syndrome (WPW). This clinical entity was first recognized as a syndrome in 1930 by Wolff, Parkinson, and White. In its full form, it is recognized by three characteristic features:

- A *short* PR interval
- The presence of *delta waves* in one or more leads
- A *widened* QRS complex

The pathophysiology of WPW is that an *accessory pathway* exists that connects one of the atria directly with its ipsilateral ventricle, bypassing the AV node. As discussed in Chapter 1 (PR Interval), during normal conduction, a substantial portion of the PR interval (up to 0.10 second) is taken up by the delay that occurs at the AV node. Therefore, an alternative pathway for conduction of the sinus impulse from the atria to the ventricles that *bypasses* the AV node will greatly accelerate conduction and result in a shortened PR interval. This is precisely what the accessory pathway does. The delta wave (the slurred upstroke of the initial portion of the QRS complex) is due to premature activation of the ventricles *(preexcitation)* by the accelerated conduction.

These events are illustrated in Fig. 6-14. Panel A shows conduction over the normal atrioventricular pathway. The PR interval is normal and the QRS complex is narrow. In Fig. 6-14B, conduction is totally down the accessory pathway—completely bypassing the AV node. Total preexcitation such as this will result in a widened and bizarre QRS complex, since the ventricles are being activated by slow, myocardial cell-to-cell conduction almost as if a premature ventricular contraction (PVC) had occurred at the point of entry of the accessory pathway into the ventricular myocardium.

In Fig. 6-14C, conduction of the sinus impulse occurs *simultaneously* down both the accessory *and* the normal atrioventricular pathway. It arrives first in the ventricles by conduction down the accessory pathway (since conduction down this pathway is accelerated). The delta wave is produced as the impulse begins its journey through the ventricles. Meanwhile, conduction down the slower, normal atrioventricular pathway finally arrives in the ventricles. Here it will meet with the depolarization wavefront that had been conducted down the accessory pathway, resulting in a *fusion* complex. The resultant wide QRS complex is actually a fusion beat with the initial upward slurred portion of this complex (the delta wave—depicted in dotted lines in Panel C) resulting from activation of the ventricles via the accessory pathway, and the final portion resulting from activation of the ventricles via the normal atrioventricular pathway. The wide QRS complex that occurs with fusion of these two depolarization wavefronts (in Fig. 6-14C) is due *not* to delay in ventricular activation (as is the case with bundle branch block), but rather to early stimulation (preexcitation) of the ventricles. *The QRS complex is widened by the amount that the PR interval is shortened.*

Finally, note that conduction down the accessory pathway may result in a marked change in appearance of the ST-T wave segment (Fig. 6-14C). Since WPW alters the sequence of ventricular activation, one might expect that repolarization will also be altered. The ST segment depicted in dotted lines in Panel C contrasts the changes produced by conduction down the accessory pathway with those of normal conduction.

Clinically with WPW, conduction may proceed entirely via the normal atrioventricular pathway (as in Panel A), entirely down the accessory pathway (as in Panel B), or simultaneously down both pathways (as in Panel C). The situation illustrated in Panel C is by far the most commonly seen.

At times, conduction may alternate between both pathways. This is shown in Fig. 6-15. Again, although this tracing superficially resembles LBBB, the three characteristic findings of WPW (short PR interval, delta wave,

Figure 6-13

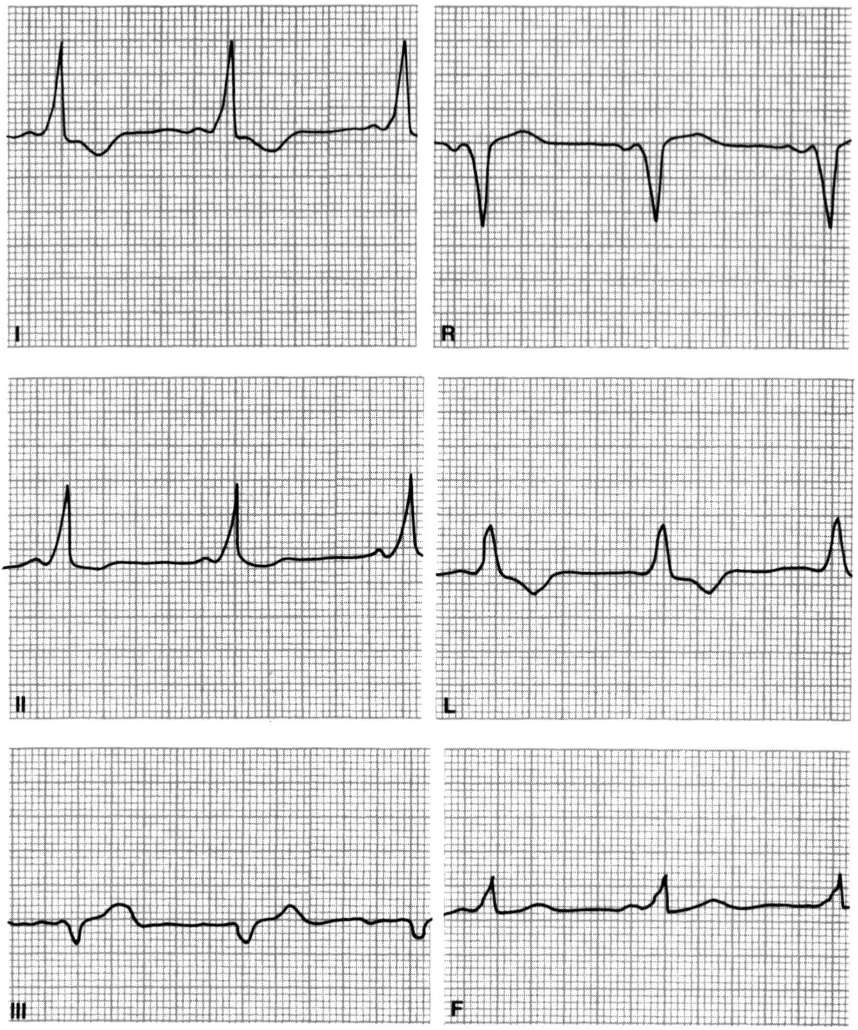

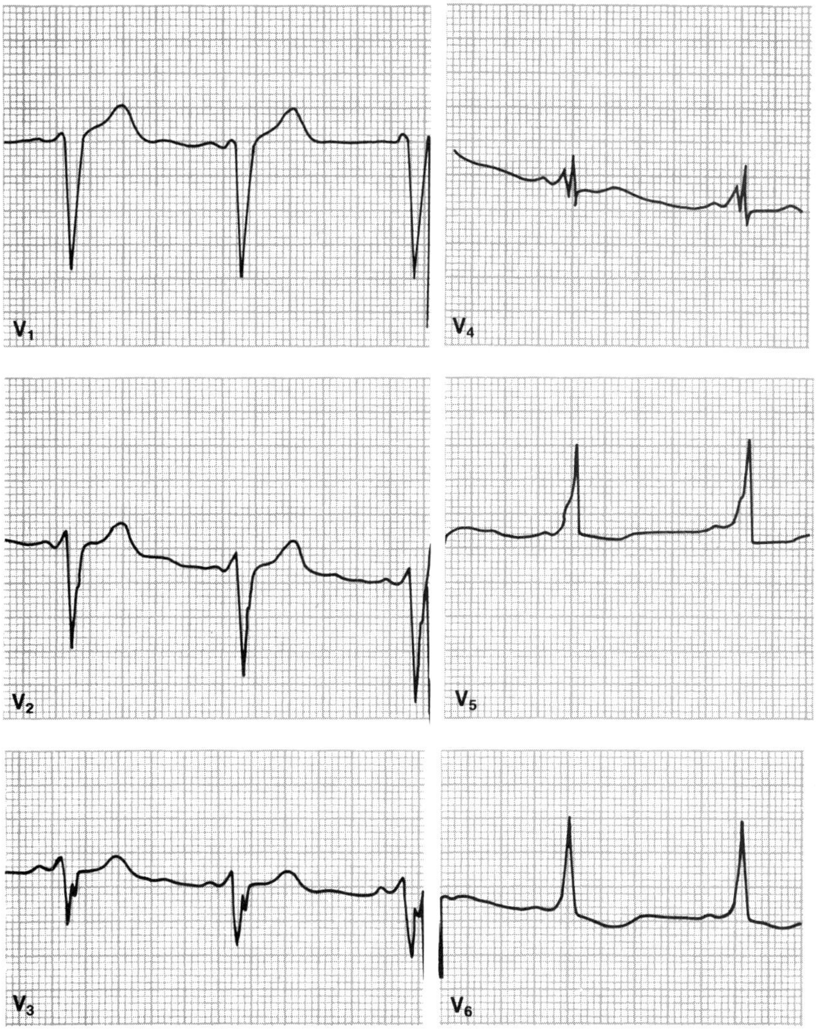
V1
V4
V2
V5
V3
V6

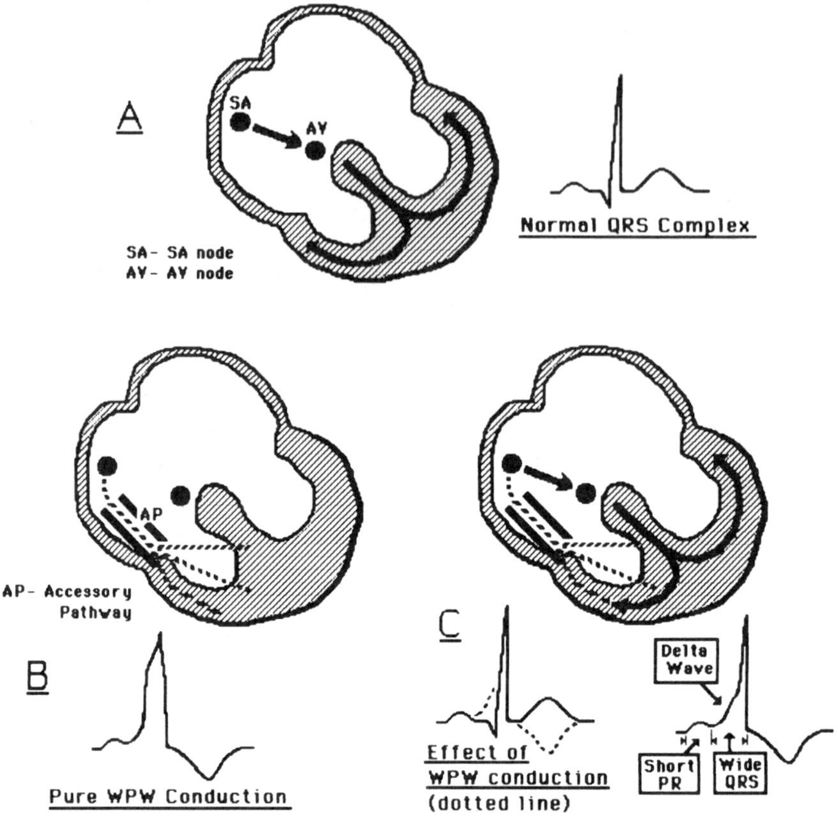

Figure 6-14. Wolff-Parkinson-White syndrome. **A.** Normal conduction of the sinus impulse to the AV node and then to the ventricles. The PR interval is normal and the QRS is narrow. **B.** Conduction of the impulse solely down the accessory pathway, resulting in a wide QRS complex. **C.** Conduction down both the accessory pathway and the AV nodal pathway. This results in a fusion complex in which the PR interval is short and the QRS complex widened by the addition of a delta wave (dotted line). Note the change in the ST segment produced by conduction down the accessory pathway (dotted ST segment).

and wide QRS complex) are easily identified in each of the lateral leads.

The rhythm strip below the ECG is taken from lead II, and demonstrates varying degrees of preexcitation *(fusion)* as conduction alternates between the normal atrioventricular pathway and the accessory pathway.

WPW has traditionally been classified into two types, A and B, based on the orientation of the delta wave and QRS complex in lead V_1. With *type A WPW,* the QRS complex is predominantly *upright* in lead V_1, whereas with *type B WPW,* it is predominantly negative. One may find it easy to remember this distinction by mentally visualizing the capital letter "A," and the *upright* sides that make up the frame of this letter. (Fig. 6-16).

PROBLEM: Review the examples of WPW that were shown in Figs. 6-13 and 6-15. Would you classify them as type A or B WPW?

ANSWER: The QRS complex is predominantly negative in lead V_1 of both of these tracings. Therefore, they would both be classified as type B WPW.

Although in the past it was thought that this classification would be helpful in identifying the location of the accessory pathway (type A WPW was thought to be due to a left-sided accessory pathway, and type B to a right-sided one), recent evidence has shown this *not* to be the case. Nonetheless, this nomenclature survives in practice.

The incidence of WPW in the general population is thought to be between 0.1 and 0.3 percent. Thus, the syndrome is *not* uncommon, and *all* health care providers probably will encounter a number of patients with this disorder during their career. Although WPW may be associated with several types of congenital heart disease, most of the time it occurs in otherwise healthy individuals without any underlying cardiac disorder.

WPW is important clinically for two principal reasons. *First,* patients with this syndrome are prone to tachydysrhythmias, particularly paroxysmal supraventricular tachycardia (PSVT). When conditions are right, the accessory pathway allows retrograde conduction to the atria, setting up a cycle whereby the impulse is conducted down the normal atrioventricular pathway and then back to the atria via the accessory pathway. Less commonly, conduction goes down the accessory pathway and is conducted retrograde via the atrioventricular pathway. In either case, a *reentry* mechanism is established that may sustain the tachycardia for long periods of time.

Second, the ECG of these patients may mimic virtually any electrocardiographic pattern! We have already seen how WPW may mimic LBBB. It may also mimic RBBB, LVH, RVH, and inferior, anterior, or posterior myocardial infarction.

Return to Fig. 6-15 and look at lead aVL. Note that the first QRS complex in this lead (the one conducted down the accessory pathway) has an R wave that satisfies the voltage criteria for LVH, and an ST-T wave segment that has the appearance of "strain." Yet the normally conducted beat (the second QRS complex in this lead) shows that true voltage in this lead is a far cry from satisfying the requirements for LVH.

Now study the second QRS complex in lead III of this tracing. The initial slurring of this negative complex is the result of a *negative* delta wave. When delta waves are oriented in a negative direction (as they are in this lead), myocardial infarction may be closely simulated.

PROBLEM: Examine the ECG shown in Fig. 6-17 obtained from an asymptomatic 30-year-old man. Is there any evidence of preexcitation?

ANSWER to Fig. 6-17: This is *not* WPW, because the QRS complex is not widened, and there are no delta waves. However, the PR interval is definitely

Figure 6-15

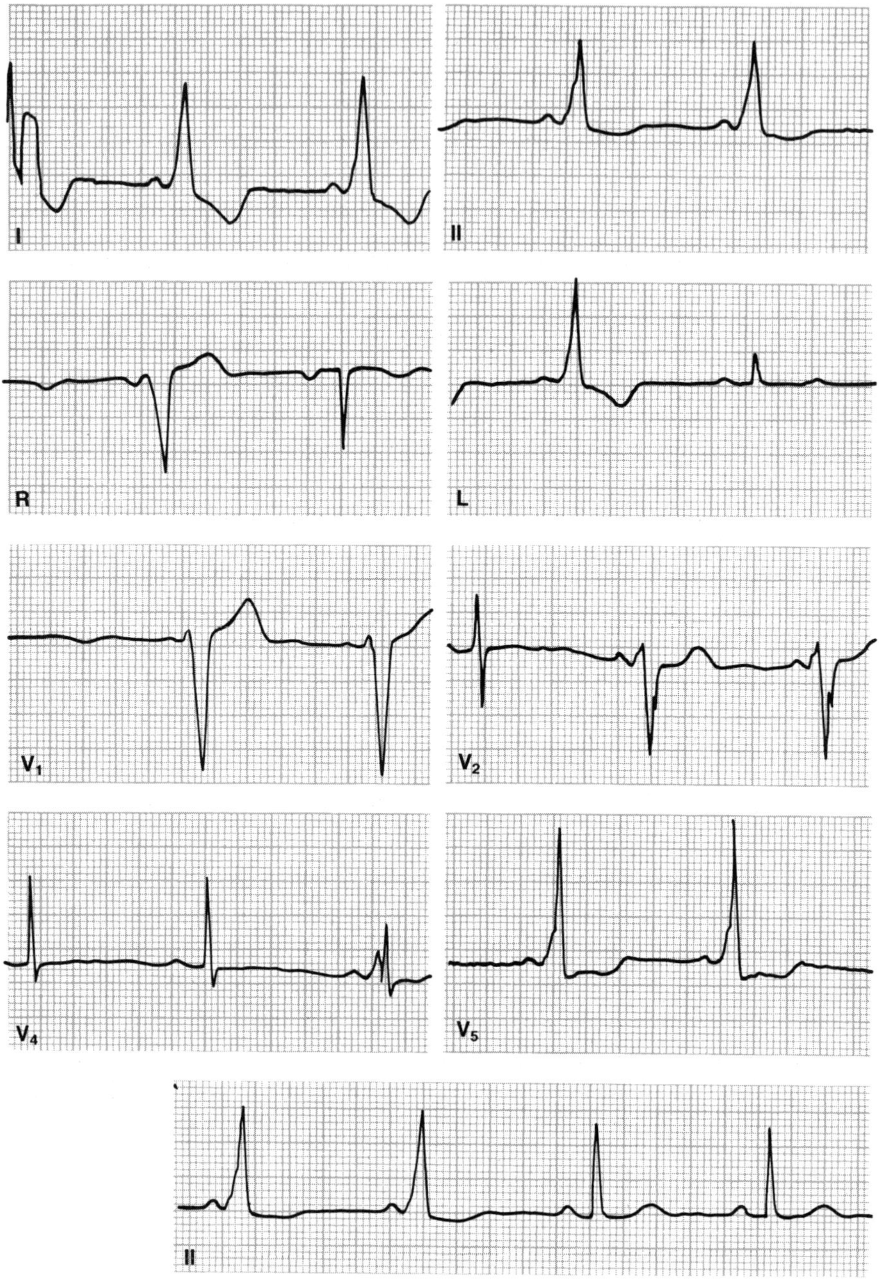

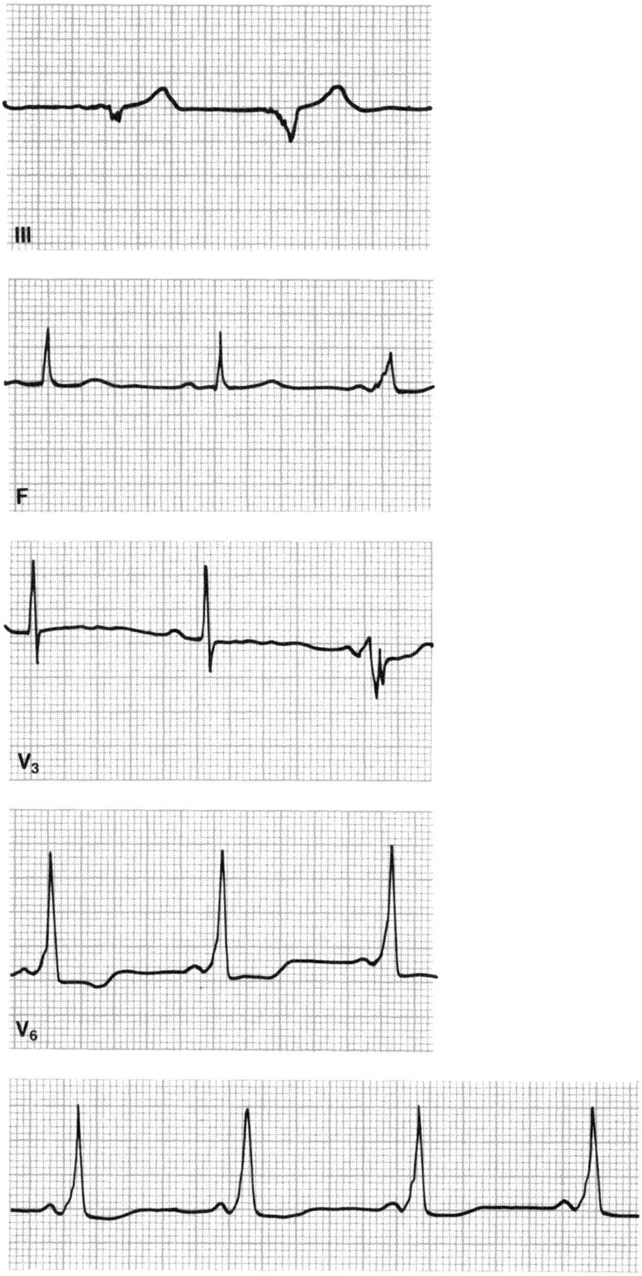
III
F
V3
V6

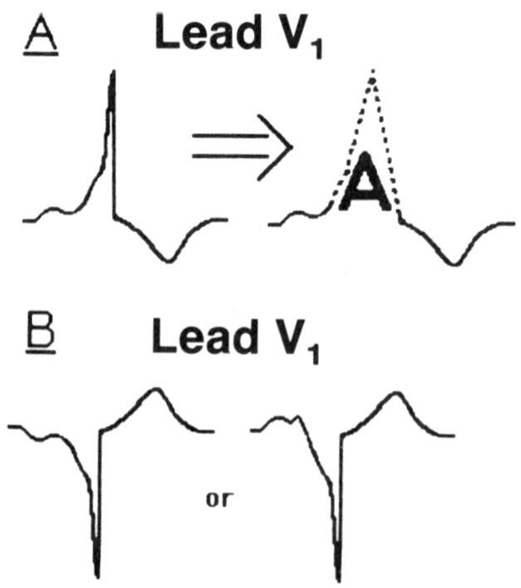

Figure 6-16 Classification of WPW based on appearance of the QRS in lead V_1. **A.** Type A WPW—predominantly upright QRS complex in lead V_1. **B.** Type B WPW—predominantly negative QRS complex in lead V_1. This classification can be remembered by mentally visualizing the *upright* sides of the letter "A."

shortened (<0.12 second) in this otherwise entirely normal tracing. Although preexcitation of the ventricles via an accessory pathway that completely bypasses the AV node is one possible explanation, there are others. A little historical background may be illustrative.

In 1952, Lown, Ganong, and Levine first described the syndrome of a short PR interval associated with normal QRS complexes *and* tachydysrhythmias (particularly PSVT). This *Lown-Ganong-Levine (LGL) syndrome* has been thought by some to be an extension of the WPW syndrome, in that an accessory pathway is thought to connect the atria to the ventricles, bypassing the AV node. Whereas the QRS complex is widened with WPW, however, it is of normal duration in LGL, because the bypass tract links the atria *directly* with the bundle of His.

As a result of the description of this syndrome, many electrocardiographers diagnosed LGL whenever a short PR interval was detected. However, a short PR interval is a common finding in the general population. It is estimated to occur in at least 1 to 2 percent of all adults. Many of these individuals are entirely asymptomatic and *never* develop any tachydysrhythmias. In them, the short PR interval is probably *not* due to an accessory pathway, but rather to rapidly conducting intranodal fibers or an anatomically normal but small AV node.

In summary, the incidental ECG finding of a short PR interval in an asymptomatic individual without a history of tachydysrhythmias should be thought of as part of the *normal* distribution and requires no additional evaluation or follow-up. Only those patients who have tachydysrhythmias associated with PR-interval shortening should be considered to have LGL syndrome.

Our suggested interpretation of the ECG shown in Fig. 6-17 from the asymptomatic 30-year-old man would therefore be:

"Sinus arrhythmia. Short PR interval. Otherwise normal ECG."

Although one could not rule out the possibility that this individual had an accessory pathway, statistically it would be more likely that he did not, and without a history of dysrhythmias, clinically there would be no need to find out.

Review

Let us conclude this chapter on intraventricular conduction delays with two review tracings.

PROBLEM: What conduction disorder(s) is (are) suggested by the ECGs shown in Figs. 6-18 and 6-19?

INTERPRETATION of Fig. 6-18

The QRS complex is wide and has the characteristic appearance of complete LBBB (absence of septal q waves with monophasic R waves in the lateral leads, predominantly negative QRS complexes in the anterior precordial leads, and appropriate-looking secondary ST-T wave changes). However, this is *not* the answer!

PROBLEM: Did you first determine the rhythm before analyzing the morphology of the QRS complexes? What electrolyte disorder might cause this type of rhythm and intraventricular conduction disturbance? (You may wish to refer to Chapter 5.)

ANSWER: The rhythm is regular at about 95 beats/min, but *no atrial activity is evident!* Possibilities include an accelerated ventricular rhythm, junctional rhythm with either preexisting LBBB or aberrant conduction, or sinoventricular rhythm with intraventricular conduction delay due to hyperkalemia.

In fact, this patient had a serum potassium of over 8.0 mEq/L! Sinus P waves returned and the QRS complex normalized over the next few days as the electrolyte disturbance was corrected.

The points to make from this example are several. First, morphology of the QRS complex is typical in *every* way of the characteristic findings of complete LBBB that were illustrated in Table 6-1 at the beginning of this chapter.

Second, the need is apparent to evaluate *all* ECGs *systematically* (preferably in a similar order to that outlined in Table 1-6), even if seemingly obvious findings jump out at you. Failure to do so will result repeatedly in

Figure 6-17

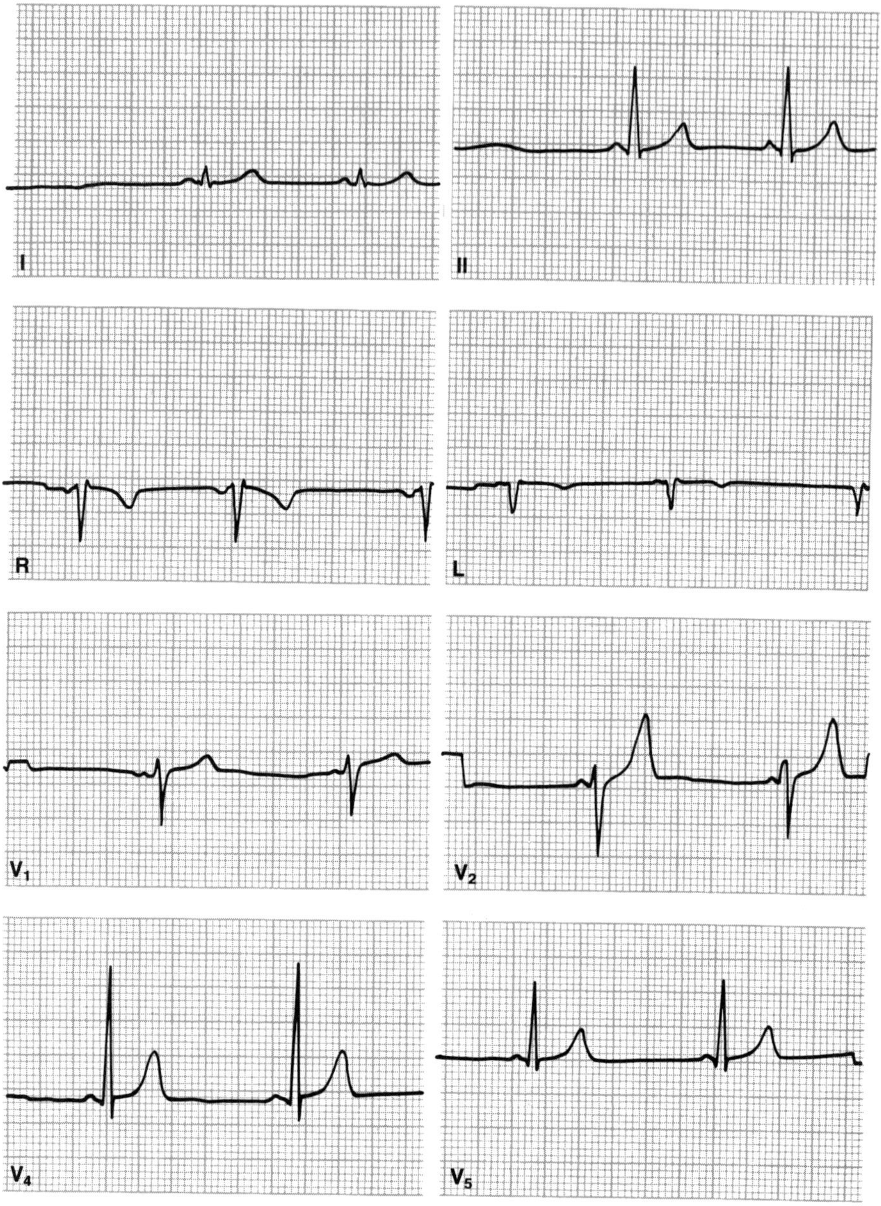

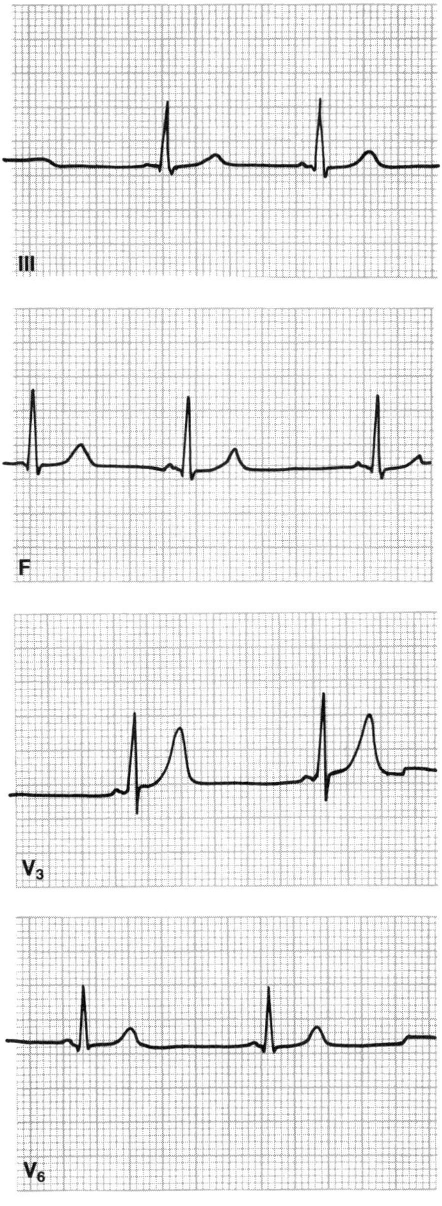
III
F
V3
V6

Figure 6-18

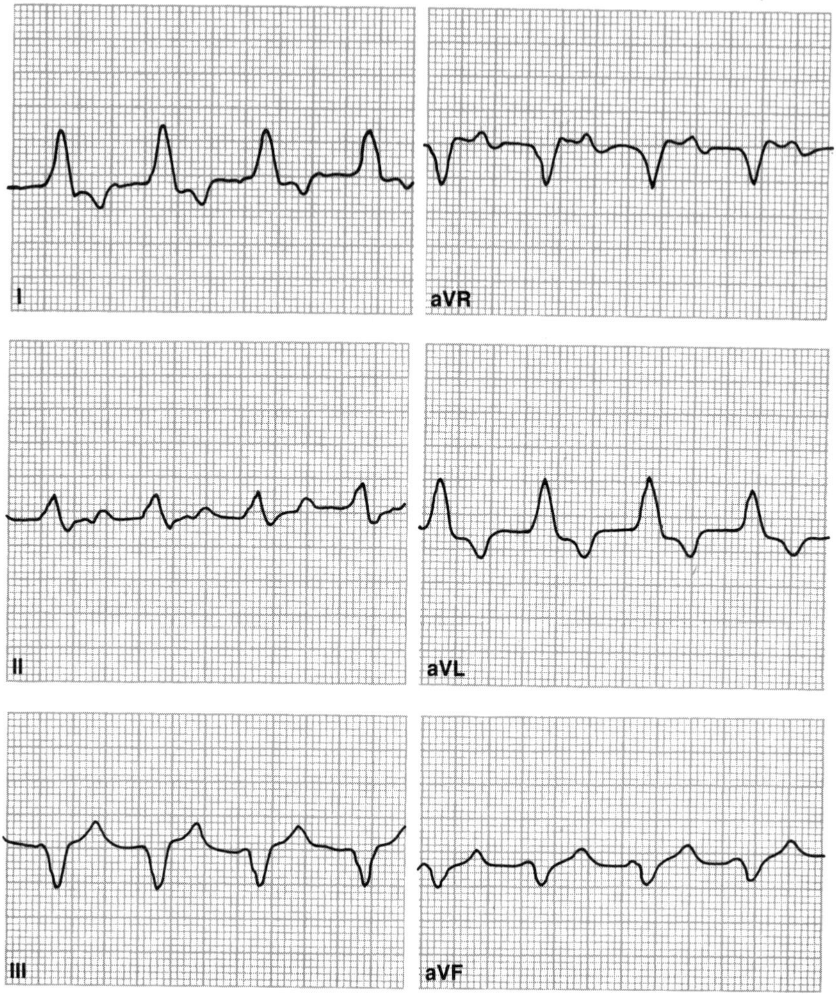

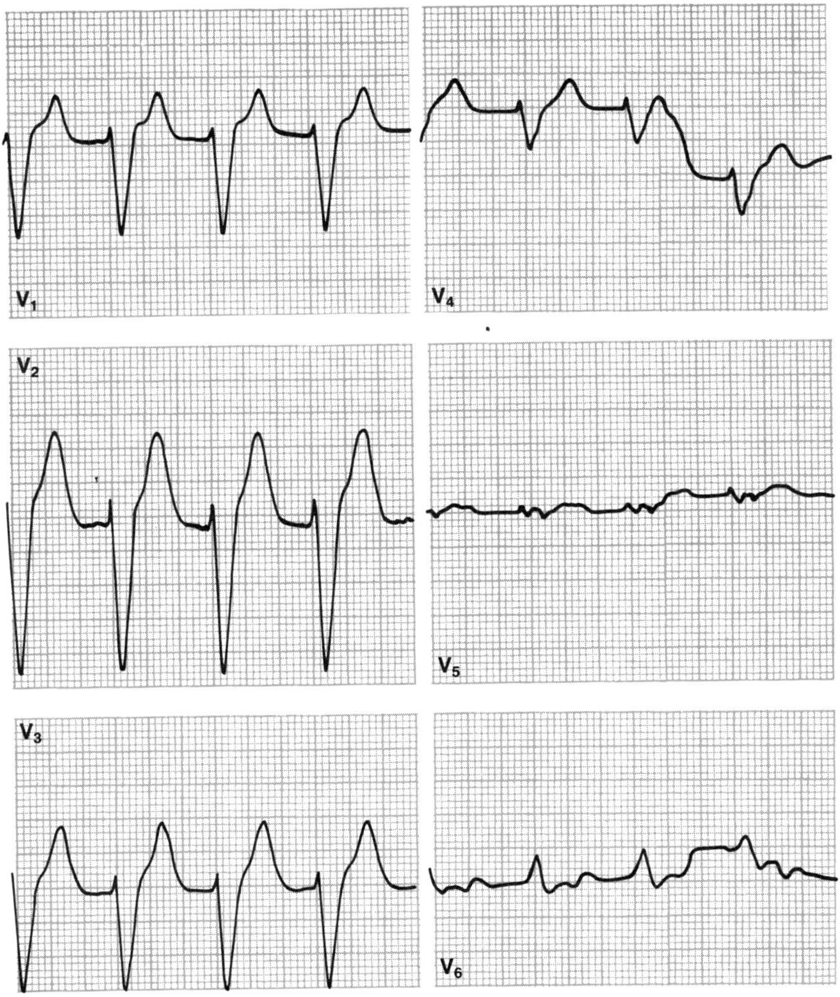
V1
V4
V2
V5
V3
V6

Figure 6-19

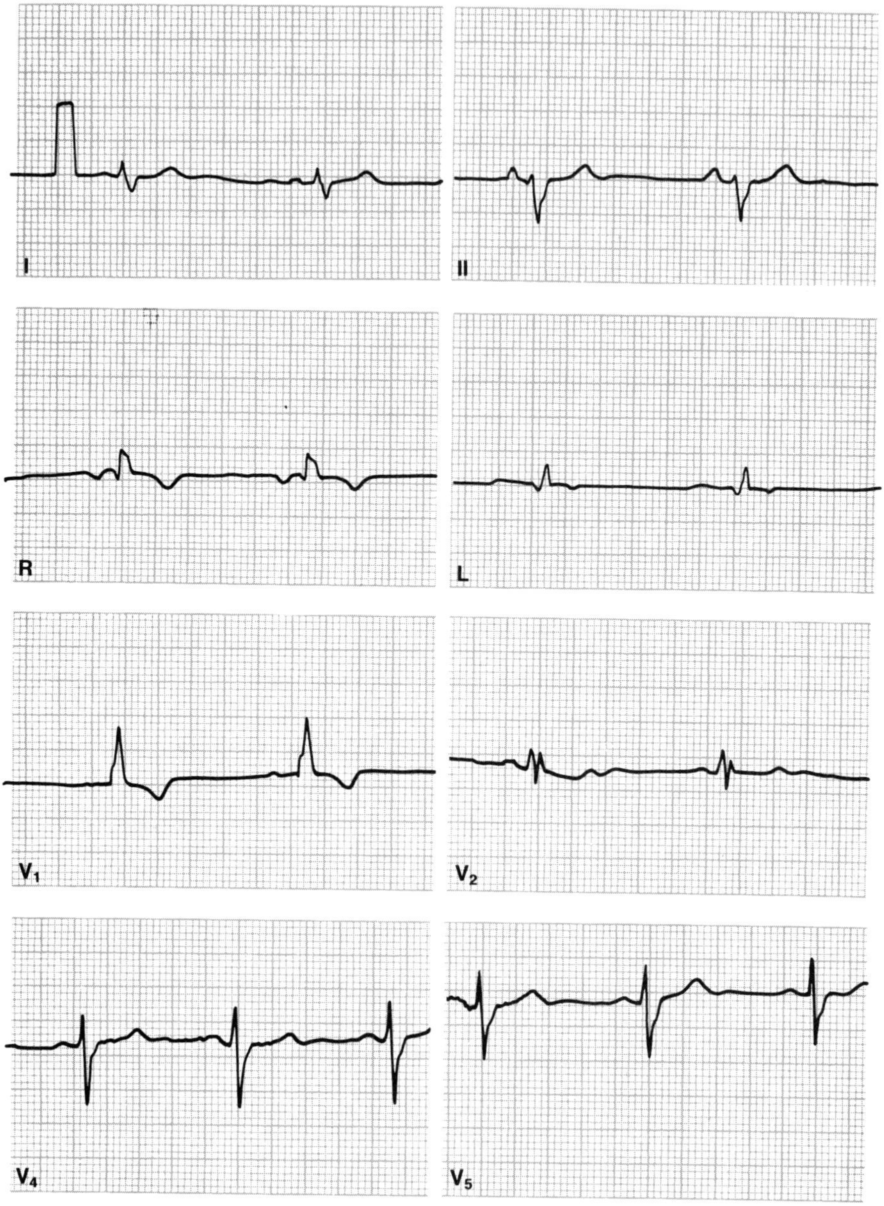

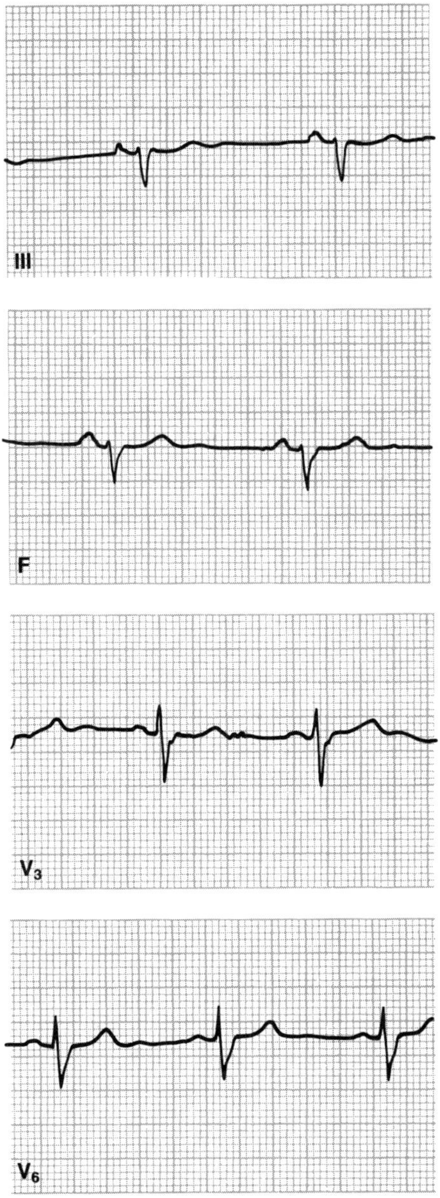
III
F
V3
V6

missing less obvious but equally important findings (such as the lack of atrial activity in Fig. 6-18).

And finally, emphasis on the need for clinical correlation and comparison of the ECG at hand with previous tracings cannot be overstated. Without knowledge of this patient's serum potassium value, or benefit of prior tracings, it would be impossible to differentiate among accelerated ventricular rhythm, junctional rhythm with preexisting LBBB, and sinoventricular rhythm with IVCD (from hyperkalemia).

INTERPRETATION of Fig. 6-19

Rate and rhythm: Sinus arrhythmia at 50 to 65 beats/min.

Intervals

PR interval: 0.16 second.

QRS interval: Prolonged (to 0.12 second). Although the QRS complex does not appear long in many leads, it takes up three little boxes (0.12 second) in lead V_6. The features of complete RBBB are present—RBBB-equivalent pattern in lead V_1 and wide S waves in the lateral leads.

QT interval: Normal.

Axis: Marked LAD (probably to at least −70°). Thus, in addition to RBBB, LAHB is also present (there is *bifascicular* block).

Chamber enlargement: None.

QRST changes: There are no Q waves. Typical ST-T wave changes of RBBB are seen in lead V_1. Otherwise, there are no acute changes.

CHAPTER 7

MYOCARDIAL INFARCTION

Evaluation of patients for acute myocardial infarction is probably the most frequently used application of the ECG. However, there are pitfalls to interpretation that make ECG recognition of infarction an extremely challenging task. In this chapter we will first review guidelines for detecting acute myocardial infarction, and then present examples to illustrate clinical application.

ECG Characteristics of Acute Myocardial Infarction

We have already introduced the three most characteristic findings of acute myocardial infarction. These are development of Q waves, ST-segment elevation and T-wave inversion.

Q waves that are produced by myocardial infarction represent an area of myocardial *necrosis* (irreversibly damaged, or dead, heart tissue). With necrosis, a certain amount of myocardial tissue becomes electrically inert and unable to generate depolarizing forces. As discussed in Chapter 4, Q waves derive from a loss of depolarizing forces over this area of necrosis (Fig. 4-10). Remaining forces of ventricular depolarization now become accentuated (since they are no longer opposed), and the resulting vector of depolarization is reoriented in a direction *away* from the zone of necrosis (in the direction of the unopposed forces). Thus, the Q wave of myocardial infarction reflects the change in direction of the initial vector of ventricular depolarization to an orientation directed *away* from the zone of electrically inert dead tissue.

In the past it was thought that an infarction had to involve the entire thickness of the myocardial wall (it had to be *transmural*) for Q waves to be generated. Infarctions that involved only a portion of the myocardial wall (most often the more vulnerable subendocardial layers—*subendocardial* infarctions), could produce a rise in cardiac enzymes and serial ST-T wave changes, but were not supposed to generate Q waves. From an anatomic viewpoint, we now know that this distinction between subendocardial and transmural infarctions is not necessarily accurate. Transmural infarctions do *not* always result in Q waves, while subendocardial infarctions sometimes *do,* even though they do not involve the entire thickness of the myocardial wall. Thus, it may really be more appropriate to designate infarctions as "Q-wave producing" and "non-Q-wave producing." Because of its persistent use among the medical community, however, we have retained the term "subendocardial," and will continue to use it to refer to those infarctions that do not produce Q waves.

Fig. 7-1 illustrates the characteristic ECG manifestations of acute myocardial infarction. The zone of *infarction* is depicted here as involving the entire thickness of the myocardial wall. It should be apparent from the above discussion that Q waves may be produced even when only a portion of the wall thickness is necrosed, since the *initial* vector of depolarization will still be oriented away from the zone of dead tissue.

A final point to emphasize regarding the genesis of Q waves is that entities other than myocardial necrosis may produce them. Small, narrow q waves are commonly seen in the lateral leads of otherwise healthy individuals, simply reflecting the fact that septal depolarization normally proceeds from left to right. Similarly, Q waves may be produced by idiopathic hypertrophic subaortic stenosis (from septal hypertrophy); LVH (from predominant left ventricular forces that overshadow anterior forces in leads V_1 to V_3); chronic obstructive pulmonary disease (resulting from posterior reorientation of depolarization forces in the transverse plane); and intraventricular conduction delays such as LAHB, LBBB, IVCD, or WPW (from the alteration in sequence of ventricular activation produced by these disorders). It is

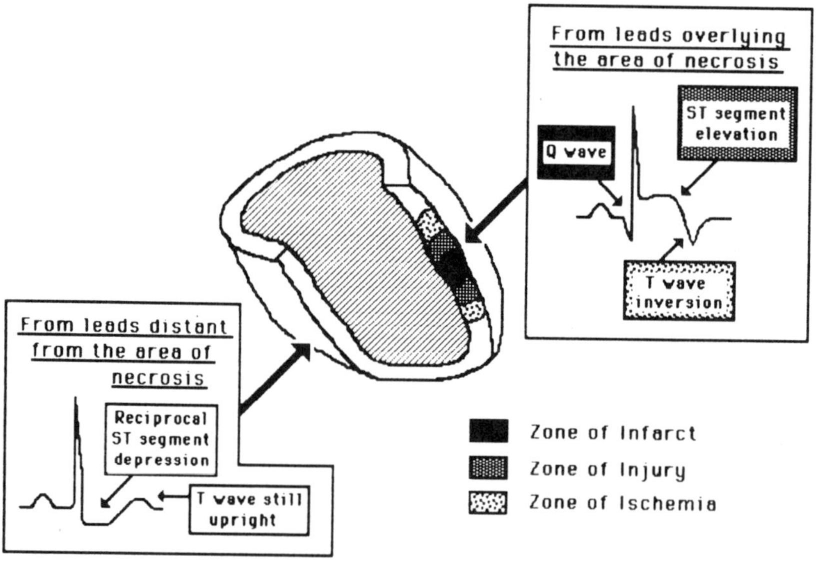

Figure 7-1. Characteristic ECG recordings of acute myocardial infarction

often difficult by appearance alone to distinguish between Q waves produced by any of these entities and those produced by myocardial infarction.

Also recorded from ECG leads overlying the area of an acute infarct are zones of injury and ischemia. Both of these zones represent areas of myocardial tissue that are inadequately perfused, but *not* yet irreversibly damaged.

While one may not be able to do anything about irreversibly lost myocardial tissue, the goal in treating acute infarction would seem to be to limit loss of myocardium from potentially reversible areas (myocardial tissue from zones of injury or ischemia) as much as possible. Conservative measures such as bed rest, improved oxygenation, and relief of pain as well as the newer invasive interventions that seek to reestablish coronary blood flow (streptokinase infusion or coronary angioplasty) all attempt to salvage myocardial tissue that has not yet necrosed.

As depicted in Fig. 7-1, the zone of *injury* lies adjacent to the zone of infarction. The zone of *injury* is thought to represent myocardial tissue with a greater degree of circulatory compromise than the more peripherally situated zone of ischemia. Electrocardiographically, acute injury results in ST-segment elevation of overlying leads. The caveat is that an almost identical picture (dramatic ST-segment elevation) may be produced by pure coronary spasm, in which blood flow through one or more of the major coronary arteries is suddenly and drastically reduced.

The zone of *ischemia* is the most peripherally located area. With diminished blood flow through the major coronary arteries (which course along the *epicardial,* or outer, surface of the heart), perfusion to the innermost layer of the myocardium (the *endocardium*) is compromised. This results in T-wave inversion on the ECG.

Infarction does not necessarily have to take place for there to be ischemia. On the contrary, ischemia is said to occur whenever blood supply to the heart is inadequate to meet demand. The clinical expression of this is angina pectoris. The ECG expression is a primary T-wave change. In the absence of associated infarction, ischemia does not affect the process of ventricular depolarization (the sequence of ventricular activation), but simply alters the process of repolarization. *Symmetric* T-wave inversion is produced. Alternatively, with pure ischemia, ST-segment depression (reflecting compromised subendocardial blood flow) may be another ECG expression.

An additional ECG characteristic that is often associated with acute myocardial infarction is recorded not from leads overlying the area of necrosis, but rather from *reciprocal* leads (leads overlying an area of myocardium that is *distant* from the acute insult). Instead of ST segments going up as they do with an acute injury current, they are *depressed* (reciprocal ST-segment depression). T waves may invert, or they may remain upright.

Reciprocal ST-T wave changes are usually most pronounced during the early hours of infarction. Their recognition sometimes provides a useful diagnostic clue that an infarction is acute. However, it may be difficult to distinguish reciprocal changes from concomitant ischemia occurring in the distant area.

PROBLEM: Apply this information in the interpretation of Fig. 7-2, taken from a 60-year-old man with chest pain. Is there evidence for myocardial infarction?

INTERPRETATION of Fig. 7-2

Rate and rhythm: Sinus rhythm at 85 beats/min. Normal PR and QRS intervals. The QT interval is prolonged. (See below.)

Axis: Normal. Probably about +30°. (See below.)

Chamber enlargement: LAA. The terminal negative component of the P wave in lead V_1 is at least a box deep and a box wide. Although P waves are somewhat prominent and peaked in the inferior leads, they do not meet the amplitude requirement of 2-1/2 mm that is needed to diagnose RAA. There is no evidence of ventricular enlargement.

QRST changes: All three indicative changes of acute myocardial infarction illustrated in Fig. 7-1 are simultaneously present in the *inferior leads* (II, III, and aVF) of this tracing: Q waves, ST-segment elevation, and T-wave inversion. In addition, reciprocal ST-segment depression is present in lead aVL, and to a lesser extent, probably also in lead I. The findings indicate acute inferior infarction.

Note that the QT interval in Fig. 7-2 is prolonged. As is the case for intraventricular conduction delays, myocardial infarction and ischemia have a significant effect on ventricular depolarization and repolarization, and, consequently, often prolong the QT interval. QT-interval determination in this setting will usually not contribute much additional information to the clinical situation.

The mean QRS axis in this tracing is probably about +30°. It is evident that accurate determination of axis in the setting of acute infarction may at times be difficult (as it is here) because of development of Q waves and ongoing ST-T wave changes that distort the baseline.

Significance of Q Waves

PROBLEM: Are the Q waves seen in the inferior leads "significant"?

ANSWER: Because of the common occurrence of small q waves in lateral (and sometimes inferior) leads of normal healthy individuals, criteria have been developed to assist in differentiating normal septal q waves from pathologic ("significant") Q waves indicative of myocardial infarction. Thus, *significant* Q waves are defined as being abnormally wide (≥0.04 seconds in duration) and/or abnormally deep (≥25 percent of the height of the R wave in a given lead). The Q waves in all three of the inferior leads in Fig. 7-2 meet these criteria.

Unfortunately, numerous exceptions exist to these criteria for "significance." A deep Q wave (and sometimes a QS complex) is frequently seen in lead III. When it occurs in isolation, it is of no special importance. Similarly, with a vertical mean QRS axis, a deep Q wave and/or a QS complex may be found also in lead aVL. Once again, it is of no special importance when seen in isolation.

Although a small r wave is present in most individuals in each of the anterior precordial leads (because of septal depolarization), the r wave may sometimes *normally* be lacking in lead V_1 or V_2. In this case, a QS complex is recorded in these leads. Errors in lead placement (applying recording electrodes an interspace too high) may also result in Q waves that mysteriously "vanish" the next day when the ECG is repeated by a different technician. Thus, unless there is strong evidence to the contrary, anterior infarction should *not* be diagnosed unless the r wave is *completely* lacking in leads V_1, V_2, and V_3.

Q waves may be *positional*. Simply standing up may result in enough of an axis shift to produce Q waves in one or more of the inferior leads. Because the inferior surface of the heart lies on the diaphragm, *deep breathing* (with its downward diaphragmatic excursion) may result similarly in Q-wave production, particularly in lead III or aVF.

Finally, although Q waves are known as the "marker of infarction" and usually persist indefinitely, this is *not* always the case. *Q waves may decrease in size with time.* One might ask how a Q wave from a previously documented infarction can "lose significance" with time? The Q wave may get smaller with time, but even though smaller, it is still the marker of the prior infarction. Clearly, small size of a q waves *in no way rules out previous infarction.* On the other hand, it is true that the deeper and wider a Q wave is, the greater the chance that infarction has occurred at some point.

PROBLEM: Is there evidence that anything other than inferior infarction is going on in the ECG shown in Fig. 7-2?

ANSWER: Although ST segments are not really elevated in the lateral precordial leads (leads V_4 to V_6), the ST segment is *coved* and T waves are symmetrically inverted in these leads. As emphasized in Chapters 1 and 5, the *shape* of ST-segment changes is often more important than the degree of elevation or depression. ST-segment coving and symmetric T-wave inversion in these leads suggest the possibility of acute lateral injury with associated ischemia.

Evolutionary Changes of Acute Myocardial Infarction

The typical sequence of evolutionary changes with acute myocardial infarction is illustrated in Fig. 7-3.

The first change to occur is development of a *hyperacute T wave.* Within the first few hours of an acute infarction, T waves overlying the area

Figure 7-2. ECG from a 60-year-old man with chest pain.

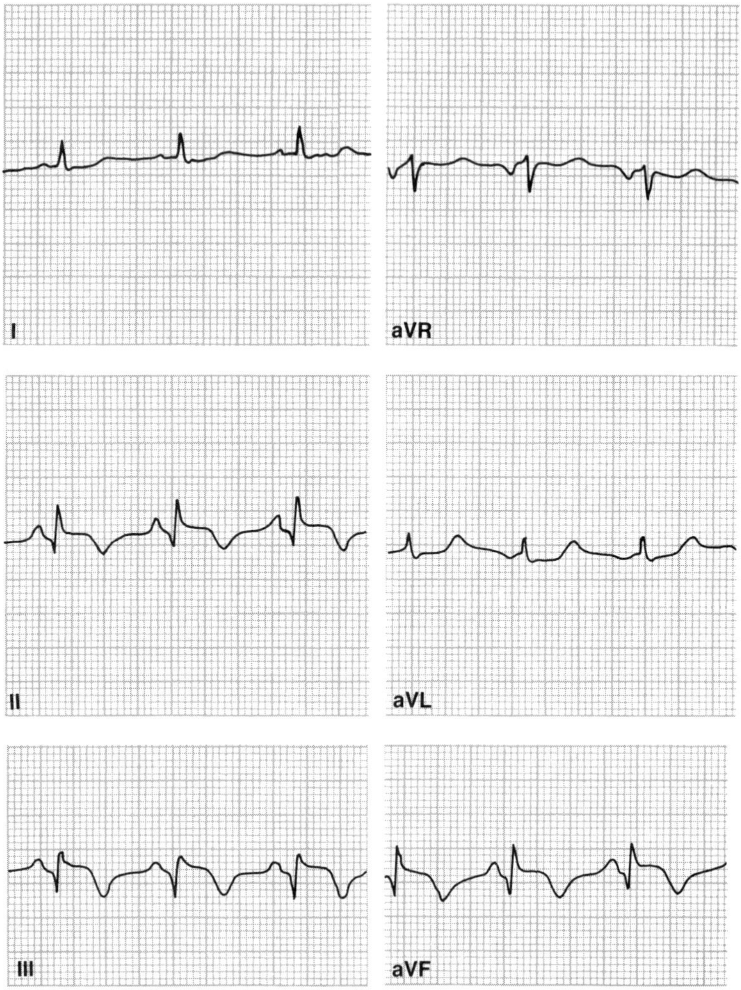

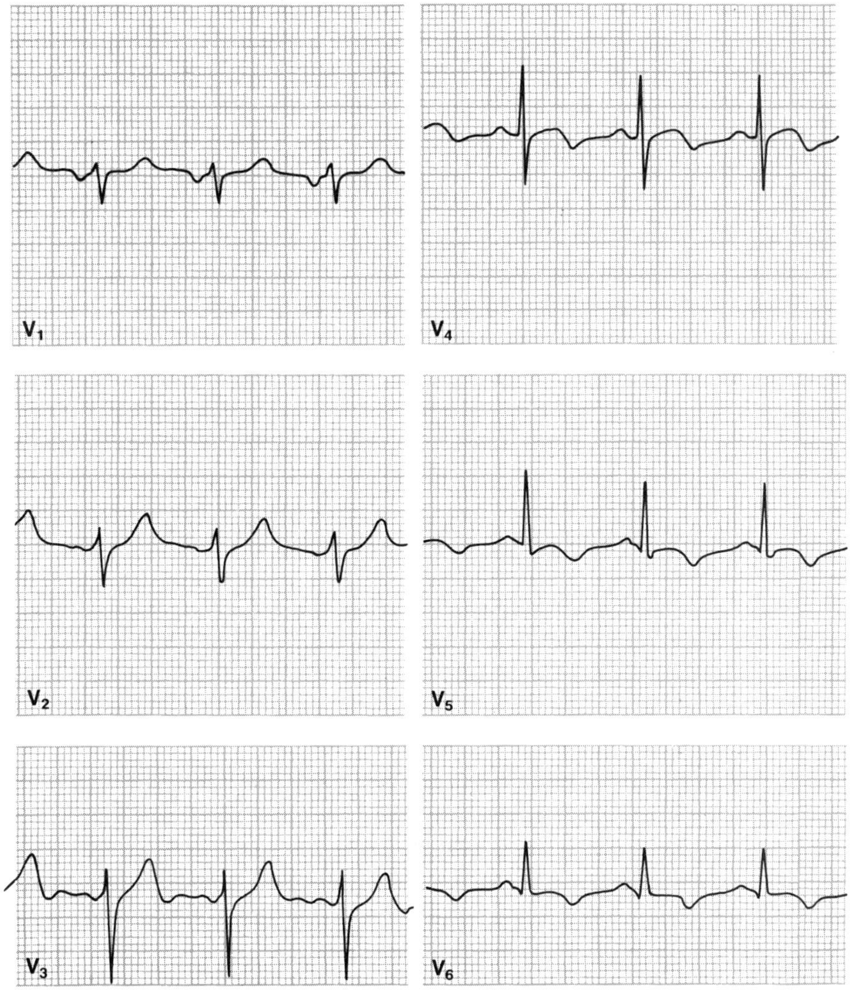
V1
V2
V3
V4
V5
V6

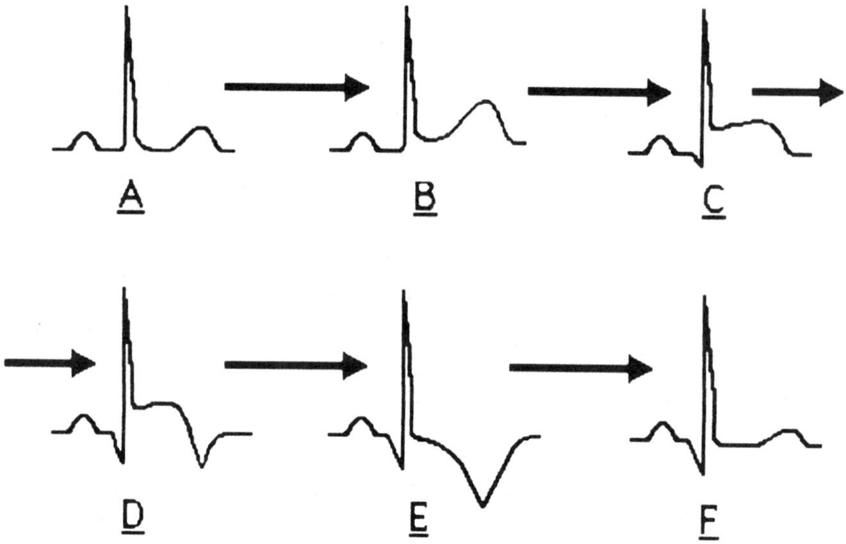

Figure 7-3. Typical evolutionary changes of acute myocardial infarction. **A.** Normal. **B.** Hyperacute T-wave change with early ST-segment elevation. **C.** Continued elevation of ST segment, which now takes on a coved appearance; development of a Q wave. **D.** Deepening of Q wave; inversion of T wave. **E.** Return of ST segment to baseline; symmetric T-wave inversion deepens. **F.** Persistence of Q wave; ST segment and T wave may almost resume normal appearance.

of acute injury often become taller and broader, almost as if they were trying to "pull up" the ST segment (Fig. 7-3B). At times, hyperacute T-wave changes can be quite subtle; they may easily pass unrecognized if an ECG is taken before the stage of frank ST-segment elevation occurs. They are also *transient,* and often have disappeared by the time the patient presents to the emergency department.

The etiology of hyperacute T-wave changes is unknown. Because elevation of the T wave is sometimes accompanied by peaking (to a much greater extent than is shown in Fig. 7-3B), it has been postulated that the hyperacute T-wave change may result from leakage of intracellular potassium from damaged myocardial cells into the extracellular spaces (producing changes similar to those of hyperkalemia, shown previously in Fig. 5-19).

Following the hyperacute T-wave stage, and sometimes "blending" into it, *ST-segment elevation* occurs (Fig. 7-3B to D). ST segments (representing the acute injury current) are usually convex up or coved in shape (they present the "frowny" configuration, previously illustrated in Fig. 1-5). At about this time, *Q waves* may develop or become deeper, implying that necrosis has occurred (Fig. 7-3C and D).

T-*wave inversion* often begins while the ST segment is still elevated (Fig. 7-3D). In a manner suggesting that the ST segment was being "pulled down," deep T-wave inversion now develops as the ST segment returns to baseline (Fig. 7-3E). Finally, ST-segment and T-wave changes may almost totally revert back to normal (Fig. 7-3F). This is *not* always the case; ST-segment elevation may persist for days, weeks, or months. (When ST segments remain elevated in leads overlying an infarct for three weeks or more, development of a *ventricular aneurysm* is suggested.) Similarly, T-wave inversion may persist for days, weeks, or months following infarction. Sometimes T-wave inversion remains indefinitely.

The "marker of infarction" (the Q wave) usually persists, but as mentioned earlier, Q waves may decrease in size with time. Occasionally, they even *disappear,* leaving no trace of a previous infarction!

PROBLEM: Examine the three sets of limb leads in Figs. 7-4, 7-5, and 7-6. These sets of limb leads were all taken from the same patient—a 67-year-old woman who was evolving an acute inferior infarction. They are out of order. Can you guess the probable correct sequence to demonstrate acute inferior infarction in evolution? Which was taken on day 1? Which on day 2? Which on day 3?

ANSWER: The actual sequence for the above sets of limb leads on this patient was

Day 1—Fig. 7-5; Day 2—Fig. 7-6; and Day 3—Fig. 7-4.

Fig. 7-5 demonstrates tall peaked *(hyperacute)* T waves with early ST-segment elevation in the inferior leads and reciprocal changes in lead aVL and, to a lesser extent, lead I. This corresponds to the stage of evolution represented by Fig. 7-3B. The ST-T wave complex in lead aVL is virtually a mirror image reflection of the inferior ST-T wave changes.

Fig. 7-6 shows that small q waves have already formed in the inferior leads. Amplitude of the QRS complex has also decreased in these leads, perhaps reflecting loss of depolarizing forces (necrosis). ST-segment elevation and hyperacute T waves are still present, although the T waves are decidely less prominent than they were in Fig. 7-5. These changes correspond to the stage of evolution represented by Fig. 7-3C. Note also that the reciprocal changes of the lateral leads have lessened, reflecting this later stage in evolution.

Fig. 7-4 demonstrates further evolution in the process. Q waves have deepened, particularly in lead III. The ST segments have returned somewhat to the baseline and assumed a more coved appearance as they are "pulled down" by the symmetrically inverting T waves. These changes correspond to stages D and E in Fig. 7-3. Reciprocal changes in the lateral leads have almost resolved.

Despite the orderly sequence of evolutionary changes described here, in practice it is often exceedingly difficult to determine the age of an infarct

Figure 7-4

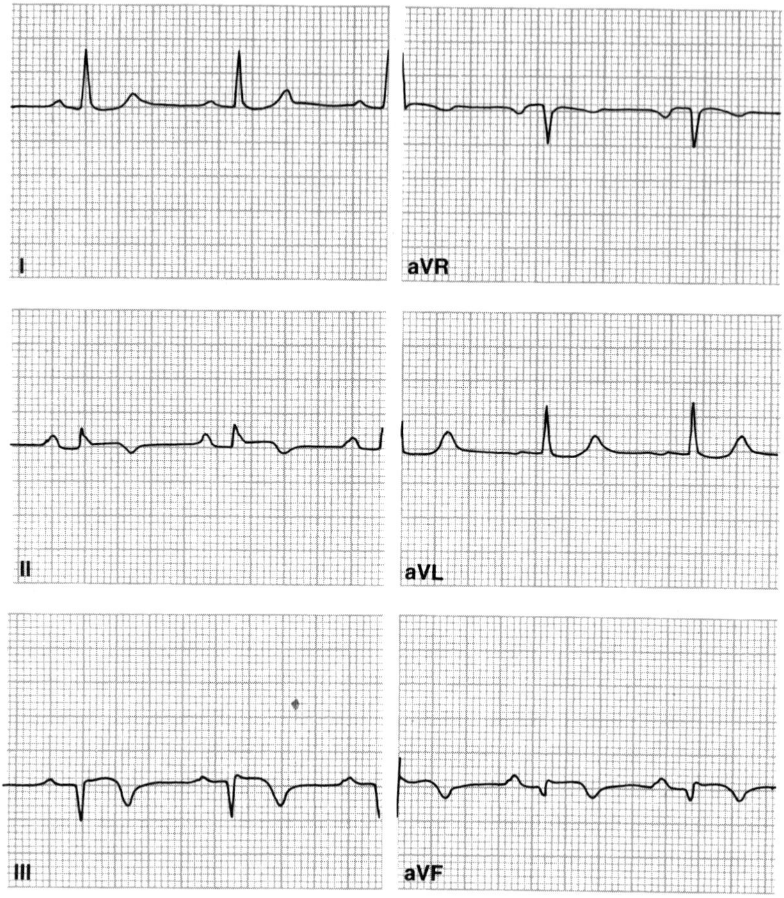

Figure 7-5

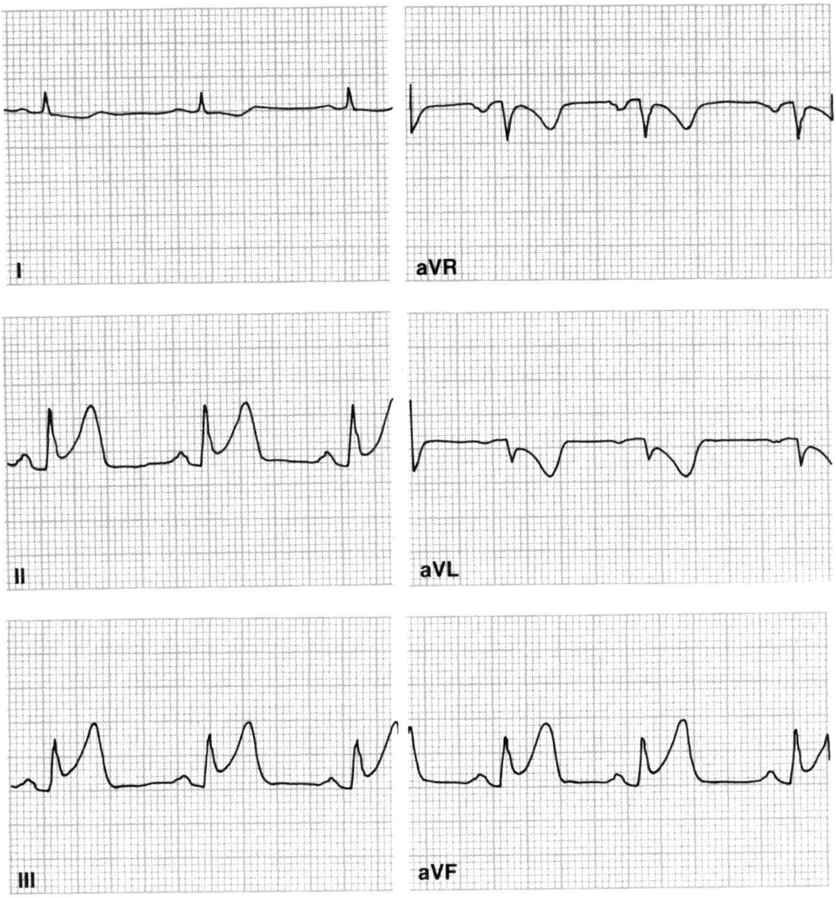

Figure 7-6

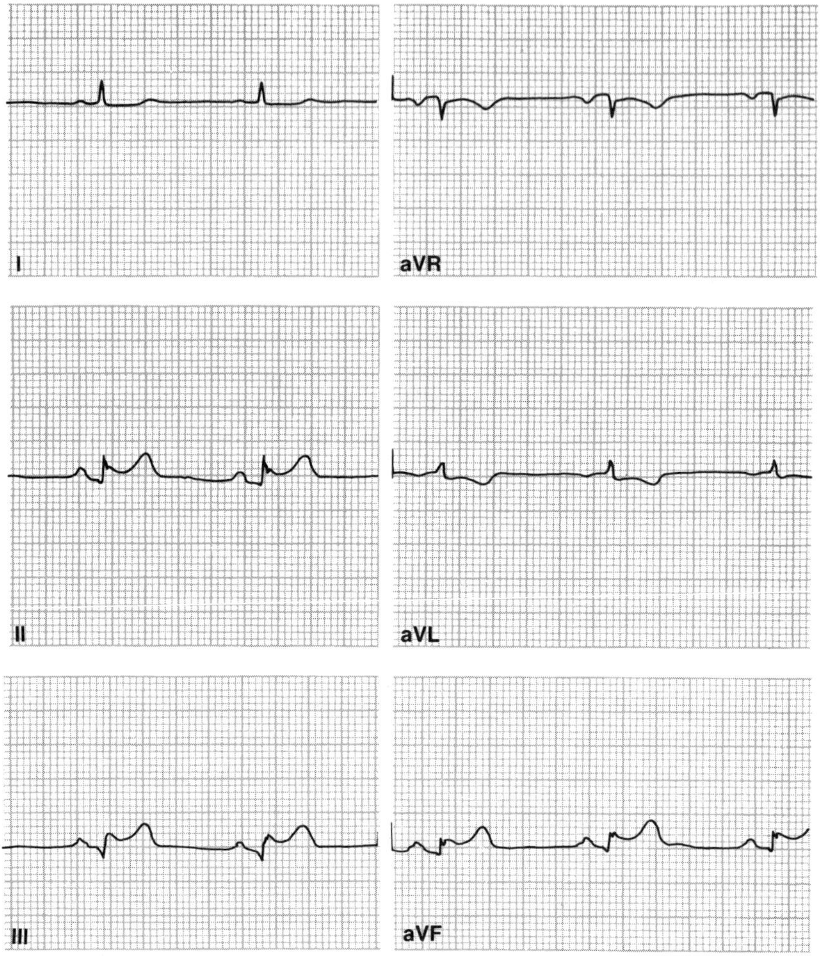

from an ECG, particularly in the absence of previous tracings or clinical history. Realistically, one often can do no better than to say than an infarction is "probably" acute, subacute, or old. *"Acute"* in this context is used to mean that the infarct has occurred within the past several hours to a day ago; *"subacute"* (or recent), that the infarct has occurred within the past few days or weeks; and *"old"* that it occurred in the more distant past.

PROBLEM: Return to the ECG shown in Fig. 7-2. How would you "date" this infarction?

ANSWER: ST-segment elevation in leads II, III, and aVF suggests that the inferior infarction shown here is *acute.* This is supported by reciprocal ST depression in lead aVL, and to a lesser extent in lead I. However, the facts that fairly deep Q waves in the inferior leads have already formed, and that T waves in these leads are deeply inverted, suggest that the infarction may be more than just hours old—it may be *subacute.*

In fact, this ECG was taken on the *second* day of this patient's acute inferior infarction. The ST-segment coving and T-wave inversion in leads V_4 to V_6 raised concern that he was now *extending* the area of injury laterally.

It should be emphasized that no definite time sequence can be assigned to the events illustrated in Fig. 7-3, and the actual order of occurrence for these changes may be quite variable. As mentioned above, hyperacute T waves are often no longer present by the time the patient presents for initial care. In addition, Q-wave development and T-wave inversion may both sometimes be seen very early, and at the same stage as ST-segment elevation.

PROBLEM: Examine the ECG shown in Fig. 7-7, taken from a 40-year-old man who was awakened from a sound sleep by the sudden onset of crushing chest pain. What areas of the heart are involved by the changes shown?

INTERPRETATION of Fig. 7-7

Rate and rhythm: Sinus tachycardia at about 100 beats/min. The PR interval is at the upper limits of normal (about 0.20 second), the QRS interval is normal, and the QT interval is prolonged.

Axis: About +75°.

Chamber enlargement: None.

QRST changes: Small q waves are present in the inferior leads and in leads V_3 to V_6. Despite their small size, these q waves are more than likely "significant." Considering the dramatic accompanying ST-T wave changes, they should probably be interpreted as a portent of what is to come.

Hyperacute T waves and marked ST-segment elevation are seen inferiorly (in leads II, III, and aVF), and in the anterolateral leads (leads V_{3-5}). Reciprocal changes are seen in leads I and aVL.

Figure 7-7. ECG from a 40-year-old man awakened from sleep by crushing chest pain.

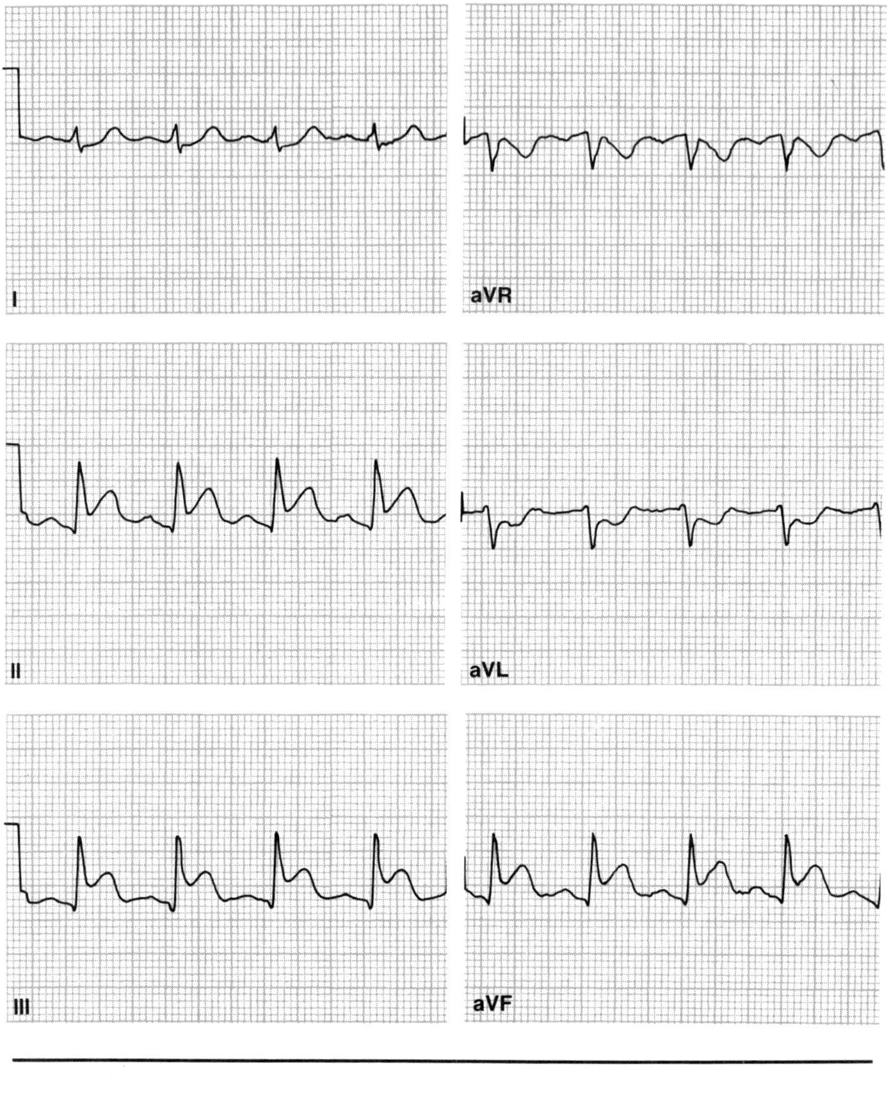

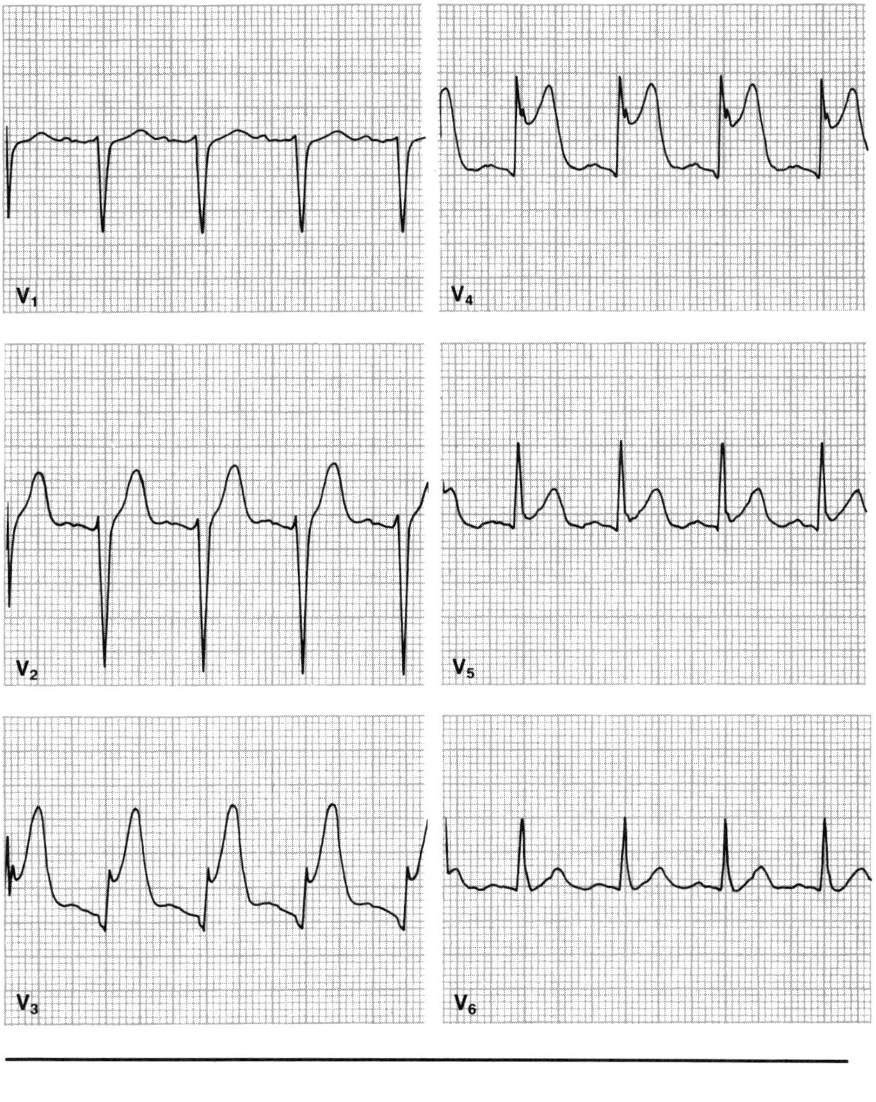
V_1
V_4
V_2
V_5
V_3
V_6

It's easy to understand why this patient was awakened from a sound sleep. The ECG and clinical story strongly suggest *acute infero-antero-lateral infarction.* Unfortunately, several hours after the tracing shown in Fig. 7-7 was taken, the patient died from cardiogenic shock, a complication of the extensive necrosis he suffered.

Localization and Prognostic Implications of Myocardial Infarction

Localization of myocardial infarction can usually be fairly accurately determined by observing which ECG leads show characteristic changes. However, determination of the *size* of infarction is not nearly as accurate. The ECG frequently *underestimates* extent of infarction. In addition, certain areas of the heart are only poorly (if at all) visualized on the ECG (they are electrocardiographically "silent"). Specifically intramural or subendocardial infarctions that are surrounded by normal myocardium may be too small to produce Q waves or ST-T wave changes. Atrial, right ventricular, posterior, and apical infarctions are other examples of areas of the heart that are often difficult to visualize electrocardiographically.

Virtually all myocardial infarctions involve the *left* ventricle. Although isolated right ventricular infarction (without accompanying left ventricular infarction) is rare, autopsy studies have shown the *right* ventricle to be involved to at least some degree in up to 25 percent of inferior infarctions. Occasionally, right ventricular infarction does produce acute right-sided congestive heart failure, however, most of the time it is unimportant clinically. Consequently, we will concern ourselves principally with infarction of the left ventricle.

Left ventricular infarctions can be divided into two main groups, depending on whether the inferior or anterior wall of the heart is primarily involved. Clinically, this distinction is important because of the different therapeutic and prognostic implications of these two types of infarctions.

In general, *anterior* infarctions tend to carry a poorer prognosis than inferior infarctions. Whereas any patient with acute infarction may develop lethal ventricular dysrhythmias, development of pump failure (cardiogenic shock) seems to be closely related to the size of the infarct. It becomes increasingly likely when more than 35 percent of total ventricular mass has been destroyed. Since anterior infarctions tend to be larger than inferior infarctions, they have a greater predisposition for developing this dreaded complication.

Severe conduction system defects (Mobitz type II 2° AV block, 3° AV block, and bundle branch blocks) are also more common with anterior infarction. Although 1° AV block and Mobitz type I 2° AV block (Wenckebach) are more common with *inferior* infarction, these conduction defects tend to be transient and do not usually require aggressive treatment. In contrast, conduction disorders that develop in association with acute anterior infarction more often require prophylactic pacemaker insertion to protect against progression to complete heart block. (Discussion of specific conduction defects and the types of infarctions that cause them was covered in detail in the section on The Coronary Circulation in Chapter 4.)

A third clinical difference between anterior and inferior infarctions is the type of autonomic nervous system dysfunction that each usually produces. Parasympathetic hyperactivity is commonly observed with acute inferior infarction. Patients often develop bradycardia, hypotension, or both. If treatment is needed, atropine is usually effective. In contrast, anterior infarction tends to result in sympathetic hyperactivity. This is often associated with sinus tachycardia and/or hypertension. Treatment differs significantly from that for inferior infarction, and may include such medications as vasodilators (nitroglycerin or sodium nitroprusside) or beta blockers. (These different autonomic effects on heart rate may be remembered by thinking of *inferior* infarction as bringing the heart rate and/or blood pressure *down*).

Figures 7-8 and 7-9 schematically show ECG lead groupings used for localization of myocardial infarction. For greater clarity, only the left ventricle is depicted in these figures. As might be inferred from Fig. 7-8, *right* ventricular infarctions would require monitoring of right-sided precordial leads (V_2R to V_4R and occasionally lead V_1) for adequate visualization. With infarction, these leads would show the same sequence of evolutionary changes illustrated in Fig. 7-3. Since right ventricular infarctions are only rarely of clinical importance, however, right-sided precordial leads (V_2R to V_4R) are rarely obtained.

The inferior (or diaphragmatic) wall of the heart, as its name implies, sits right on top of the diaphragm. *Inferior myocardial infarctions* involve ECG leads II, III, and aVF. In the past, the terms "inferior" and "posterior" were sometimes used interchangeably. Both areas are usually supplied by the same right coronary artery. To avoid confusion with terminology, we prefer use of the term *inferior* to designate infarctions confined to the diaphragmatic surface of the heart, whereas the term *posterior* implies involvement higher up on the posterior surface of the heart (Figs. 7-8 and 7-9). None of the standard ECG leads directly view the posterior wall. However, since the anterior wall lies directly opposite, *posterior wall infarctions* can be visualized *indirectly* by observing the anterior precordial leads, which provide an upside-down mirror image of the posterior wall. (Recognition of posterior infarctions will be discussed in more detail later.) Clinically, posterior infarctions are most often associated with inferior infarctions.

Anterior infarctions may involve the septum, the anterior wall proper, or both. They can even extend out to the lateral wall. Pure *septal infarctions* are recognized by development of QS complexes in leads V_1 and V_2. The small initial r wave that normally represents septal depolarization is lost. *Isolated anterior infarctions* produce changes in leads V_2 to V_4, while *lateral infarctions* involve leads V_4 to V_6, I and aVL. Extensive anterior infarctions (anterolateral infarctions) may involve all of these leads.

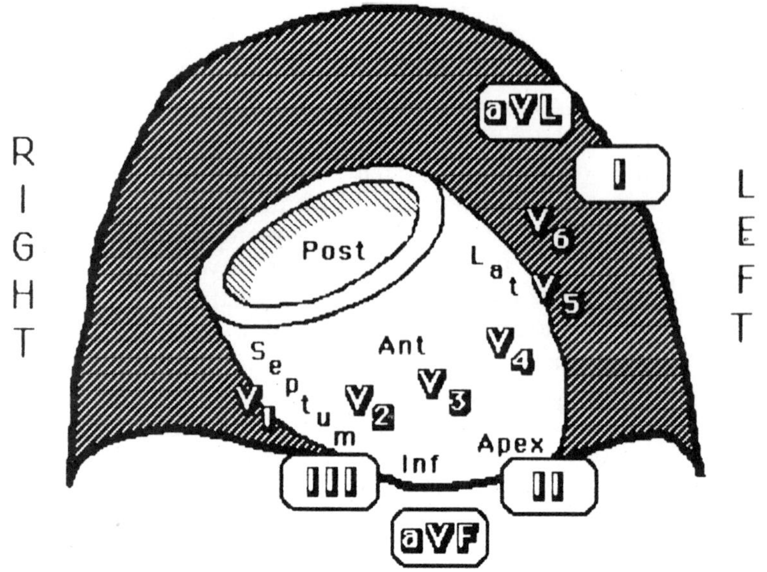

Septum- septal leads = V_{1-2}
Ant- anterior leads = V_{2-4}
Lat- lateral leads = V_{4-6}
Inf- inferior leads = II, III, aVF
Apex- apical leads = II, III, aVF, V_{2-4}
Post- posterior leads = V_{1-3} (mirror image)

Figure 7-8. Lead localization with acute myocardial infarction (AP view).

Note that there is significant *overlap* between the precordial lead groupings:

- Septal leads: V_1 to V_2
- Anterior leads: V_2 to V_4
- Lateral leads: V_4 to V_6.

PROBLEM: Return for a moment to Fig. 7-7. Acute infero-antero-lateral infarction was said to be occurring. Is the *septum* likely to be involved?

ANSWER: Although q waves have developed in leads V_3 to V_6 of this tracing, the small initial r waves that represent septal depolarization are still present in leads V_1 and V_2. This implies that, despite the extensive anterolateral involvement, the septum is still intact!

As much of the interventricular conduction system is contained within the septum, whcther or not this structure is involved with acute infarction may become very important clinically in some cases.

Distinction is sometimes made between the lateral precordial leads (V_4 to V_6) and the lateral limb leads (I and aVL). The latter are often referred to as

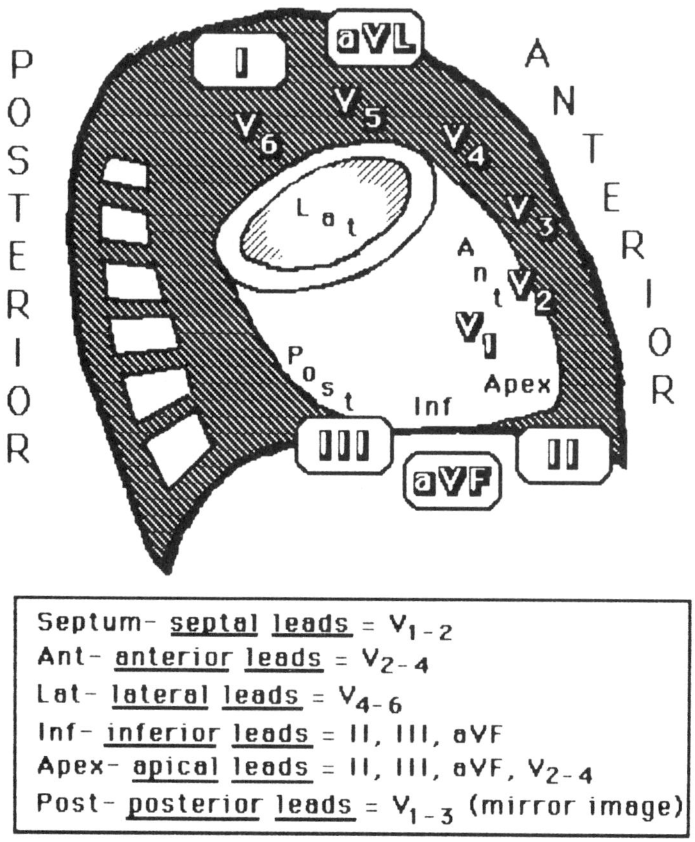

Figure 7-9. Lead localization with acute myocardial infarction (lateral view).

"high lateral leads." This distinction may be remembered easily by thinking of lead aVL as viewing the heart from the left shoulder, which is above (at a *higher* location) where the lateral precordial recording electrodes (leads V_4 to V_6) are placed on the chest.

An often neglected area is the ventricular apex. *Apical infarctions* may involve leads II, III, aVF, and V_2 to V_4. When new Q waves and/or ST-T wave changes are seen in this combination of leads, a *single* infarction involving the cardiac apex should be thought of rather than separate infarctions of the inferior and anterior walls.

As stated above, infarctions of the apex are often electrocardiographically "silent." Two factors may account for this. First, the myocardium of the apex is involved only minimally in the generation of initial forces. Consequently, infarction of the apex may not generate Q waves. Second, there is relatively little ventricular muscle diametrically opposed to the cardiac apex (Figs. 7-5 and 7-6). Thus, there will be relatively few opposing forces available to generate an initial opposing vector (a Q wave) if the apex is infarcted (if the apex becomes electrically inert).

Subtle Changes of Infarction

The ECGs that we have discussed previously have exhibited exceedingly obvious changes. Let's look at a few tracings that show more subtle findings.

PROBLEM: Examine the ECG shown in Fig. 7-10, obtained from a 58-year-old man with atypical chest pain. The patient had been initially evaluated at an urgent care center, and then referred to the emergency department. Fig. 7-10 represents the tracing obtained on his arrival in the emergency department. Based on this ECG, would you admit him to the hospital?

INTERPRETATION of Fig. 7-10

Rate and rhythm: Sinus rhythm at 70 beats/min. All intervals are normal.

Axis: About +40°.

Chamber enlargement: None.

QRST changes: Very small and narrow q waves are present in the inferior leads. Although subtle, the ST segment is definitely elevated in these leads, and manifests a coved appearance. A similar picture (small q waves and coved ST-segment elevation) is seen in leads V_5 and V_6. Equally subtle reciprocal changes are seen in a number of leads, (ever-so-slight ST-segment depression in leads I, aVL, V_2, and V_3). Without the benefit of a previous tracing for comparison, one would have to be suspicious of acute inferolateral infarction.

PROBLEM: The patient was immediately admitted to the coronary care unit. Shortly thereafter, the ECG arrived that had been done several hours *earlier* while he was at the urgent care center. It is shown in Fig. 7-11. How would you interpret this tracing?

INTERPRETATION of Fig. 7-11

Rate and rhythm: Sinus bradycardia at 56 beats/min. All intervals are normal.

Axis: About 60° to 70°.

Chamber enlargement: None.

QRST changes: Although this tracing is not of good technical quality (significant baseline artifact is present in leads V_1 and V_4 to V_6), it demonstrates dramatic changes of acute *inferolateral injury* and *probable infarction.* ST segments are markedly elevated in the inferior leads and culminate in hyperacute T waves. Tiny q waves are beginning to form. In leads V_4 to V_6, even though ST-segment elevation is lacking, hyperacute changes are probably also present, as the T waves appear broadened and peaked. Finally, mirror-image reciprocal changes are seen in lead aVL and the anterior precordial leads.

These two tracings provide a superb example of how a follow-up ECG obtained only hours into an acute myocardial infarction may sometimes look much less abnormal than the initial tracing. Little doubt of the diagnosis can exist from inspection of Fig. 7-11. Although not normal by any means, the ECG shown in Fig. 7-10 demonstrates much more subtle findings. The point to emphasize is that an ECG may look *relatively* or even *entirely normal* despite ongoing acute infarction! When evaluating patients for chest pain, one should never be lulled into a false sense of security by a normal tracing, but should remember that:

- ECG findings of acute infarction can sometimes be delayed for several hours.
- Infarction of "electrocardiographically silent" areas of the heart may not produce any ECG changes at all.
- The ECG in question may be an *intermediate* tracing obtained in between the stage of ST-segment elevation and the one of T-wave inversion. If ST segments have almost returned to the baseline and significant Q waves have not yet formed (as in Fig. 7-10), then the ECG may not look particularly abnormal.

For patients with chest pain, the history is *more* important than the ECG in determining the need for admission to the hospital. An adult with a history suggestive of acute myocardial infarction should be admitted to the hospital *regardless* of what the ECG shows.

Two final points should be made from Fig. 7-11. The first is that the sinus bradycardia in this tracing is typical of the parasympathetic hyperactivity that is so common during the initial stages of acute inferior infarctions.

The second deals with the location of reciprocal changes. As discussed earlier, reciprocal ST-T waves changes are seen in leads *distant* from the acute infarction. Because of the cylindrical structure of the left ventricle (schematically depicted in Figs. 7-8 and 7-9), the anterior, posterior, lateral, and inferior walls of the heart are all almost *equidistant* from each other. As a result, when changes of acute infarction occur in one of these walls of the heart, any or all of the remaining walls may demonstrate reciprocal changes. Thus, in Fig. 7-11, reciprocal changes of the acute inferior infarction are seen in both the high lateral and anterior precordial leads.

PROBLEM: Imagine the ECG shown in Fig. 7-12 is presented to you for review. You are told that it had been obtained a day earlier from a 55-year-old man, but no other clinical history is given. How would you interpret this tracing? Clinically, what would you do?

INTERPRETATION of Fig. 7-12

Rate and rhythm: Sinus rhythm at about 65 beats/min. All intervals are normal.

Axis: About +40°.

Chamber enlargement: None. A terminal negative component to the P wave

Figure 7-10. ECG from a 58-year-old man with chest pain.

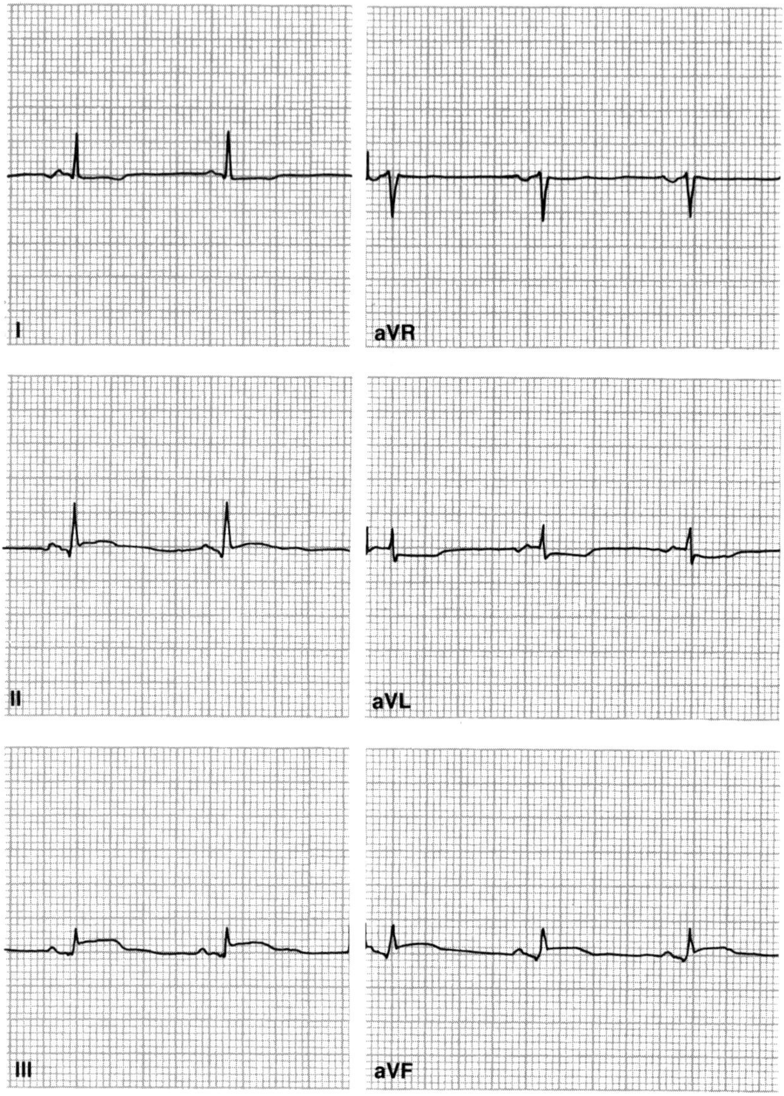

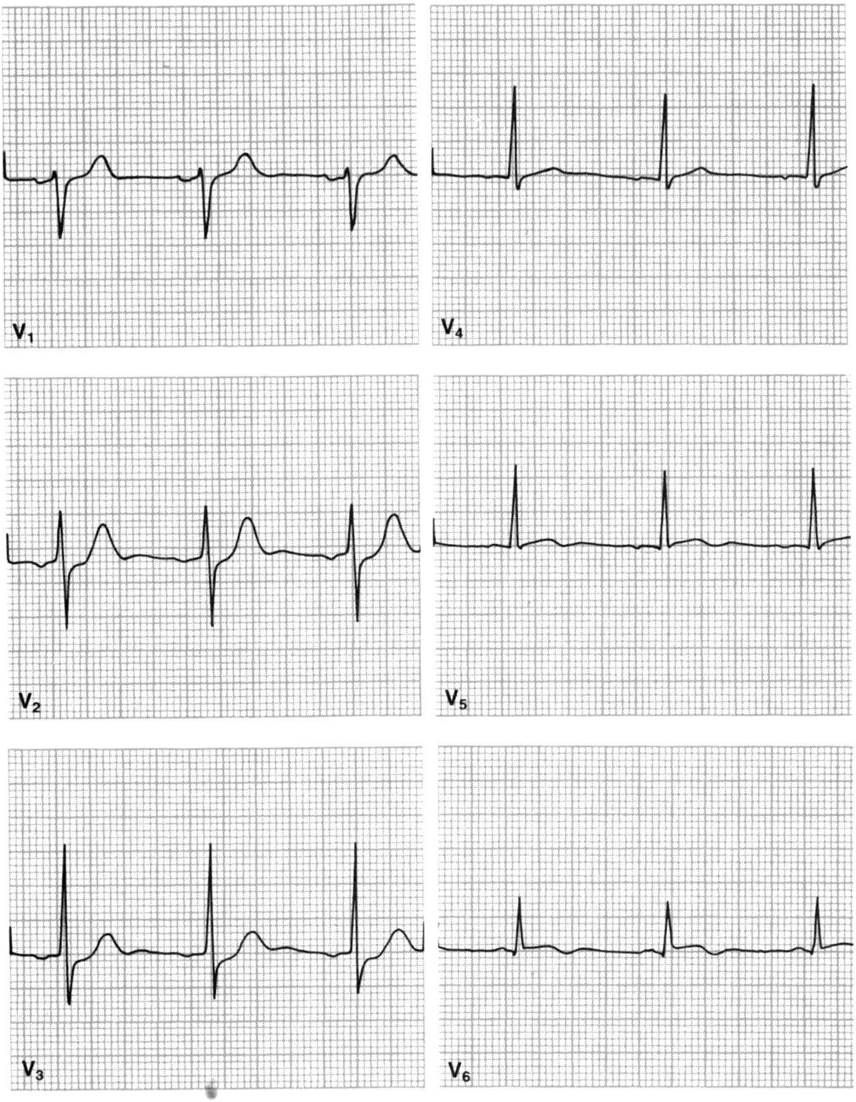
V1
V4
V2
V5
V3
V6

Figure 7-11. ECG from the 58-year-old man. This tracing had been obtained several hours *prior* to the ECG shown in Fig. 7-10.

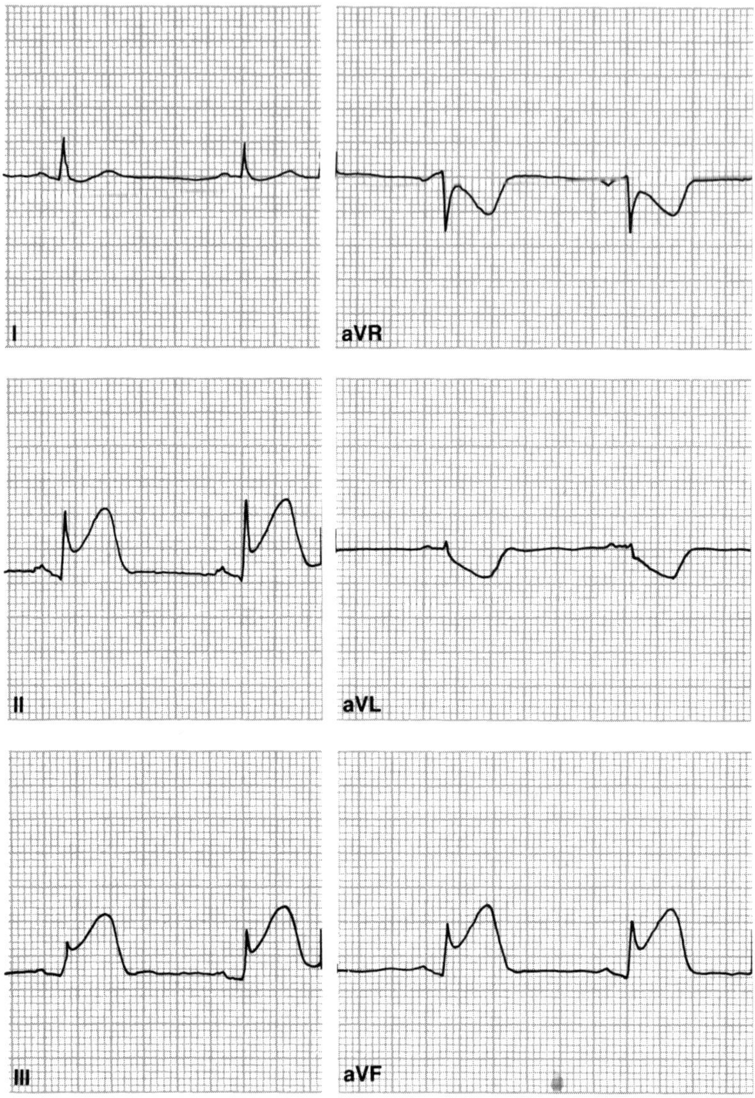

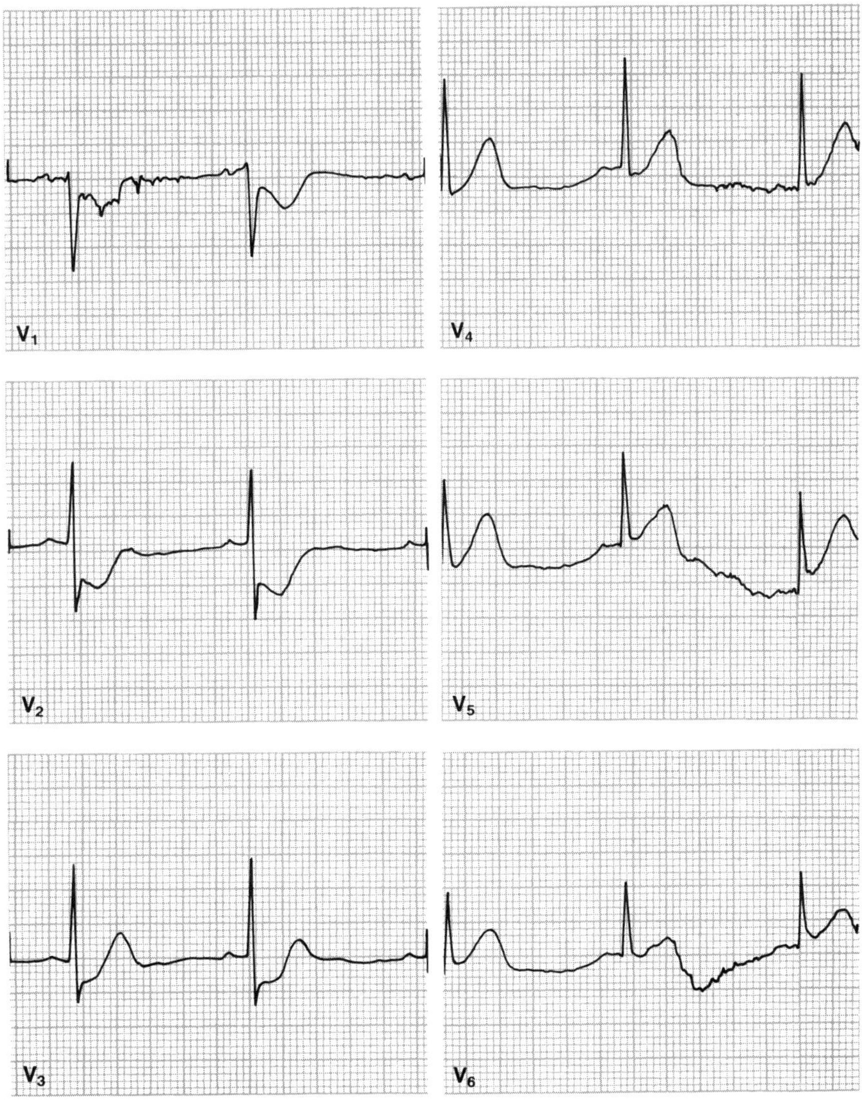
V1
V4
V2
V5
V3
V6

Figure 7-12. ECG from a 55-year-old man.

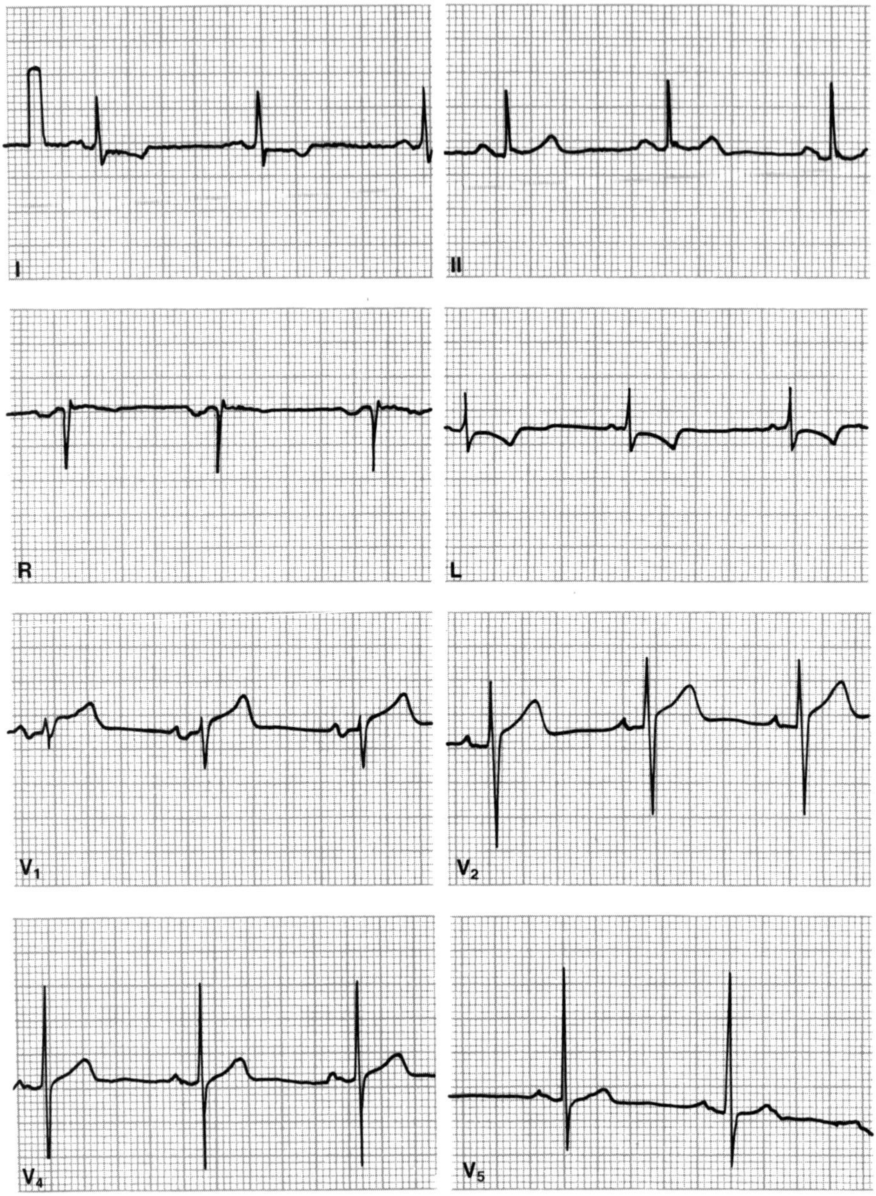

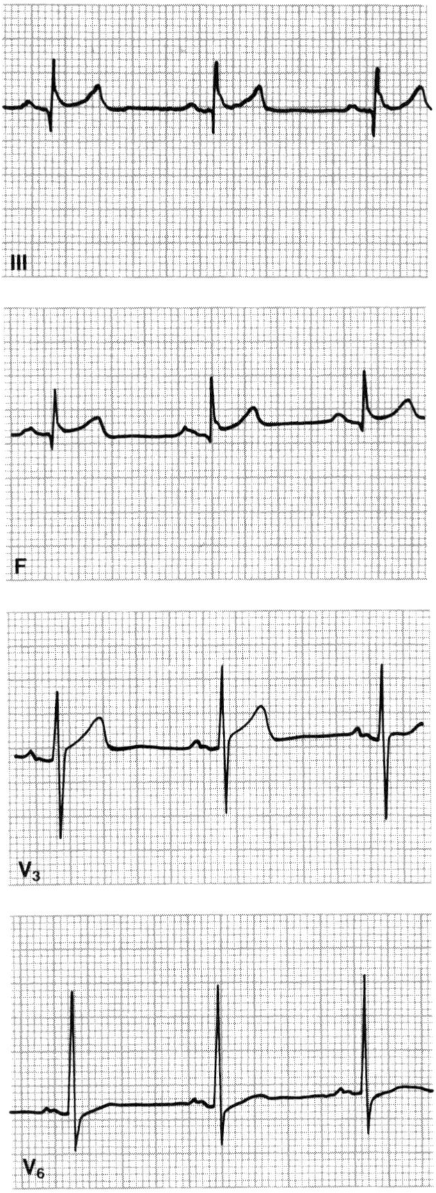
III
F
V_3
V_6

is present in lead V_1, but it probably falls short of the criteria for LAA (that this terminal negative component be a little box deep and a little box wide).

QRST changes: A small, narrow q wave is present in lead aVF. There is a deeper but still narrow Q wave in III. ST-segment elevation with an upward concavity (a "smiley") is seen in these leads, and to a lesser extent in lead II. Despite the *upward-sloping* contour of ST segments in the inferior leads (which often implies a benign process such as early repolarization) and the lack of a q wave in the third inferior lead (lead II), in a middle-aged man (even without a known history of chest pain), one would have to consider the possibility of inferior infarction that *may* be acute.

PROBLEM: Is there any other finding on this tracing that suggests possible acute infarction?

ANSWER: ST-segment depression and T-wave inversion (the mirror-image of the ST-T wave complex in the inferior leads) are present in leads I and aVL. These may be reciprocal changes, and should increase your suspicion for acute infarction.

Two key pieces of information are missing here: clinical history and a previous ECG. In fact, this tracing was obtained as a "routine" follow-up ECG, and the patient was *not* having any symptoms at the time it was recorded. Review of the patient's chart revealed that he had suffered an inferior infarction a number of years earlier, and that the ECG shown in Fig. 7-12 was *identical* to previous tracings.

The points to emphasize here are several. First, in the absence of comparison tracings and clinical history, one *must* strongly consider the possibility of acute infarction from the ECG shown in Fig. 7-12. One would be even more suspicious if a q wave were also present in lead II, and if ST segments were more coved in appearance, but the onus of proof should always be that a patient is *not* infarcting, rather than the other way around.

Second, given the QRST configuration in the inferior leads, the ST-segment depression and T-wave inversion seen in the lateral leads should substantially increase one's suspicions of an acute process.

Finally, an ECG is merely electrical activity recorded on a piece of paper. Interpretation in a clinical void can be a perilous venture. Unfortunately, in the real world it happens all the time. In this particular case, the moment previous ECGs on this patient were reviewed it became obvious that none of the findings on his present ECG were acute.

The next patient is a 78-year-old woman with a history of diabetes mellitus and congestive heart failure (previously controlled with digitalis and diuretics), who presented to the emergency department because of an increase in pedal edema over the past week. She had *not* had any chest pain at all during this time period. An ECG performed in the emergency department (Fig. 7-13) was interpreted as follows:

"Sinus rhythm at 80 beats/min.
1° AV block.
Axis = +70°.
LAA.
LVH and strain and/or digitalis effect."

PROBLEM: Do you agree with the interpretation? The patient's pedal edema was attributed to an exacerbation of her congestive heart failure, and she was treated with additional furosemide before being discharged home. Do you agree with the diagnosis and management?

ANSWER: In general, the above interpretation is correct, with one very important exception.

INTERPRETATION of Fig. 7-13:

Rate and rhythm: Sinus rhythm at 80 beats/min. 1° AV block (PR interval = 0.22 second) is present; the QRS and QT intervals are normal.

Axis: +70°.

Chamber enlargement: The P wave is notched and prolonged (to 0.12 second) in lead II, consistent with LAA. QRS voltage is markedly increased (S waves in leads V_1 and V_2 are recorded at *half* sensitivity), suggesting LVH.

QRST changes: Small, probably insignificant q waves are present in the inferior and lateral precordial leads. Down-sloping ST-segment depression in leads I, II, III, and aVF, in conjunction with the marked increase in QRS voltage is consistent with *strain* and/or *digitalis effect.*

PROBLEM: What about R-wave progression? Do you see anything in the precordial leads that might explain the patient's symptoms (increased pedal edema over the past week)?

ANSWER: Although an initial small r wave is present (as it should be) in leads V_1 and V_2 (implying that the septum is intact), it is *lost* after that! A QS complex appears in lead V_3, and a deep, wide Q wave follows this in V_4. Careful inspection of the ST segments in the anterior precordial leads reveals that they are elevated in V_2 to V_4. What is of even more concern, however, is the *shape* of the ST-segment elevation, particularly in lead V_4 (and to a lesser extent in leads V_5 and V_6) where it is *coved!* The overall picture is very suggestive of *antero-lateral infarction* in the not-too-distant past *(subacute).*

Comparison of Fig. 7-13 with an ECG done on this patient a year earlier (Fig. 7-14) confirms the above suspicions. Note that R-wave progres-

Figure 7-13. ECG from a 78-year-old woman presenting with an increase in pedal edema over the past week. No chest pain.

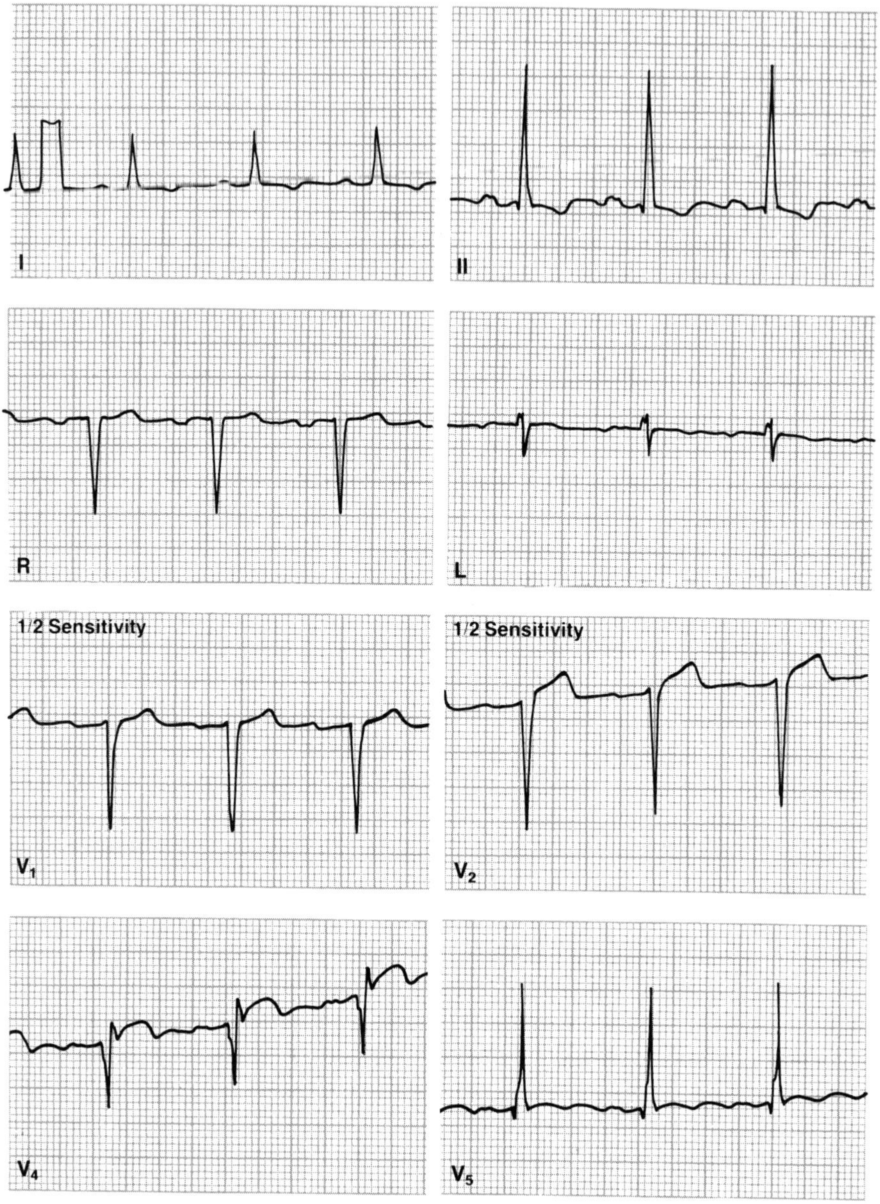

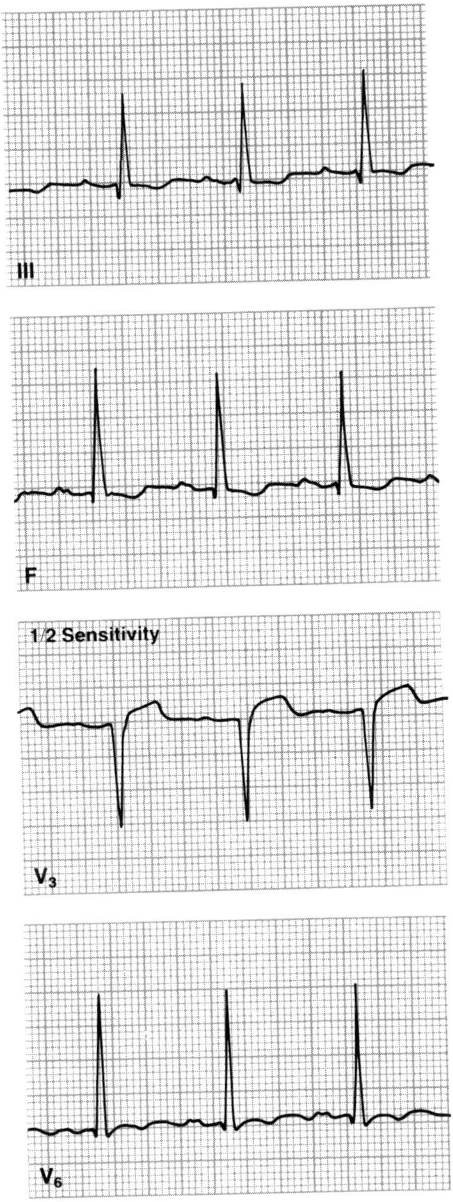
III
F
1/2 Sensitivity
V3
V6

Figure 7-14. ECG from this same 78-year-old woman obtained a year before the tracing shown in Fig. 7-13 was done.

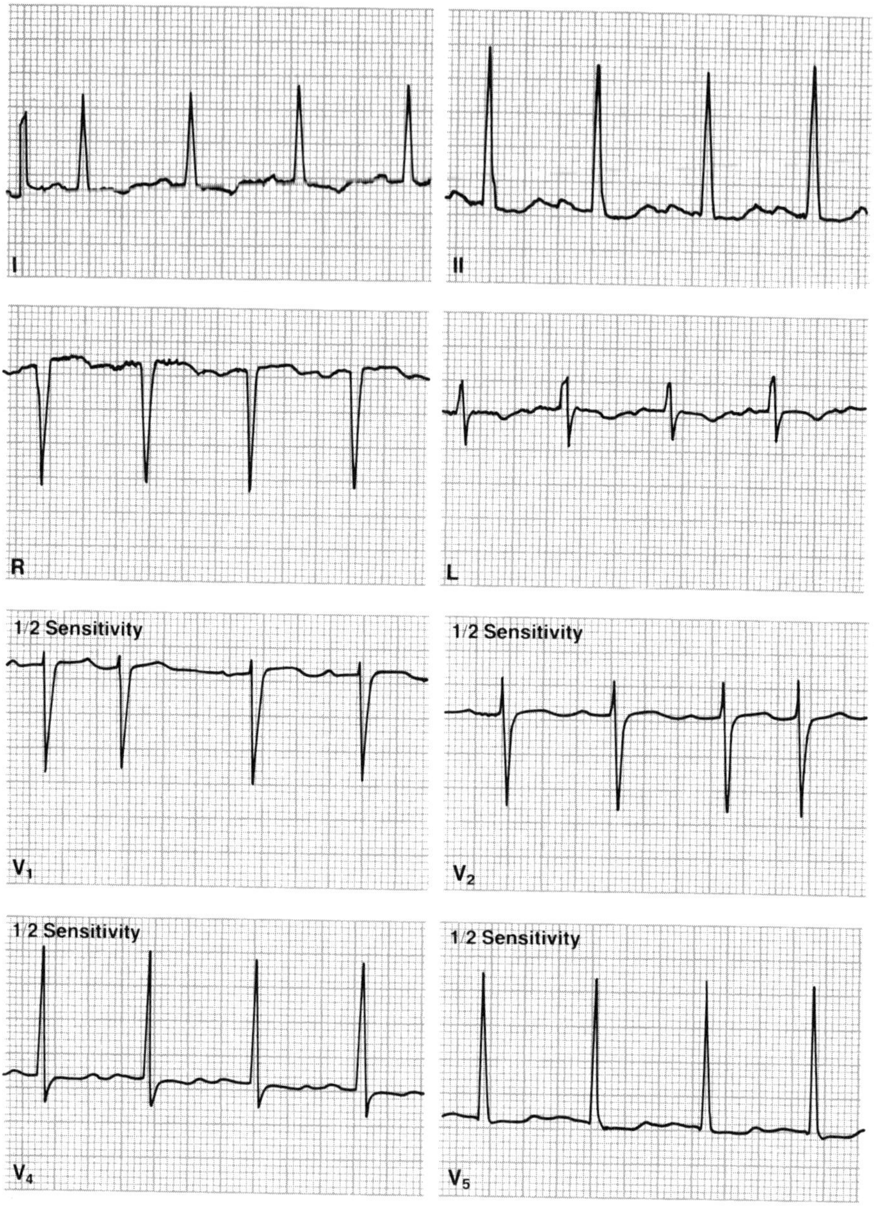

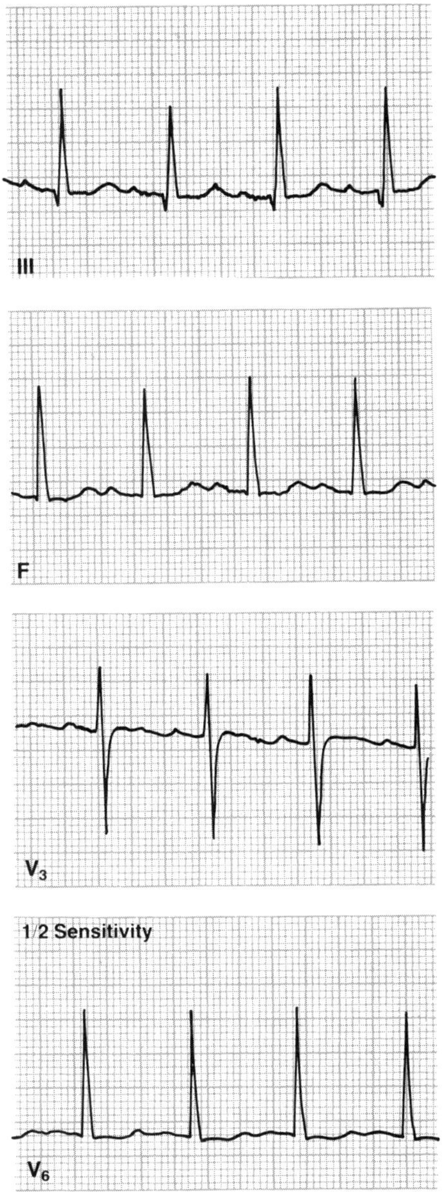
III
F
V3
1/2 Sensitivity
V6

sion in this previous tracing was normal. The coved ST-segment elevation seen in Fig. 7-13 is all new.

Although *loss of R-wave progression* as occurs in Fig. 7-13 may be caused by faulty precordial lead placement, it is often a sign of anterior infarction. In addition, wide, slurred, or notched Q waves such as those in lead V_4 of Fig. 7-13 are also suggestive of infarction.

Silent Myocardial Infarction

"Silent" myocardial infarction is a much more common clinical entity than is generally appreciated. Up to 20 percent of *all* infarctions are thought to be "silent"—without chest pain at all or with atypical symptoms. Much of the time, the diagnosis is only made retrospectively, when an ECG obtained for some unrelated reason (routine preoperative ECG, health maintenance, etc.) demonstrates Q waves that had not been present on a previous tracing.

Silent myocardial infarction seems to be more common among diabetics and the elderly. Both groups may have decreased perception of pain — the former due to neuropathy, and the latter as a result of the aging process. But silent myocardial infarction occurs also in otherwise healthy middle-aged adults, and the diagnosis needs to be entertained whenever patients present with unexplained physical findings that might possibly result from infarction. The elderly patient with stroke, syncope, new onset of a cardiac dysrhythmia, or a sudden change in mentation may have had a silent myocardial infarction as the precipitating factor.

The patient in this case was both elderly and diabetic. She presented with increased pedal edema that was attributed to an exacerbation of her congestive heart failure. However, congestive heart failure should always be regarded as a symptom, *not* as a diagnosis. Given the above history, it is likely that this patient's congestive failure was aggravated by the *acute myocardial infarction* that she suffered at home the week before the ECG shown in Fig. 7-13 was done.

Causes of Anterior ST-Segment Depression

PROBLEM: Return to the ECG shown in Fig. 7-11. This tracing was interpreted as being highly suggestive of acute inferolateral infarction. Is any other area of the heart likely to be involved? Can you think of three possible causes of the ST-segment depression seen in the anterior precordial leads?

ANSWER: The *posterior* wall of the heart may also be involved. Three possible reasons for ST-segment depression in the anterior precordial leads are:

- *Reciprocal ST-segment depression* from the acute inferior infarction.
- *Concomitant anterior ischemia.* Inferior infarction is almost always the result of occlusion of the right coronary artery. Concomitant anterior ischemia (in the distribution of the left anterior descending branch of the left coronary artery) has also been shown to result in ST-segment depression in leads V_1 to V_3. (These aspects of the coronary circulation were discussed in Chapter 4.)
- *Posterior wall infarction.*

Posterior Wall Infarction

As discussed earlier in this chapter, none of the standard ECG leads directly view the posterior wall of the heart (Figs. 7-8 and 7-9). Were one to extend precordial lead placement to include leads V_{7}, $_{8}$, $_{9}$, and $_{10}$ (where lead V_{10} would be in the fifth intercostal space in the midline of the back), leads V_9 and V_{10} would then look directly at the posterior wall of the heart. With posterior infarction, these leads would now demonstrate the sequence of evolutionary changes discussed previously.

Since leads V_7 to V_{10} are usually not obtained (the patient would have to assume the prone position for this), diagnosis of posterior wall infarction is usually made *indirectly* by observing the anterior precordial leads. Since the anterior wall of the heart lies directly opposite to the posterior wall, it provides us with an upside-down *mirror image* of the posterior wall. By applying the mirror test (illustrated in Fig. 7-15), we can detect posterior infarction by the changes it produces in the anterior leads.

Fig. 7-15A shows the Q wave and ST-segment elevation typically seen with acute infarction. If one turns this QRS complex upside down and looks at its *mirror image,* an RS complex with significant ST-segment depression is obtained (Fig. 7-15B). When QRS complexes with this appearance are observed in the anterior precordial leads, posterior involvement should be strongly considered.

Panels C and D illustrate how the test is applied to an ECG. In C, the ECG is held upright. Leads V_2 and V_3 show QRS complexes that look similar to the pattern noted in Panel B. If the ECG is *turned over* (so as to obtain the lead configuration shown in Panel D) and held up to the light, a Q wave and ST-segment elevation is now observed in the anterior precordial leads. This is a *positive* test.

Any of the anterior precordial leads (leads V_1, V_2, or V_3) may show these findings. Note that the taller the R wave in the upright ECG (as in lead V_3 in Panel C), the deeper the Q wave in the turned-over ECG (as in upside-down V_3 in Panel D). Thus, the finding of a tall R wave in anterior precordial leads, *especially* when found in lead V_1, should prompt one to think of posterior infarction.

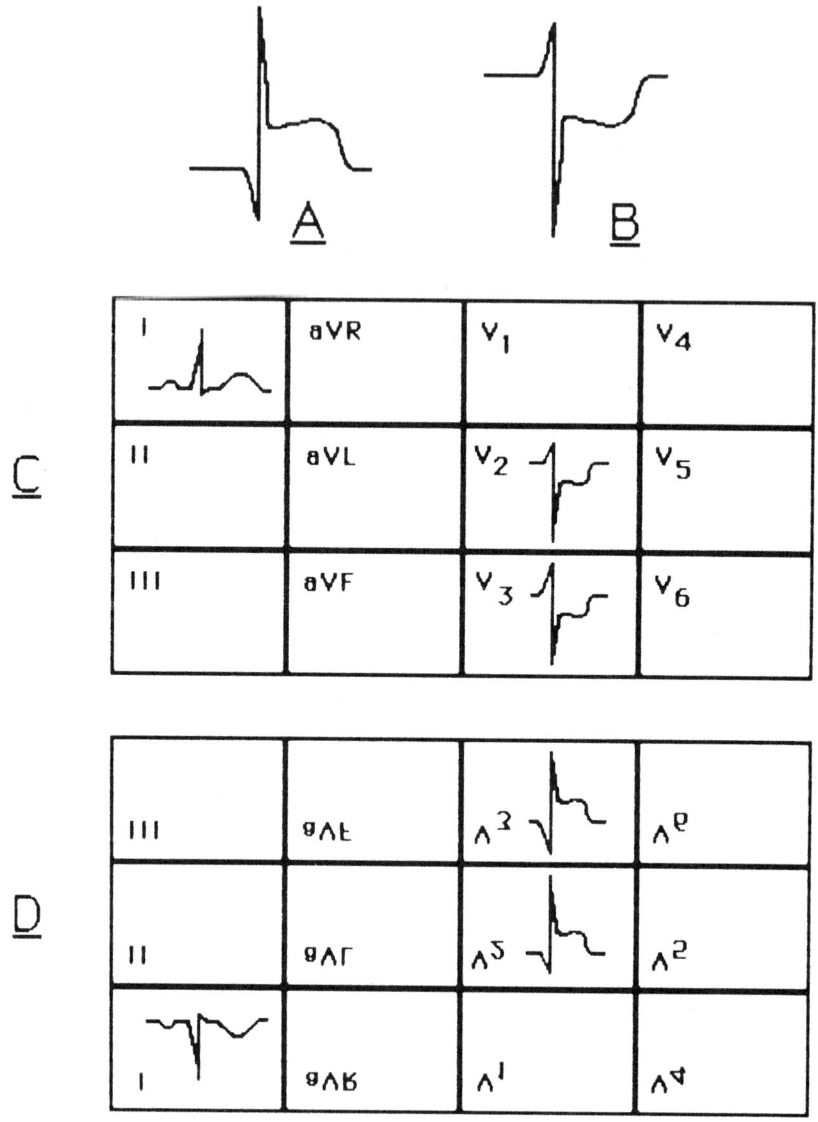

Figure 7-15. Mirror test for posterior wall injury. **A.** Typical pattern of infarction, with Q wave and ST-segment elevation. **B.** Upside-down mirror image of A. **C.** Normally mounted ECG showing anterior ST-segment depression in a pattern similar to B. **D.** Method of turning ECG over to demonstrate pattern of A. Note that the taller the R wave in the upright ECG (C), the deeper the Q wave in the turned over ECG (D).

A virtual prerequisite of diagnosing posterior infarction is evidence of *inferior* infarction elsewhere on the tracing. The reason is that these two areas of the heart are almost always supplied by the same right coronary artery. As a corollary to this, the clinical importance of posterior involvement in *addition* to inferior infarction is that it implies a more extensive infarction and consequently a greater risk of complications.

Returning to Fig. 7-11, in addition to the acute inferior infarction, significant ST-segment depression is noted in the anterior precordial leads. Transition occurs early (relatively tall R waves are present in leads V_2 and V_3), and turning this ECG over and holding it up to the light would result in a *positive mirror test.* Posterior extension of the inferior infarction should therefore be considered as a possible explanation for the anterior ST-segment depression. Reciprocal ST-segment depression, concomitant anterior ischemia, or any combination of the above may also account for this finding.

PROBLEM: Apply this information in the interpretation of the ECG shown in Fig. 7-16, taken in the office from a middle-aged man who complained of "indigestion" the night before. No previous tracing is available. Should the patient be given some antacid and sent home?

INTERPRETATION of Fig. 7-16

Rate and rhythm: Sinus bradycardia and arrhythmia. All intervals are normal.

Axis: −40° (LAHB).

Chamber enlargement: None. Although amplitude of the R wave equals that of the S wave in lead V_1, there is no other suggestion of RVH (normal QRS axis, no RAA, no "strain" in the right procordial leads, and no persistence of S waves across the precordium). One would *not* diagnose RVH on the basis of the relatively tall R wave alone.

QRST changes: Small (probably normal) septal q waves are present in the lateral leads. As noted above, transition occurs early (between leads V_1 and V_2). ST segments in the inferior leads appear to be elevated ever so slightly. In addition, in lead III there is a hint of an upward *convexity* (coving) to the ST segment, with the suggestion that the T wave is "trying to invert." These subtle changes raise the possibility of acute inferior injury as the etiology of this patient's "indigestion" the night before.

PROBLEM: Bearing this in mind, to what might you attribute the relatively tall R waves in the anterior precordial leads?

ANSWER: One should *always* consider posterior infarction in the differential of a tall R wave in lead V_1, *especially* when there is suspicion of associated inferior infarction (as there is in this case).

Applying the mirror test (turning the ECG over and holding it up to the light) transforms the relatively tall R waves into Q waves, and the subtle,

Figure 7-16. ECG from a middle-aged man complaining of "indigestion" the night before. No previous tracing available.

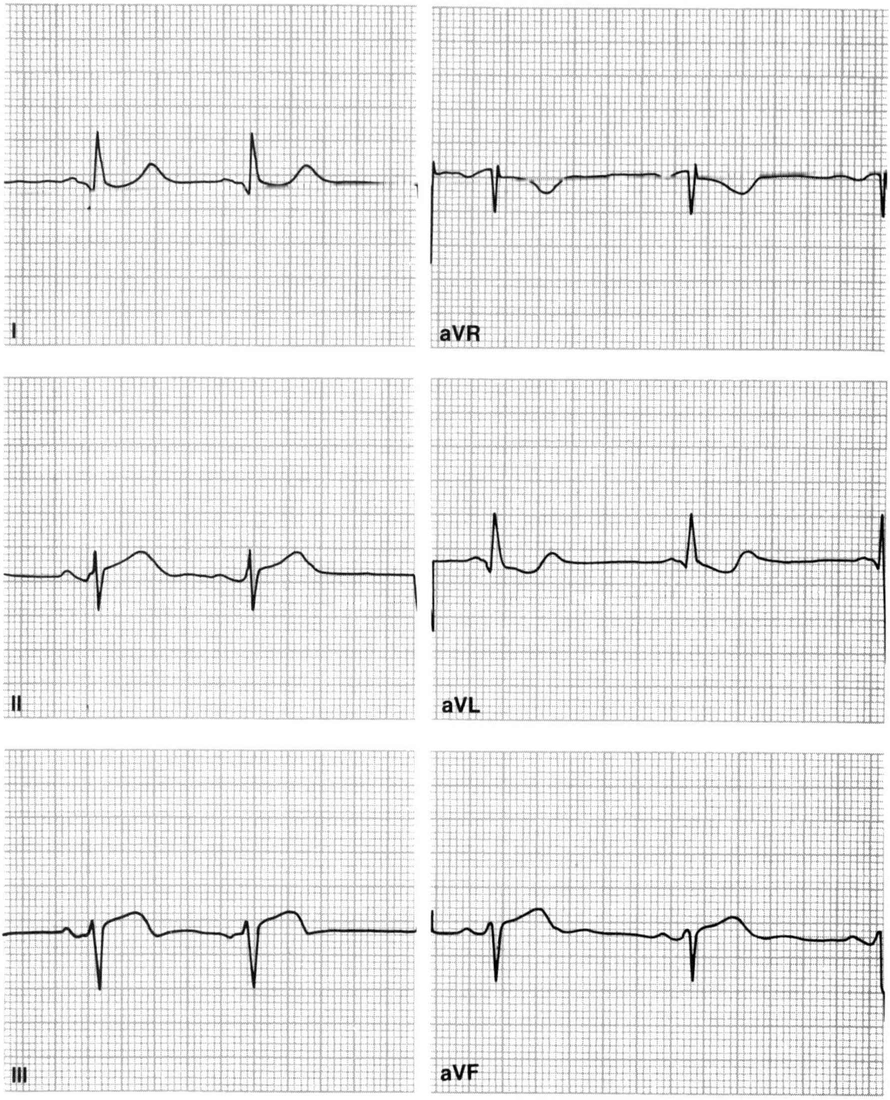

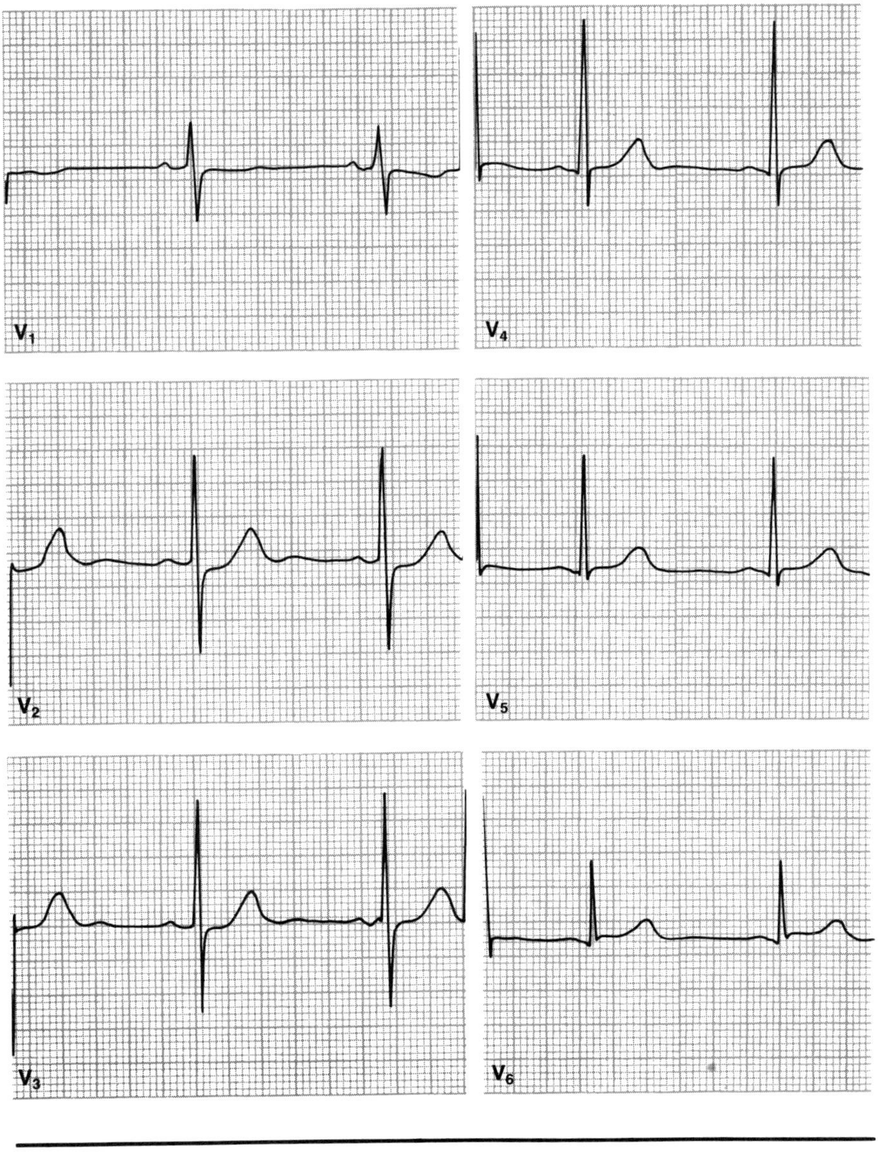
V1
V4
V2
V5
V3
V6

ST-segment depression in leads V_2 and V_3 into ST-segment elevation—a *positive* test.

The ECG obtained on the next day (Fig. 7-17) left little doubt as to the diagnosis.

Deep, symmetric T-wave inversion is now present in the inferior leads. In addition, relative R-wave amplitude (compared to respective S-wave amplitude in a given lead) has increased, particularly in leads V_1 and V_2 where R waves are now clearly greater than S waves. Finally, amplitude of the QRS complex in the lateral precordial leads (V_4 to V_6) has decreased, suggesting loss of depolarizing forces (lateral necrosis). Consistent with this finding is the coved ST-segment and symmetric T-wave inversion now present in lead V_6. The total picture here *suggests evolving infero-postero-lateral infarction.*

One should remember that the inferior (diaphragmatic) surface of the heart, as its name implies, sits right on top of the diaphragm. Consequently, it is not at all uncommon for patients with acute inferior infarction to present complaining *only* of epigastric discomfort. Occasionally there is excess belching and/or "heartburn". Often these symptoms are attributed to "gas" or "indigestion," no ECG is taken, the patient is given a "GI cocktail" and then sent home. This was the sequence of events in this case. The patient had self-diagnosed himself as having "indigestion," and didn't seek medical attention until the next day when his pain was still present.

Inferior Infarction, LAHB, or Both?

A final, *subtle* point to bring out from the tracings in Figs. 7-16 and 17 is that although on the follow-up ECG (Fig. 7-17) R-wave amplitude has decreased in lead II, no Q waves have formed. Instead, the pattern of left anterior hemiblock (LAHB) persists.

A dilemma exists in electrocardiography when predominantly negative QRS complexes are seen in leads II, III, and aVF (an LAHB pattern). The presence of this conduction disturbance may occasionally *mask* the simultaneous occurrence of inferior infarction. As discussed in Chapter 4 (Left Anterior Hemiblock), the presence of LAHB causes the electrical impulse to begin activation of the left ventricle via the intact left posterior hemidivision of the left bundle branch. Since this conduction fascicle is directed rightward and *inferiorly,* initial activation of the electrical impulse should also be directed in this orientation. In contrast, uncomplicated inferior infarction produces the opposite effect. As a result of inferior necrosis, initial activation is directed *away* from the electrically inert infarcted tissue, or in a *superior* orientation.

If both LAHB and inferior infarction are present simultaneously, an unpredictable composite effect will occur. If, as in this case, the initial forces resulting from the LAHB predominate, initial activation will be in the direction of the intact left posterior hemibranch and rS complexes will be seen in the inferior leads. If, on the other hand, the initial forces due to the inferior infarction predominate, initial activation will be *away* from the infarction (superiorly directed), and Q waves will be seen in the inferior leads. *Thus, the presence of either LAHB* or *inferior infarction may mask the presence of the other condition.*

Vectorcardiography

Vector loops were described and illustrated in Chapter 4. (R-Wave Progression). A vector loop simply traces the spread of ventricular depolarization as it varies from instant to instant during a single cardiac cycle. With the recording of a *vectorcardiogram,* vector loops in three dimensions (the frontal, transverse, and sagittal planes) are obtained.

The advantages that vectorcardiography offers over electrocardiography are the ability to closely examine the direction of the *initial* vector of ventricular depolarization, and then to follow spread of the activation wavefront in *three* dimensions. Thus, in Fig. 4-8, anterior infarction is suggested by loss of initial anterior forces in the transverse vector loop. Vector 1 in this figure is immediately directed posteriorly as a result of the infarction. On the other hand, with left ventricular hypertrophy (Fig. 4-9), initial forces (vector 1 in this figure) are normally directed in an anterior and rightward orientation. Although anterior infarction might be simulated by the ECG picture of poor R-wave progression in leads V_1 to V_4, normal orientation of the initial vector of depolarization on the vectorcardiogram would make this much less likely.

In a similar manner, vectorcardiography may assist in evaluation of the initial vector of depolarization in patients with suspected inferior infarction. It may thus be helpful in determining whether small q waves in the inferior leads are indicative of prior myocardial infarction. In addition, it may shed light on the problem posed in the previous section, namely, whether predominantly negative QRS complexes in the inferior leads represent inferior infarction, LAHB, or both.

Initially, vectorcardiograms were greeted with enthusiasm by the medical community. With time, however, much of this enthusiasm has waned. Drawbacks to performing vectorcardiography include the need for special equipment and the extra time required by the technician to apply the recording electrodes to the patient.

Interpretation of vectorcardiograms is much more difficult than interpretation of 12-lead ECGs, so that vectorcardiography can truly be looked upon as an art unto itself. The intricacies of the field extend well beyond the scope of this book. Practically speaking, it is probably enough for the primary-care provider to be aware of the principal clinical settings in which obtaining a vectorcardiogram may help in evaluation of otherwise equivocal ECG findings (Table 7-1).

Figure 7-17. ECG obtained the next day on the middle-aged man in follow-up to Fig. 7-16.

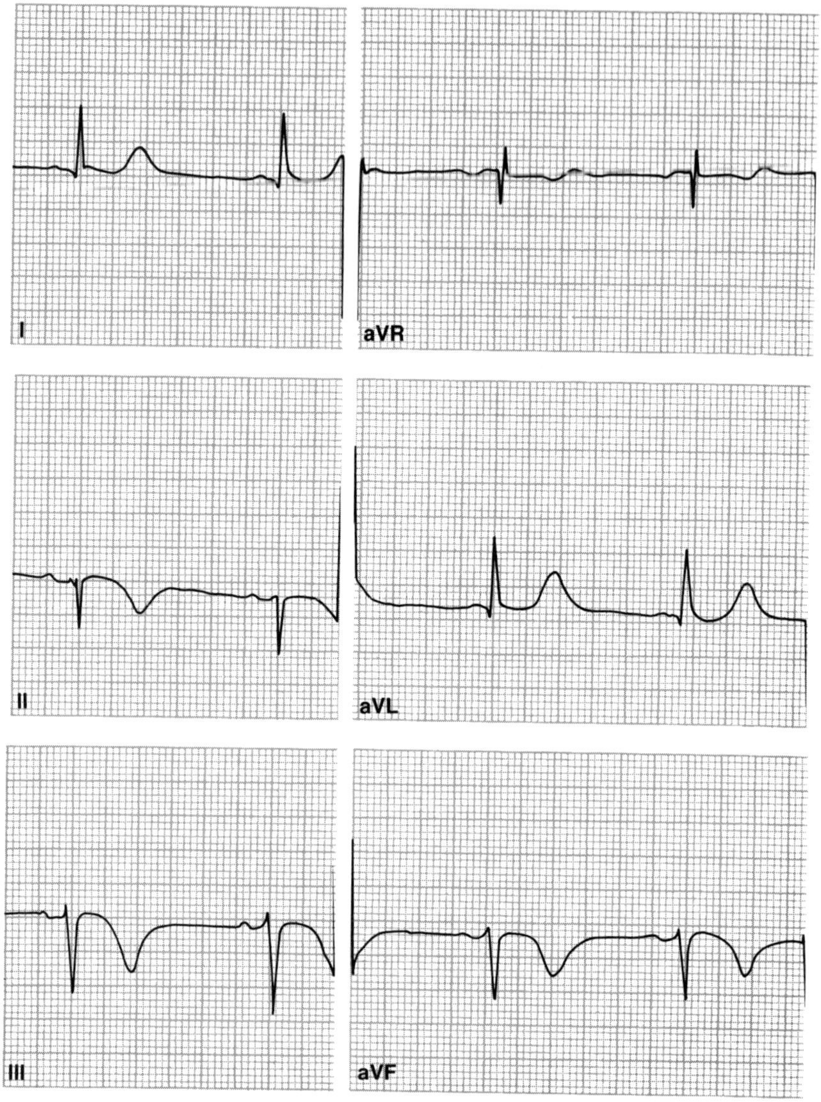

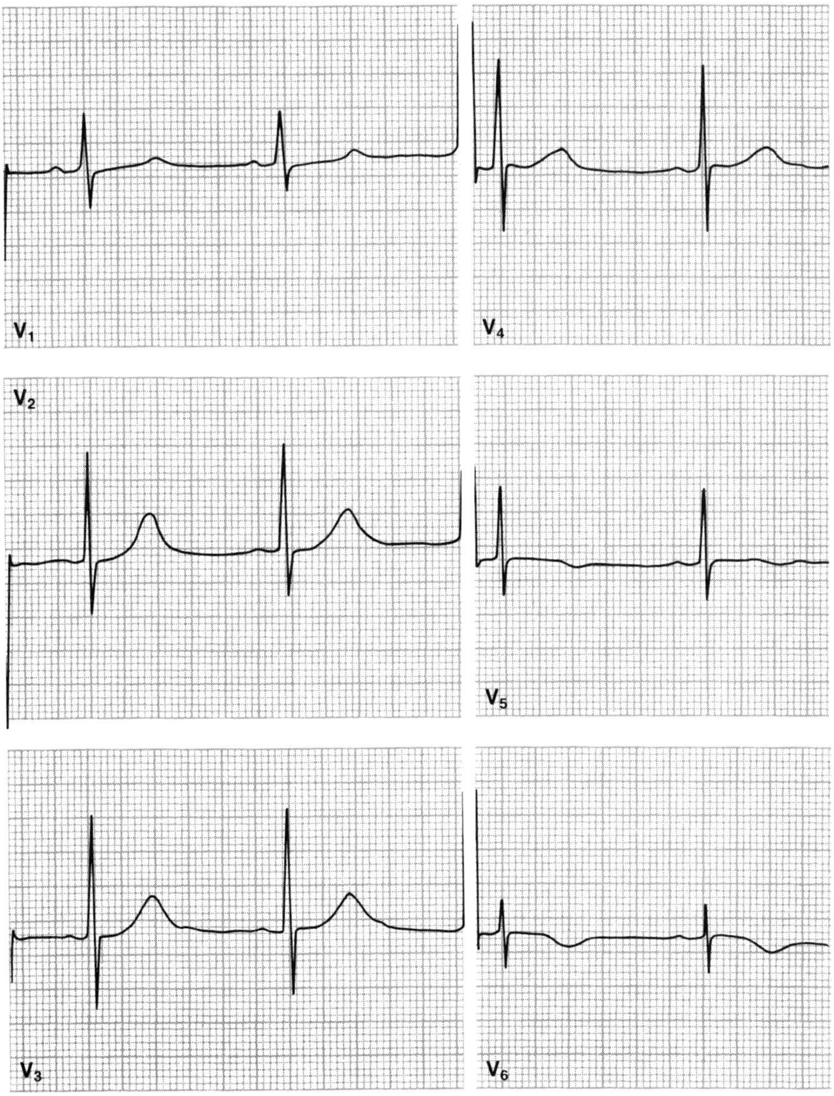

V_1
V_4
V_2
V_5
V_3
V_6

TABLE 7-1

Most useful clinical applications of vectorcardiography
• Detection of types A, B, and C RVH
• Differential diagnosis of the tall R wave in lead V_1: -RVH -RBBB -Posterior myocardial infarction -WPW -Normal variant
• Evaluation of poor R-wave progression: -Anterior (or anteroseptal) myocardial infarction -COPD, type C RVH, or both -LVH -None of the above
• Determination of inferior infarction: -Are small q waves in II, III, and/or aVF indicative of prior inferior infarction? -Is predominantly negative QRS complex in inferior leads due to LAHB, inferior infarction, or both?

Subendocardial Infarction

At the beginning of this chapter we acknowledged that since subendocardial infarctions *have* been shown at times to produce Q waves, use of this term should *not* be taken as synonymous with the more anatomically accurate designation of "non-Q-wave-producing infarction." Despite this limitation, and the fact that we now know transmural infarctions do *not* always produce Q waves, the potentially misleading terms *transmural* and *subendocardial* have remained in popular use. We will, therefore, continue to employ these terms to indicate infarctions that do and do not (respectively) produce Q waves.

PROBLEM: How does one diagnose subendocardial infarction? Is one present in either of the ECGs shown in Figures 7-18 and 7-19?

INTERPRETATION of Fig. 7-18

Rate and rhythm: Sinus rhythm at 85 beats/min. The PR and QRS intervals are normal. The QT interval is prolonged.

Axis: About +30°.

Chamber enlargement: None.

QRST changes: There are no Q waves, and R-wave progression is normal. Deep, symmetric T-wave inversion is present in most leads.

Although this ECG is certainly suggestive of *ischemia,* diagnosis of acute subendocardial infarction *cannot* be made on the basis of any one tracing alone. This is because the ST-segment and T-wave abnormalities associated with acute subendocardial infarction are too nonspecific. At times, they are easily confused with conditions such as acute ischemia, coronary spasm, left ventricular strain, pericarditis, electrolyte disturbance, digitalis effect, and metabolic disorders.

To diagnose acute subendocardial infarction definitively, one must combine the picture of *evolutionary* ECG changes with clinical history and serial cardiac enzyme abnormalities. In fact, the ST-T wave changes shown in Fig. 7-18 did not evolve, and were *not* the result of acute infarction.

INTERPRETATION of Fig. 7-19

Rate and rhythm: Sinus rhythm at 70 beats/min. The PR and QRS intervals are normal. The QT interval is probably prolonged.

Axis: +105° (RAD, and possibly even LPHB).

Chamber enlargement: None.

QRST changes: Small, narrow (and probably insignificant) q waves are evident in the inferior leads. R-wave progression is normal. Nonspecific ST-segment flattening is seen inferiorly, and fairly deep, symmetric T-wave inversion is present in the anterolateral leads. While not as impressive as the picture in Fig. 7-18, this ECG is still strongly suggestive of *ischemia.*

Fig. 7-20 is one of the follow-up ECGs obtained on the patient whose initial tracing was shown in Fig. 7-19. In contrast to the first patient, this 63-year-old woman *did* infarct. Fig. 7-20 shows an evolutionary pattern of the ST-T wave complex, particularly in the anterolateral leads where much of the T-wave inversion has resolved. CPK isoenzyme elevation confirmed the diagnosis.

Note that although the area of transition in the precordial leads remained the same in both ECGs (between leads V_3 and V_4), QRS amplitude is definitely less in the later tracing. While this may simply be the result of a technical error (resulting from slightly different electrode lead placement on the patient's chest), it may also be a real finding indicative of a loss in depolarizing forces from the infarction. Some infarctions, instead of producing Q waves, manifest by a reduction in R-wave amplitude. As one might imagine, it is often extremely difficult to determine if such changes in R-wave amplitude are truly significant, because of the normal variations in QRS voltage that occur from day to day in normal persons, and the inevitable variation in precordial lead placement that occurs when serial ECGs are taken on successive days by different technicians.

In the past, clinical significance had been attributed to the differentiation between subendocardial and transmural infarctions. Since less of the myocardial wall was thought to be involved in the former (the non-Q-wave -producing infarction), one expected long-term prognosis to be correspondingly better. However, recent studies have shown long-term prognosis for these two entities to be quite similar. Although initial mortality for transmural infarction may be somewhat greater, subendocardial infarction is a more unstable entity with a much higher recurrence rate of infarction during the first few months following hospital discharge.

Figure 7-18. ECG from a 50-year-old woman with new-onset chest pain.

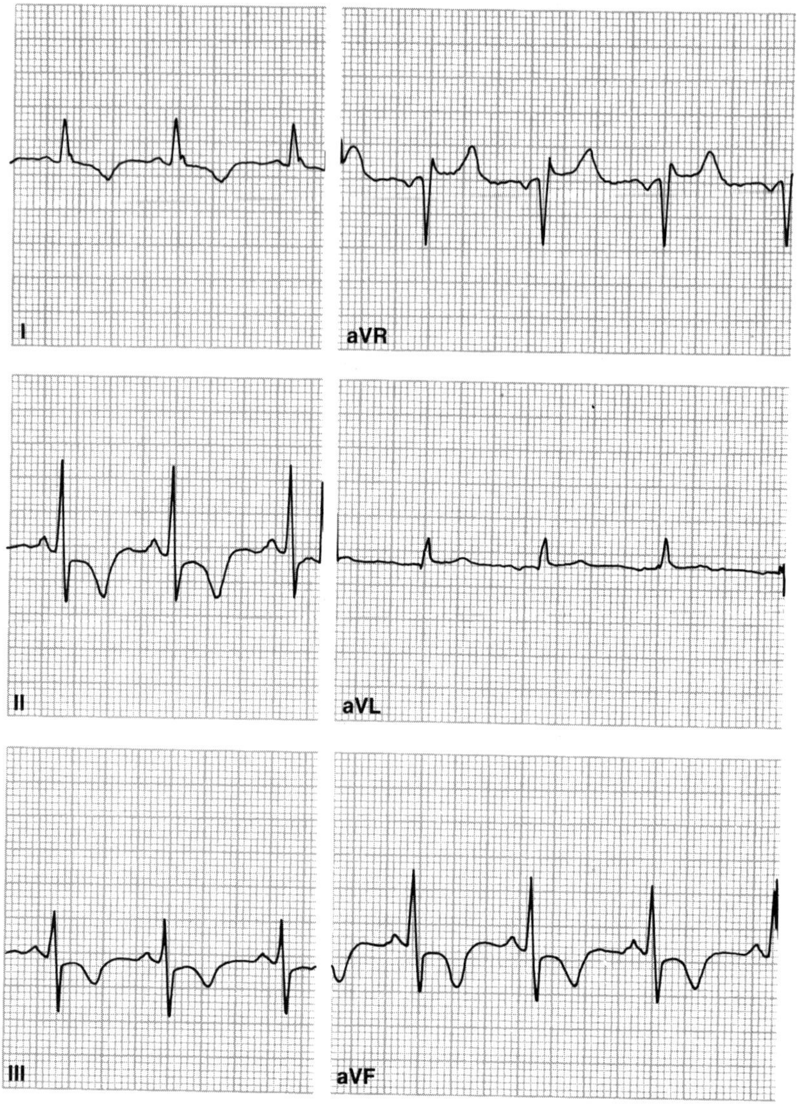

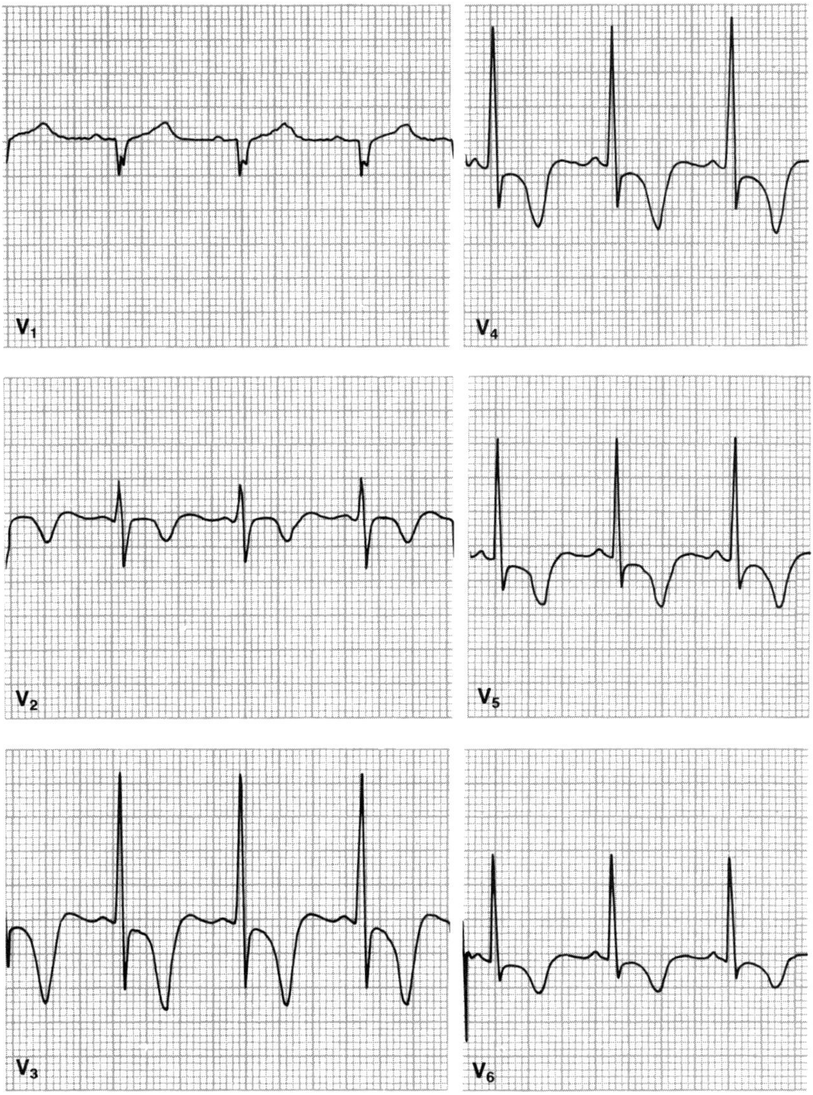
V1
V4
V2
V5
V3
V6

Figure 7-19. ECG from a 63-year-old woman with new-onset chest pain.

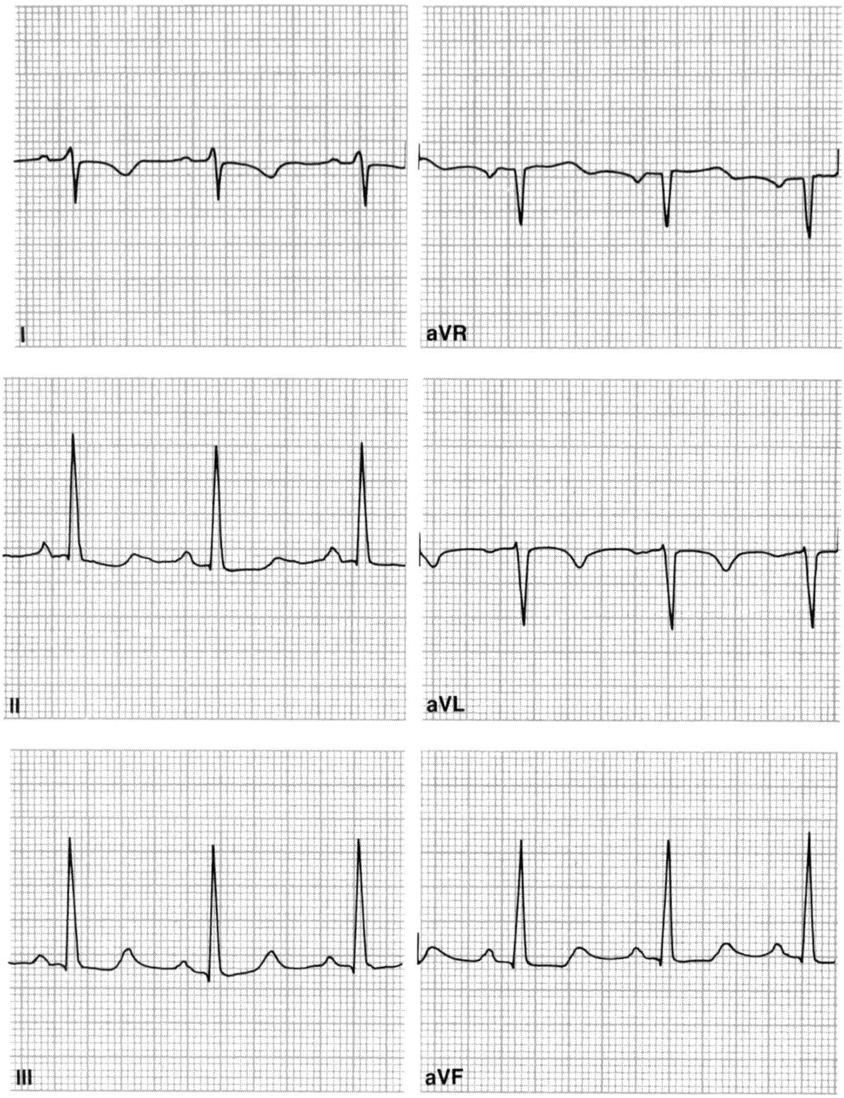

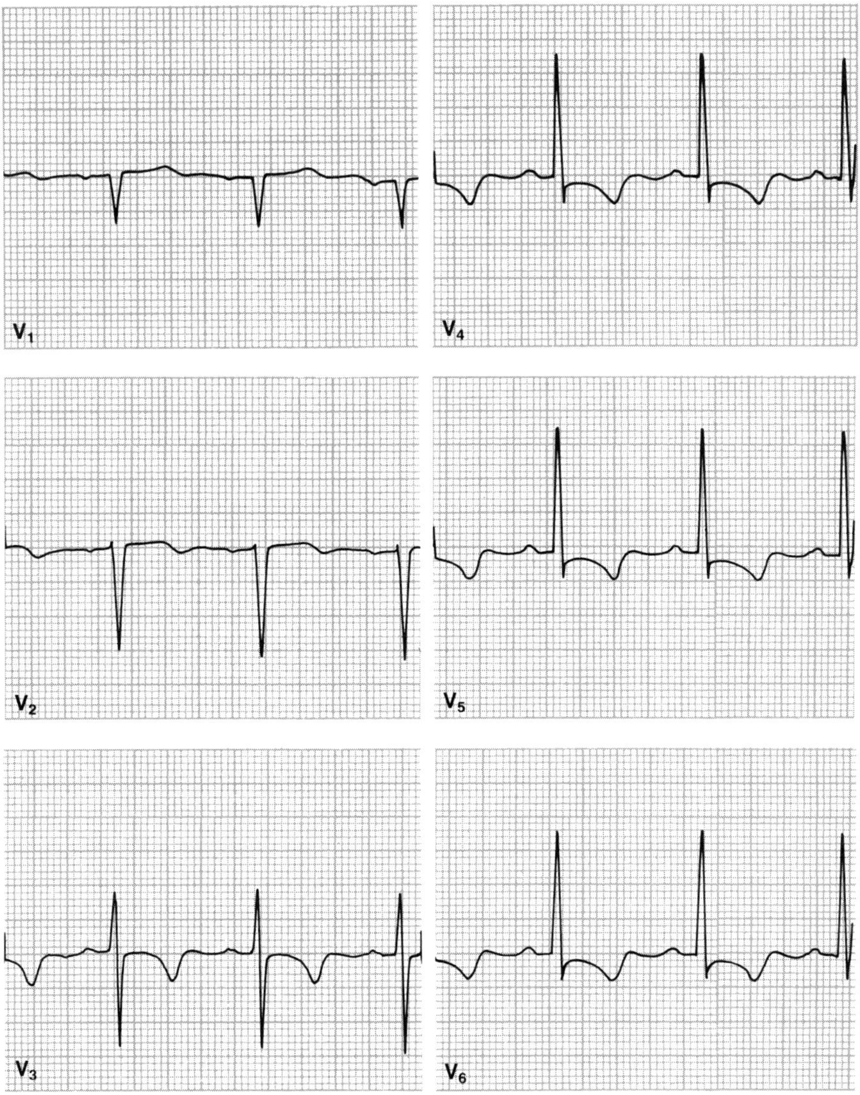
V1
V2
V3
V4
V5
V6

Figure 7-20. Follow-up ECG on the 63-year-old woman obtained several days after the ECG shown in Fig. 7-19 was done.

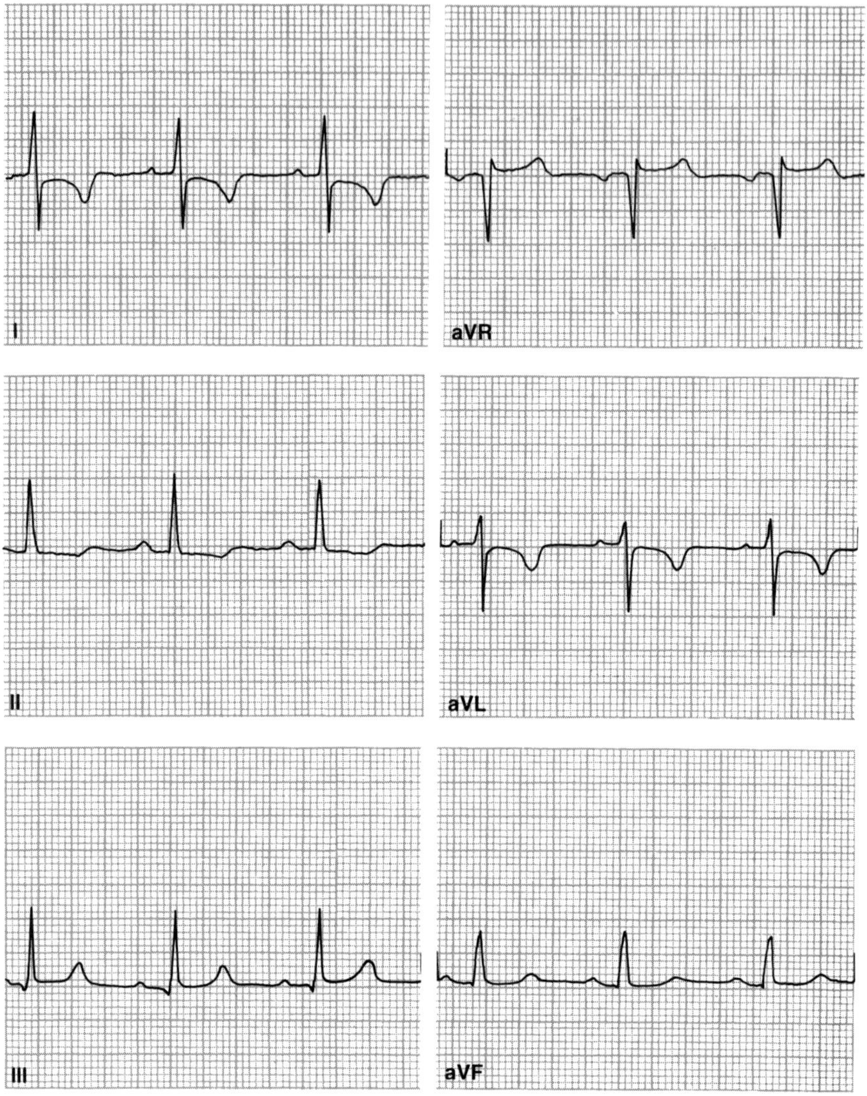

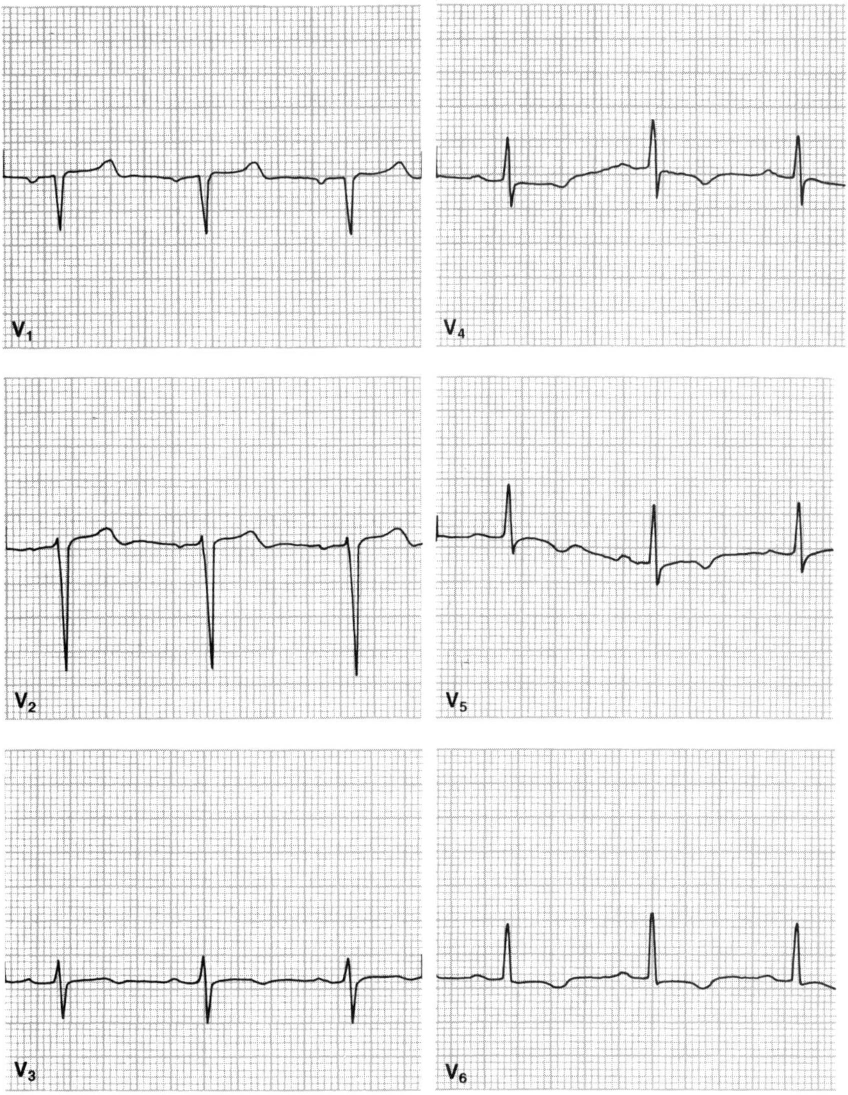
V1
V4
V2
V5
V3
V6

PROBLEM: Examine the ECG shown in Fig. 7-21, taken from a previously healthy 30-year-old-woman with new onset of pleuritic-type chest pain. Is she likely to be having an infarction?

INTERPRETATION of Fig. 7-21

Rate and rhythm: Sinus tachycardia at 130 beats/min. One PVC is seen in the simultaneously recorded anterior precordial leads (the fourth complex in leads V_1, V_2, and V_3). The PR and QRS intervals are normal. The rate is too fast to say anything about the QT interval.

Axis: About +70°.

Chamber enlargement: None.

QRST changes: Diffuse ST-segment elevation is seen virtually everywhere!

Pericarditis

Although it would be impossible to rule out acute myocardial infarction from the ECG shown in Fig. 7-21, *acute pericarditis* is a much more likely diagnosis. The first hint is in the history. While acute myocardial infarction seems to be occurring in younger and younger individuals, it is still quite uncommon among otherwise healthy young adults. On the other hand, sudden onset of *pleuritic-type* chest pain in this age group should at least suggest pericarditis as a possible diagnosis. Pain is usually the principal presenting complaint of this disorder. While at times the pain may closely mimic that of ischemic heart disease, it more often is positional and/or pleuritic in nature.

Electrocardiographically, it would be unusual (though not impossible) for acute myocardial infarction to produce changes as *diffuse* as are shown here. More commonly, ST-segment elevation is limited to one or two areas of the heart. Q waves usually develop with acute infarction, and areas distant to the acute insult frequently shown reciprocal ST-T wave changes. None of these findings are present here.

An additional finding of acute pericarditis that is often overlooked or misinterpreted is *PR-segment depression.* To the unwary, it is easy to mistake PR-segment depression for ST-segment elevation. This is illustrated in Fig. 7-22.

At first glance, one might be tempted to call the ST segment of the QRS complex in Panel B elevated. In fact, it is *isoelectric;* the PR segment is *depressed,* giving the illusion that the ST segment is elevated.

In Chapter 1 (The ST Segment), we advised that the PR segment be used as the baseline and reference point for judging ST-segment deviations *except* for a few special situations. Conditions such as pericarditis that can produce PR-segment deviations make up one of those special situations. Rather than choosing the PR segment as the baseline and reference point in this circumstance, the *TP segment* should be used instead.

Thus, in Panel A of Fig. 7-22, *both* the PR segment and the ST segment are isoelectric (even the baseline as determined by the TP segment). As mentioned above, in Panel B the PR segment is depressed, but the ST segment is isoelectric. In Panel C, only the ST segment is deviated (elevated) from the baseline. Finally, in Panel D, both the PR *and* the ST segments are deviated from the baseline (with respect to the TP segment). The former is depressed, and the latter is elevated.

PROBLEM: Reexamine the ST-T wave segments in Fig. 7-21. Are the ST segments elevated, or are the PR segments depressed?

ANSWER: The ST segments are clearly elevated in virtually all leads of this tracing except for aVR, aVL, and V_1. At least in the inferior leads, PR-segment depression is also present.

PR segment depression is thought to be due to atrial involvement in the pericardial process. At times it may be the *only* electrocardiographic sign of acute pericarditis. (PR segment depression may also be seen with atrial infarction [which is rare] and occasionally in normal individuals [especially during exercise], so, unfortunately, this sign is *not* specific for pericarditis.)

More typically, acute pericarditis undergoes a four-stage evolutionary sequence. In the first stage, ST segments in virtually *all* leads are elevated. This is thought to be due to the generalized subepicardial involvement of the ventricles that occurs with the pericardial process. In the third stage, virtually all of the leads that demonstrated ST-segment elevation during stage I now show T-wave inversion. In the final stage, resolution of ST-T wave changes occurs.

PROBLEM: If ST segments are diffusely "up" in stage I, and T waves diffusely "down" in stage III, what appearance would you predict for the ST-T wave during stage II?

ANSWER: Stage II is a *transition* stage. As such, it might be expected to produce intermediate changes between those seen in stage I and those of stage III. The ST-T wave may thus appear almost normal ("pseudonormalization") during this stage, despite ongoing evolution of acute pericarditis.

The principal ECG manifestations of the four stages of acute pericarditis are illustrated in Fig. 7-23.

The stage of diffuse ST-segment elevation (stage I illustrated in Panel A) is the most characteristic ECG sign of acute pericarditis. When present in its typical form (as it is in Fig. 7-21), it is almost diagnostic. ST segments are usually *concave up* in shape (as they are in leads I, II, III, aVF, and V_6 in Fig. 7-21). Occasionally they are straightened (as in leads V_2 to V_5 in Fig. 7-21). They are almost never coved (as occurs with acute myocardial infarction). The T wave is upright. It is almost as if one took a normal ST segment and a normal T wave and moved them together as a unit up on the QRS complex.

Figure 7-21. ECG from a previously healthy 30-year-old woman with new-onset pleuritic-type chest pain.

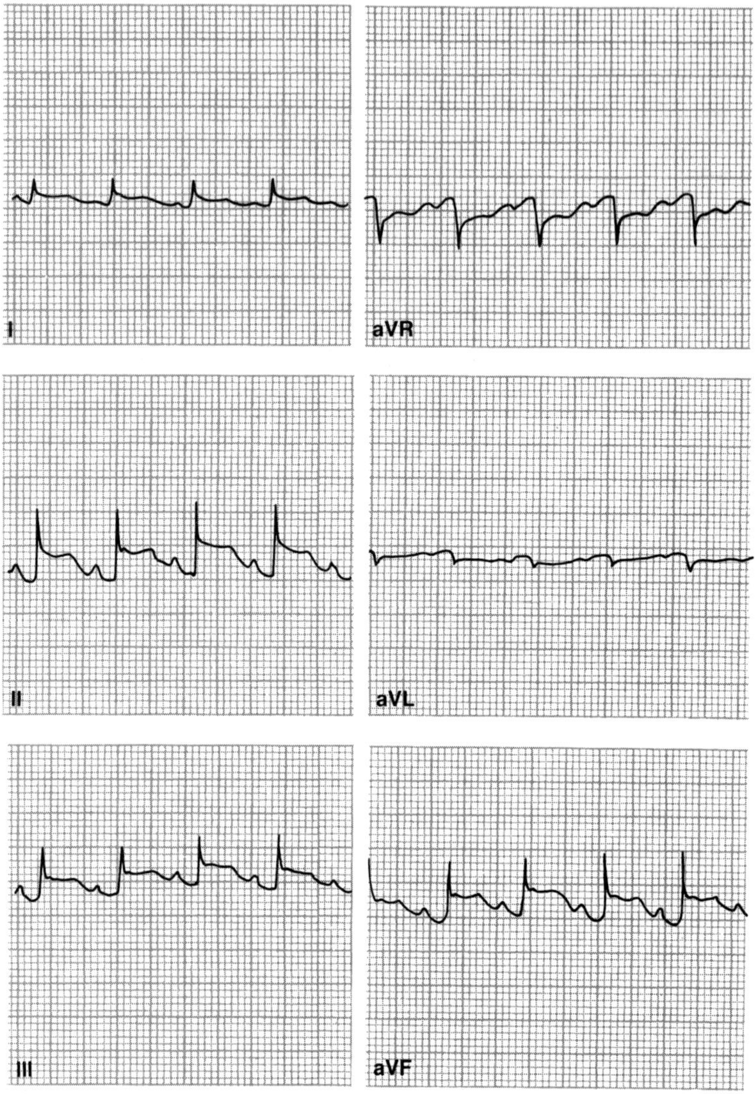

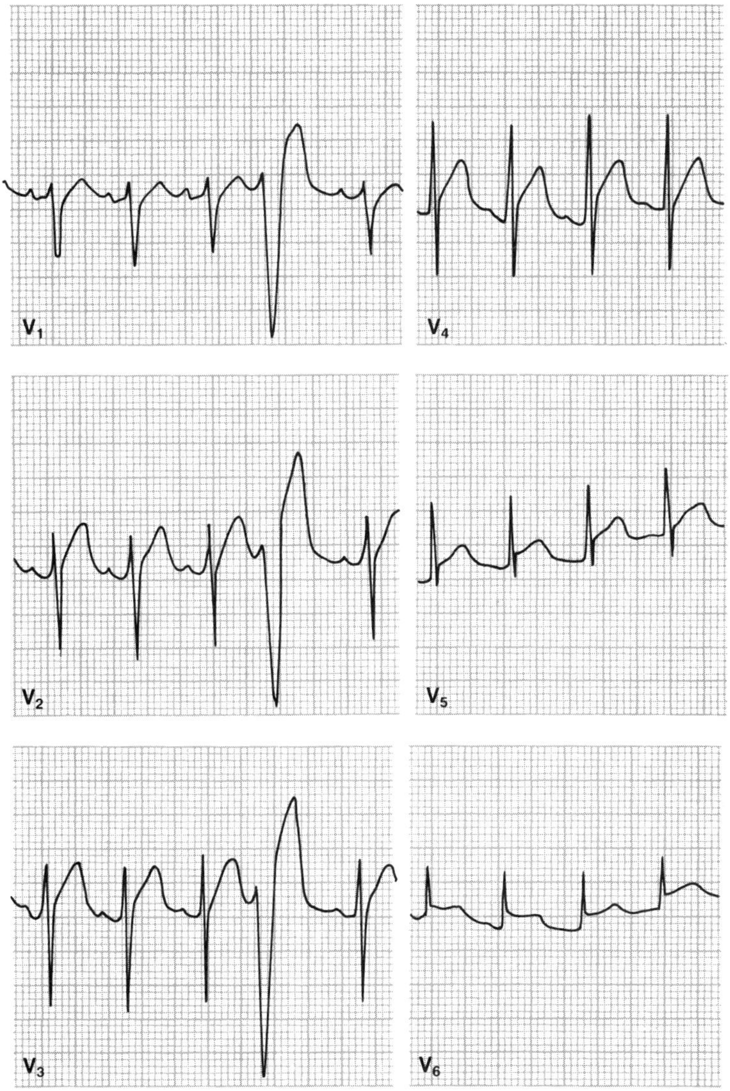

V1
V4
V2
V5
V3
V6

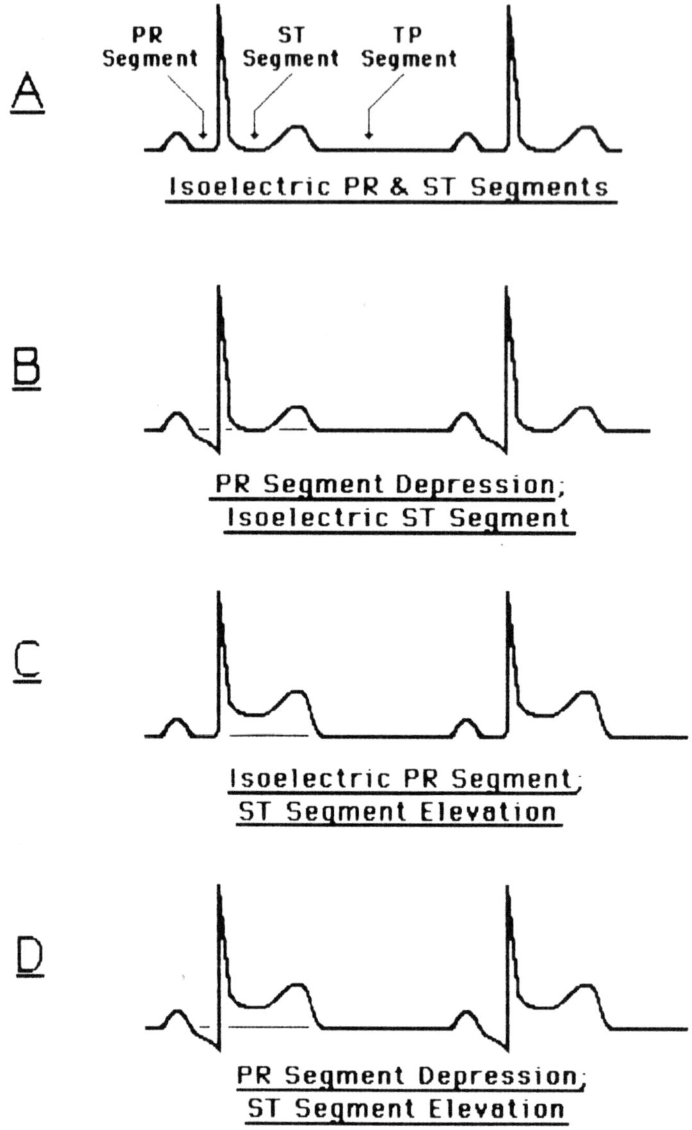

Figure 7-22. PR and ST segment deviations.

The one lead that should never show ST-segment elevation with acute pericarditis is lead aVR. Instead, ST-segment depression is the rule. Leads aVL, III, and V_1 are variable and may show ST-segment elevation, an isoelectric ST segment, or ST-segment depression. All other leads should clearly demonstrate ST-segment elevation.

As mentioned above, stage II pericarditis (Panel B) is a stage of transition between the ST-segment elevation of stage I and the T-wave inversion of stage III. Consequently, the ECG may look deceptively normal during this stage.

In stage III (Panel C), virtually all of the leads that had demonstrated ST-segment elevation now show symmetric (and often fairly deep) T-wave inversion. A key distinguishing feature between pericarditis and myocardial infarction is that the ST segment tends to return to the baseline *before* the T wave inverts in pericarditis, whereas with myocardial infarction, T-wave inversion commonly occurs while the ST segments are still elevated.

In the final stage (stage IV illustrated in Panel D), the ST-T wave abnormalities resolve.

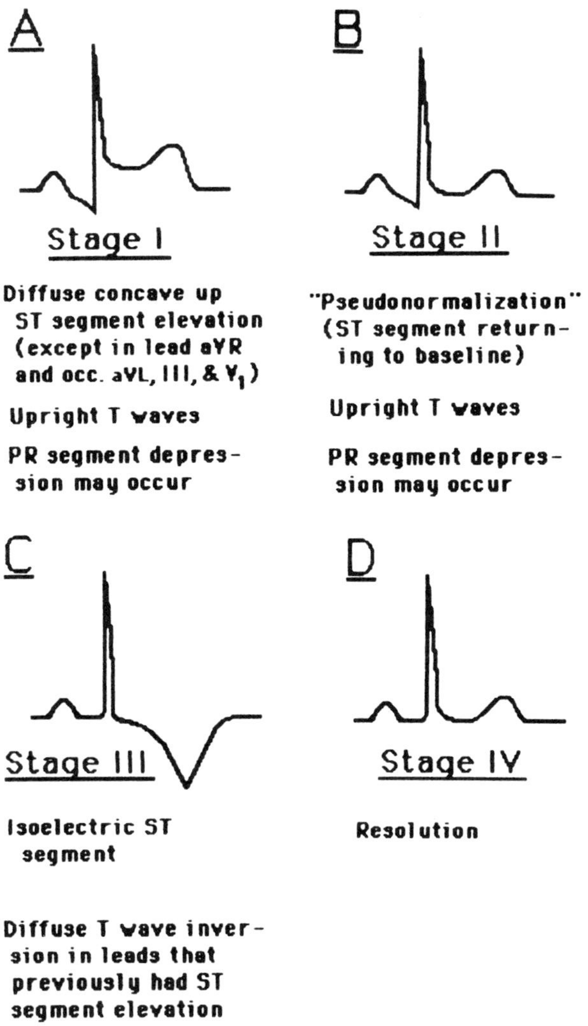

Figure 7-23. The four typical stages of pericarditis.

The time sequence of these four evolutionary stages is *highly* variable. They may occur over hours, days, weeks, or months. Not all patients progress through all four stages. Some may skip one or more of the stages. In others, the diffuse ST-T wave abnormalities of stage III *never* resolve.

It is important to emphasize that the ECG is diagnostic of pericarditis *only* during stage I. During stages II and IV, the ECG is fairly unremarkable and may pass for a normal tracing. The diffuse, symmetric T-wave inversion of stage III may look very much like the ECG that we presented in Fig. 7-18. Such a picture is not at all specific for pericarditis, and may be virtually impossible to differentiate from myocardial ischemia.

Table 7-2 summarizes our discussion so far by highlighting the principal distinguishing characteristics between the changes of typical stage I acute pericarditis and acute myocardial infarction. Application of this information should leave little doubt about the etiology of the diffuse ST-segment elevation that we saw in Fig. 7-21.

The problem arises when the typical course is not followed. Unfortunately, a substantial percentage (up to 40%) of patients with acute pericarditis undergo an *atypical* evolutionary pattern. (See Bruce and Spodick, 1980.) Some of these patients *never* develop any ST-segment elevation at all.

TABLE 7-2

Changes of typical stage I acute pericarditis and acute myocardial infarction

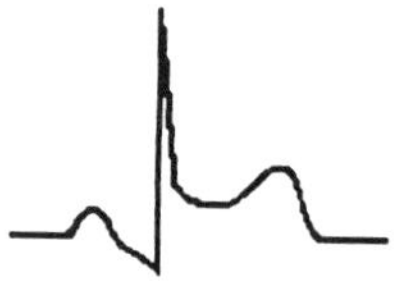

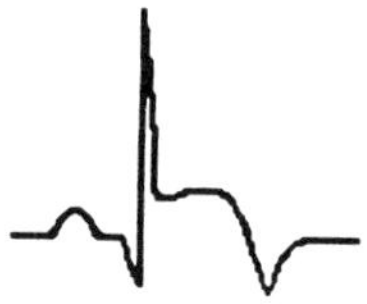

Acute Pericarditis (Typical Stage I)	**Acute Myocardial Infarction**
No Q waves (Unless patient had Q waves before or pericarditis complicates acute myocardial infarction)	*New Q waves*
Concave-up ST-segment elevation ST segments elevated diffusely with the following exceptions: aVR—ST depression usual III, V_1—ST may be isoelectric Reciprocal ST-T wave changes *not* seen	*Coved ST-segment elevation* Localized to leads overlying the infarction Reciprocal ST-T wave changes seen in other areas
Upright T waves in stage I (T waves usually don't invert while ST segment still elevated)	*Symmetric T-wave inversion* May occur while ST segment still elevated
PR segment may be depressed	*PR segment isoelectric*

In them, the only way to make the diagnosis is by detection of a pericardial friction rub. This often seems to be the case in patients with uremic pericarditis. In others with atypical evolutionary patterns, only *localized* ECG changes are observed. (ST-segment elevation occurs in only a few ECG leads rather than being generalized.) It then becomes extremely difficult to differentiate between the ST-segment elevation of acute *localized* pericarditis and that of acute infarction. Localized involvement appears to be especially prevalent when pericarditis complicates acute myocardial infarction. Because of this, the ECG is usually *not* of much assistance in detection, and diagnosis of pericarditis in the setting of acute myocardial infarction almost always has to be made by hearing a rub. (See Krainin and Flessas, 1985.)

PROBLEM: Examine the ECG shown in Fig. 7-24, taken from an asymptomatic 46-year-old man. Is the ST-segment elevation in the precordial leads likely to represent *asymptomatic* pericarditis?

INTERPRETATION of Fig. 7-24

Rate and rhythm: Sinus rhythm at about 60 beats/min. All intervals are normal.

Axis: $+35°$.

Chamber enlargement: There is voltage for LVH ($SV_1 + RV_5 \geq 35$ mm).

QRST changes: Small (normal) septal q waves are seen in the lateral leads. Transition occurs early (between V_1 and V_2). ST-segment elevation with an upward concavity is present in most of the precordial leads. It is particularly marked in lead V_2, where the J point is elevated at least 3 mm above the baseline.

This tracing illustrates an exceedingly common problem in general practice, namely, differentiation of the pattern of early repolarization shown here from more serious conditions. *Early repolarization* is frequently encountered in the general population. Although more often observed in young black male athletes, it is also *commonly* seen in Caucasians, women, and older individuals. Elevated ST segments typically manifest an upward concavity that may closely resemble the ST-segment elevation of typical stage I acute pericarditis. PR segments on occasion may be depressed. However, as opposed to pericarditis, the changes in early repolarization are generally *limited* to one or two areas of the heart, rather than being generalized.

Nonetheless, the ECG shown in Fig. 7-24 poses a true dilemma. There is *no way* to rule out pericarditis on the basis of this one tracing alone! Although ST segments are not significantly elevated in the limb leads, one could conceivably be catching acute pericarditis just *before* such elevation was about to occur—or perhaps at the moment when the patient was evolving into stage II (transition), and ST segments were returning to the baseline before T-wave inversion occurred. *History and comparison with prior tracings* are all-important here. In an asymptomatic patient, particularly an

Figure 7-24. ECG from an asymptomatic 46-year-old man.

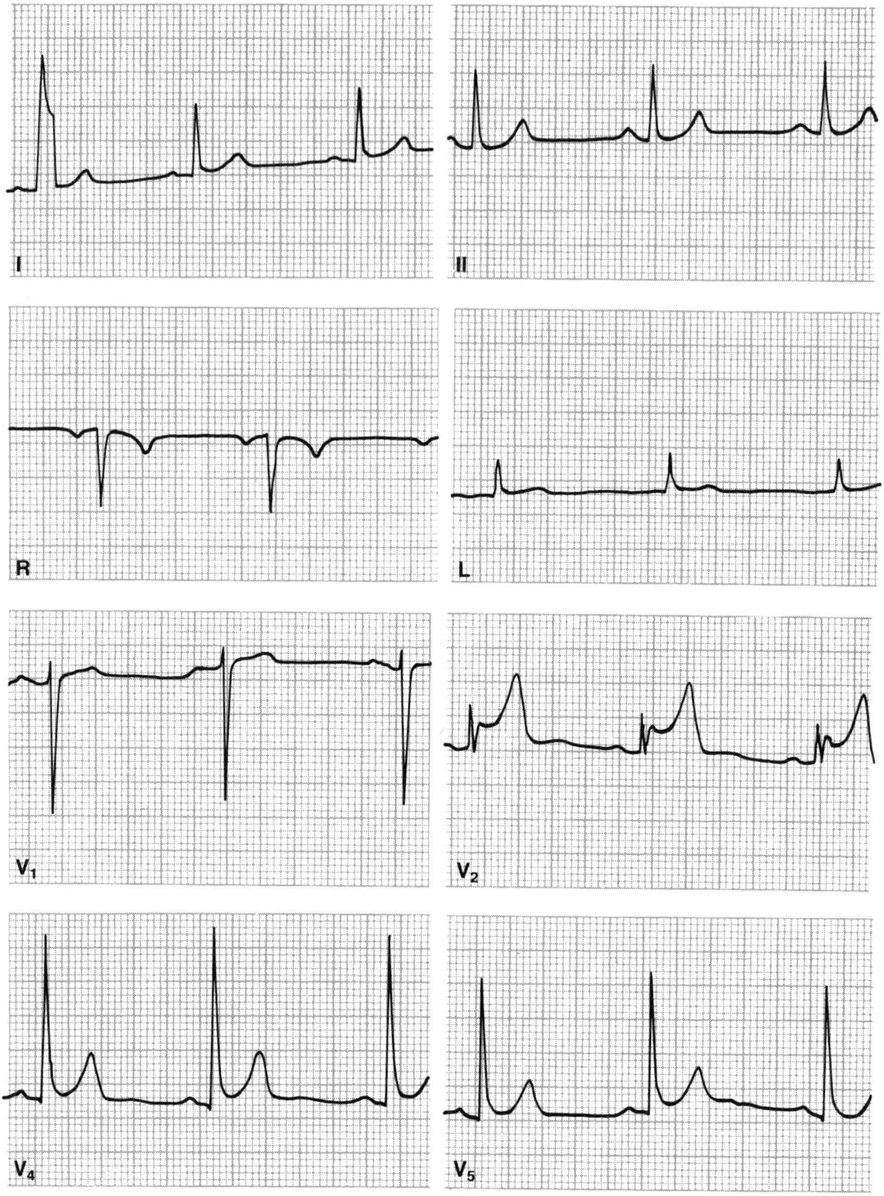

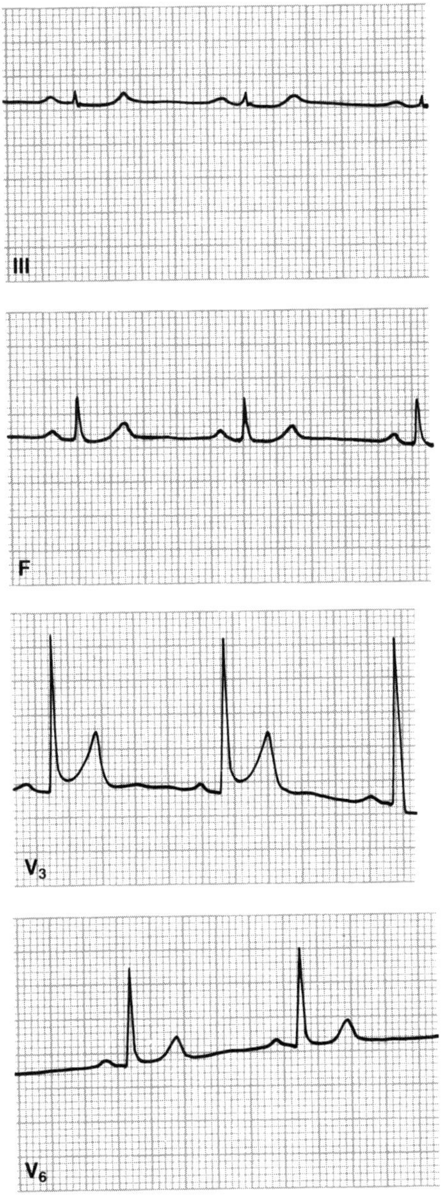
III
F
V_3
V_6

otherwise healthy young adult, the odds would overwhelmingly favor early repolarization as the etiology of the ST-segment elevation. Access to a previous ECG showing an identical pattern would be confirmatory.

The other important consideration that should be brought to mind from inspection of this ECG (especially since it is from a 46-year-old man), is the possibility that the ST-segment elevation could represent acute myocardial infarction (an acute injury current) coronary spasm, or both. And while none of the features of acute myocardial infarction that were illustrated in Table 7-1 are present here (there are no significant Q waves, ST segments are not coved, no reciprocal changes are present, and T waves are not inverted), the earliest stage of acute infarction (the *hyperacute* T-wave stage) could present a very similar picture to that shown in Fig. 7-24.

In deference to the above limitations of the ECG as a diagnostic tool, the written interpretation for this ECG might read as follows:

> "Sinus rhythm at 60 beats/min.
> Axis = +35°.
> Voltage for LVH.
> J-point ST-segment elevation in the precordial leads, *probably* due to early repolarization. *Strongly* suggest clinical correlation, and/or comparison with a prior tracing."

If the patient were known to you, or the history were included on the ECG request form, no more follow-up might be required. In the absence of this knowledge or a prior tracing, it becomes the electrocardiographer's *responsibility* either to alert the primary-care provider or to determine this information himself or herself to assure that a potentially serious condition is not overlooked.

The importance of having access to previous ECGs for comparison should be evident from the examples presented in this chapter. Unfortunately, comparison tracings are often not *available* when needed. In anticipation of this problem, one might consider making *wallet-sized* reproductions of baseline ECGs for selected patients. For example, ready availability of the baseline ECG shown in Fig. 7-24 might be extremely helpful in preventing unnecessary admission to the hospital should this 46-year-old man ever present to an emergency department with a history of atypical chest pain.

Review: Are These Patients Infarcting?

PROBLEM: As a review of this chapter, examine the following ECGs, taken from adults complaining of new-onset chest pain. Which of these patients do you suspect may be infarcting?

INTERPRETATION of Fig. 7-25

Rate and rhythm: Sinus rhythm at about 70 beats/min. All intervals are normal.

Axis: 60°.

Chamber enlargement: None.

QRST changes: There is the suggestion of tiny q waves in the inferior and lateral leads. Transition occurs somewhat early, with a fairly prominent R wave being seen in lead V_2. Worrisome ST-segment elevation with hyperacute T waves is evident in the infero-lateral leads, and reciprocal ST-segment depression is seen in leads aVL, V_2 and V_3. The overall picture suggests probable *acute inferolateral infarction,* with *possible posterior extension.* (This ECG is actually the intermediate tracing obtained in between the ECGs shown in Figs. 7-11 and 7-10.)

INTERPRETATION of Fig. 7-26

Rate and rhythm: Sinus rhythm at 70 beats/min. The PR interval is normal. The QRS interval is prolonged (to 0.14 second) in the pattern of *complete LBBB.*

Axis: About −20°. (Left axis is definitely present since the QRS complex in lead aVF is predominantly negative. Although the *amplitude* of the R wave in lead II is about equal to that of the S wave in that lead, the R wave appears to be *wider.* Therefore, the net deflection of the QRS complex in this lead is *positive,* and the mean QRS axis will be *less* than −30°, or about −20°.)

Chamber enlargement: No atrial enlargement. Although LVH is difficult to call in the presence of LBBB, the tremendously deep S wave in lead V_2 (about 30 mm deep) suggests that it probably is present.

QRST changes: A Q wave is evident in leads III and V_1. R-wave progression is poor, with predominantly negative complexes persisting up until lead V_5. Although at first glance this might suggest anterior infarction, no such diagnosis should be made in the presence of LBBB. Finally, typical ST-T wave changes of complete LBBB are seen in the appropriate leads. Interpretation of this ECG should read:

> "Sinus rhythm at 70 beats/min. Complete LBBB."

Infarction may be occurring, but it *cannot* be detected from this ECG.

INTERPRETATION of Fig. 7-27

Rate and rhythm: The rhythm is regular at 85 beats/min. However, the P wave is *not* upright in lead II.

Axis: −90°. (The QRS complex is isoelectric in lead I at 0°. The mean QRS axis is thus perpendicular to this lead. To determine whether the mean axis is at +90° or −90°, one can look at leads II and III. Since both of these leads are predominantly negative, left axis deviation [to −90°] is present.)

Figure 7-25. From a middle-aged adult with new-onset chest pain.

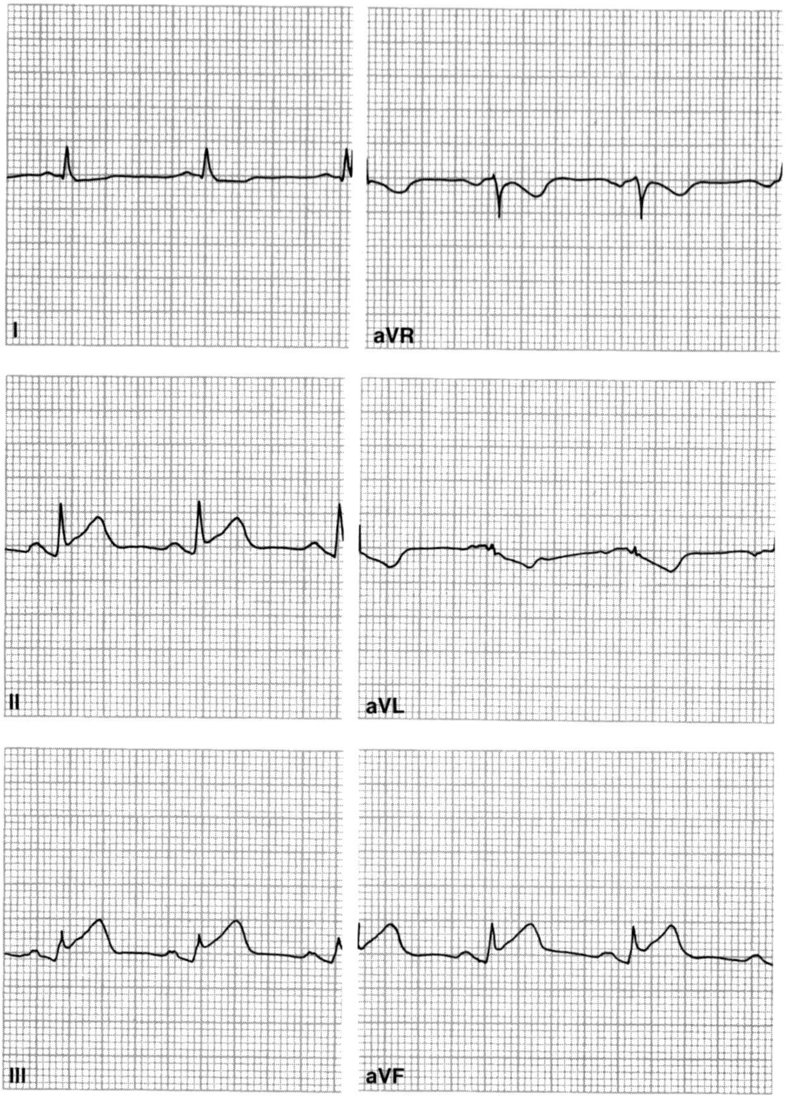

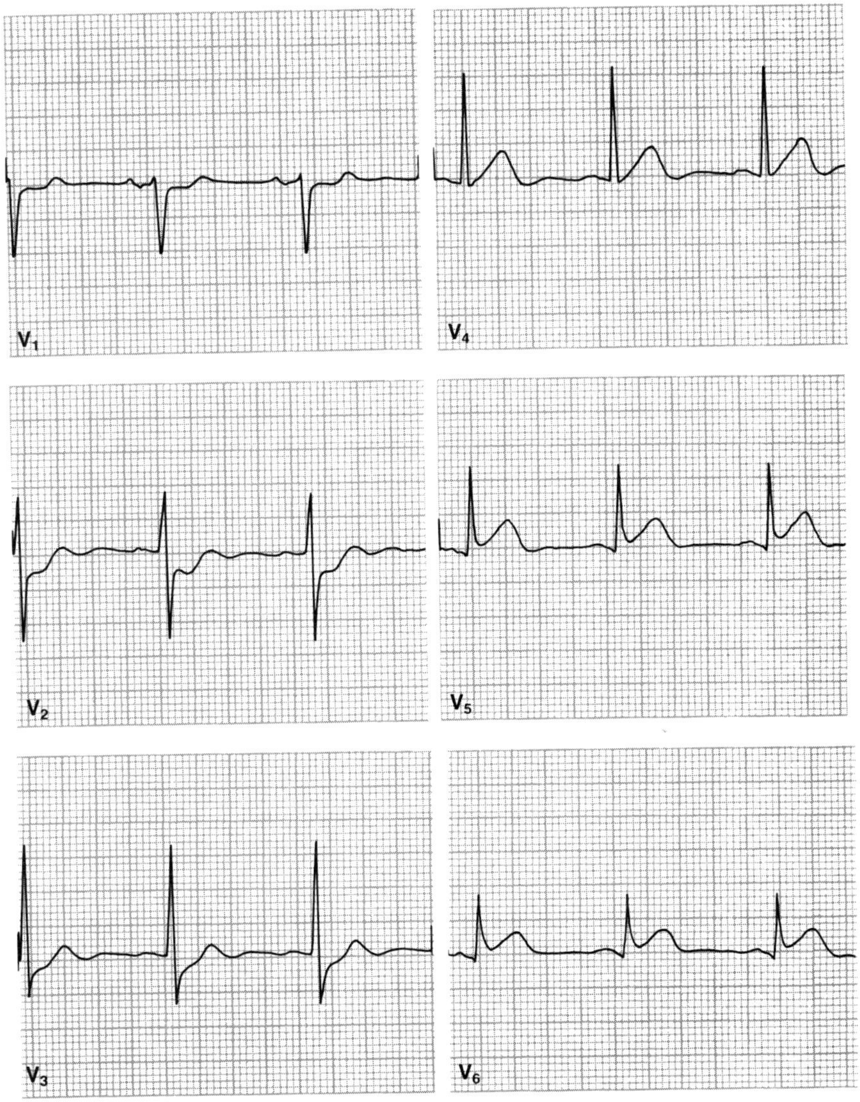
V1
V4
V2
V5
V3
V6

Figure 7-26. From a middle-aged adult with new-onset chest pain.

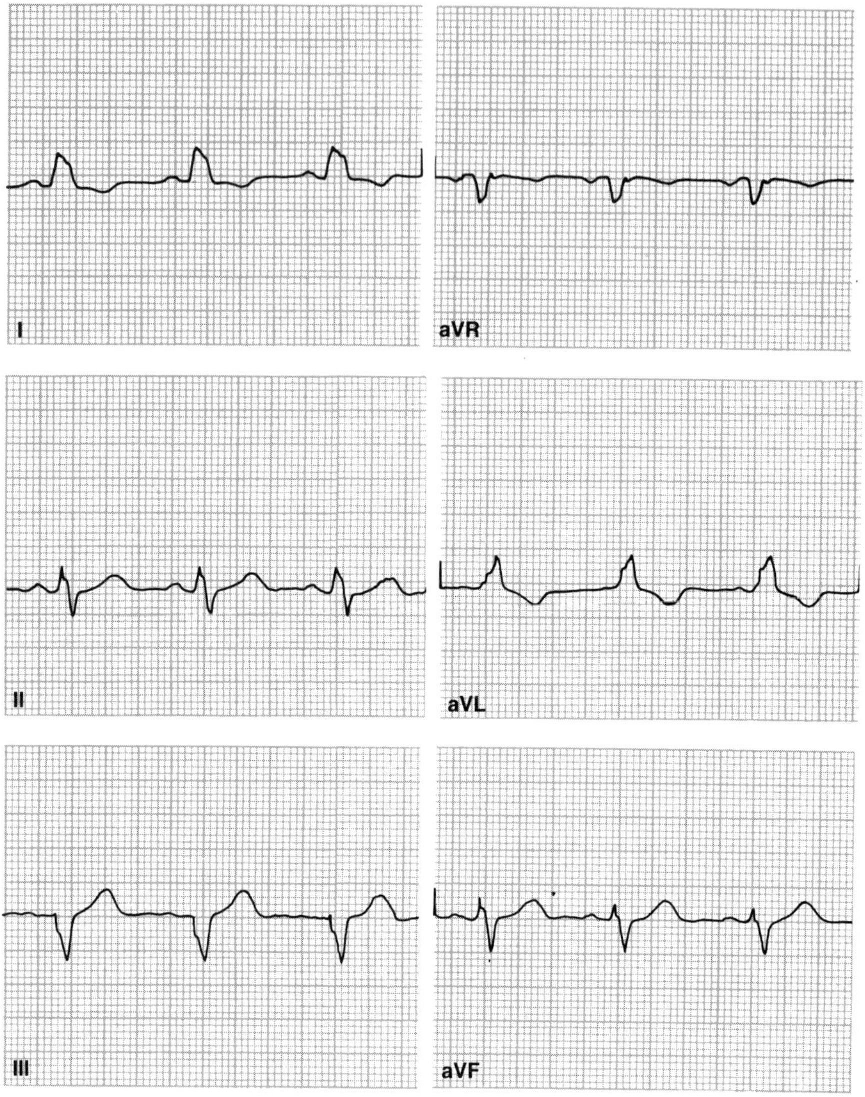

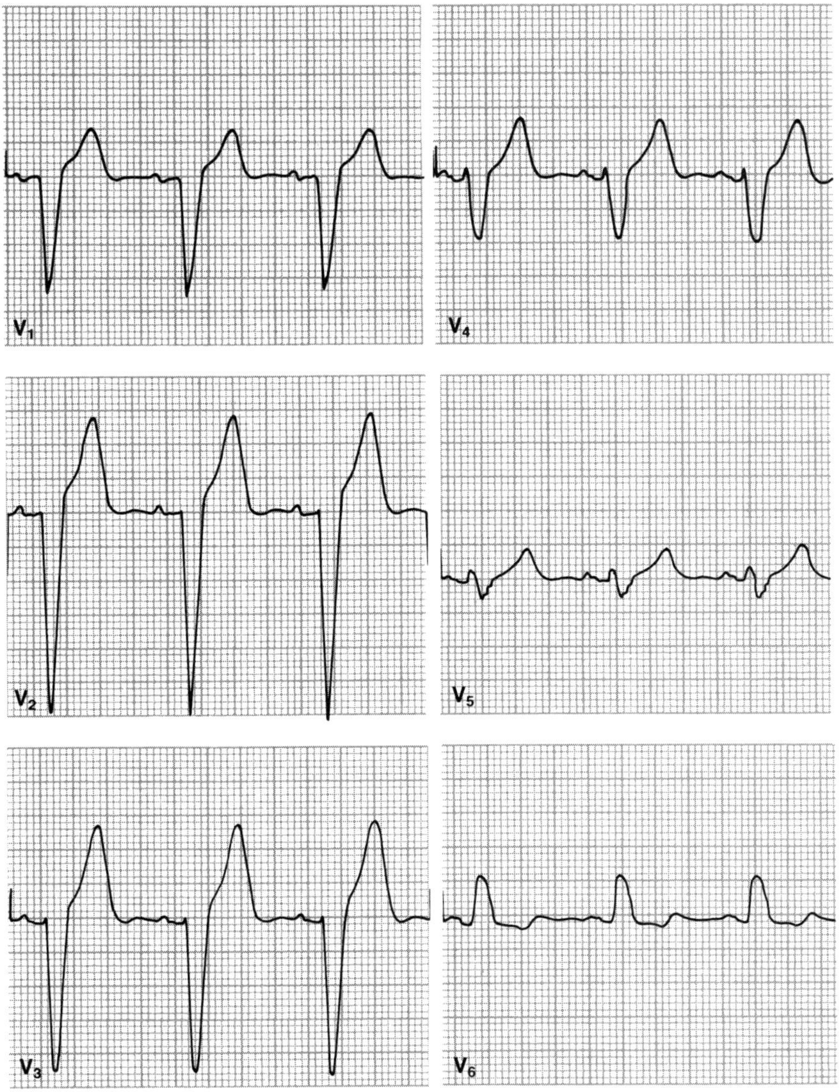
V1
V4
V2
V5
V3
V6

Figure 7-27. From a middle-aged adult with new-onset chest pain.

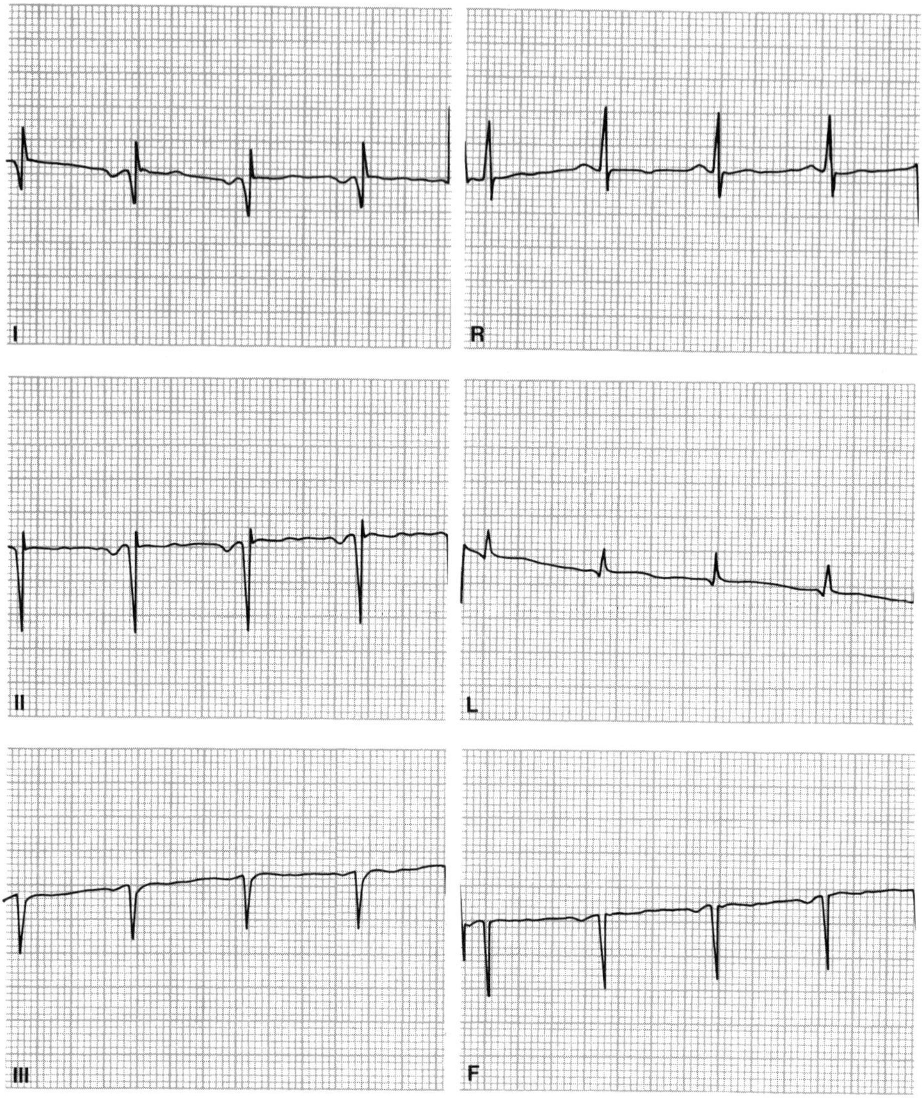

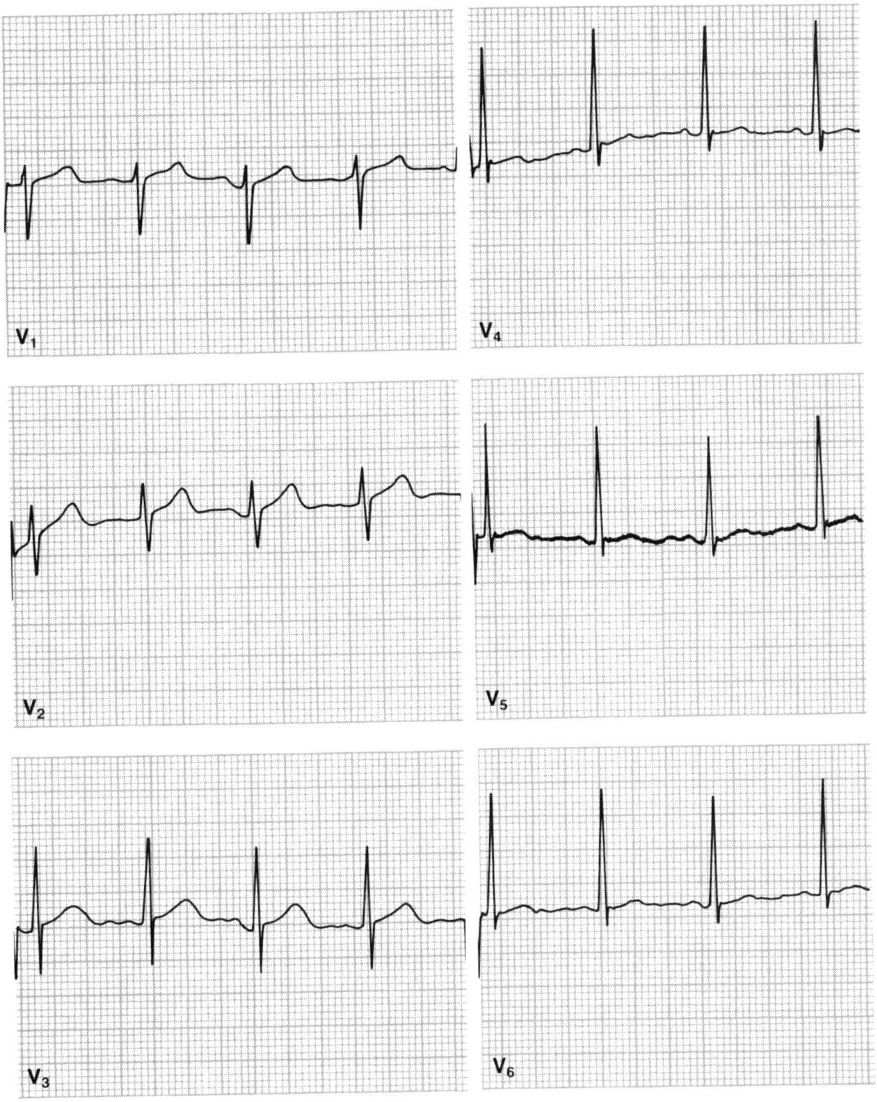
V1
V4
V2
V5
V3
V6

Figure 7-28. Follow-up ECG the next day on the patient whose admission tracing was shown in Fig. 7-27. Note that the P wave is now upright in lead II, there is global negativity in lead aVR, and the QRS complex is upright in lead I.

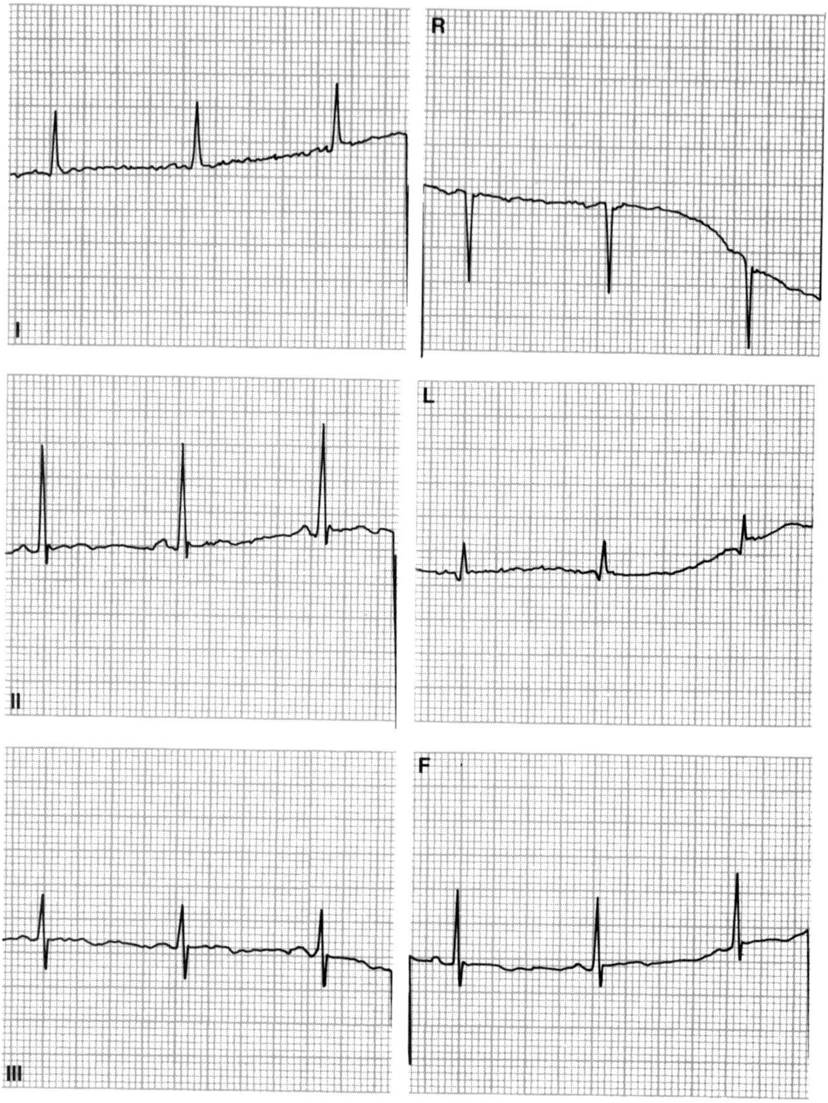

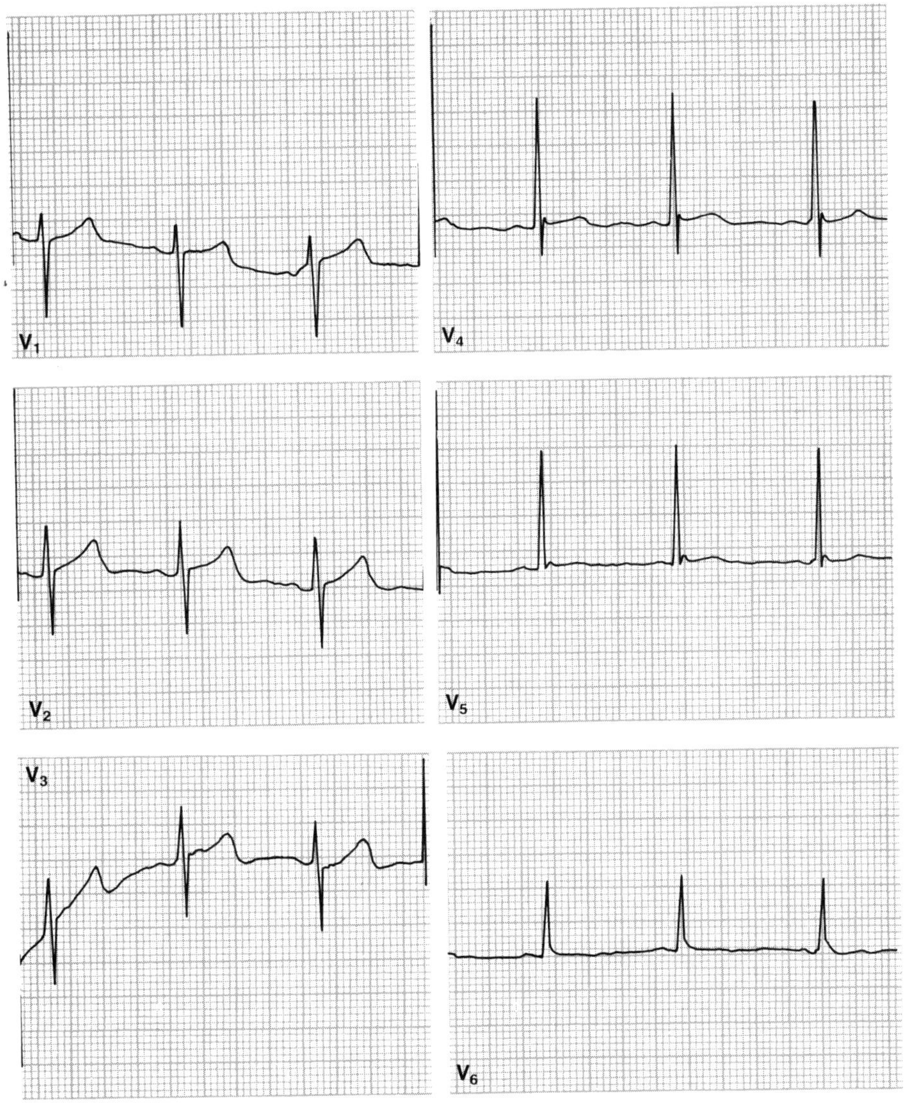
V1
V2
V3
V4
V5
V6

Figure 7-29. From a middle-aged adult with new-onset chest pain.

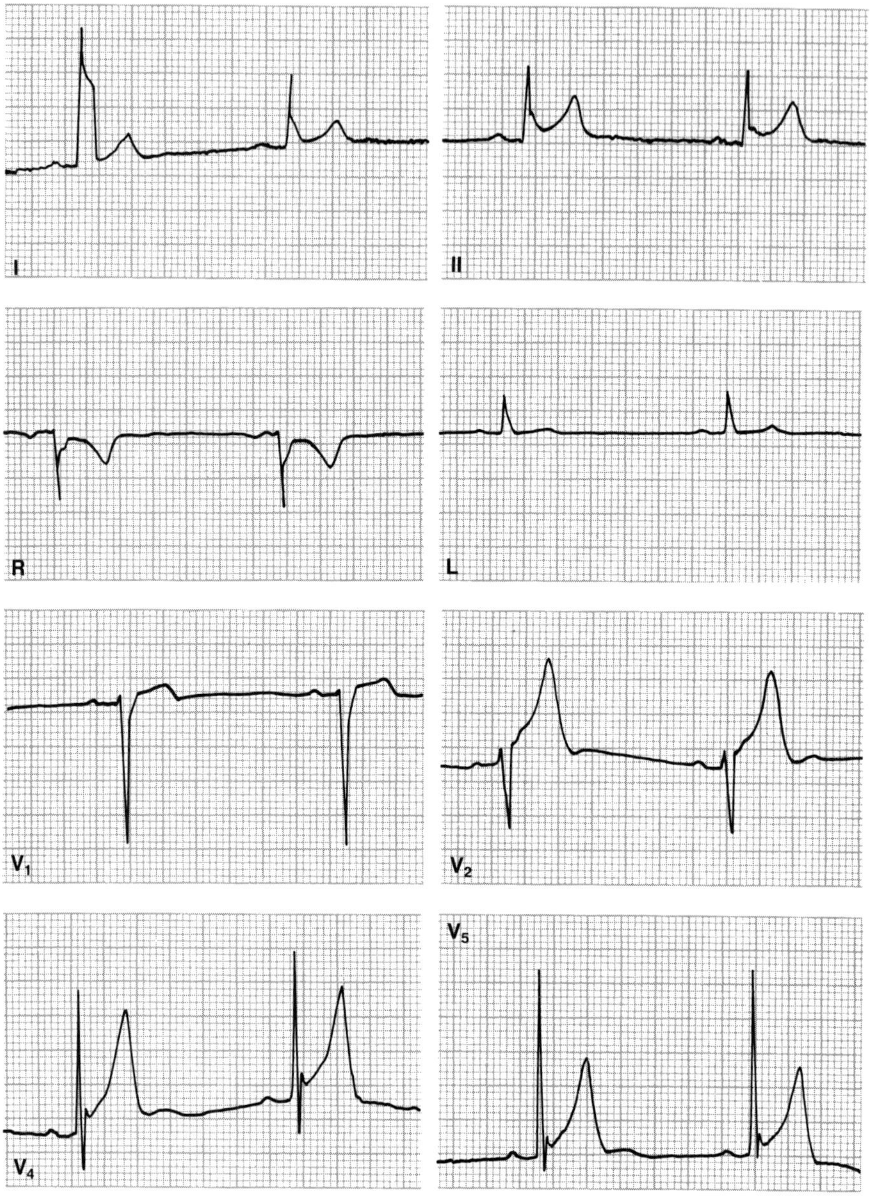

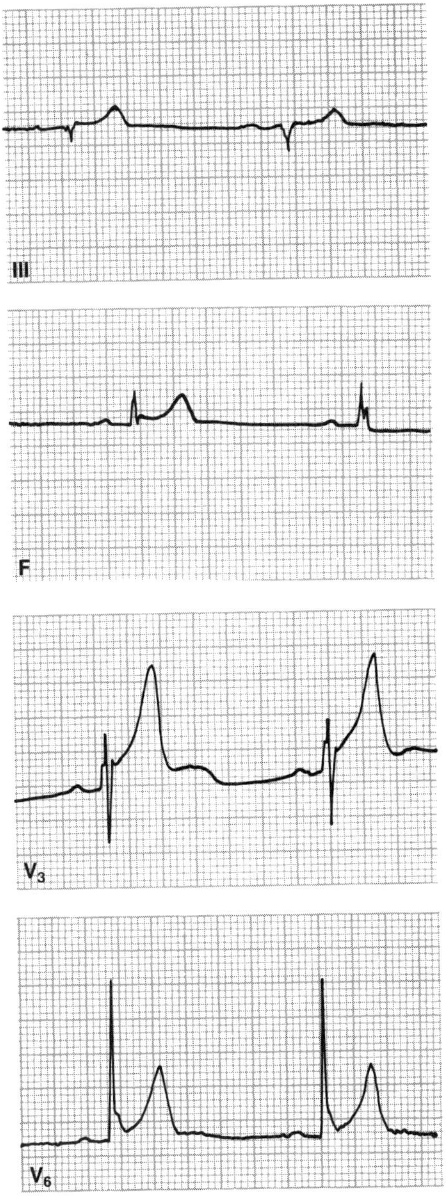
III
F
V_3
V_6

Chamber enlargement: None.

QRST changes: Deep Q waves are present in leads I, II, III, and aVF. There is a smaller q wave in lead aVL.

The temptation is to say that this patient has sustained an inferolateral infarction. In fact, this patient was admitted to the hospital with this diagnosis as a direct result of this ECG.

PROBLEM: Can you guess what his ECG looked like the next day?

ANSWER: The next day's ECG on this patient is shown in Fig. 7-28.

INTERPRETATION of Fig. 7-28

Rate and rhythm: Sinus rhythm at 70 beats/min. All intervals are normal.

Axis: +45°.

Chamber enlargement: None

QRST changes: Non-specific ST-T wave abnormalities.

The next day's ECG (Fig. 7-28) shows absolutely no evidence of myocardial infarction. The reason that deep Q waves had been seen in most limb leads of the admission tracing (Fig. 7-27) is that the *limb leads were reversed!* The right arm and left leg recording electrodes were interchanged in a manner similar to that previously discussed in Fig. 3-26.

Limb-lead reversal is not common, but it definitely *does* occur. Failure to recognize it is embarrassing, and may lead to false diagnosis of myocardial infarction and the unnecessary admission that resulted in this case. Several clues generally suggest its presence:

1. ***Under usual circumstances, with normal sinus rhythm the P wave is always upright in lead II.*** If the P wave is negative, it either means that a low atrial or junctional rhythm is present, or that something *unusual* is occurring. The negative P wave in Fig. 7-27 should therefore provide the first clue that some *unusual* circumstances (limb-lead reversal or dextrocardia) may be in effect.

2. ***Global negativity of the P wave, QRS complex, and T wave is virtually always seen in lead aVR.*** Even when a substantial R wave is present in aVR (as may be seen in some cases of RVH), the first deflection in this lead is almost always *negative* (a Q wave). The Rs pattern seen in Fig. 7-27 is distinctly atypical, and should provide the second clue that something is wrong.

3. ***A predominantly positive QRS complex with no more than a small septal q wave is usually seen in lead I.*** If there is global negativity in lead I (if the P wave, QRS complex, and T wave are all negative), or, as occurs in this case, if the P wave is inverted and a deep Q wave is seen in this lead, one should suspect that something may be amiss.

INTERPRETATION of Fig. 7-29

Rate and rhythm: Sinus bradycardia at about 48 beats/min. All intervals are normal.

Axis: +25°.

Chamber enlargement: Voltage for LVH.

QRST changes: ST segment elevation with an upward concavity is noted in almost every lead except aVR, where the ST segment is slightly depressed. Three diagnostic entities could cause this picture:

1. ***Acute myocardial infarction.*** The age of the patient and the presenting complaint should make this a prime concern. Sinus bradycardia might be a reflection of increased parasympathetic tone from acute inferior infarction. The Q wave in lead III would be consistent with this, although in isolation a Q wave in this lead is of questionable significance.

2. ***Acute pericarditis.*** As discussed in the previous section of this chapter, diffuse ST-segment elevation of the type seen here should suggest this possibility. This picture would be perfectly consistent with the changes of typical stage I acute pericarditis.

3. ***Early repolarization.*** Statistically, this might be the most common of these three diagnostic entities, but diagnosis of early repolarization should *always* be a diagnosis of *exclusion.* Although ST-segment elevation with early repolarization is usually not to the degree shown here (the ST segments are almost elevated by 4 mm in lead V_3), and changes are most often more localized, the shape of the ST segments (their upward concavity) and the very prominent J points seen in leads V_4 and V_5 are very characteristic of early repolarization.

On closer questioning, it was learned that this patient's chest pain had actually been going on for several days and sounded more gastrointestinal in nature. Physical examination was unremarkable (no pericardial friction rub was heard on careful auscultation), and a prior ECG showing a similar pattern was found hidden away in his chart. Thus, by exclusion, the changes manifest in the ECG shown in Fig. 7-29 could be more confidently attributed to *early repolarization.*

References

Bruce MA, Spodick DH: Atypical electrocardiogram in acute pericarditis: Characteristics and prevalence. *J Electrocardiol* 1980; 13:61–66.

Krainin FM, Flessas AP: Infarction-associated pericarditis: Rarity of diagnostic electrocardiogram. *N Engl J Med* 1985; 311:1211–1214.

CHAPTER 8

CHAMBER ENLARGEMENT

Electrocardiography is one of the principal modalities used to detect chamber enlargement. In this chapter, we will discuss the strengths and weaknesses of the various ECG criteria used to diagnose enlargement of each of the four cardiac chambers, and review their clinical application.

Cardiac Enlargement and Hypertrophy

When the heart is subjected to an increased workload, individual cardiac chambers respond by either increasing the thickness of their walls *(hypertrophy),* or by increasing their overall dimensions *(enlargement).* The thin-walled atria characteristically dilate and enlarge. Minimal *thickening* of the atrial wall occurs. The ventricular response to an increased workload is more complex. Initially, there is increase in thickness of the ventricular wall. However, actual chamber enlargement *(dilatation)* may not occur until later when the ventricle begins to fail.

Cardiac enlargement is easily seen on chest X-ray films. The heart is said to be enlarged when the cardiac silhouette exceeds one-half the widest thoracic diameter on a PA chest film. Hypertrophy is harder to determine. Because *thickness* but not necessarily overall chamber size is increased, significant left ventricular hypertrophy may not be apparent on chest X-ray. Thus, cardiac *enlargement* and *hypertrophy* are two very different entities. While they both may be present simultaneously, more often than not, one or the other process predominates.

PROBLEM: Examine the ECG shown in Fig. 8-1, taken from a 67-year-old woman with new-onset congestive heart failure (CHF). Is there ECG evidence for LVH on this tracing?

INTERPRETATION of Fig. 8-1

Rate and rhythm: The rhythm is irregularly irregular, and P waves are absent. This is *atrial fibrillation* with a *controlled ventricular response.*

The QRS interval is normal. Due to the indistinctness of the T wave, the QT interval cannot be determined. The third QRS complex in lead II is wide and bizarre in morphology. It is a PVC.

Axis: +10°.
Chamber enlargement: None.
QRST changes: There are no Q waves. R-wave progression is normal. Nonspecific ST-T wave flattening is present diffusely.

The chest X-ray from this patient is shown in Fig. 8-2. Cardiac enlargement, consistent with her clinical history of new onset CHF, is definitely present. Yet LVH *cannot* be diagnosed from the tracing shown in Fig. 8-1 by any ECG criteria!

It has been shown that the prevalence of cardiac enlargement on chest X-ray *(cardiomegaly)* at any age is at least twice that of LVH on ECG. When subjects with cardiomegaly by chest X-ray are followed over a 10-year period, less than 20 percent of them develop LVH on ECG. Yet among subjects with LVH on ECG, less than 50 percent have coexistent cardiomegaly by chest X-ray. Thus the two modalities are *not* mutually exclusive, and they must measure somewhat different parameters!

Types of LVH

Let's look at these two processes in more detail. Fig. 8-3 illustrates how they act in the different types of ventricular hypertrophy. With increased pressure load states (increased *afterload*) as occurs with aortic stenosis and systemic hypertension, the interventricular septum and left ventricular free wall thicken in a symmetric manner. Since there is little change in left ventricular cavity size, this type of hypertrophy is called *concentric hypertrophy* (Panel B in Fig. 8-3). Mild-to-moderate degrees of left ventricular hypertrophy do not necessarily exert an adverse effect on left ventricular function. Up to 50 percent of all patients with mild essential hypertension have increased left ventricular mass, yet have normal or even better than normal left ventricular function. Similarly, athletes who participate in isometric exercise (wrestlers and weight lifters) also place an increased afterload on the left ventricle, and consequently develop concentric hypertrophy to a varying degree. At the extreme, left ventricular mass may more than *double* in certain power-trained athletes. In these highly trained individuals, the increased myocardial mass usually has a beneficial effect that enables the left ventricle to function more efficiently.

Initially then, a mild-to-moderate degree of left ventricular hypertrophy seems to serve an *adaptive* purpose. It is usually well tolerated, and often beneficial. A more advanced degree of left ventricular hypertrophy is definitely detrimental and predisposes the patient to increased risk of cardiovascular morbidity and mortality.

Progression of left ventricular hypertrophy is almost always a clinically *silent* event. At some point a *critical mass* is reached at which left ventricular hypertrophy ceases to be adaptive (beneficial) and becomes detrimental (pathologic). Unfortunately, there is no good way to determine this point.

Figure 8-1. ECG from a 67-year-old woman with new-onset congestive heart failure.

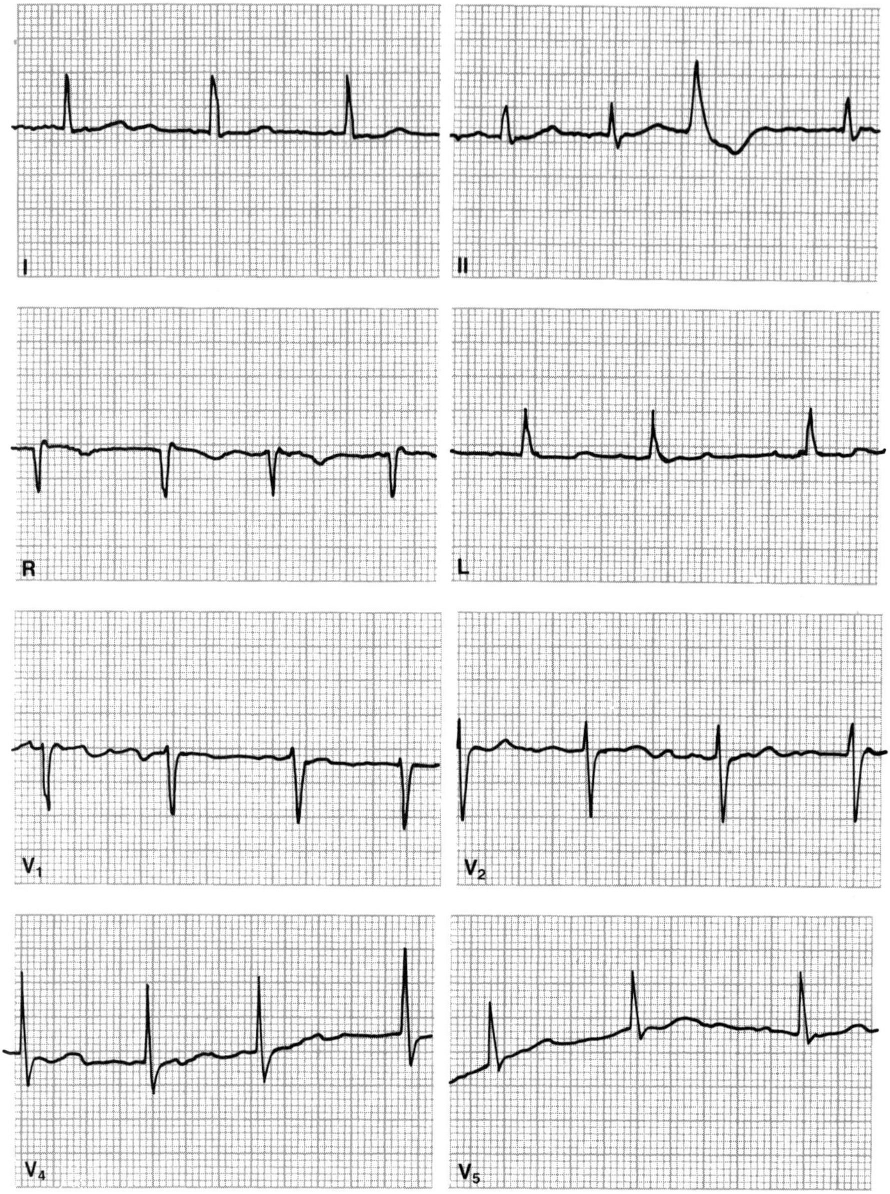

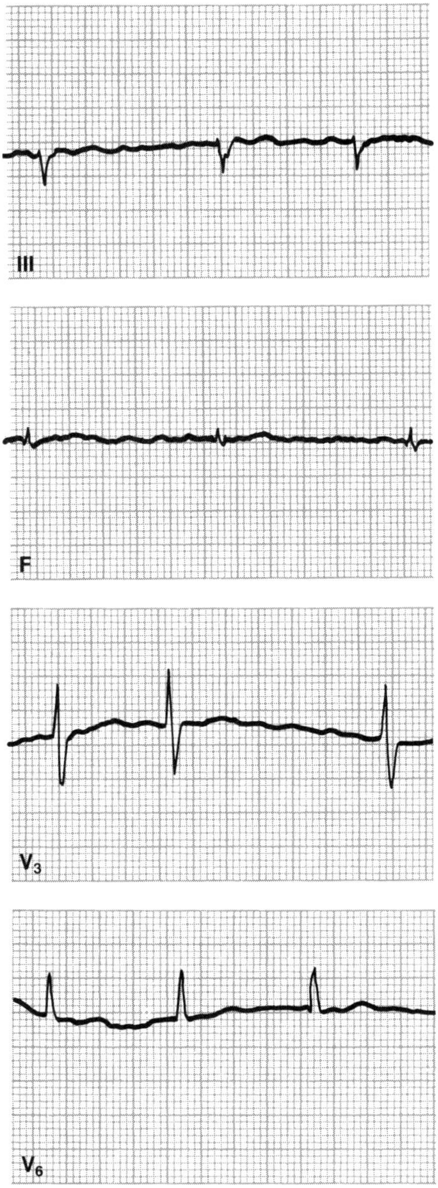
III
F
V_3
V_6

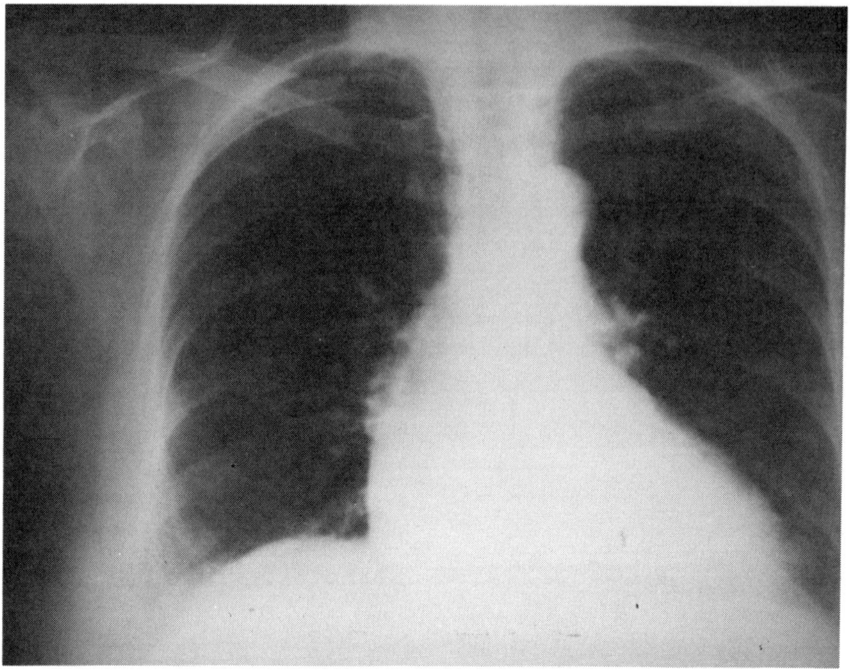

Figure 8-2. Chest X-ray film of the 67-year-old woman whose ECG was shown in Fig. 8-1.

Many investigators feel that by the time ST-T wave repolarization abnormalities ("strain") become evident on the ECG, critical mass has been exceeded.

In contrast to the concentric hypertrophy that results from increased pressure-load states, the heart responds differently to increased volume-load states. Clinically, increased volume load (increased *preload*) occurs with valvular regurgitant lesions such as aortic and mitral insufficiency. It is also seen in obese individuals in whom increased body mass is associated with a larger circulating blood volume. To accommodate an increased preload state, the left ventricular cavity expands (dilates). Force of contraction—and hence, stroke volume—increase to the extent needed to eject the additional volume load. Characteristically, the left ventricular free wall thickens more than the interventricular septum, which is the reason this type of ventricular hypertrophy is known as *eccentric hypertrophy* (Fig. 8-3D).

As was the case for subjects with concentric hypertrophy, mild degrees of eccentric hypertrophy may initially be beneficial. Such is the case with athletes who perform endurance exercise (running, bicycling, swimming, etc.) in whom increased venous return from daily conditioning results in enlargement of the left ventricular cavity with compensatory hypertrophy. In long-standing pathologic conditions (aortic or mitral regurgitation), however, the heart eventually will become unable to keep up with the additional volume load. When this happens, further dilation occurs without compensatory hypertrophy, and left ventricular function deteriorates.

Several additional types of ventricular hypertrophy are illustrated in Fig. 8-3. Panel C represents *asymmetric septal hypertrophy,* commonly known as idiopathic hypertrophic subaortic stenosis (IHSS). The interventricular septum thickens to a much greater extent than the left ventricular free wall, without any increase in left ventricular cavity size. Obstruction of the left ventricular outflow tract may occur during systole when the anterior

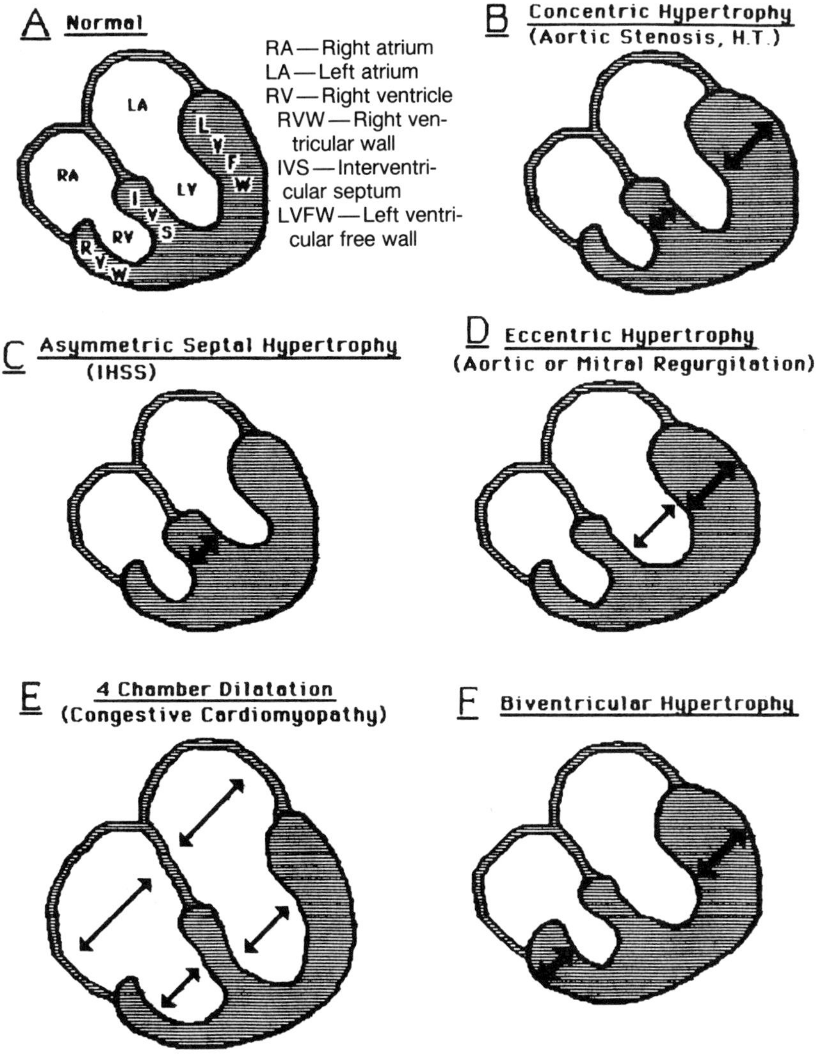

Figure 8-3. Types of ventricular hypertrophy.

leaflet of the mitral valve abuts on the greatly hypertrophied septum. Hence the other name for this entity is hypertrophic obstructive cardiomyopathy.

The picture of *congestive cardiomyopathy* is shown in Panel E. All four cardiac chambers eventually dilate. Compensatory hypertrophy does *not* occur, and cardiac contractility is extremely poor. Resulting stroke volume is greatly reduced in these patients.

In general, increases in voltage on the ECG correlate better with left ventricular *mass* than with left ventricular cavity size. Thus, a patient who develops concentric hypertrophy (Panel B) should be more likely to demonstrate increased voltage on the ECG than one who develops congestive cardiomyopathy (Panel E). In practice, a combination of factors that increase *both* preload *and* afterload commonly exists, so that the processes of left ventricular cavity enlargement and ventricular wall hypertrophy often occur together (Panel D). It is exceedingly hard to separate the effects of each on the ECG. With *biventricular hypertrophy* (Panel F), another problem arises. Combined ventricular hypertrophy increases the electrical potential of both the right and left heart. These effects frequently counteract each other. As a result, biventricular hypertrophy is surprisingly difficult to detect by ECG.

One should remember that there are other ways to determine cardiac enlargement. Commonly overlooked is the physical examination. The finding of a sustained apical impulse is a highly sensitive sign for left ventricular *hypertrophy* in patients with a normal chest wall. An apical impulse that is diffuse (palpable in more than one interspace) and laterally displaced is highly specific for cardiac *enlargement.* Assessment of cardiac size by physical examination loses its sensitivity with obese individuals and patients with emphysema.

Perhaps the most sensitive and specific noninvasive method for determining enlargement of each of the four cardiac chambers is echocardiography. Minimal increases in atrial size, ventricular thickness, or both, can usually be detected long before ECG signs become apparent.

Criteria for ECG Diagnosis of LVH

In Chapter 4, we introduced a number of *voltage* criteria for the ECG diagnosis of LVH. These and other criteria are listed in Table 8-1.

The two major voltage criteria to remember from this table are enclosed within the solid rectangle:

i. Sum of deepest S wave in lead V_1 and V_2 + tallest R wave in lead V_5 and $V_6 \geq 35$ mm

ii. R wave in lead aVL ≥ 12 mm.

The first criterion (i) is by far the best known and the most helpful. If one were to remember only *one* number for the ECG diagnosis of LVH, it should be 35!

The second criterion (ii) is most useful in subjects with a horizontal

TABLE 8-1

Criteria for ECG diagnosis of LVH

VOLTAGE CRITERIA

i) Sum of deepest S wave in lead V_{1-2} + tallest R wave in lead V_{5-6} ≥35 mm.
ii) R wave in lead aVL ≥12 mm

iii) Deep S waves in V_1 or V_2 ≥25 mm.
iv) Tall R waves in V_5 or V_6 ≥25 mm.
v) Sum of tallest precordial lead R wave + deepest precordial lead S wave ≥45 mm.

vi) R wave in V_6 > R wave in V_5.
vii) Sum of R wave in lead I + S wave in lead III ≥25 mm.
viii) R wave or S wave in any limb lead ≥20 mm.

ASSOCIATED MINOR CRITERIA

LAE

Left axis deviation

AGE OF PATIENT

≥35 years of age

REPOLARIZATION CHANGES

"Strain"

Strain equivalent

axis. Since precordial leads are applied to the chest wall at the level of the fourth or fifth intercostal space, they will *not* be directly in the plane of the heart's electrical activity if the mean QRS axis is shifted upward (when there is left axis deviation). In this situation, a lead such as aVL that looks *down* at the heart from the left shoulder will be in a far better position to determine the relative magnitude of left ventricular forces.

PROBLEM: Examine the ECG shown in Fig. 8-4. Is LVH present?

INTERPRETATION of Fig. 8-4

Rate and rhythm: Sinus rhythm at 70–75 beats/min. All intervals are normal.

Axis: +75°

Chamber enlargement: Voltage for LVH would seem to be easily satisfied, since the sum of the deepest S wave in leads V_1 or V_2 + the tallest R wave in leads V_5 or V_6 easily exceeds 35 mm.

QRST changes: Small septal (normal) q waves are seen in the inferolateral leads. R-wave progression is normal. T waves are prominent and peaked in most of the precordial leads. Although this pattern superficially resembles hyperkalemia, the base of the T wave is broader than

Figure 8-4. ECG from an asymptomatic 29-year-old man.

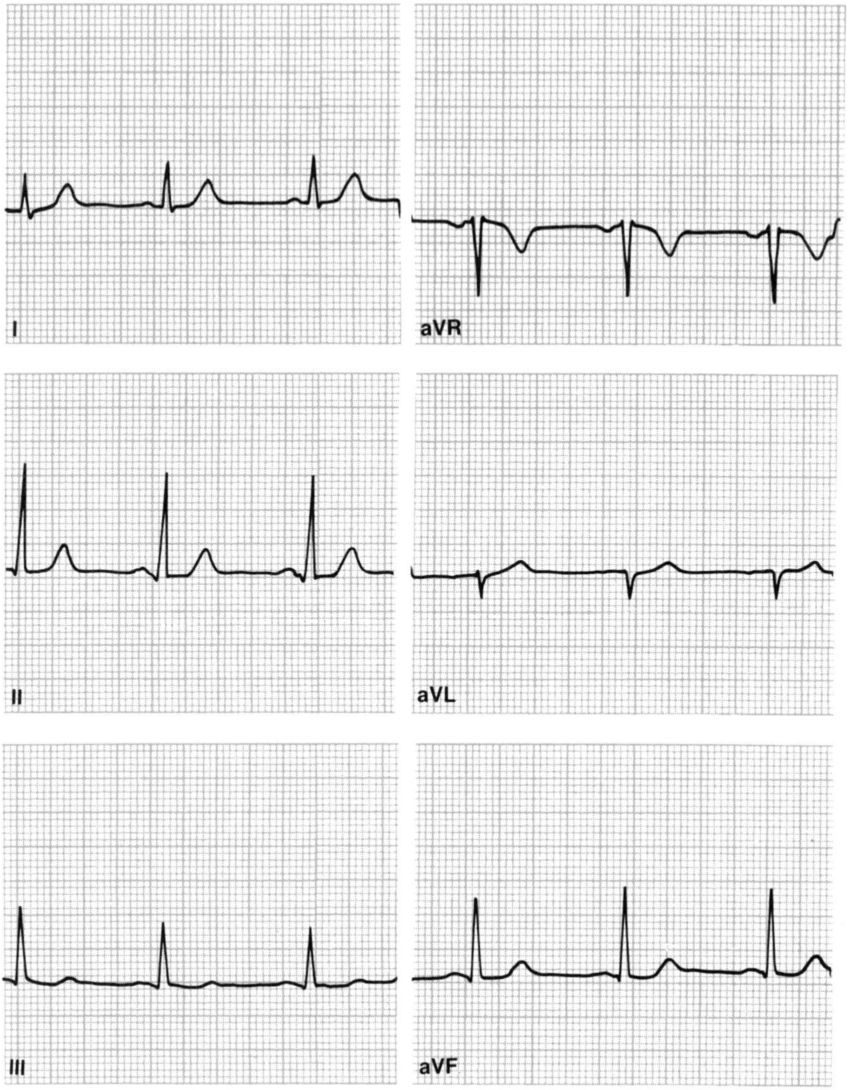

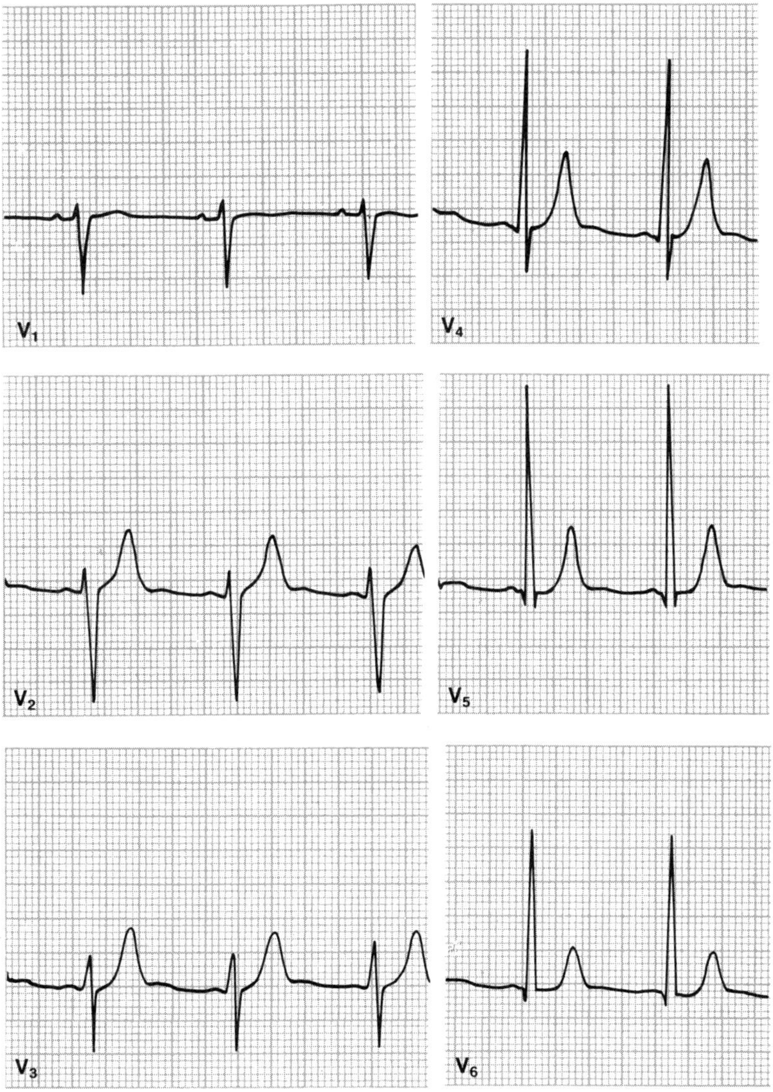
V1
V4
V2
V5
V3
V6

one would expect with this electrolyte abnormality. In an asymptomatic young adult, such T-wave morphology most likely represents a normal *repolarization variant.* (Differentiation between hyperkalemia and this type of repolarization variant was covered in detail in Chapter 5 (Hyperkalemia).

Despite ample voltage, there are *two* reasons one should *not* diagnose LVH from this tracing. The first is the patient's *age.* Young adults commonly manifest increased voltage, and all of the criteria listed in Table 8-1 are much less meaningful in subjects under 35 years of age.

Remembering the number 35 thus serves a dual purpose—it is the standard for the most important voltage criterion, and it recalls that a patient should be at least 35 years old for this standard to be valid. As a ballpark figure, the digits may be *reversed* to provide a standard for voltage in an individual under 35. That is, the sum of the deepest S wave in leads V_1 or V_2 + tallest R wave in leads V_5 or V_6 should be ≥ 53 before one can confidently say that voltage criteria are satisfied in this age group.

Even if this patient were over 35, LVH still should *not* be diagnosed from this tracing, because repolarization abnormalities are lacking! In the absence of characteristic ST-T wave repolarization abnormalities ("strain"), voltage alone is an extremely *insensitive* indicator of true LVH. Undue reliance on this parameter will result in a large number of false-positive diagnoses.

When voltage criteria for LVH are satisfied in a patient over 35 in whom repolarization changes are absent, we suggest the designation "voltage for LVH" be written as part of the interpretation. Doing so acknowledges that while there may truly be LVH, the specificity for determining this electrocardiographically is poor without the presence of repolarization changes.

PROBLEM: Eight voltage criteria for the ECG diagnosis of LVH are listed in Table 8-1. Actually, more than 30 sets of voltage criteria have been reported in the literature. Can you imagine why so many criteria have been proposed?

ANSWER: The reason so many sets of voltage criteria have been proposed is simply that *none* of them are very accurate. Studies correlating antemortem ECGs with left ventricular mass determined at autopsy have shown *sensitivity* for detecting LVH by ECG to be less than 60 percent, regardless of the standard chosen.

Sensitivity for detecting LVH by ECG may be improved slightly by using a *combination* of voltage criteria. Those listed in the table are the ones we have found most helpful. *The overwhelming majority of subjects who fulfill some measure of increased voltage will satisfy one or both of the criteria enclosed within the solid rectangle.* Simply remembering these two major voltage criteria should allow one to identify most patients with LVH who can be detected on ECG.

Remembering additional criteria is a bonus. The three additional criteria that we have found most helpful are enclosed within the dashed rectangle. Occasionally one of these will identify a subject with increased voltage who was not picked up by either of the two major criteria. For example, in some patients with significant LVH, orientation of electrical forces in the horizontal plane is shifted so posteriorly that transition is delayed beyond the V_6 lead. In such cases, the increased R-wave amplitude that one would expect to see in leads V_5 and V_6 doesn't occur. Instead, *deep* S waves (≥ 25 mm) are present in leads V_1, V_2, or both (criterion iii in the table). Such deep S waves reflect significant forces directed away from these right-sided leads (toward the enlarged left ventricle).

In other patients with LVH, the opposite occurs. Instead of relatively deep S waves in leads V_1 and V_2, only shallow S waves are apparent. In this case, R-wave amplitude may be greatly increased in the lateral precordial leads. Finding an R wave ≥ 25 mm in lead V_5 or V_6 satisfies voltage criteria (criterion iv), even if the sum of the deepest S wave in lead V_1 or V_2 + the tallest R wave in lead V_5 or V_6 is less than 35 mm.

Finally, in some patients with an early transition, tall R waves will be seen in leads V_3 or V_4 rather than in V_5 and V_6. In such cases, if the sum of the tallest precordial-lead R wave and the deepest S wave is ≥ 45 mm, voltage criteria for LVH are satisfied (criterion v).

The last three voltage criteria (vi, vii, and viii, Table 8-1) that we have found helpful are:

vi. Finding an R wave in lead V_6 that is taller than the R wave in lead V_5

vii. Sum of the R wave in lead I + S wave in lead III ≥ 25 mm

viii. R wave or S wave in any limb lead ≥ 20 mm

Practically speaking, it is rare for any of these criteria to be present without there being other evidence of increased voltage on the tracing.

In addition to voltage criteria, two ECG findings have been *associated* with LVH. They are left atrial enlargement (LAE) and left axis deviation (LAD). LAE and LAD have been proposed as *minor* criteria for the ECG diagnosis of LVH. Of the two, we have found the former to be much more helpful. Detection of LAE in a tracing with borderline voltage greatly increases the likelihood that true LVH is present.

Simplified Criteria for ECG Diagnosis of LVH

One may easily feel overwhelmed by the abundance of criteria enumerated for the ECG diagnosis of LVH. Fortunately, these criteria may be simplified considerably without much sacrifice in sensitivity (Table 8-2).

TABLE 8-2

Simplified criteria for ECG diagnosis of LVH

Voltage Criteria
- Sum of deepest S wave in lead V_{1-2} + tallest R wave in lead V_{5-6} ≥35 mm.
- R wave in lead aVL ≥12 mm (with leftward axis).

Age of Patient

≥35 years of age

Repolarization Changes

"Strain"

PROBLEM: Examine the ECG shown in Fig. 8-5, taken from a 67-year-old man with hypertension. With what degree of certainty would you diagnose LVH?

INTERPRETATION of Fig. 8-5

Rate and rhythm: Sinus rhythm at 70 beats/min.

PR interval: 0.19 second

QRS interval: 0.10 second (upper limits of normal).

QT interval: Normal.

Axis: About +50°.

Chamber enlargement: Tremendous voltage is present in the precordial leads. The S wave in lead V_2 alone is 35 mm. R-wave amplitude in leads V_5 and V_6 exceeds 25 mm, and sum of the deepest S wave in lead V_1 or V_2 + the tallest R wave in lead V_5 or V_6 is over 60 mm!

Although the P wave is biphasic in lead V_1, the terminal negative component in this lead is *not* a box wide and a box deep. Therefore, criteria for LAE are not met.

QRST changes: A narrow but fairly deep Q wave is present in lead aVL. Since it occurs in isolation (none of the other lateral leads manifest Q waves), it is probably of no significance. Tiny, insignificant q waves are seen in leads V_1 and V_2.

R-wave progression is slightly delayed because transition doesn't occur until lead V_4 to V_5. Since the left ventricle enlarges to the left and *posteriorly,* delayed transition is not at all unusual with LVH.

Typical repolarization abnormalities of "strain" are evident in the lateral precordial leads. Nonspecific ST-segment depression is seen in the limb leads.

Of incidental note, U waves are present in leads V_2 and V_3 as a broad, low-amplitude upright deflection between the T wave and the P wave. Although most often considered a sign of hypokalemia, U waves are also commonly seen with bradycardia, LVH, or both.

Whereas sensitivity of the criteria for LVH is poor, *specificity* of these criteria is much better. If *any* of the voltage requirements listed in Table 8-1 are met in an adult *over 35* who manifests the *typical* repolarization abnormalities of strain, LVH may be diagnosed with greater than 90 percent accuracy. The more voltage criteria that are satisfied, the more certain the diagnosis. Similarly, the greater the magnitude of voltage for any particular requirement, the more accurate the criteria. Excessive voltage to the degree shown in Fig. 8-5 in an adult with typical repolarization abnormalities makes diagnosis of LVH a virtual certainty.

Two additional *subtle* findings are present in this tracing. The first is that the septal q waves that one usually sees in lateral precordial leads are absent. This finding is commonly noted when voltage is markedly increased. It has been attributed to either septal fibrosis or a conduction defect (incomplete LBBB).

Second, QRS duration is slightly prolonged (to 0.10 second), though still within the upper limits of normal. Slight prolongation of QRS duration should be expected when left ventricular mass is increased because of the greater amount of myocardium that the impulse must activate.

PROBLEM: In contrast to the marked voltage that was seen in the previous tracing, examine the ECG shown in Fig. 8-6. Would you diagnose LVH?

INTERPRETATION of Fig. 8-6

Rate and rhythm: Sinus rhythm at 70 beats/min. All intervals are normal.

Axis: +70°

Chamber enlargement: LAE is suggested by the deep terminal negative component of the P wave in lead V_1. The S wave is 16 mm deep in lead V_1 and 15 mm deep in lead V_2. R-wave amplitude is 18 mm in lead V_5, and 17 mm in lead V_6. Sum of the deepest S wave in lead V_1 or V_2 (=16 mm) + tallest R wave in lead V_5 or V_6 (=18 mm) therefore falls just shy of the 35-mm voltage requirement.

QRST changes: Small (probably insignificant) q waves are seen in the inferolateral leads. Despite the fact that transition occurs normally (between leads V_3 and V_4), R-wave progression is poor. Although one can't rule out previous anterior infarction, this diagnosis should probably not be made without other supporting evidence since small (but definite) r waves *are* present in leads V_1 to V_3.

ST-segment sagging with slightly asymmetric T-wave inversion is present in the inferolateral leads. While these changes might represent ischemia, they are more characteristic of strain.

Perhaps the best way to interpret this ECG would be:

"Sinus rhythm at 70 beats/min.
LAE.
Probable LVH and/or ischemia."

Although strict criteria for LVH are *not* met, LVH is *probably* present

Figure 8-5. ECG from a 67-year-old man with hypertension.

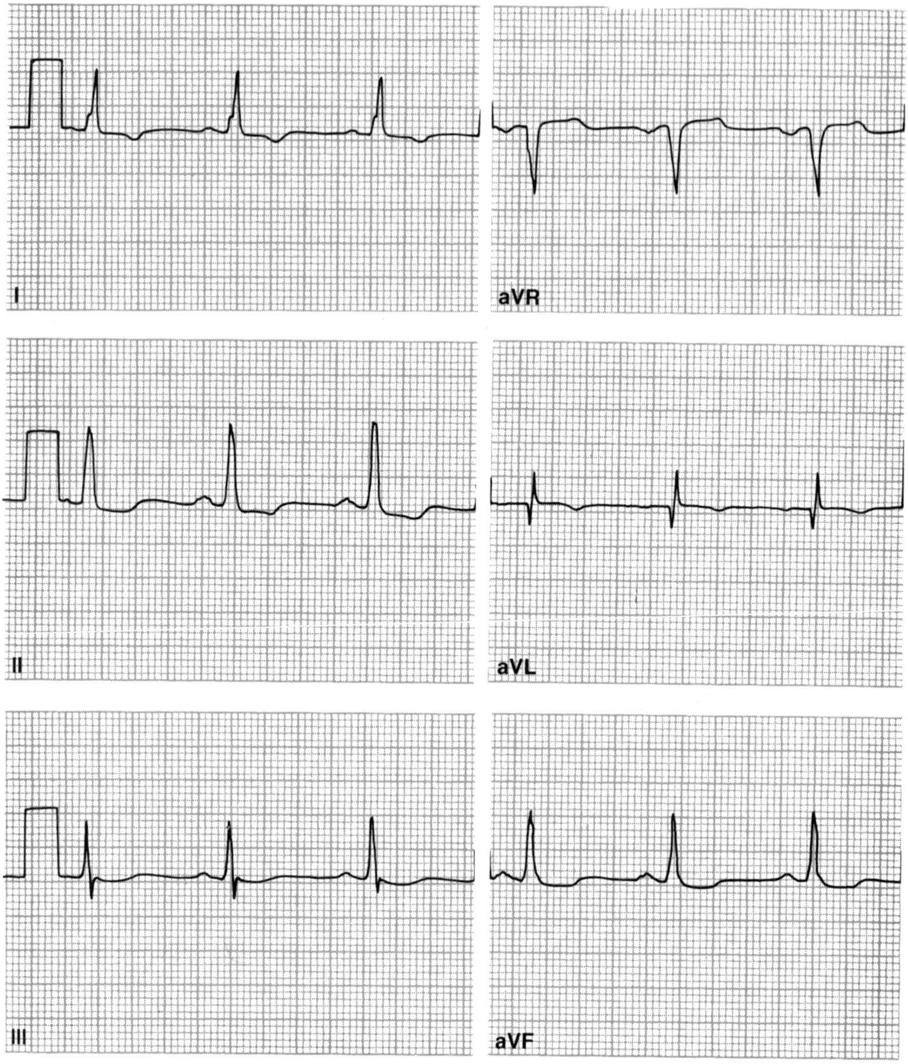

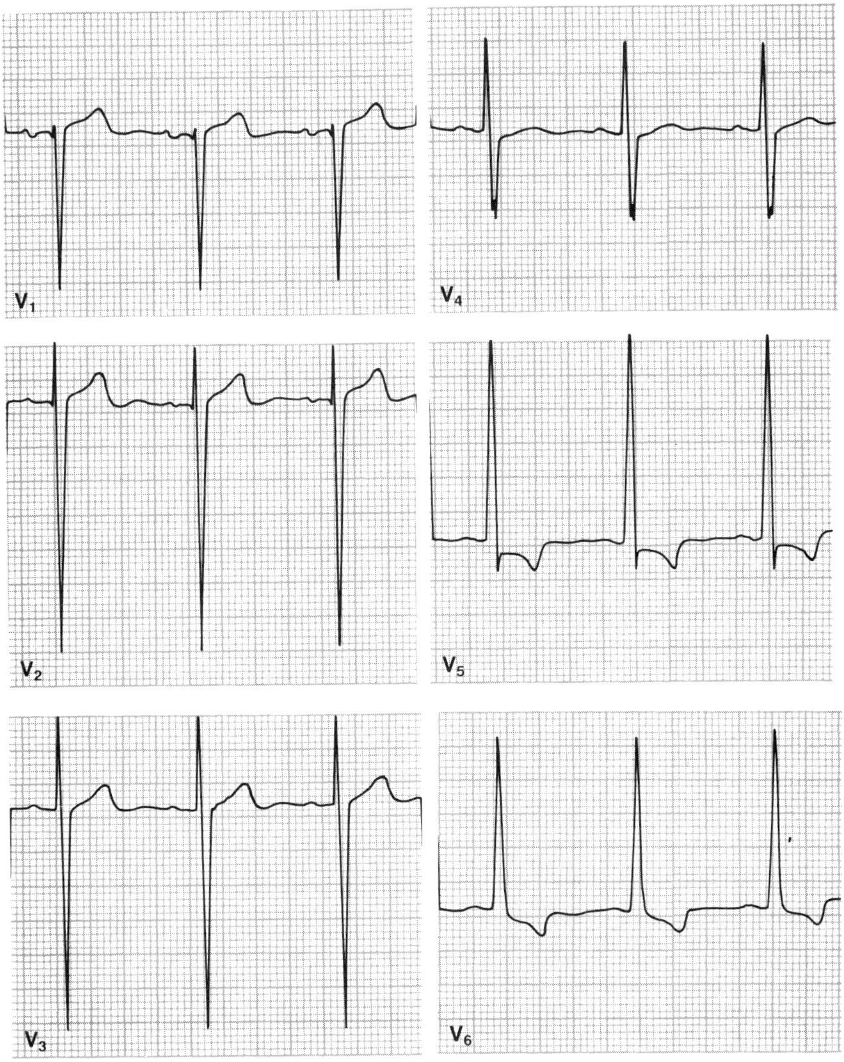
V_1
V_4
V_2
V_5
V_3
V_6

Figure 8-6. ECG from a 52-year-old man with hypertension and ischemic heart disease.

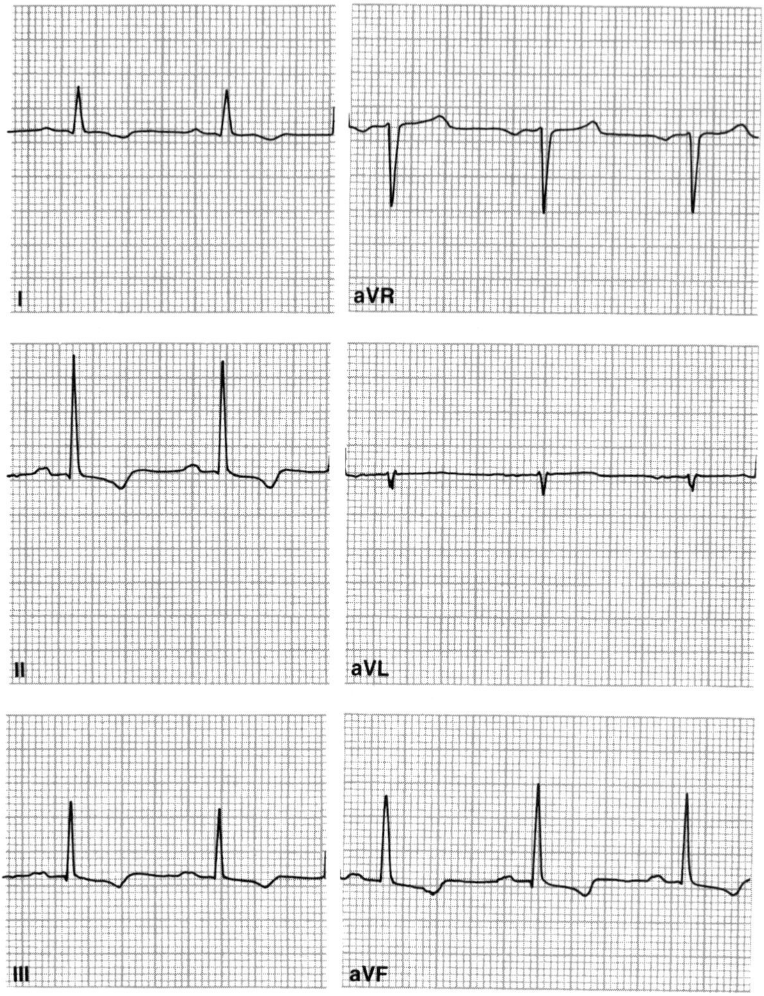

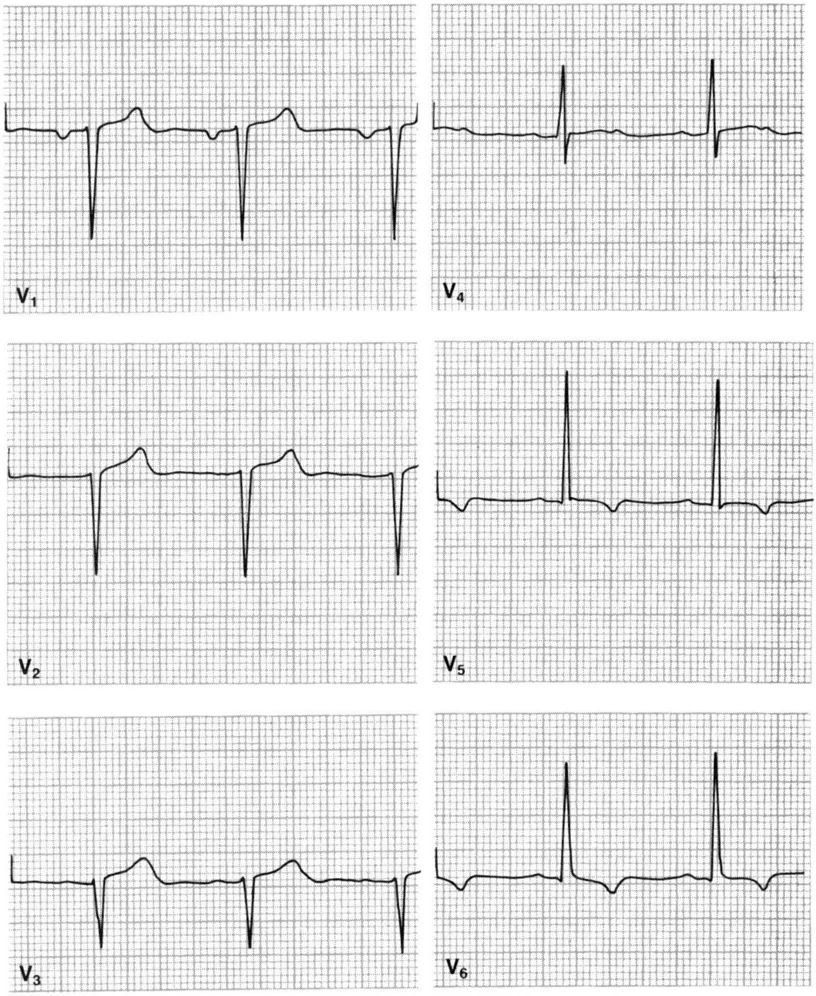
V1
V2
V3
V4
V5
V6

considering the patient's age, clinical diagnoses (hypertension and ischemic heart disease), the presence of LAE, borderline voltage *and* repolarization abnormalities consistent with strain.

Pitfalls in the ECG Diagnosis of LVH

Electrocardiographic voltage is a much more precarious index of left ventricular mass than is generally appreciated. Significant variation in precordial lead voltage (in the range of 10 to 20%) has been shown to occur when serial ECGs are performed on a given individual. Even when identical precordial lead position is assured on serial tracings by marking the patient's chest, day-to-day variation in QRS amplitude of up to 10 percent still occurs.

Changes in position may also have a significant effect on voltage. Mean QRS axis in the frontal plane can shift dramatically from a baseline supine tracing when a patient sits up or stands. Since QRS amplitude in the precordial leads is influenced by position of the heart relative to the chest wall and distance from the recording electrodes, diaphragmatic excursion (as occurs with respiration) or even turning slightly in bed may affect voltage readings.

Taking these factors into account, and considering the associated findings of LAE and strain (assuming the patient was not taking digitalis), the borderline voltage seen in Fig. 8-6 is probably significant. A follow-up ECG on this same patient might well demonstrate more than adequate voltage to fulfill the strict criteria.

It is well to remember that in addition to young adults, individuals with thin chest walls commonly manifest increased QRS amplitude, particularly in the precordial leads. This is simply due to the fact that with a thin chest wall, distance between the heart and the recording electrode is correspondingly decreased. On the other hand, obese individuals or power-trained athletes with thick chest musculature may register falsely low voltages in the precordial leads due to the increased space between recording electrodes and the heart.

Pitfalls other than variability in voltage exist in the ECG diagnosis of LVH. A number of them are listed in Table 8-3. First, reliability of diagnostic criteria is open to question. No universally accepted "gold standard" exists for defining LVH. While autopsy determination of left ventricular wall thickness and heart weight would seem to be the ideal standard, it too has drawbacks. Dissection technique varies. Due to loss of muscle tone, ventricular wall thickness in death may differ from what it was during life when the ECG was recorded. Even the question of what heart weight to choose as the dividing point between a ventricle that is "normal" in size and one that is hypertrophied remains controversial. How to factor in body weight, age, sex, and race of the patient further complicates the issue.

Over 30 sets of voltage criteria have been proposed for the ECG diagnosis of LVH. All of them suffer from a lack of sensitivity. Disagreement among different cardiologists about which criteria should be used is never-

TABLE 8-3

Pitfalls in the ECG diagnosis of LVH

Questionable Reliability of Diagnostic Criteria
- Multiplicity of criteria for ECG diagnosis of LVH
  - Poor sensitivity of criteria
  - Inter- and intraobserver variability in interpretation
- Lack of suitable "gold standard"
- Abruptness of cutoff point for making diagnosis
- Effect of age, sex, race, physical conditioning, and body habitus on baseline voltage

Variability in QRS Amplitude Measurements
- Day-to-day variability in voltage
- Effect of positional change on voltage
- Effect of precordial lead placement on voltage

Presence of Competing Conditions
- Conduction defects (RBBB, LBBB, IVCD)
- Myocardial infarction
- Chronic obstructive pulmonary disease
- Coexistent RVH

ending. Since no one can really "prove" which criteria are best, individual preferences are retained and *interobserver* variability (among different cardiologists reading the same tracing) is inevitable. *Intraobserver* variability (between the first and second readings of the same ECG by the same cardiologist) has also been shown to occur (in the range of 10 to 20%).

Competing conditions may disguise ECG diagnosis of LVH. Conduction defects alter QRS amplitude by affecting the path of depolarization. Loss of lateral forces from infarction may mask LVH, whereas loss of anterior forces may actually simulate LVH by deepening S waves in the anterior precordial leads. Chronic obstructive pulmonary disease with hyperinflation and increased AP thoracic diameter dampens QRS amplitude by increasing distance between the heart and the chest wall. Finally, biventricular hypertrophy surprisingly often masks ECG diagnosis of LVH and RVH because of the canceling out effect of the increased forces from each hypertrophied ventricle.

Recognition and Importance of Strain

Left ventricular strain has been shown to be an extremely important factor in making the ECG diagnosis of LVH. Even without supportive voltage criteria, the presence of strain *alone* (in a patient not taking digitalis) is highly correlated with the existence of LVH.

In Chapter 5 we described the ECG changes that occur with strain. Typically, there is ST-segment depression with asymmetric T-wave inversion. The gradual descent of the sagging ST segment blends imperceptibly with the first portion of the T wave. The final ascending portion of the T wave has a much more rapid upslope as it returns to the baseline. This picture is illustrated in Fig. 8-7B.

ECG changes of strain are usually best seen in monitoring leads that view the left ventricle (I, aVL, V_5, and V_6). In a given tracing, one or more of

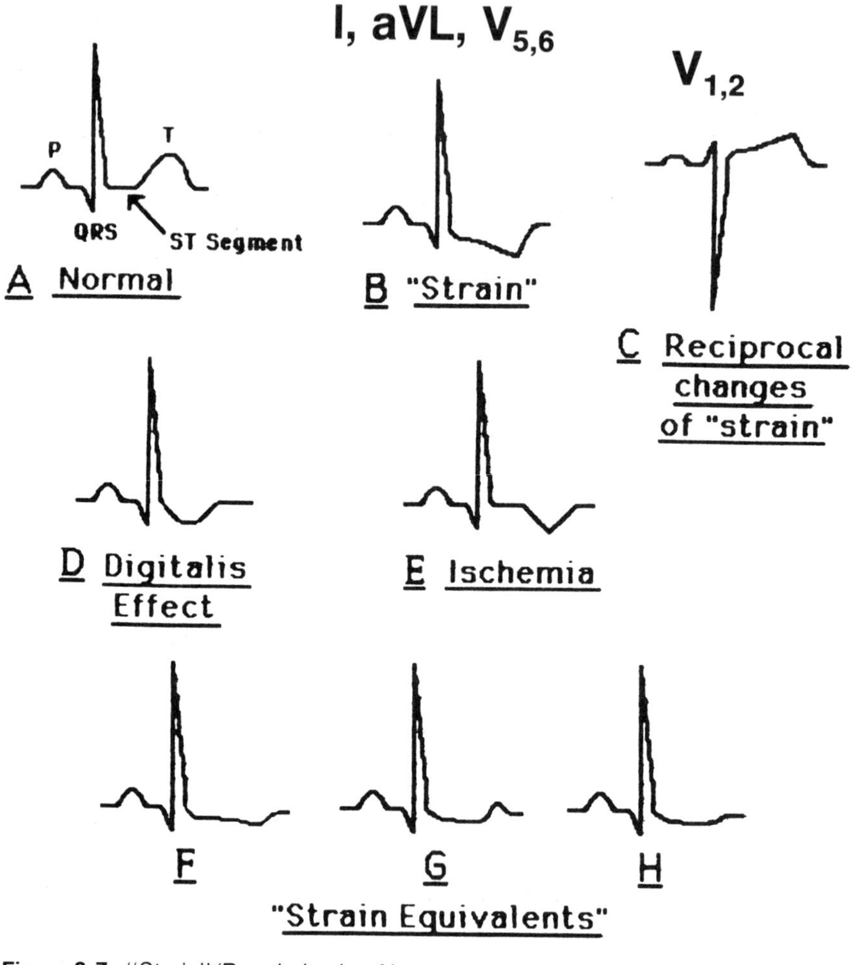

Figure 8-7. "Strain" (Repolarization Abnormalities) of LVH **A.** Normal ST-T wave **B.** Left ventricular "strain": ST-segment depression and asymmetric T-wave inversion with a gradual descent and a more rapid ascent back to the baseline. Strain is most often seen in the left ventricular leads (I,aVL,V_{5-6}). **C.** Reciprocal ST-T wave changes of "strain": ST-segment elevation with an upright T wave may reflect "reciprocal" changes of strain in the anterior precordial leads. **D.** Digitalis effect: Scooped ST-segment depression with shortening of the QT interval. [Digitalis may also produce ST-T wave changes identical to strain (B)]. **E.** Ischemia: Symmetric T-wave inversion. Strain may sometimes be masked by ischemia. **F, G,** and **H.** "Strain equivalents".

these leads may manifest such changes. Occasionally when the heart has a vertical electrical axis, typical repolarization abnormalities will be observed in the inferior leads.

Reciprocal repolarization changes may often be seen in the anterior precordial leads of patients with LVH. Instead of ST-segment depression and asymmetric T-wave inversion, T waves will be upright and the ST segments are elevated (Fig. 8-7C).

A number of conditions may produce ST-T wave changes that closely resemble those of strain. Two that are commonly encountered are digitalis use and ischemia. As discussed in Chapter 5, digitalis may affect the resting ECG in one of two ways ("digitalis effect"). In some patients, ST-segment depression and asymmetric T-wave inversion indistinguishable from strain is produced. In others, QT-interval shortening with a scooping or "hockey stick" deformity of the ST segment is seen (Fig. 8-7D). The discriminating value of ST-T wave changes in the ECG diagnosis of LVH is diminished in patients taking digitalis.

Ischemia characteristically produces *symmetric* T-wave inversion. Accompanying ST-segment depression may or may not be present. At times, the primary T-wave change of ischemia may mask secondary repolarization changes of strain. The reverse may also occur.

Finally, mention should be made of *"strain equivalents."* While not of the same diagnostic value as the typical changes of strain, ST-T wave flattening, depression, or both (Panels F, G, and H of Fig. 8-7) in association with increased voltage increases the likelihood that LVH is present.

PROBLEM: Examine the tracings shown in Figs. 8-8 and 8-9. Is LVH present? If so, with what confidence level would you make this diagnosis?

INTERPRETATION of Fig. 8-8

Rate and rhythm: Sinus rhythm at 78 beats/min. All intervals are normal.

Axis: $+50°$.

Chamber enlargement: Although decreased in amplitude, the P wave is notched and prolonged in duration (to 0.13 second) in lead II. Thus, LAE is present. Deep S waves are evident in lead V_1 and particularly in lead V_2. Voltage criteria for LVH are easily met.

QRST changes: Scooped ST-segment depression is seen in multiple leads. T waves are generally diminished in amplitude, but still upright.

In the context of the marked increase in QRS amplitude observed in this tracing, this type of ST-T wave change qualifies as a "strain equivalent" (Fig. 8-7G). Considering the patient's age, clinical history, marked increase in voltage, and associated findings of LAE and repolarization abnormalities, confidence in the diagnosis of LVH should be high.

INTERPRETATION of Fig. 8-9

Rate and rhythm: Sinus tachycardia at 120 beats/min. The PR and QRS

Figure 8-8. ECG from an 80-year-old man with aortic stenosis.

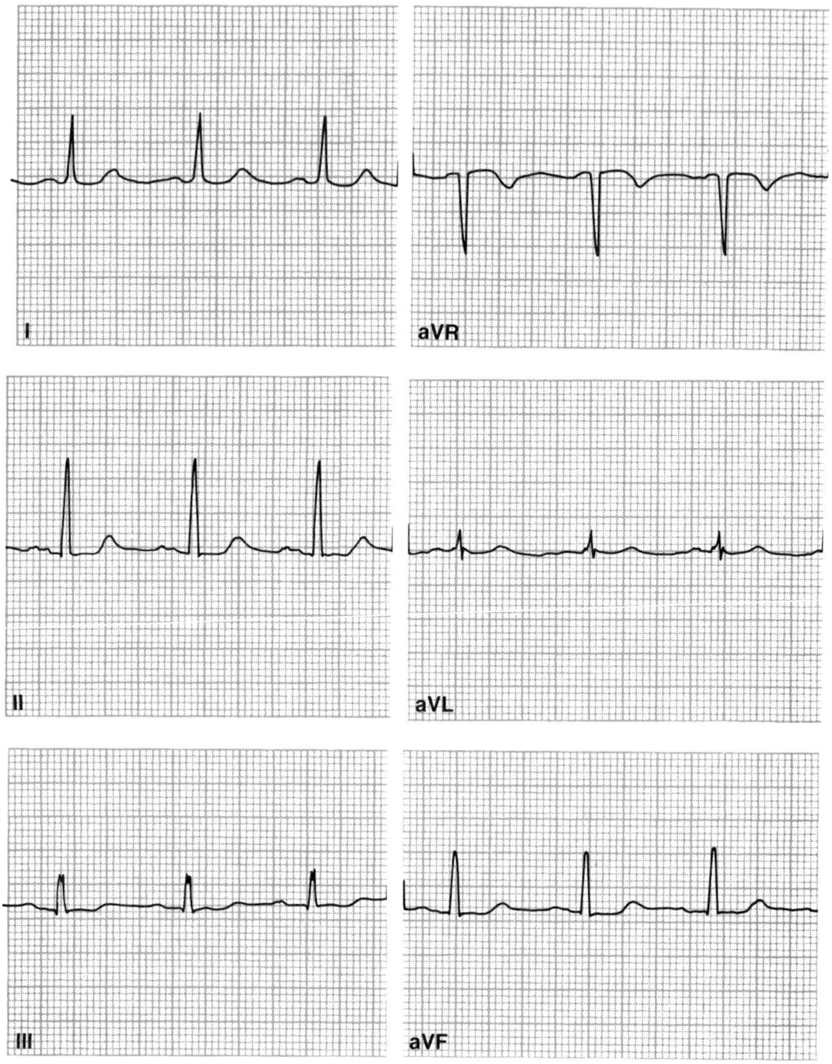

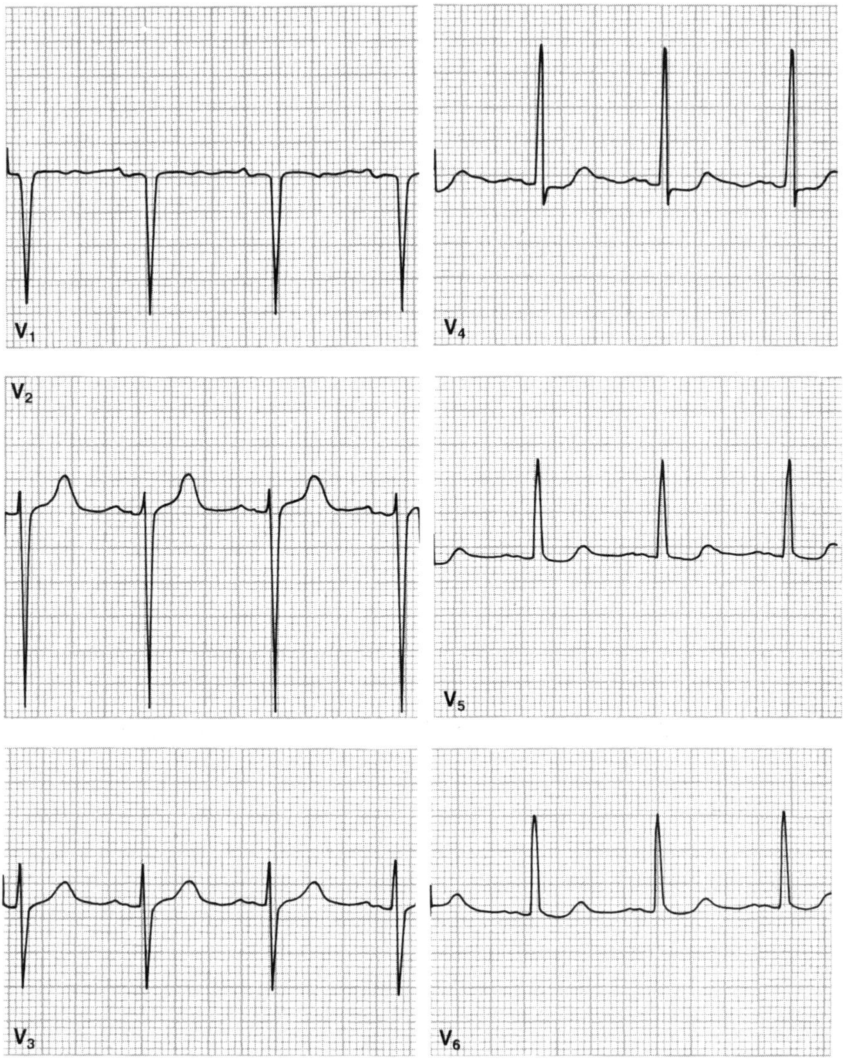
V1
V2
V3
V4
V5
V6

Figure 8-9. ECG from a 77-year-old woman with hypertension and congestive heart failure.

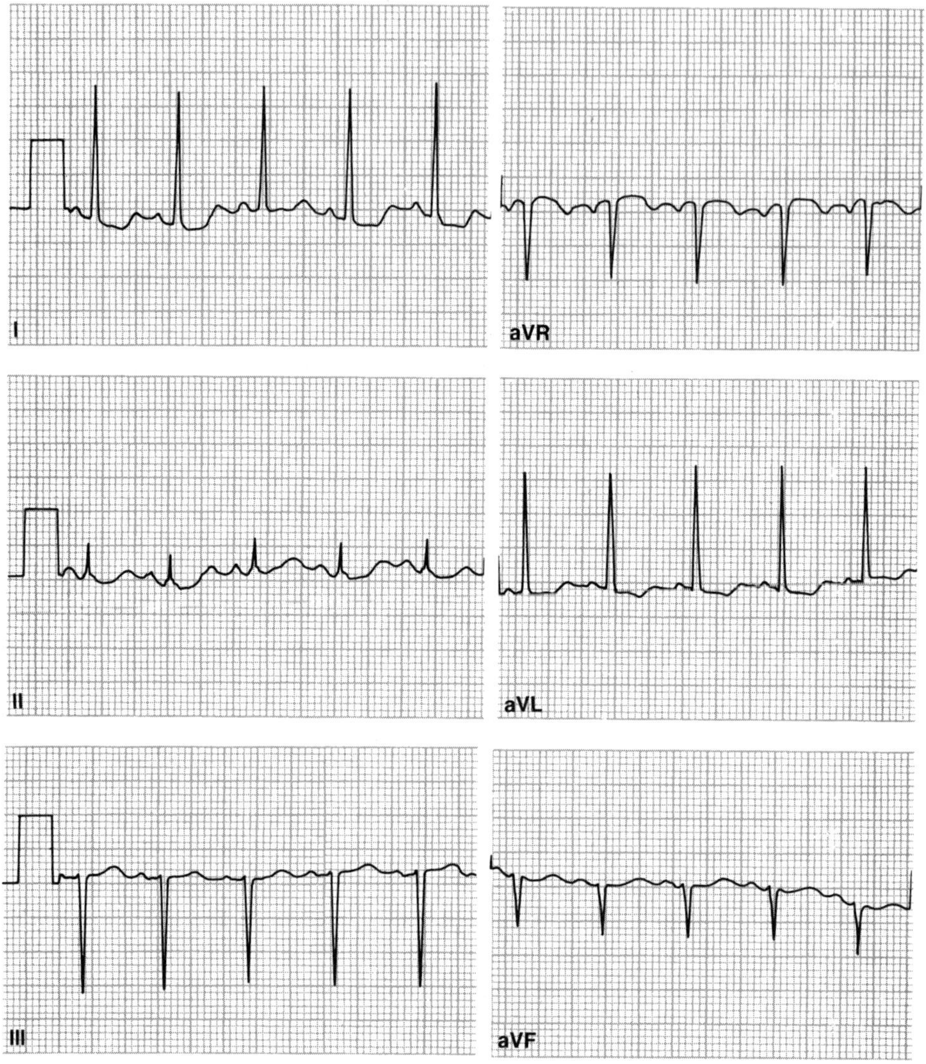

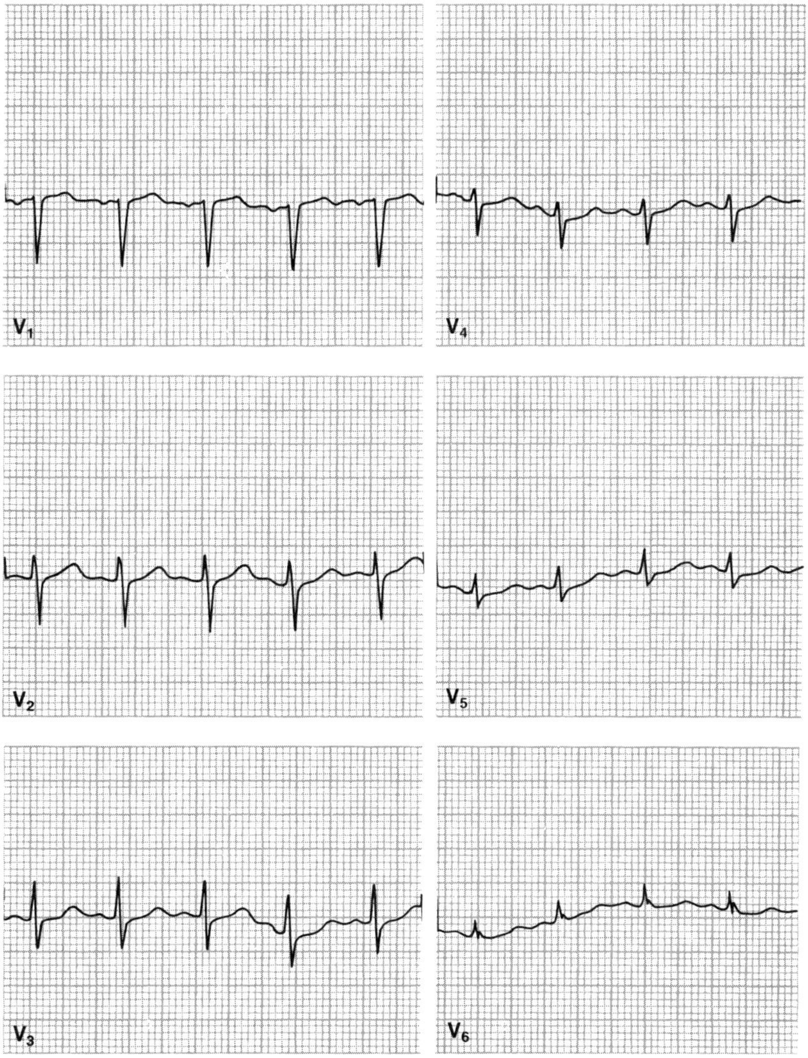
V1
V4
V2
V5
V3
V6

intervals are normal. Calculation of the QT interval is less reliable at this rate.

Axis: $-15°$.

Chamber enlargement: LVH (R in aVL ≥ 12 mm; also sum of R wave in lead I + S wave in lead III ≥ 25 mm).

QRST changes: Consistent with strain in the limb leads. Nonspecific ST-T wave abnormalities are present in the precordial leads.

This ECG offers a nice example of how with a leftward axis the typical changes of LVH and strain may be present in lead aVL, but totally absent in the precordial leads. Again the patient's age, clinical history, marked increase in limb-lead voltage, and characteristic repolarization abnormalities make confidence in the diagnosis of LVH extremely high.

Clinical Implications of LVH

Most of the patients whose ECGs we have examined in this chapter have had underlying hypertension. One point to emphasize is that development of LVH *and* strain in patients with hypertension is an *ominous* rather than incidental finding! It more than doubles the risk of morbidity and mortality from hypertension alone. Once LVH has set in, cardiovascular mortality from stroke, congestive heart failure, ischemic heart disease, and peripheral vascular disease increases about eightfold. Within five years, 30 percent of these patients will have a major cardiovascular event.

In contrast, the presence of voltage criteria for LVH *without* the associated ST-T wave abnormalities of strain carries a much lower risk of cardiovascular morbidity and mortality. As we alluded to in the beginning of this chapter, development of strain may signal the point when *critical mass* is exceeded and left ventricular function has begun to deteriorate.

Clinical implications of the ECG diagnosis of LVH are summarized in Table 8-4.

A question that frequently arises is whether to obtain a chest X-ray, ECG, or both in the routine evaluation of patients with essential hypertension. The Joint National Committee on Detection and Treatment of Hypertension recommends an ECG unless aortic coarctation is suspected. Although at any age the prevalence of cardiac enlargement on chest X-ray is at least twice that of LVH on ECG, the prognostic information that a chest X-ray provides for hypertensive patients is much more limited than that gathered from an ECG. While one should never be lulled into a false sense of security when the ECG of a patient with hypertension is normal, the finding of LVH *and* strain should alert the primary-care provider to the immediate need for aggressive antihypertensive therapy in an attempt to avert serious complications. Finding voltage for LVH without strain, on the other hand, does *not* put the patient at any greater risk of cardiovascular morbidity and mortality than the hypertension alone. Nevertheless, it should serve as a

TABLE 8-4

Clinical implications of LVH

LVH and Strain
- 8X ↑ in mortality from cardiovascular disease (stroke, CHF, IHD, peripheral vascular disease)
- More than doubles the risk of H.T. alone
- Within 5 years, 30% of these patients will have a major cardiovascular event
- After an acute MI, development of ECG LVH results in 4X ↑ in mortality
- After onset of angina pectoris, development of ECG-LVH results in 4X ↑ in mortality

Voltage for LVH alone
- Risk is similar to that of H.T. alone, and less than half that of ECG-LVH

Cardiac Enlargement on Chest X-ray Films
- Risk is less than half that of ECG-LVH

CHF—congestive heart failure
IHD—ischemic heart disease
H.T.—hypertension
Acute MI—acute myocardial infarction

warning that development of strain and its ominous implications may be forthcoming unless blood pressure is lowered. If blood pressure control can be achieved and maintained, encouraging recent evidence suggests that even established LVH may be reversed (at least in part), and the risk of complications correspondingly lessened.

Atrial Abnormality

PROBLEM: Examine the ECG shown in Fig. 8-10. Is there evidence of atrial enlargement?

INTERPRETATION of Fig. 8-10

Rate and rhythm: Sinus tachycardia at 115 beats/min. The PR and QRS intervals are normal.

Axis: About +20°.

Chamber enlargement: Biatrial enlargement. LVH.

QRST changes: Nonspecific ST-T wave abnormalities are present in the limb leads. Leads V_5 and V_6 manifest ST-segment depression and asymmetric T-wave inversion consistent with left ventricular strain.

One should also be concerned about the appearance of the ST segments and T waves in the anterior precordial leads. The ST-segments are coved and slightly elevated in leads V_1 to V_3. In the latter two leads, the T wave is beginning to invert. By lead V_4, it is deeply and symmetrically inverted. Considering the patient's clinical presentation, these changes suggest possible anterior ischemia, infarction, or both.

Figure 8-10. ECG from a 63-year-old man who presented in hypertensive crisis and fulminant pulmonary edema.

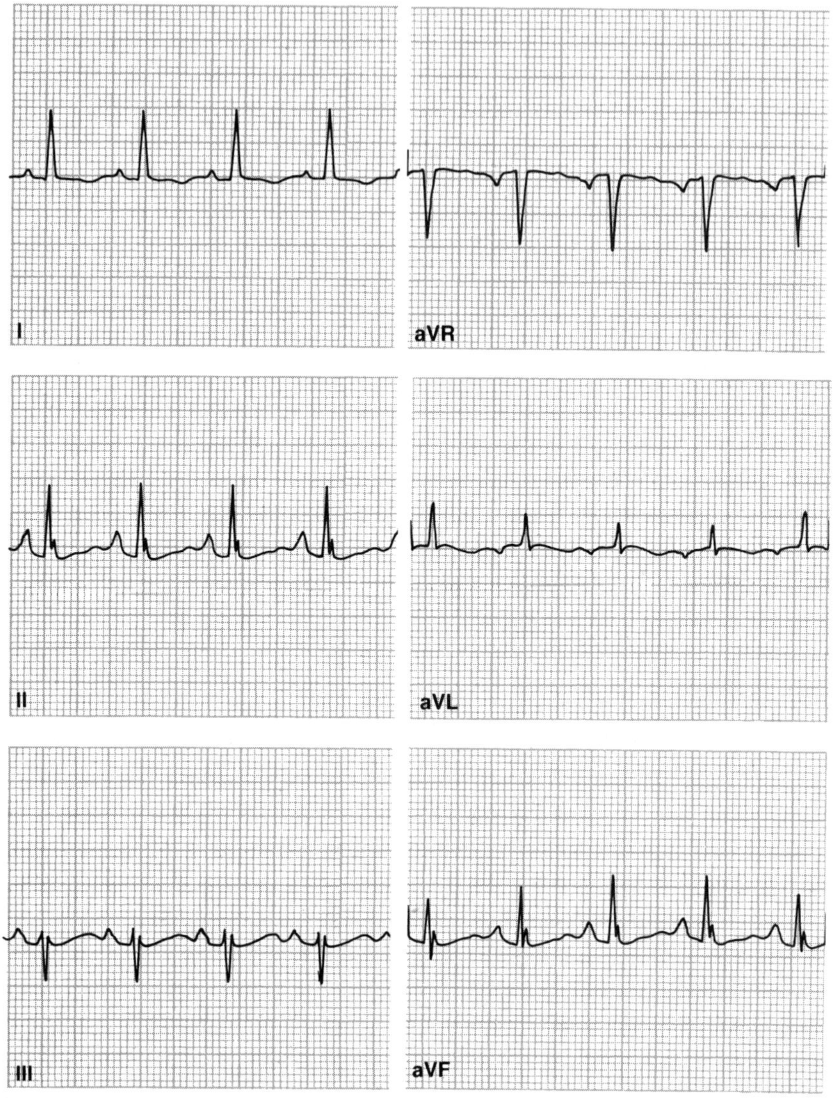

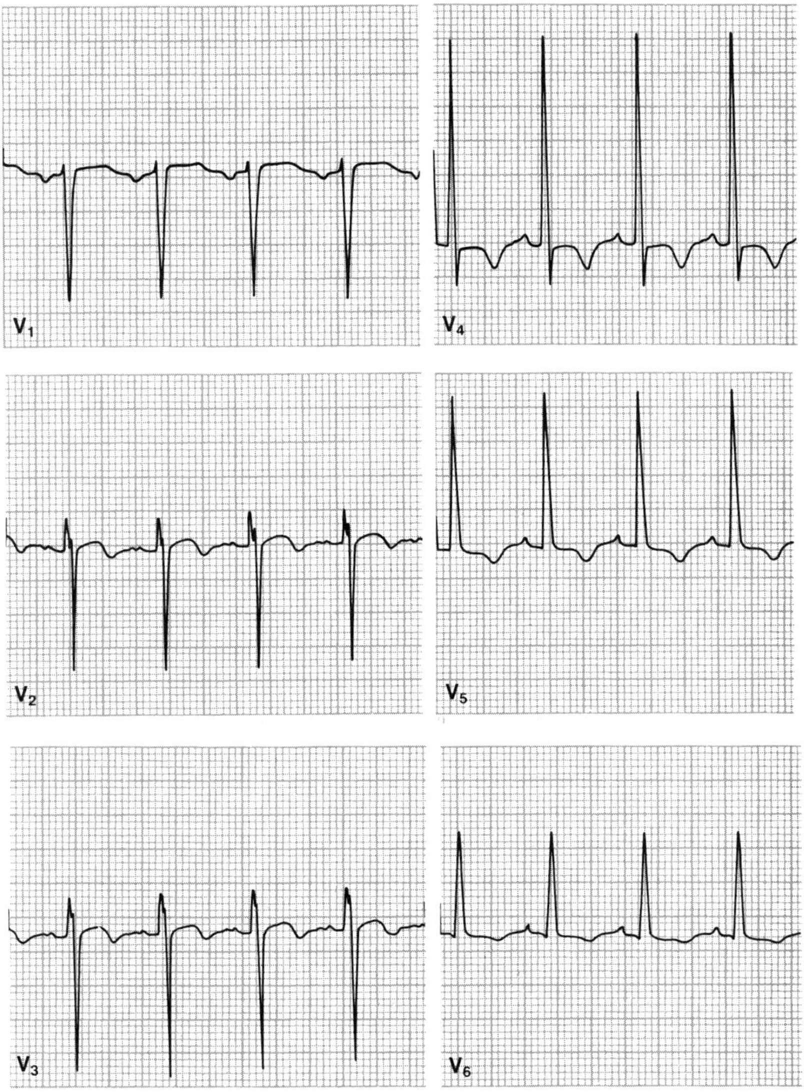
V1
V2
V3
V4
V5
V6

In addition to definite LVH and strain, *biatrial enlargement* is suggested by the tall, peaked P waves in the inferior leads (RAE), and the deep terminal negative component of the P wave in lead V_1 (LAE).

Derivation of the changes one might expect to occur in P wave morphology with atrial enlargement was discussed in Chapter 4. Table 8-5 consolidates this information.

Sensitivity and specificity of the ECG criteria for atrial enlargement are disappointing. No P-wave abnormality is observed in many patients with documented atrial enlargement. Conversely, many patients with anatomically normal atria demonstrate abnormal P waves.

Many conditions other than atrial enlargement cause alterations in P-wave morphology. Principal among these are *intra-atrial conduction defects.* Disease of the internodal or interatrial conduction pathways may result in notching, peaking, and/or prolongation of the P wave in a similar manner to the way that disease of the ventricular conduction system causes IVCD and bundle branch block.

Because the atria share a common septum and internodal conduction pathway, P-wave alterations suggesting RAE *(P-pulmonale)* may be seen with anatomically pure left-atrial enlargement. Similarly, LAE (M-mitrale) may be seen with anatomically pure right-atrial enlargement.

Other conditions that may alter P-wave morphology in the absence of true atrial enlargement are indicated in Table 8-6. Acute increases in intra-atrial pressure may sometimes produce dramatic alteration in P-wave morphology. Thus the pattern of LAE (with marked deepening of the terminal negative component of the P wave in lead V_1) sometimes develops with acute left ventricular failure, while that of RAE may be seen with acute pulmonary

TABLE 8-5

Atrial enlargement

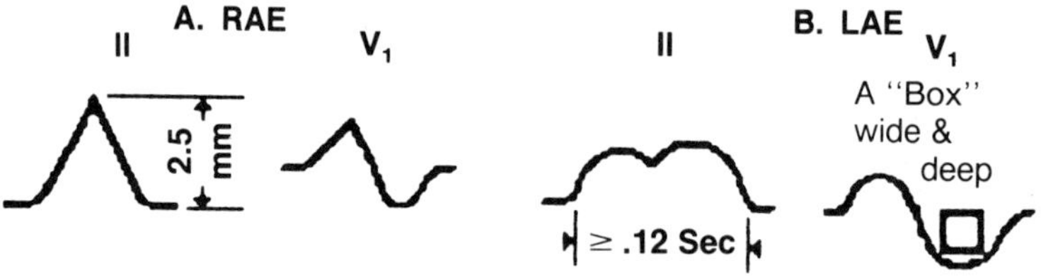

P Pulmonale
- Tall P waves
- Peaked P waves
- Rightward P axis

P-wave amplitude must be ≥2.5 mm in lead II, III, or aVF

P Mitrale
- P-wave duration of ≥0.12 sec
- Notched P wave in lead I, aVL, or II
- Large terminal negative deflection in lead V_1

embolism or accelerated pulmonary hypertension. With correction of the underlying disorder, P-wave morphology often reverts back to normal.

For unknown reasons, P waves frequently become tall and peaked in the inferior leads with hypokalemia ("pseudo P-pulmonale"). Similarly, tachycardia and/or a vertical electrical axis may also produce a pattern that suggests RAE when there is none. Finally, some patients without any underlying disorder simply manifest unusual P-wave morphology.

Because of the numerous causes of altered P-wave morphology that are totally unrelated to atrial size, use of the terms RAE, LAE, P-pulmonale, and M-mitrale is potentially misleading, and should probably be discouraged. Instead, the newer noncommital terms *right-atrial abnormality (RAA)* and *left-atrial abnormality (LAA)* should be preferred. However, the older terms still pervade the literature, and we have continued to use them throughout this book. In general, we employ the terms RAE or P-pulmonale in those cases when true right-atrial enlargement is strongly suspected on clinical grounds, from associated findings on the ECG, or both. LAE or M-mitrale is employed when true left-atrial enlargement is strongly suspected. On the other hand, when abnormal P-wave morphology occurs as an isolated finding in a patient without known reason to have atrial disease, we prefer the designations RAA and LAA.

PROBLEM: Examine Fig. 8-11, which shows leads II and V_1 from a patient with valvular heart disease. Is enlargement of one or both atria suggested?

ANSWER: The P wave is tall and peaked in lead II, suggesting RAA. It is

TABLE 8-6

Pitfalls in the ECG diagnosis of atrial enlargement

Poor Sensitivity and Specificity of Criteria

Echocardiography much more accurate

Other conditions may cause alterations in P-wave morphology

- interatrial conduction defect
- increased intraatrial pressure
- hypokalemia
- tachycardia
- "vertical heart"
- normal variant

"M-mitrale" may be seen in patients with pure RAE

"P-pulmonale" may be seen in patients with pure LAE

Biphasic P wave in lead V_1 and notched P waves may be normal

Inter- and Intraobserver Variability in Interpretation

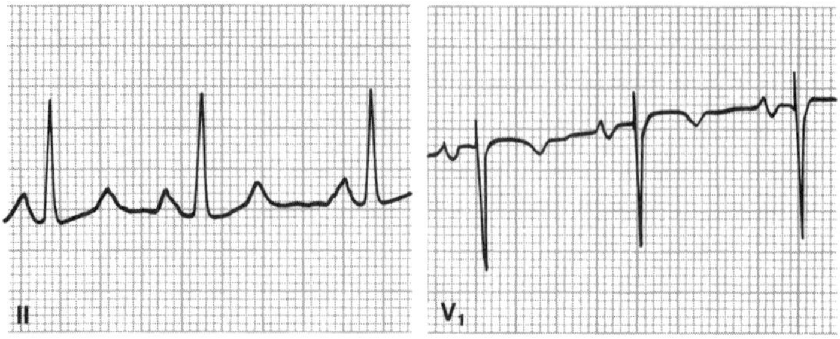

Figure 8-11. Selected leads from a patient with valvular heart disease. Is enlargement of one or both atria suggested?

biphasic in lead V_1 with a particularly prominent terminal negative component that suggests LAA. The correct ECG *interpretation* of these findings is *biatrial abnormality.* This patient turned out to have severe mitral stenosis, for which she was operated on. Her right atrium was anatomically normal.

This example highlights the lack of specificity of the ECG for atrial enlargement. Despite evidence for a "P-pulmonale" pattern (prominent, pointed P waves in lead II), this patient had no right-atrial disease. On the other hand, not even "pure" and severe mitral stenosis was enough to produce the P-wave *notching* ("M-mitrale" pattern) that supposedly typifies this disorder.

Echocardiography is far more sensitive and specific than electrocardiography for evaluating atrial disease. Two-dimensional (2-D) echocardiography provides indirect visualization of both the left and right atria, allowing early detection of chamber enlargement. In addition, ventricular function may be assessed and correlated with atrial findings. Standard M-mode echocardiography permits precise measurement of left-atrial size. M-mode and 2-D echocardiography are so sensitive at picking up mitral stenosis that one is safe in saying that a normal echocardiogram virtually excludes this disorder.

Because of the poor sensitivity and specificity of the ECG in evaluating atrial size (and the vast superiority of the echocardiogram), we prefer to *undercall* ECG signs of atrial abnormality. Thus, P wave amplitude in at least one of the inferior leads *must* fully attain 2-1/2 mm to satisfy criteria for RAA. Similarly, to satisfy criteria for LAA, the P wave in lead II must be at least 0.12 seconds in duration and/or the terminal negative component of the P wave in lead V_1 must be deep enough and wide enough to contain a 1-mm box.

Right Ventricular Hypertrophy

PROBLEM: Interpret the ECG shown in Fig. 8-12.

INTERPRETATION of Fig. 8-12

Rate and rhythm: Sinus tachycardia at about 110 beats/min. Occasional PACs (in leads I, III, and aVL).

PR interval: 0.15 second.

QRS interval: 0.10 second (upper limits of normal). IRBBB is present (rSR′ in lead V_1 and S waves in leads I and V_6, but only *minimal* prolongation of the QRS complex).

Axis: The QRS complex is predominantly *negative* in all of the limb leads. Its appearance in leads II and III suggests marked LAD. But the predominantly negative complex in lead I suggests RAD. Since it is impossible to *determine* whether marked left or right axis deviation exists, we say the mean QRS axis is *indeterminate.*

Chamber enlargement: RAA is suggested by the prominent, peaked P waves in the inferior leads, and LAA by the deep, terminal negative component of the P wave in lead V_1.

QRST changes: Although there are no Q waves, there is extremely *poor R-wave progression.* Transition never occurs. There are nonspecific ST-T wave abnormalities.

PROBLEM: Is there evidence for RVH?

ANSWER: Perhaps more than any other entity in electrocardiography, diagnosis of RVH must usually be made deductively by putting together a constellation of supportive findings into a cohesive picture. This is the case for Fig. 8-12.

At first glance, one might suspect that the poor R-wave progression in this tracing represented anterior infarction, and that a bifascicular conduction defect (LAHB and IRBBB) is present. Instead, all of the findings on this tracing can be put together into *one* unifying diagnosis: *type C RVH.*

We have previously discussed the ECG derivation of the different types of RVH in Chapter 4. Horizontal-plane vector loops and ECG criteria for types A and C RVH are again summarized in Table 8-7.

Type A RVH is thought to reflect severe pressure overload states. It is most commonly seen in children with congenital heart disease such as pulmonary stenosis, tetralogy of Fallot, or Eisenmenger's syndrome. Type A RVH is *rare* in adults, and is usually seen only with end-stage pulmonary disease or pulmonary hypertension. In contrast, type C RVH is frequently seen in adults. It is most often associated with chronic obstructive pulmonary disease.

Figure 8-12. ECG from a 70-year-old man with chronic obstructive pulmonary disease who presented with increasing dyspnea.

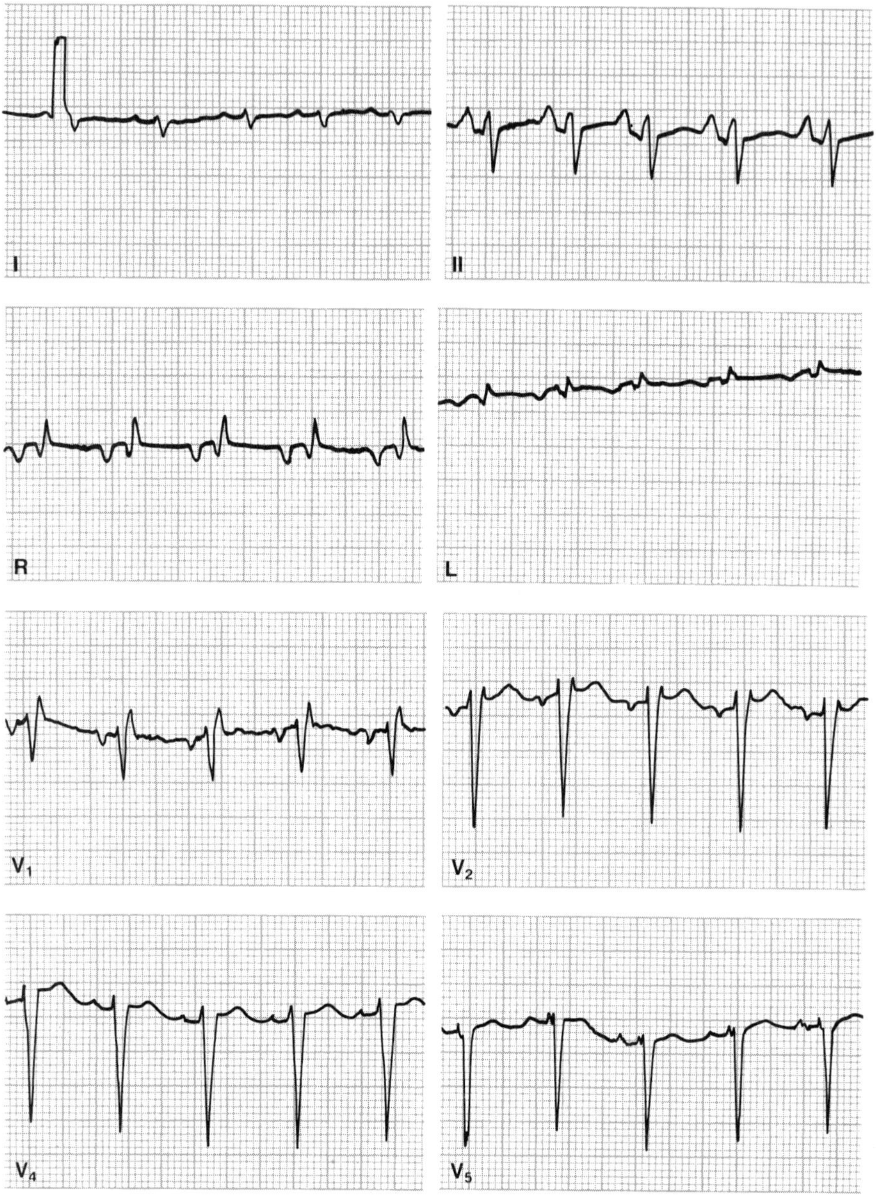

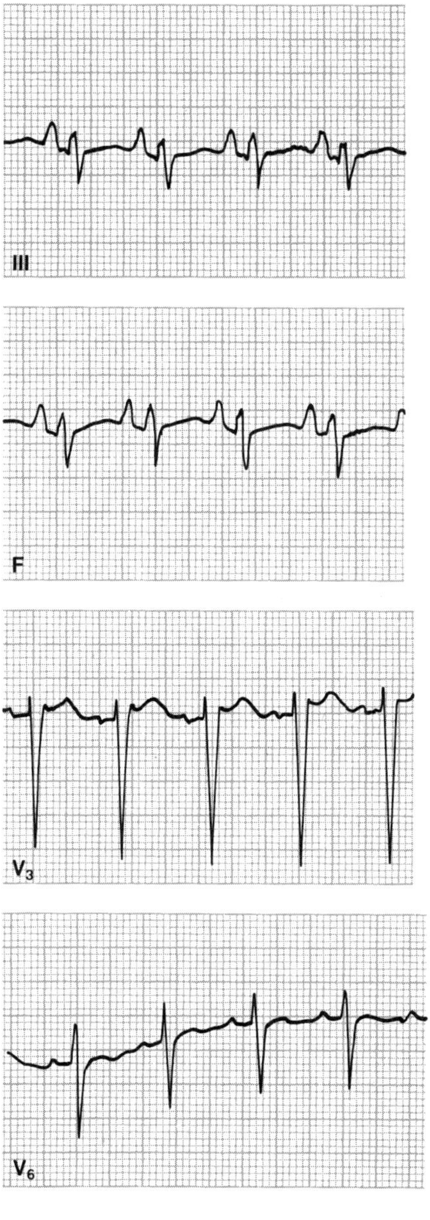
III
F
V_3
V_6

Virtually all of the findings of *type C RVH* listed in Table 8-7 are found in Fig. 8-12. QRS amplitude in the limb leads is relatively decreased (although admittedly not fulfilling strict criteria for low voltage). Indeterminate mean QRS axis, S waves in leads I, II, and III, and persistence of S waves across the precordial leads are all characteristic findings of patients with pulmonary disease, and are evident in this tracing. In addition, IRBBB is present. Development of this conduction disturbance in patients with pulmonary disease often indicates that right ventricular enlargement, increased pulmonary artery pressure, or both have become superimposed.

Finally, peaked P waves in the inferior leads indicate RAA. We have already discussed the lack of specificity that RAA has when it occurs as an isolated finding in otherwise healthy individuals. However, when RAA occurs in the context of other suggestive signs for pulmonary disease (as seen here), it becomes much more likely that this alteration in P-wave morphology represents true right atrial enlargement. With the possible exception of tricuspid stenosis, it is extremely rare for any heart disorder to produce true

TABLE 8-7

Right ventricular hypertrophy

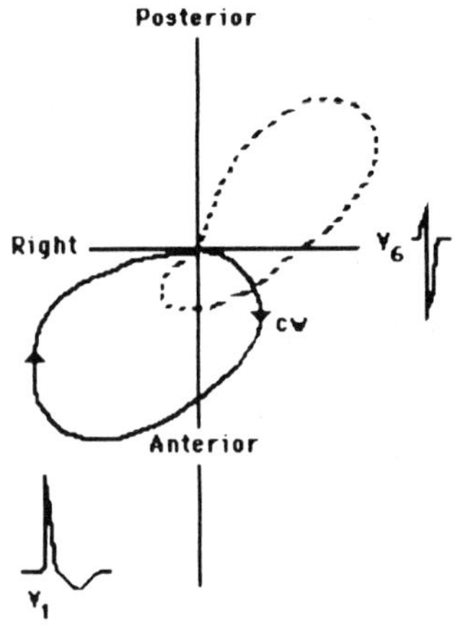

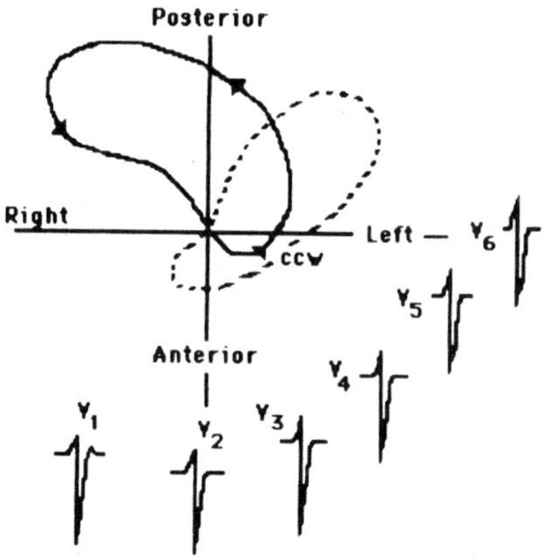

Type A RVH*
Predominant R wave in lead V_1
"Strain" pattern in inferior and/or anterior precordial leads
RAE
Right axis deviation
Deep S waves in leads V_{5-6}

Type C RVH
Low voltage in the limb leads
IRBBB
RAE
Right axis deviation or indeterminate axis
Persistence of S waves across the precordium
S waves in leads I, II, and III

**Type B RVH is a less common intermediate form. Distinction of it from type A RVH may be difficult without a vectorcardiogram.*

right atrial enlargement without also affecting the right ventricle. Consequently, detection of RAE is an important deductive sign that RVH is also probably present.

In contrast, specificity of LAA for true left atrial enlargement markedly diminishes when seen in the context of pulmonary disease. At times the right atrium may become so enlarged that it actually develops a *posterior* orientation, accounting for a deep terminal negative component to the P wave in lead V_1. This patient turned out to have pure right-sided heart disease (end-stage cor pulmonale) with an anatomically normal left atrium. Electrocardiographically, it would be impossible to know this, and the correct interpretation of P-wave morphology would have to be *biatrial abnormality*.

In summary, rather than to postulate the existence of bifascicular block, biatrial enlargement, *and* anterior infarction, it intuitively makes more sense to search for *one* unifying diagnosis: type C RVH.

PROBLEM: Examine the ECGs shown in Figs. 8-13 and 8-14. Is RVH present in one or both of these tracings?

INTERPRETATION of Fig. 8-13

Rate and rhythm: Sinus tachycardia at about 100 beats/min. The PR and QRS intervals are normal. The QT interval is probably prolonged.

Axis: About +100° (RAD).

Chamber enlargement: P-wave morphology suggests biatrial abnormality: prominent, peaked P waves in the inferior leads (RAA), and deep terminal negative component to the P wave in lead V_1 (LAA). There is also RVH.

QRST changes: A qR complex is present in lead V_1. ST-segment depression and T-wave inversion are seen in the inferior leads and across the precordium.

This ECG demonstrates *all* of the characteristic findings of *type A RVH* (Table 8-7):

- Predominant R wave in lead V_1
- Right ventricular "strain" pattern
- RAE
- Right axis deviation
- Deep S waves in leads V_5 and V_6

At first glance, one might be tempted to diagnose diffuse ischemia due to the ST-segment depression and T-wave inversion that is seen in multiple leads. Once again, however, it is the *constellation* of findings that suggests the correct diagnosis. While a number of clinical entities may produce a tall R wave in lead V_1, the associated findings of RAE, RAD, and persistent S waves in leads V_5 and V_6 overwhelmingly favor RVH as the underlying cause. In this context, the diffuse ST-T wave changes that are seen almost certainly represent right ventricular "strain." While right ventricular strain is most often seen in the anterior precordial leads (V_1 to V_3) and/or in the

Figure 8-13. ECG from a 43-year-old woman who presented with increasing dyspnea.

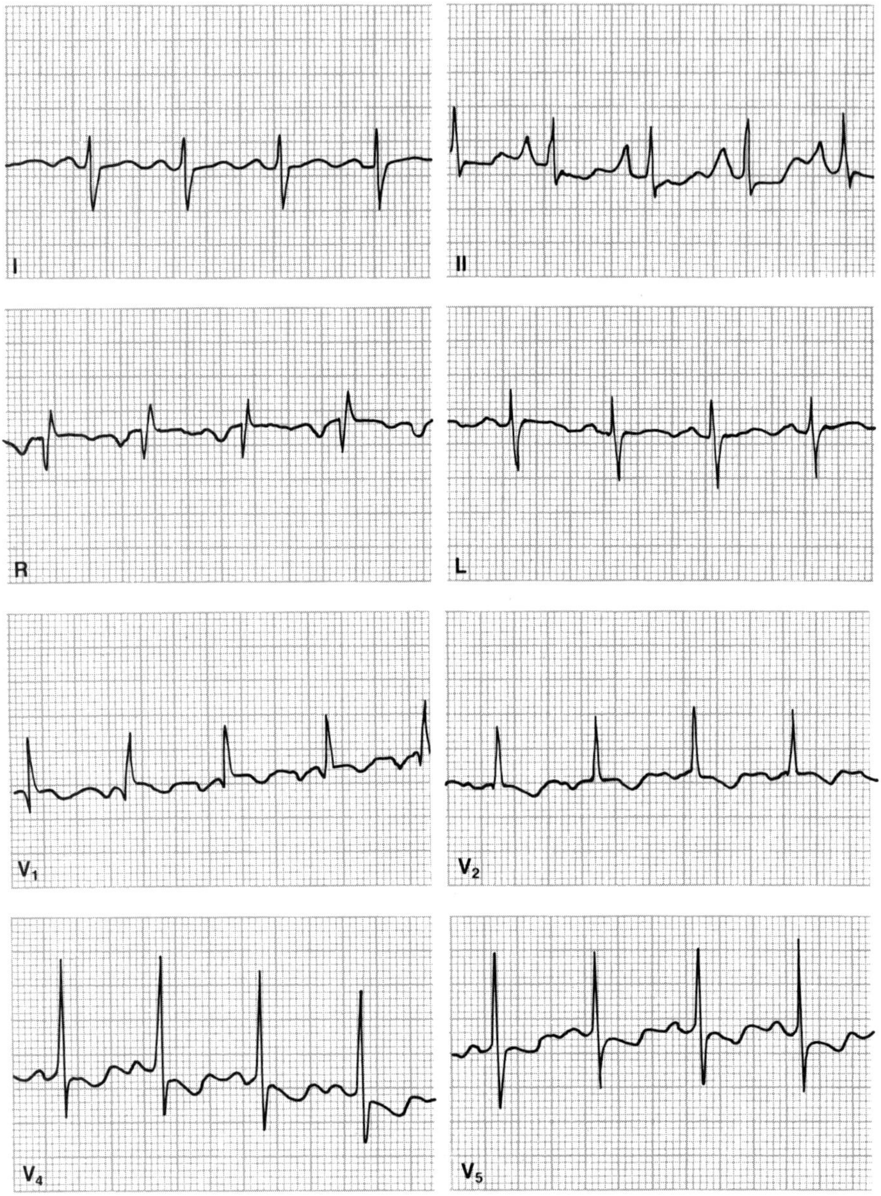

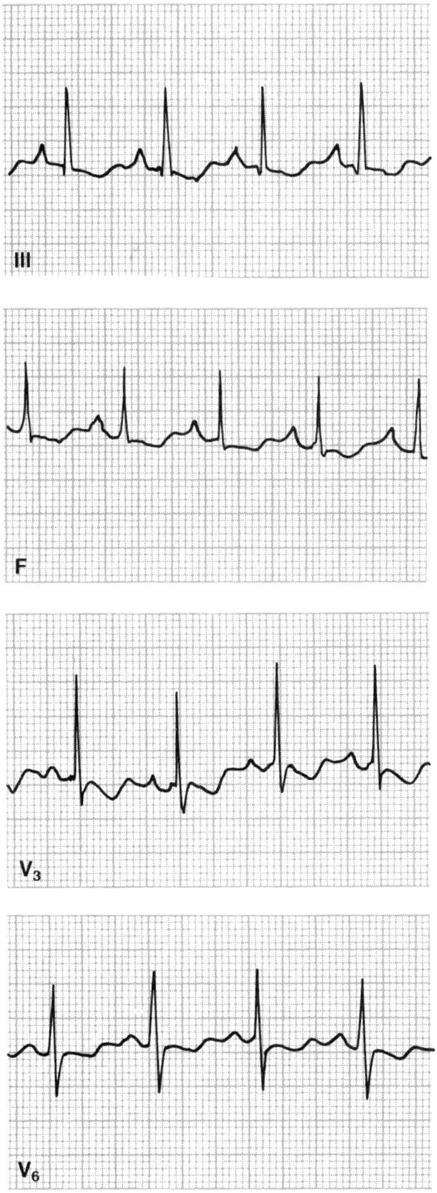
III
F
V_3
V_6

Figure 8-14. ECG from a 79-year-old man who presented with congestive heart failure.

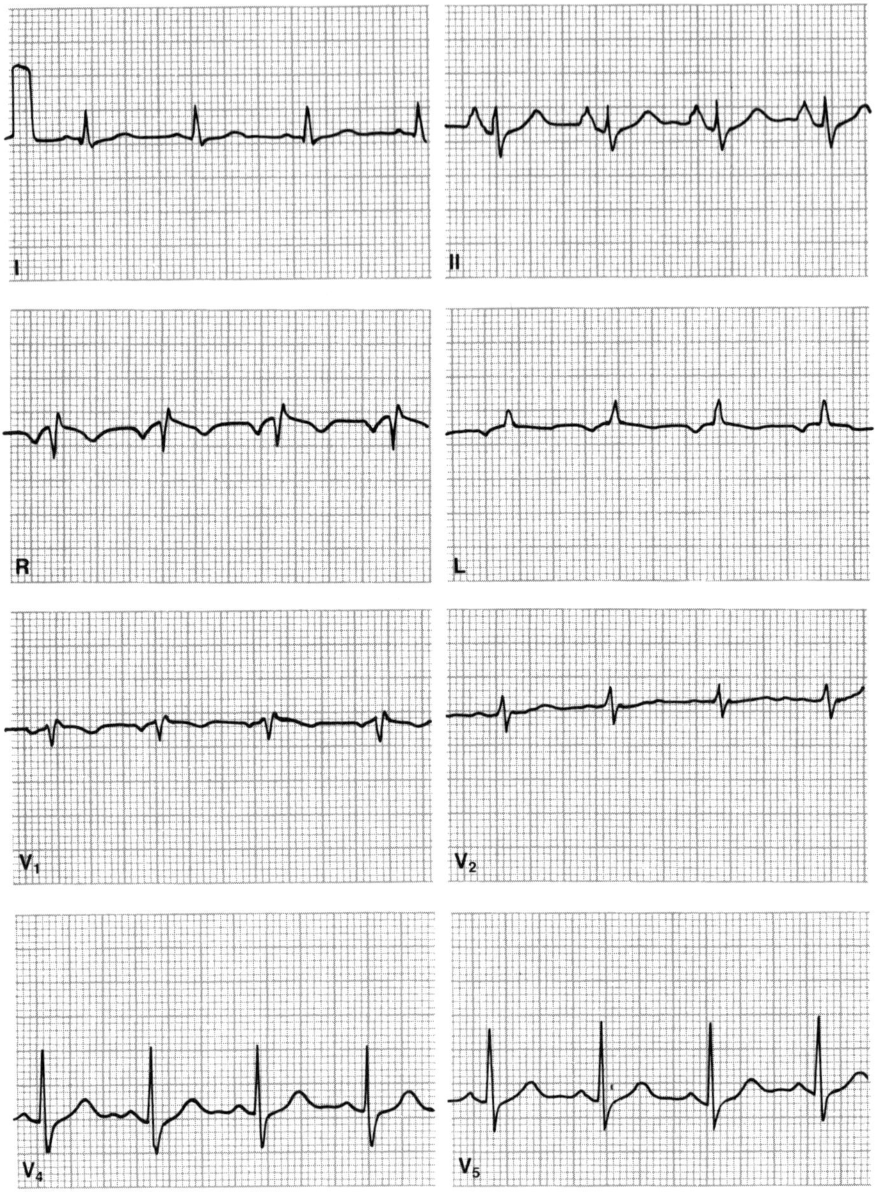

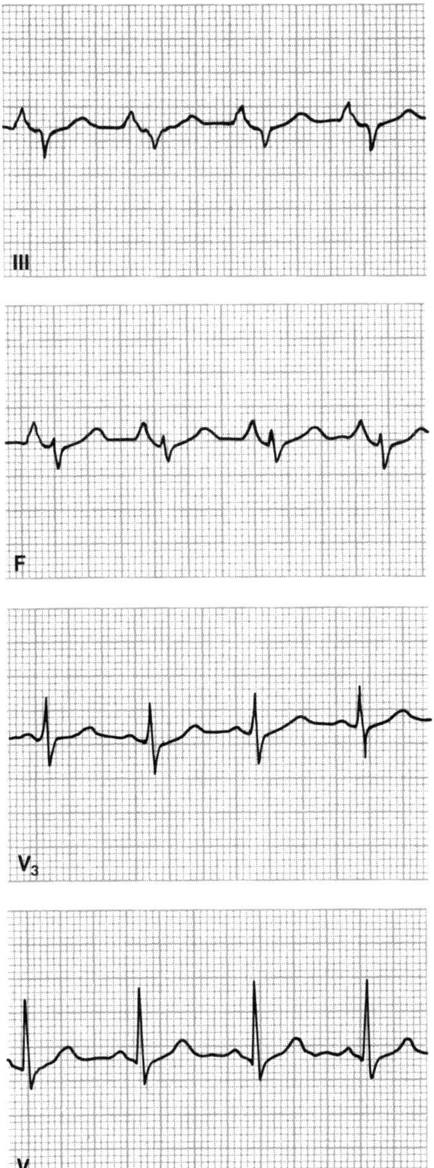
III
F
V_3
V_6

inferior leads (II, III, and aVF), it may occasionally involve the lateral precordial leads as well (as it does here).

This patient turned out to have primary pulmonary hypertension. She had markedly elevated right-sided pressures, but normal left-sided pressures and an *anatomically normal left atrium* (despite the deep terminal negative component to the P wave in lead V_1). Her condition rapidly deteriorated, and unfortunately she died within a few weeks of this tracing.

A final *subtle* point to make from this ECG regards the qR configuration that is noted in lead V_1. When seen with RVH, this morphology is often associated with a markedly elevated pulmonary artery pressure. Derivation of the qR configuration in lead V_1 has been attributed to *rotation* of the interventricular septum which causes the initial vector of septal depolarization to shift from its usual left-to-right orientation to a more *posterior-anterior* orientation (directed *away* from lead V_1, hence producing a q in V_1.

INTERPRETATION of Fig. 8-14:

Rate and rhythm: Sinus rhythm at 90 beats/min. All intervals are normal.

Axis: −30° (LAD).

Chamber enlargement: RAA.

QRST changes: A Q wave of unknown significance is present in lead III. Transition occurs early between leads V_1 and V_2. Minimal nonspecific ST-T wave abnormalities are evident.

While one might be hard pressed to say that type C RVH is definitely present on this tracing, a number of findings do suggest *pulmonary disease.* QRS amplitude is relatively decreased in both limb and precordial leads (although once again strict criteria for low voltage in the limb leads are not met), an rSr′ pattern (IRBBB) is present in lead V_1, S waves persist throughout the precordium, and RAE is present.

PROBLEM: Examine the ECG shown in Fig. 8-15. Is RVH present?

INTERPRETATION of Fig. 8-15

Rate and rhythm: Sinus tachycardia at 90 to 140 beats/minute, depending on which leads you examine.

PR interval: Seemingly short (<0.12 second).

QRS interval: Normal.

Axis: About + 10°.

Chamber enlargement: Seemingly RVH with strain if the patient were an adult.

PROBLEM: Are any of these findings abnormal when one considers that they come from a 22-month-old infant?

ANSWER: This ECG is entirely normal considering the age of the patient.

Detecting Chamber Enlargement in Children

Although interpretation of pediatric ECGs is a specialty in itself, discussion of some easily remembered ground rules may be helpful to the primary-care provider who occasionally is called on to read ECGs in children.

Sinus arrhythmia with heart rates exceeding 100 beats/min (as in Fig. 8-15) is commonplace in infants. The mean heart rate of children under 8 years old is about 100 beats/min, and a heart rate of up to 115 beats/min is still within the normal range. Clearly, the definitions for sinus bradycardia and tachycardia do *not* hold up for infants and children.

Similarly, PR and QRS intervals are often much *shorter* in duration for infants and children than they are in adults. One should therefore *not* become concerned with the short PR interval seen in Fig. 8-15. A PR interval as short as 0.08 second is still normal for children up to 3 years of age. However, a PR interval of 0.18 second would constitute first-degree AV block for that same child.

Due to the predominant role of the right ventricle during the prenatal period, right ventricular forces commonly exceed left ventricular forces at birth. Thus, more than half of all newborn infants have an ECG pattern that resembles type A RVH. An R/S ratio >1 in lead V_1 (R wave greater than S wave in this lead) frequently persists for the first few years of life. Marked right axis deviation (RAD) is also common at birth. Most infants develop a normal mean QRS axis by 6 months of age, but, RAD of up to 120° may still be a normal finding in infants up to 1 year of age.

By the age of 5, most children show an R/S ratio <1 in lead V_1 and a mean frontal plane axis of less than 100°.

Although one may be struck by the prominent R wave in lead V_1 of Fig. 8-15, an R/S ratio >1 is acceptable in this age group. None of the associated findings that one usually expects to see with RVH are present in this tracing. Mean QRS axis is normal, RAE is not present, and S waves in the lateral precordial leads are relatively small. One might, therefore, suspect that the ECG was normal for this age group.

When in doubt, one should *never* hesitate to consult a table of pediatric norms before making the diagnosis of ventricular enlargement in children.

For reference purposes, we have simplified two such tables. Table 8-8 indicates the minimum, mean, and maximum QRS axes acceptable for infants and children; Table 8-9 indicates mean and maximum QRS amplitudes for R waves and S waves in leads V_1, V_5, and V_6.

Using these tables and referring back to Fig. 8-15, it becomes apparent that all measurements on this tracing are within normal limits. For a 22-month-old infant, the mean QRS axis in the frontal plane is 55°. Up to 100° is acceptable. An R wave of up to 18 mm is acceptable in lead V_1. Note that the mean R/S ratio for this group is 1.3. That is, in most infants this age the R wave is still greater than the S wave.

Figure 8-15. ECG from a 22-month-old infant.

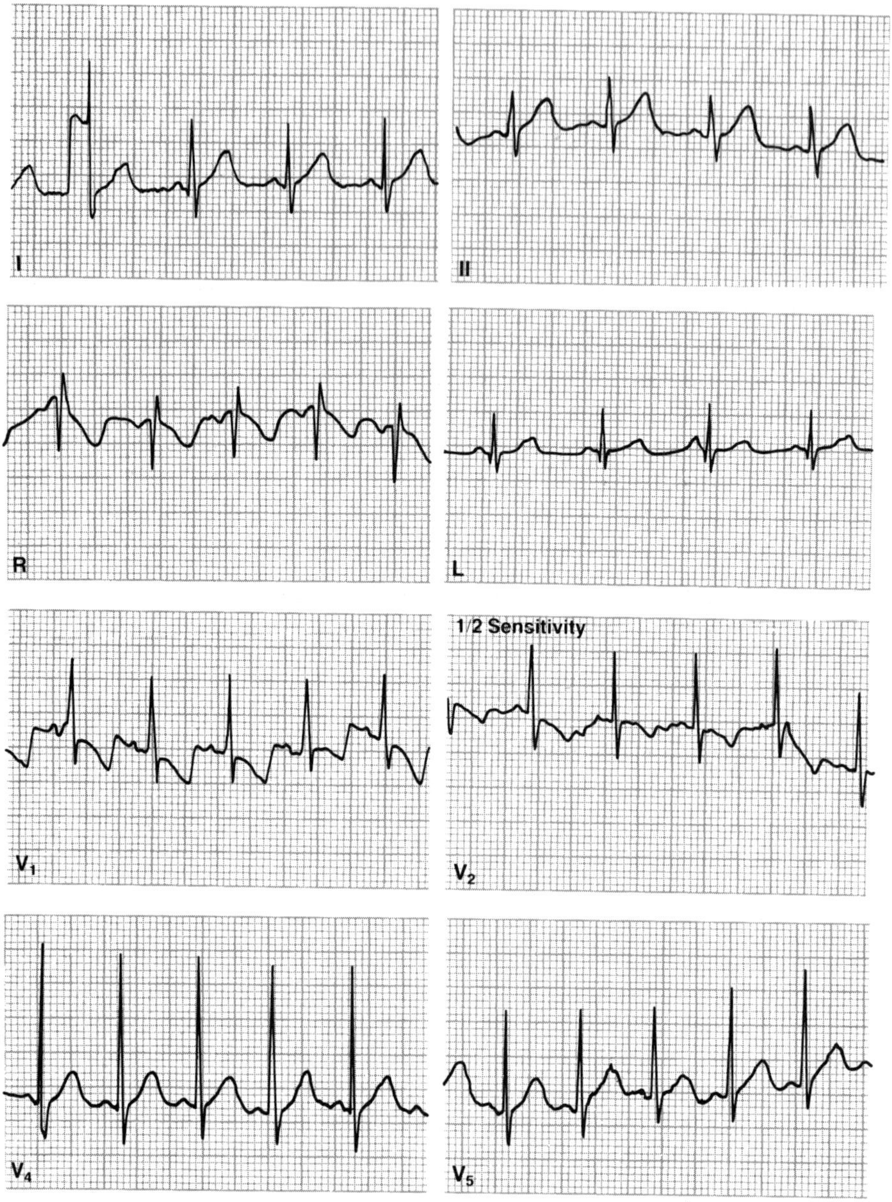

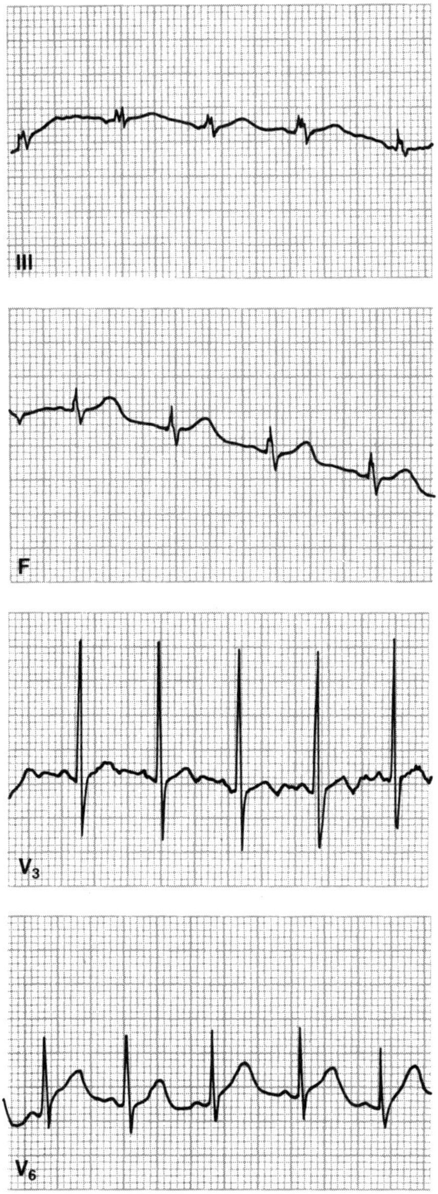
III
F
V3
V6

TABLE 8.8

Mean QRS axis (frontal plane)

	Minimum	Mean	Maximum
0–24 hours	60°	135°	180°
1–7 days	60°	125°	180°
8–30 days	0°	110°	180°
1–3 months	20°	80°	120°
3–6 months	40°	65°	100°
6–12 months	20°	65°	120°
1–3 years	0°	55°	100°
3–5 years	0°	60°	80°
5–8 years	−20°	65°	100°
8–12 years	0°	65°	120°
12–16 years	−20°	65°	100°

Table adapted from Harris LC, Feinstein E: Understanding ECGs in Infants and Children. *Boston, Little, Brown & Co, 1979.*

Tall R Wave in Lead V_1

One of the most common problems encountered in evaluating ECGs for the presence of RVH is determining the cause of a tall R wave in lead V_1. We have discussed a number of entities that may produce this finding.

PROBLEM: Study Fig. 8-16. Can you name *five* common causes of a tall R wave in lead V_1?

ANSWER: Five common conditions should *always* be considered in the differential diagnosis whenever a prominant R wave is seen in lead V_1 of an *adult.*

A. *WPW*
B. Posterior myocardial infarction.
C. Right ventricular hypertrophy (type A)
D. *RBBB*
E. Normal variant

Less common causative factors include certain types of cardiomyopathy (IHSS, Friedrich's ataxia) and dextrocardia.

Identification of a short PR interval with delta waves and QRS prolongation suggests the *Wolff-Parkinson-White syndrome (WPW).* As alluded to in Chapter 6 (Accessory Pathways), the principal importance of recognizing this entity is that it not be mistaken for RBBB, RVH, or myocardial infarction.

Posterior myocardial infarction is almost always associated with inferior infarction, since both areas of the heart are usually supplied by the same right coronary artery. Thus, a prerequisite for diagnosing posterior infarction is to find evidence of inferior infarction on the tracing. Applying the *mirror test* (Fig. 7-15) may help establish whether the relatively tall R wave and ST-segment depression in the anterior precordial leads result from posterior infarction.

Type A RVH is diagnosed by the finding of a tall R wave in lead V_1 and an ST-T wave pattern of strain in the anterior precordial leads. Other supportive findings are RAD, RAE, and deep S waves in leads V_5 and V_6.

Diagnosis of *RBBB* is usually readily apparent when the characteristic rSR′ pattern is seen in lead V_1. It may be more difficult to recognize if one of

TABLE 8-9

Amplitudes in lead V_1 (mm)

	R Wave		S Wave		Mean R/S
	Mean	Max.	Mean	Max.	Ratio
0–24 hours	15	21	9	29	2.2
1–7 days	18	30	10	26	2.5
8–30 days	11	27	5	19	3.0
1–3 months	9	21	6	20	2.3
3–6 months	11	18	7	14	2.3
6–12 months	7	18	6	17	1.6
1–3 years	9	18	11	29	1.3
3–5 years	7	18	12	35	0.8
5–8 years	7	21	13	26	0.7
8–12 years	6	18	14	26	0.5
12–16 years	5	18	13	26	0.5

Amplitudes in lateral leads V_5 and V_6 (mm)

	V_5 R Wave		V_5 S Wave		V_6 R Wave		V_6 S Wave	
	Mean	Max.	Mean	Max.	Mean	Max.	Mean	Max.
0–24 hours	10	24	12	32	3	8	5	14
1–7 days	11	28	7	20	5	17	3	14
8–30 days	12	36	5	14	7	26	2	10
1–3 months	14	24	5	14	8	14	2	7
3–6 months	18	28	4	17	10	17	2	6
6–12 months	17	28	3	11	12	20	1	4
1–3 years	18	40	2	11	11	26	1	5
3–5 years	19	36	2	8	12	23	1	4
5–8 years	20	40	2	11	13	26	1	6
8–12 years	22	36	2	11	14	23	1	4
12–16 years	17	36	2	8	13	20	1	6

Table adapted from *Harris LC, Feinstein E:* Understanding ECGs in Infants and Children. *Boston, Little, Brown & Co, 1979.*
Garson A: The Electrocardiogram in Infants and Children. *Philadelphia, Lea & Febiger, 1983.*

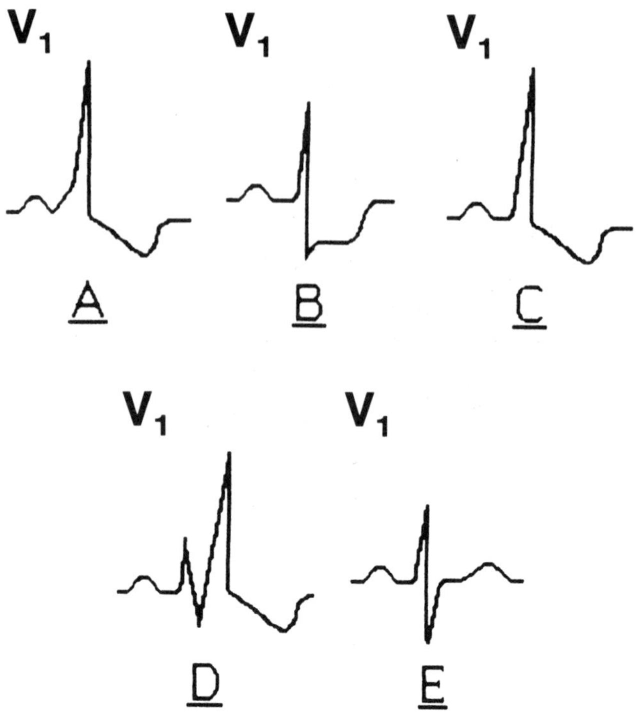

Figure 8-16. Five common causes of a tall R wave in lead V_1. Can you name them?

the "RBBB-equivalent" patterns (Table 6-2) is present in lead V_1 instead. Associated findings of RBBB include secondary ST-T wave changes in the anterior precordial leads, QRS prolongation to at least 0.11 second, and wide terminal S waves in lateral leads I and V_6.

Finally, the *normal variant pattern* should be a diagnosis of *exclusion* to be made *only* after the other four conditions have been ruled out. It should be suspected when the patient is a young adult who is asymptomatic and has normal PR and QRS intervals without right axis deviation, RAE, or evidence of inferior infarction.

Fig. 8-17 summarizes the key points to remember in considering the differential diagnosis of a tall R wave in lead V_1.

PROBLEM: Examine the ECG shown in Fig. 8-18, taken from a middle-aged adult who presented with the sudden onset of dyspnea and pleuritic chest pain. What do you suspect is going on?

INTERPRETATION of Fig. 8-18

Rate and rhythm: Sinus tachycardia at 115 beats/min.

PR interval: 0.17 second.

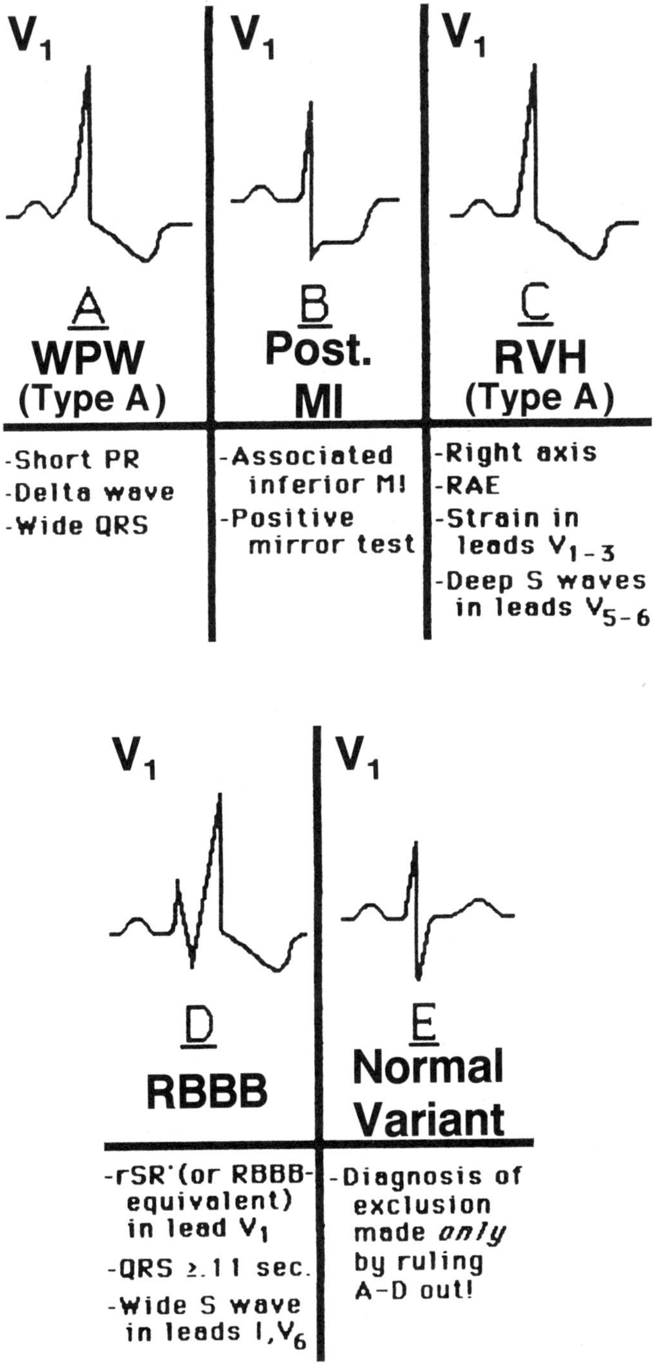
V1
V1
V1
A
WPW
(Type A)
B
Post.
MI
C
RVH
(Type A)
-Short PR
-Delta wave
-Wide QRS
-Associated inferior MI
-Positive mirror test
-Right axis
-RAE
-Strain in leads V1-3
-Deep S waves in leads V5-6
V1
V1
D
RBBB
E
Normal Variant
-rSR' (or RBBB-equivalent) in lead V1
-QRS ≥.11 sec.
-Wide S wave in leads I, V6
-Diagnosis of exclusion made *only* by ruling A-D out!

Figure 8-17

Figure 8-18. ECG from a middle-aged adult complaining of the sudden onset of dyspnea and pleuritic chest pain.

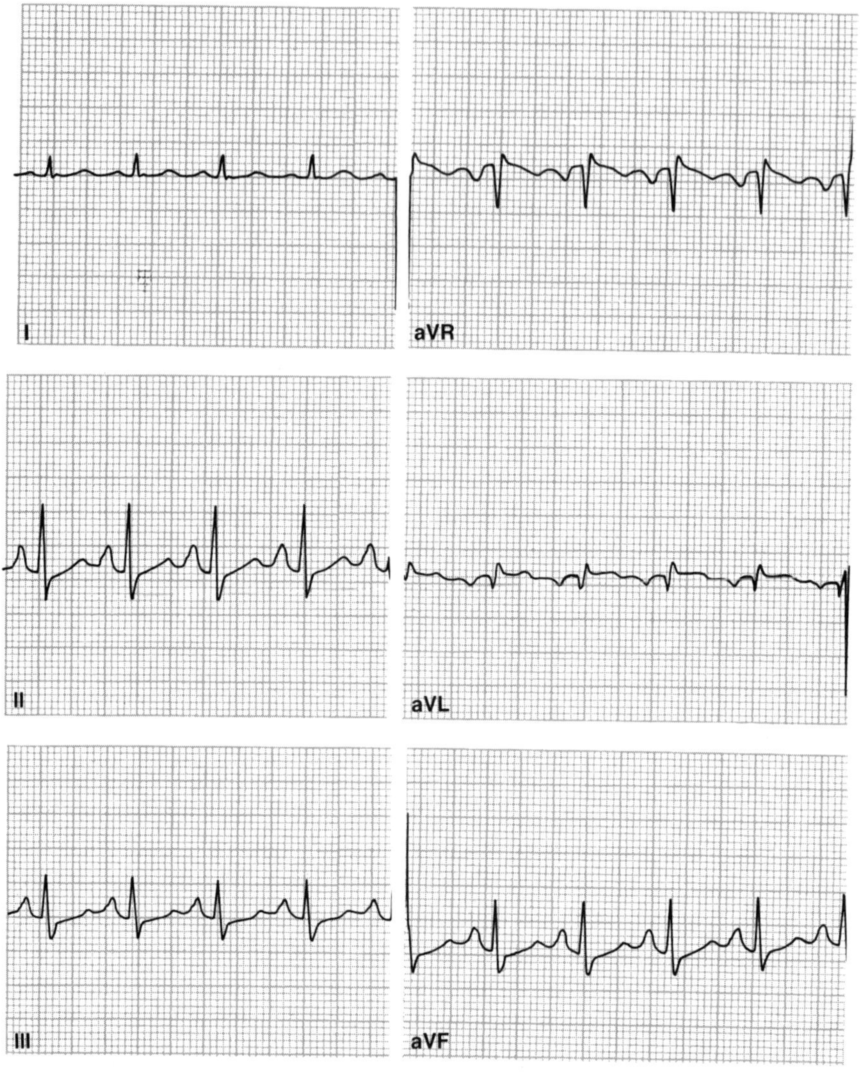

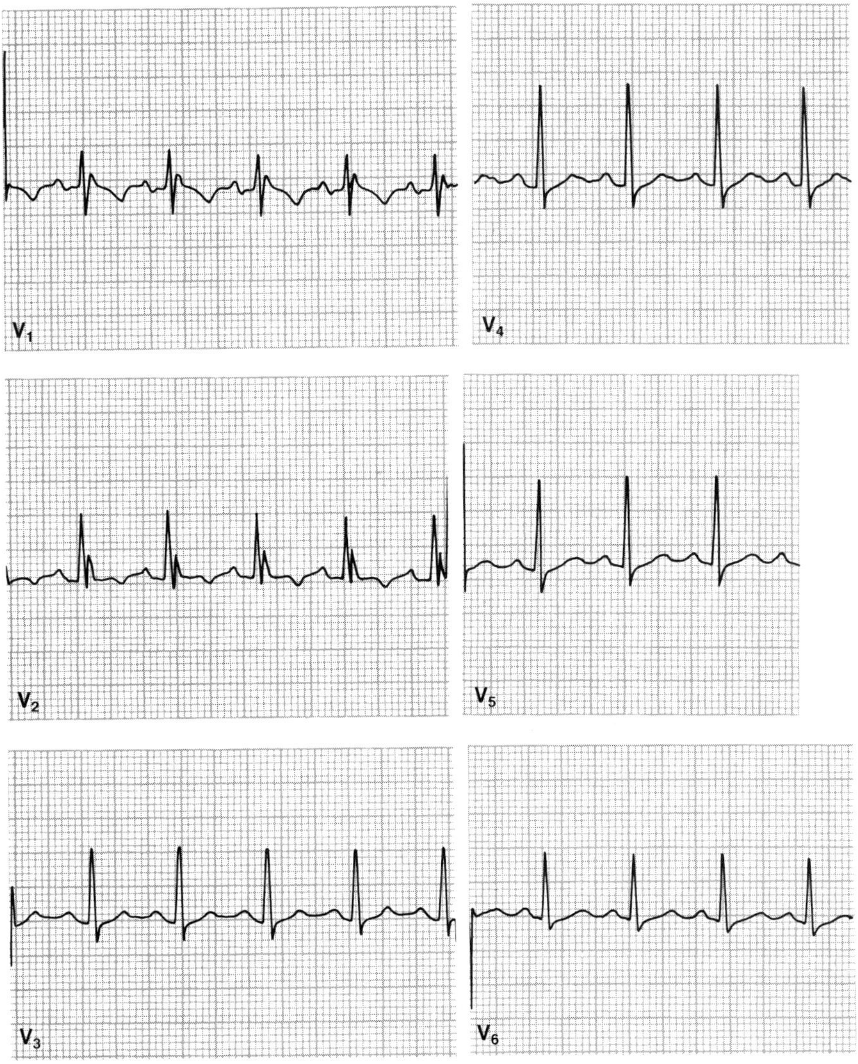
V1
V4
V2
V5
V3
V6

QRS interval: 0.10 second (upper limits of normal). IRBBB is present (Rsr′ in lead V_1, narrow S wave in lead V_6).

Axis: About + 60°.

Chamber enlargement: RAA.

QRST changes: A Q wave and ST-segment elevation are seen in lead aVL. Although one might initially be concerned about the possibility of acute high lateral infarction, this finding is probably *not* significant because it is isolated to this lead and out of context with the rest of the tracing.

Elsewhere, minimal nonspecific ST-segment depression is seen in inferior and lateral precordial leads. There is T-wave inversion in leads V_1 and V_2 that is consistent with secondary ST-T wave changes of IRBBB.

Taken together, the clinical history and ECG of this patient should suggest *acute pulmonary embolism.*

Pulmonary Embolism

Acute pulmonary embolism is still one of the most frequently overlooked diagnoses in the clinical practice of medicine. Since treatment is usually most effective if started early, the importance of prompt recognition of this disorder cannot be overstated.

The ECG has long been counted among the diagnostic modalities used to evaluate patients with suspected pulmonary emboli. When characteristic ECG findings are present, this tool may indeed be very helpful in suggesting the diagnosis. Unfortunately, even though a *majority* of patients with significant pulmonary emboli demonstrate ECG abnormalities, most of the time these changes are *nonspecific* and offer little assistance in making the diagnosis. Table 8-10 indicates the most characteristic ECGs changes of acute pulmonary embolism.

Sinus tachycardia is probably the most common finding. It is unusual for a patient with a significant pulmonary embolism to have a heart rate of under 100 beats/min. Other typical rhythm changes include atrial fibrillation (usually with a fairly rapid ventricular response), and premature atrial contractions (PACs) and/or premature ventricular contractions (PVCs).

The ECG changes most suggestive of pulmonary embolism are those of "acute right heart strain" *(acute cor pulmonale).* This may be reflected by a dramatic rightward shift of the mean QRS axis. Complete or incomplete RBBB (which is often transient) may be seen. Other evidence of acute right-heart strain may become manifest, including new-onset RAE and RVH with an accompanying right ventricular strain pattern in the inferior and/or anterior precordial leads.

Much has been written about the "SI-QIII-TIII" pattern (Fig. 8-19). Although in the past this sign was touted as being highly diagnostic of pulmonary embolism, it is rarely helpful clinically. The SI-QIII-TIII pattern

TABLE 8-10

ECG changes of acute pulmonary embolism

Rate and Rhythm
- Sinus tachycardia
- Atrial fibrillation
- PACs/PVCs

Acute Right Heart Strain
- Acute right axis deviation
- RAE
- Incomplete or complete RBBB
- New tall R wave in lead V_1
- Right ventricular strain pattern
- S_I-Q_{III}-T_{III} pattern

QRST Changes
- Nonspecific ST-T wave abnormalities

is seen in only about 10 percent of cases. Even when it does occur, the sign is usually transient (often lasting less than an hour), and suffers from a lack of specificity.

In summary, while a majority of patients with significant pulmonary emboli will demonstrate sinus tachycardia, nonspecific ST-T wave abnormalities, or both, and a few will develop an ECG picture that strongly suggests the diagnosis, most of the time the ECG will be of little assistance. Lung scan and pulmonary angiography remain the "gold standards."

Review: Is There Chamber Enlargement?

PROBLEM: Examine the ECGs shown in Figs. 8-20 and 8-21. Is there evidence of chamber enlargement?

INTERPRETATION of Fig. 8-20

Rate and rhythm: Sinus tachycardia at 115 beats/min. The PR and QRS intervals are normal.

Axis: +80°.

Chamber enlargement: The ECG suggests biatrial abnormality and LVH.

QRST changes:

Q waves: A QS complex is seen in lead aVL. In the context of markedly increased voltage and a relatively vertical QRS axis, the isolated occurrence of this Q wave is more than likely of no clinical significance.

R wave progression: Early transition.

ST-T wave changes: ST-segment sagging and T-wave inversion are seen, particularly in the leads that demonstrate the greatest R-wave

Figure 8-19. S_I-Q_{III}-T_{III} pattern from a patient with suspected pulmonary embolism. When this sign occurs as an isolated finding (as it does here in this otherwise normal ECG), it is not of much assistance in making the diagnosis.

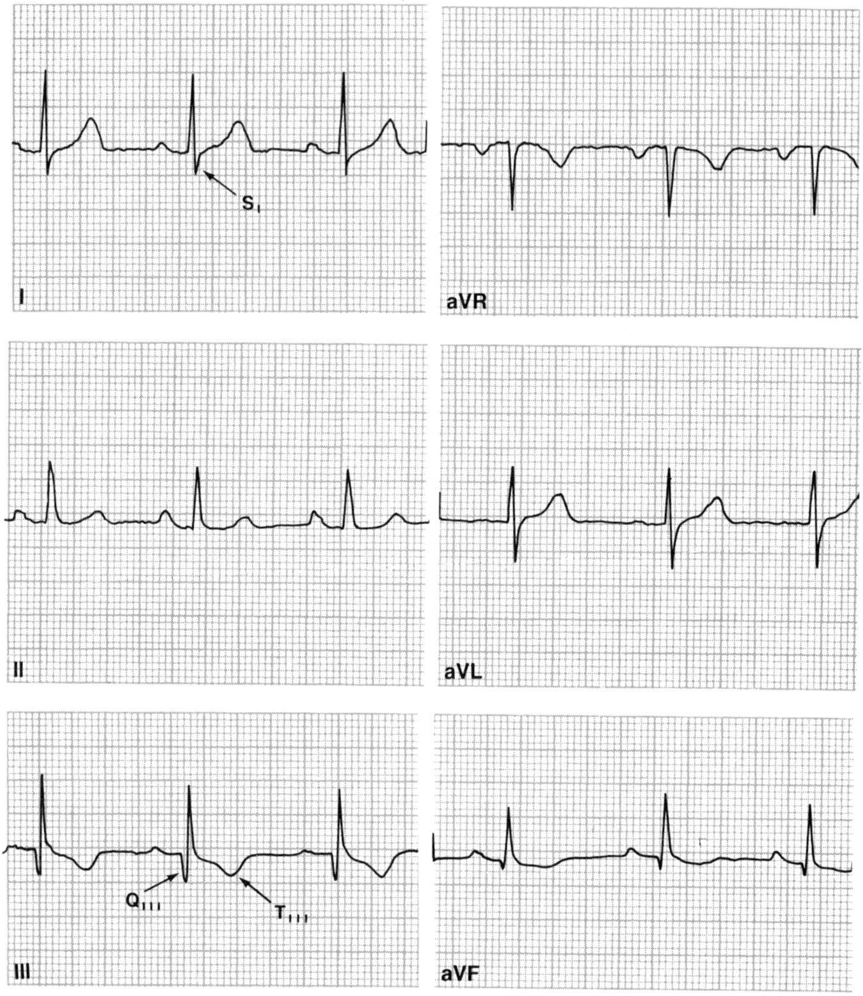

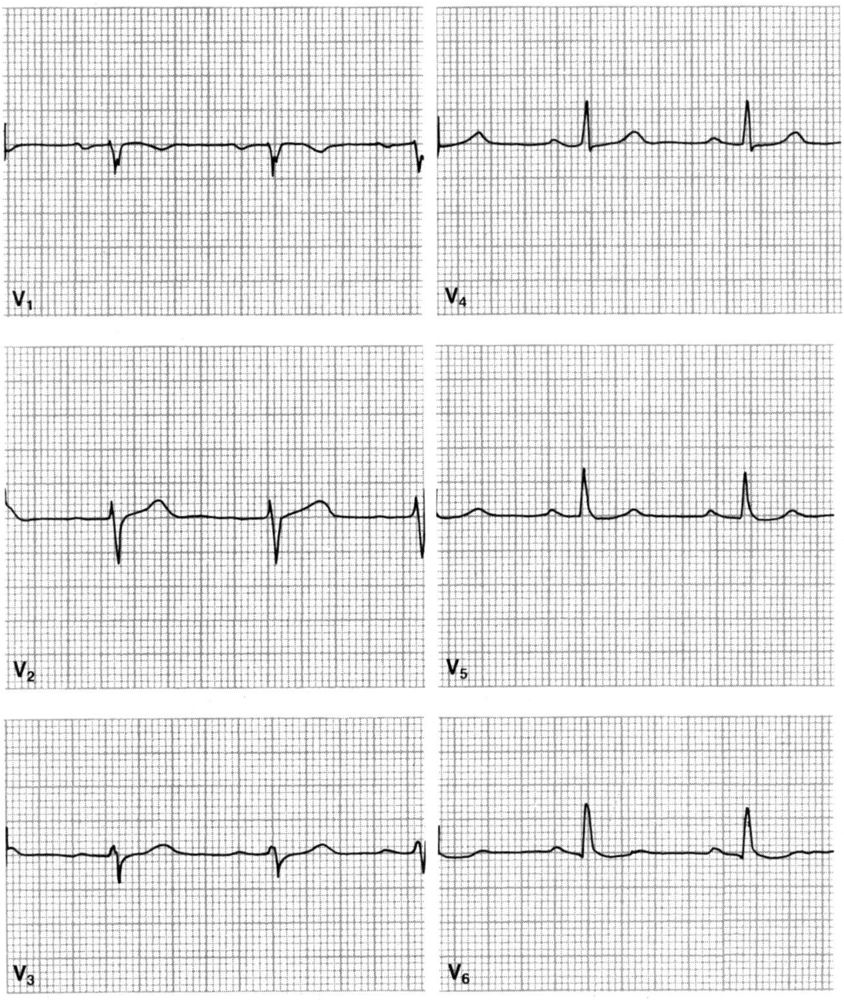
V1
V4
V2
V5
V3
V6

Figure 8-20. ECG from a 57-year-old man admitted for gastrointestinal bleeding.

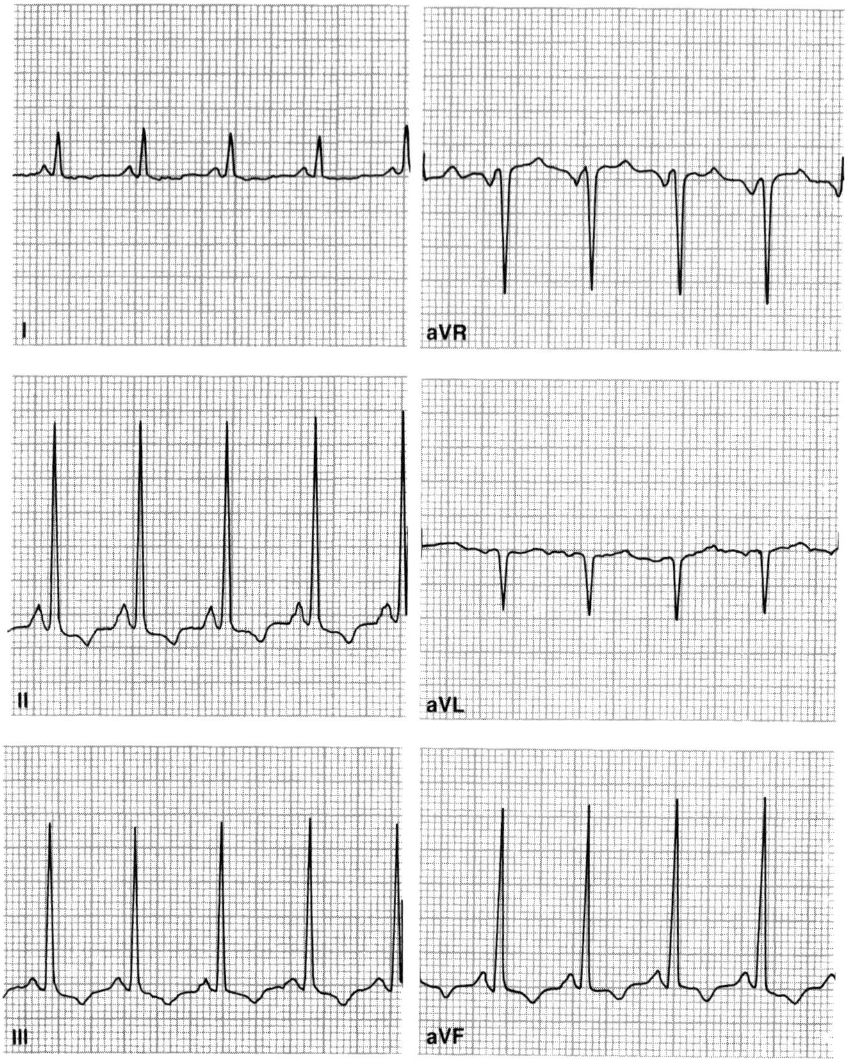

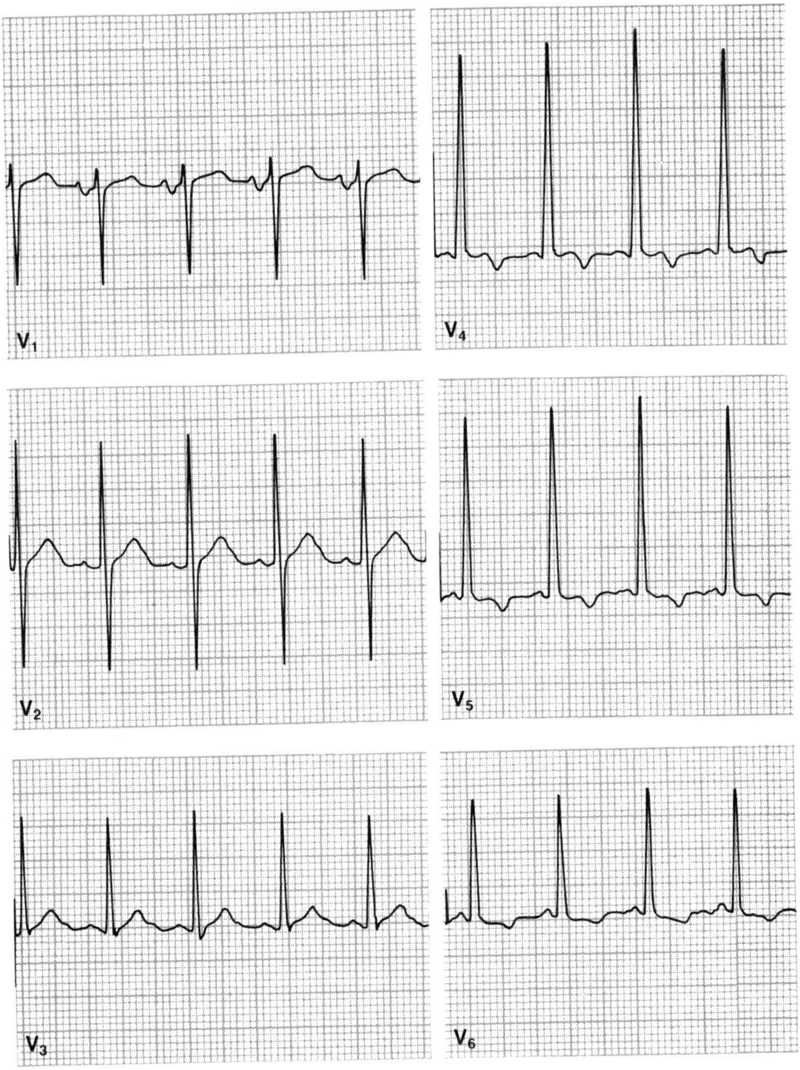
V1
V4
V2
V5
V3
V6

Figure 8-21. ECG from a 49-year-old woman admitted for chest pain.

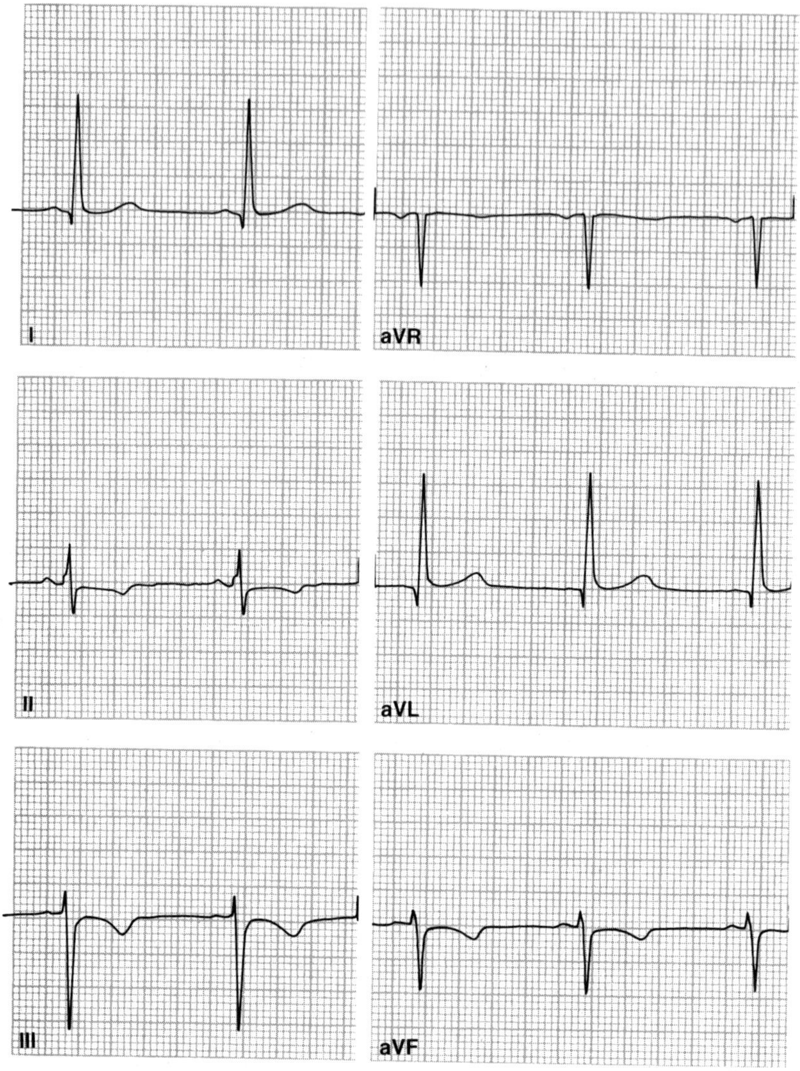

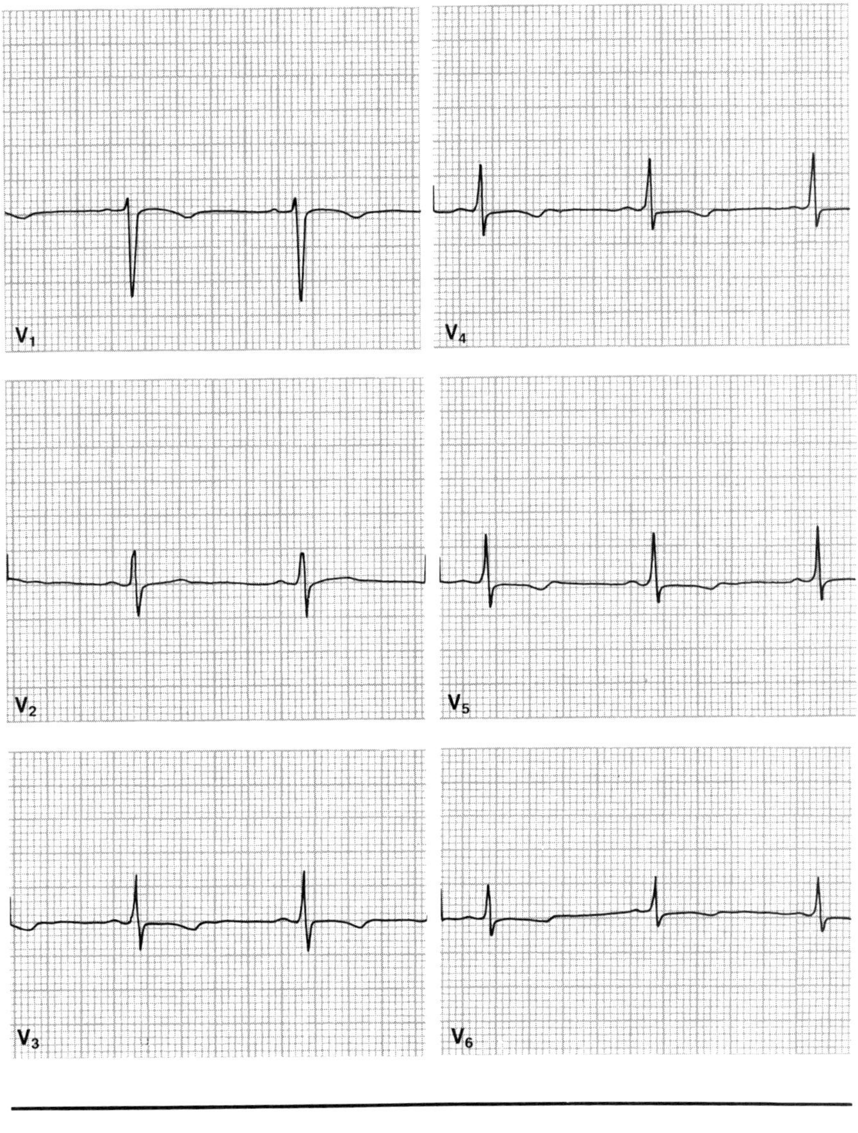
V1
V4
V2
V5
V3
V6

deflections. For the most part, this T-wave inversion is asymmetric, and consistent with secondary repolarization abnormalities (strain) from the increased voltage. It would be difficult to totally exclude superimposed ischemia.

One might write the interpretation of this tracing as follows:

"Sinus tachycardia at 115 beats/min.
Axis = +80°.
RAA.
LAA (or LAE).
LVH and strain and/or ischemia."

In the setting of the tremendously increased voltage seen here, the deep terminal negative deflection of the P wave in lead V_1 most likely represents *true* LAE (this finding is of *high* specificity in this setting). On the other hand, unless there was clinical evidence to suggest otherwise, specificity of the prominent, peaked P waves in the inferior leads of this ECG would not be nearly as high. Thus, RAA might be a more appropriate designation than RAE.

The level of confidence for diagnosing true LVH from the tracing approaches 100 percent.

INTERPRETATION of Fig. 8-21

Rate and rhythm: Sinus rhythm at 65 beats/min. The QRS interval is borderline prolonged (about 0.10 second). The PR and QT intervals are normal.

Axis: About −25° (LAD, but *not* LAHB).

Chamber enlargement: There is voltage for LVH (R in lead aVL ≥ 12 mm; also sum of R wave in lead I + S wave in lead III ≥ 25 mm).

QRST changes: Narrow, 2 to 3-mm deep q waves are seen in leads I and aVL. Associated with this, there appears to be a slight amount of ST-segment elevation with an upward concavity in these leads.

R-wave progression is normal.

Symmetric T-wave inversion is seen in the inferior leads, and nonspecific ST-segment flattening with shallow T-wave inversion in the precordial leads.

This tracing is *difficult* to interpret without additional clinical information or prior tracings for comparison. One might attempt to document the findings as follows:

"Sinus rhythm at 65 beats/min. Axis = −25° (LAD). *Voltage for LVH.* Small q waves in leads I and aVL with slight ST-segment elevation—most likely due to early repolarization, but cannot rule out acute injury. Symmetric T-wave inversion in the inferior leads and to a lesser extent in many of the precordial leads—possibly reflecting ischemia. Strongly suggest clinical correlation and comparison with previous tracings."

Compared with Fig. 8-20, the presence of *true* LVH would be much less certain in this case, due to the absence of repolarization abnormalities.

Suggested Readings

Devereux RB, Reichek N: Repolarization abnormalities of left ventricular hypertrophy: Clinical, echocardiographic and hemodynamic Correlates. *J Electrocardiology* 1982; 15:47-54.

Devereux RB, Casale PN, Eisenberg RR, Miller DH, Kligfield P: Electrocardiographic detection of left ventricular hypertrophy using echocardiographic determination of left ventricular mass as the reference standard. *J Am Col Cardiol* 1984; 3:82-87.

Freis ED: Electrocardiographic changes in the course of antihypertensive treatment. In Messerli FH, Schlant RC (eds): Proceedings of the Symposium Left Ventricular Hypertrophy in Essential Hypertension, New Orleans, Louisiana, April 23-24, 1982. *Am J Med* 1983; 75(3A):111-115.

Kannel WB: Prevalence and natural history of electrocardiographic left ventricular hypertrophy. In Messerli FH, Schlant RC (eds): Proceedings of the Symposium Left Ventricular Hypertrophy in Essential Hypertension, New Orleans, Louisiana, April 23-24, 1982. *Am J Med* 1983; 75(3A):4-11.

Larkin H, Hunyer SN: Precordial voltage variation in the normal electrocardiogram. *J Electrocardiol* 1980; 13:347-352.

Lynch P, Webb-Peploe MM: The P terminal vector in lead V_1 of the electrocardiogram in cor pulmonale. *J Electrocardiol* 1982; 15:205-208.

Messerli FH, Devereux RB: Introduction: Left ventricular hypertrophy—Good or evil? In Messerli FH, Schlant RC (eds): Proceedings of the Symposium Left Ventricular Hypertrophy in Essential Hypertension, New Orleans, Louisiana, April 23-24, 1982. *Am J Med* 1983; 75(3A):1-3.

Romhilt DW, Bove KE, Norris RJ, Conyers E, Conradi S, Rowlands DT, Scott RC: A critical appraisal of the electrocardiographic criteria for the diagnosis of left ventricular hypertrophy. *Circulation* 1969; 40:185-195.

PART THREE

Review: Exercises in ECG Interpretation

EXERCISE A

METABOLIC DISTURBANCES

Interpret the ECGs shown in Figs. A1 to A6. A metabolic disorder was suspected in each. Can you surmise what kind? (The only clinical history available is indicated above each tracing.)

Figure A-1. ECG from a 79-year-old woman with a history of hypertension who is admitted for syncope. She is on multiple medications.

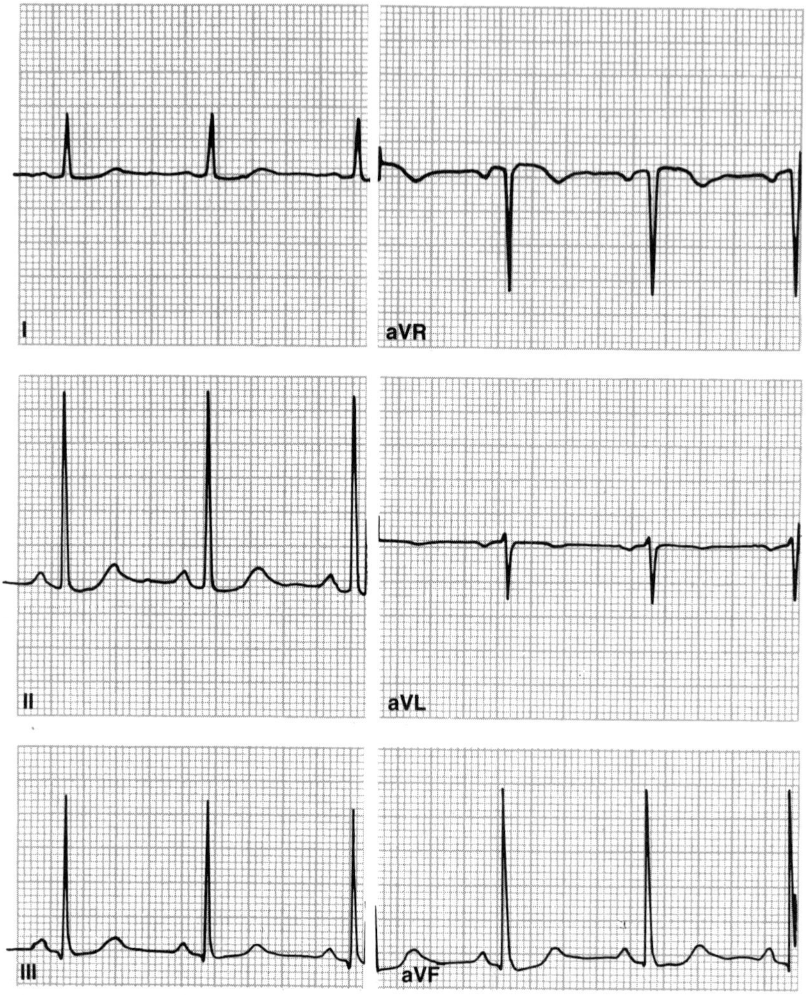

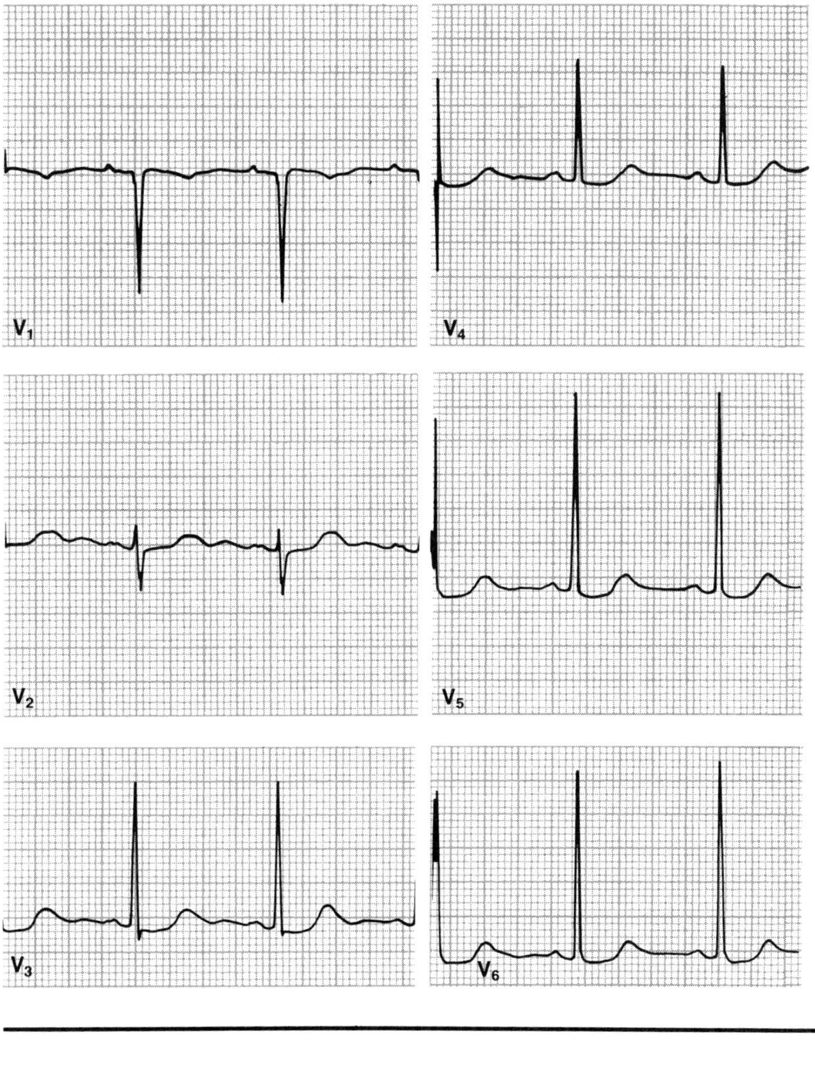
V1
V2
V3
V4
V5
V6

Figure A-2. ECG from a 53-year-old woman with renal failure.

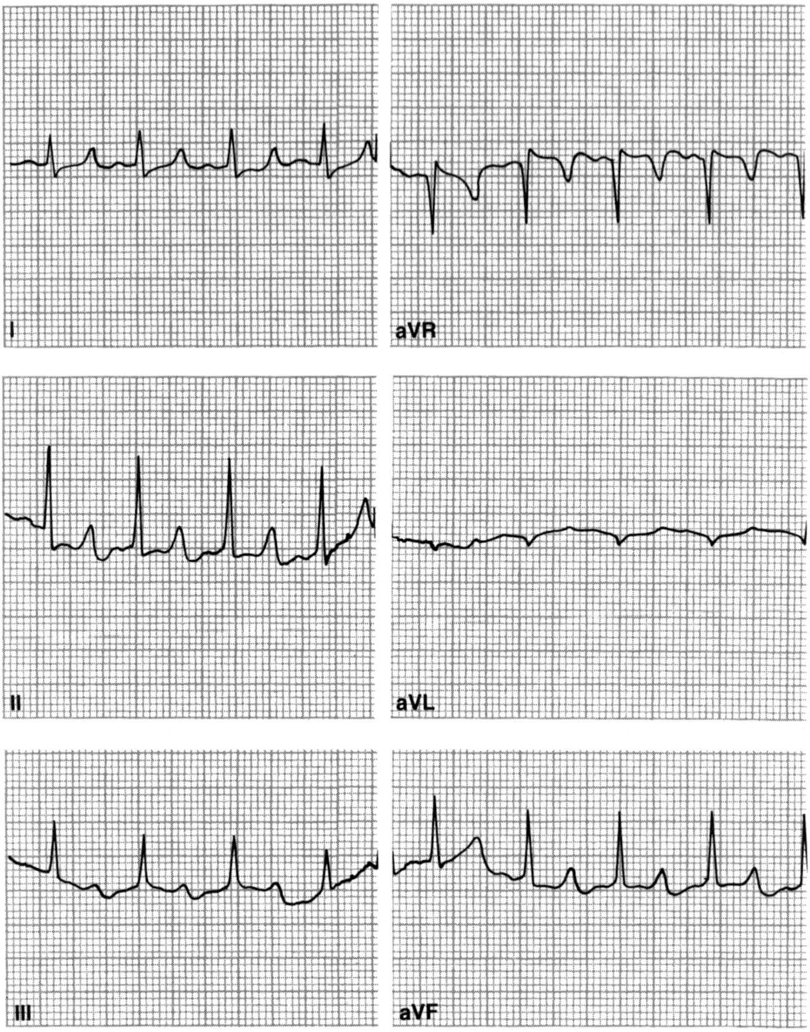

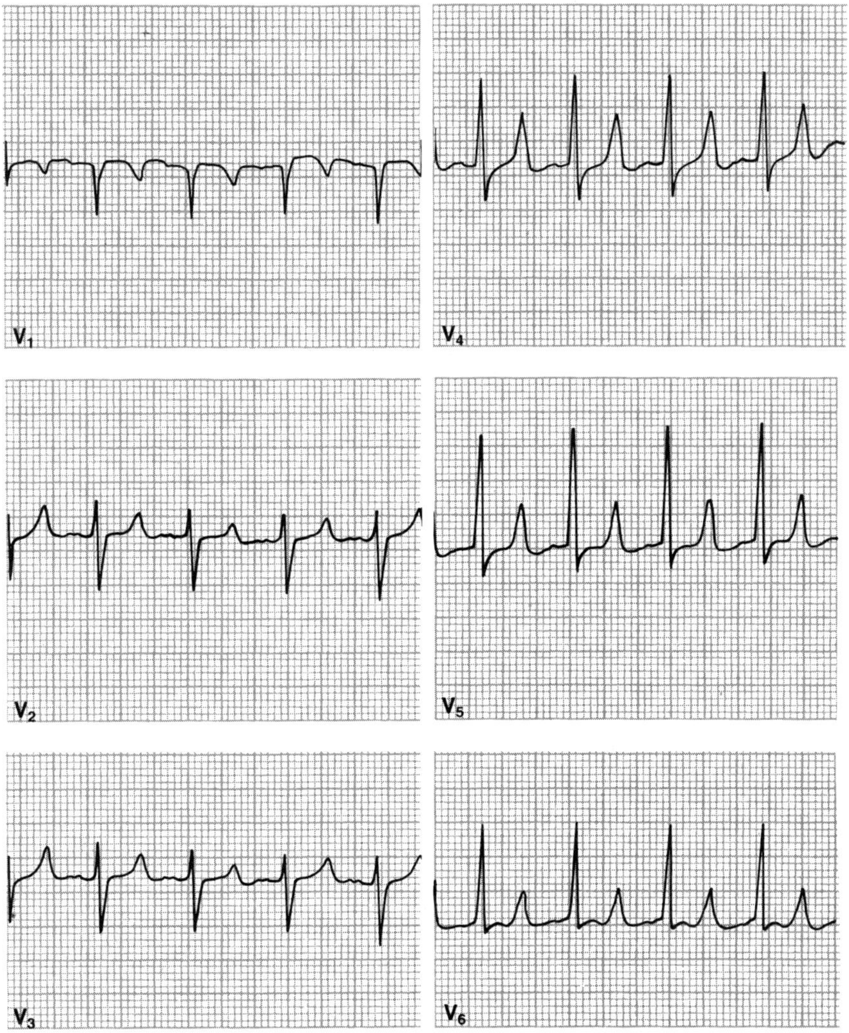
V1
V4
V2
V5
V3
V6

Figure A-3. ECG from an asymptomatic 39-year-old man with hypertension.

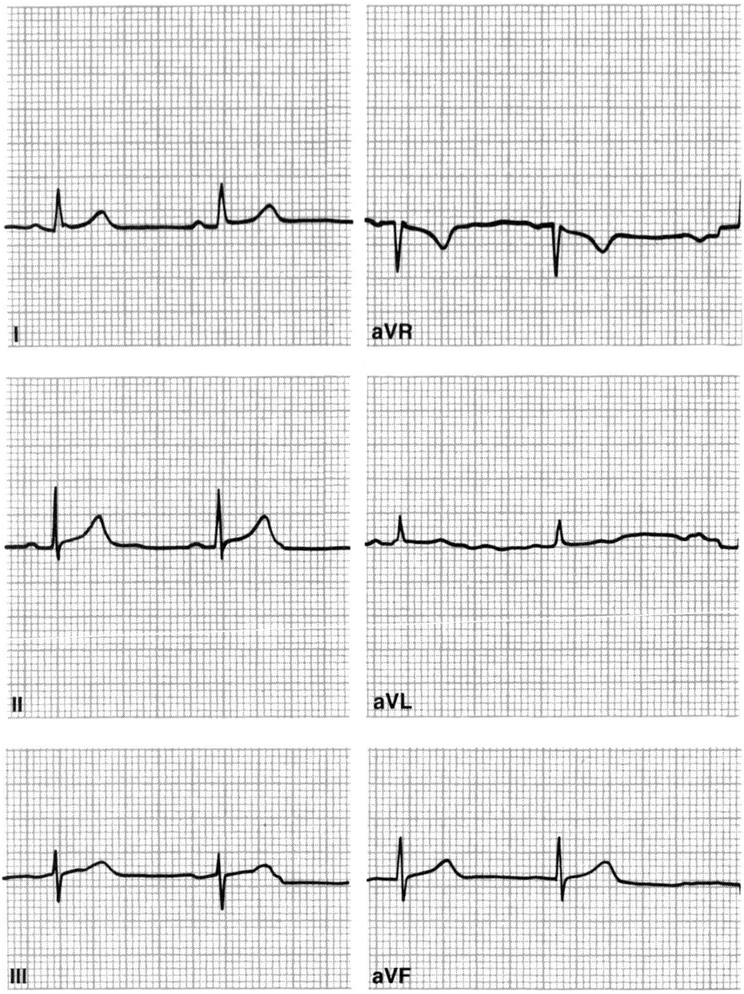

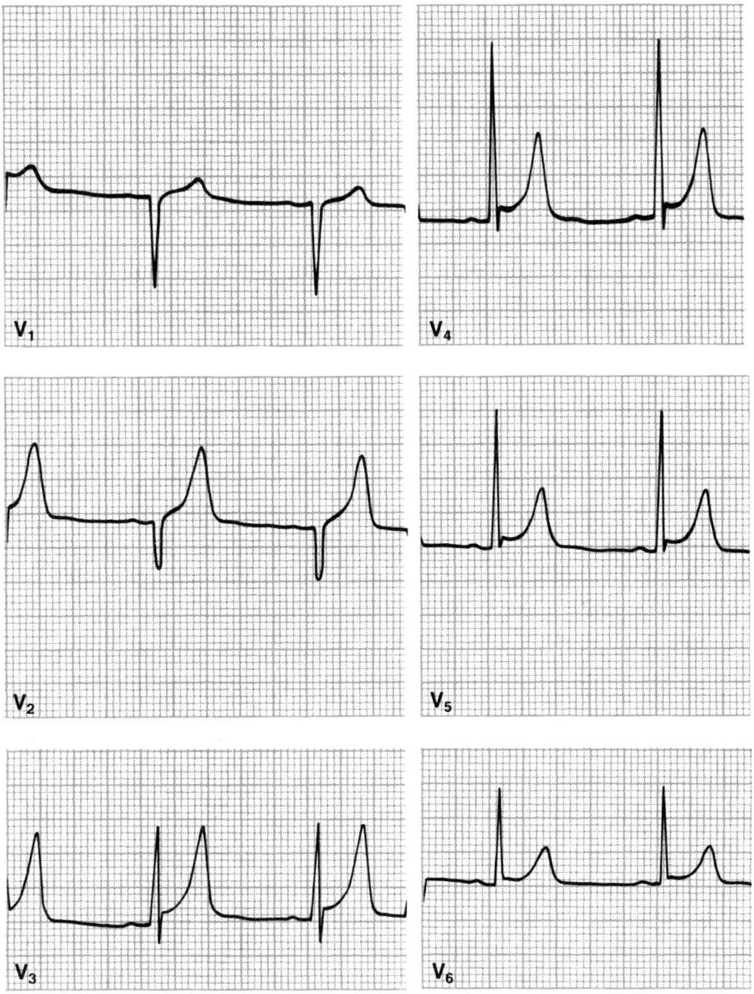
V1
V4
V2
V5
V3
V6

Figure A-4. ECG from a 79-year-old woman with a history of breast cancer who presented to the emergency department in a comatose condition.

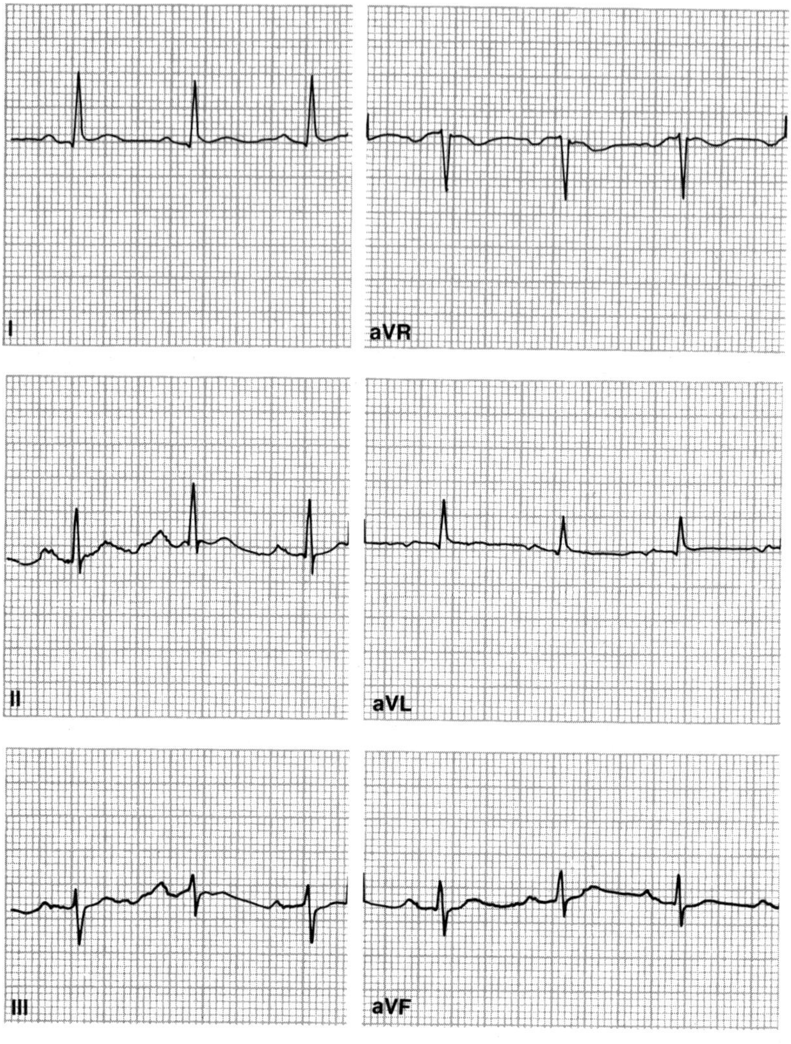

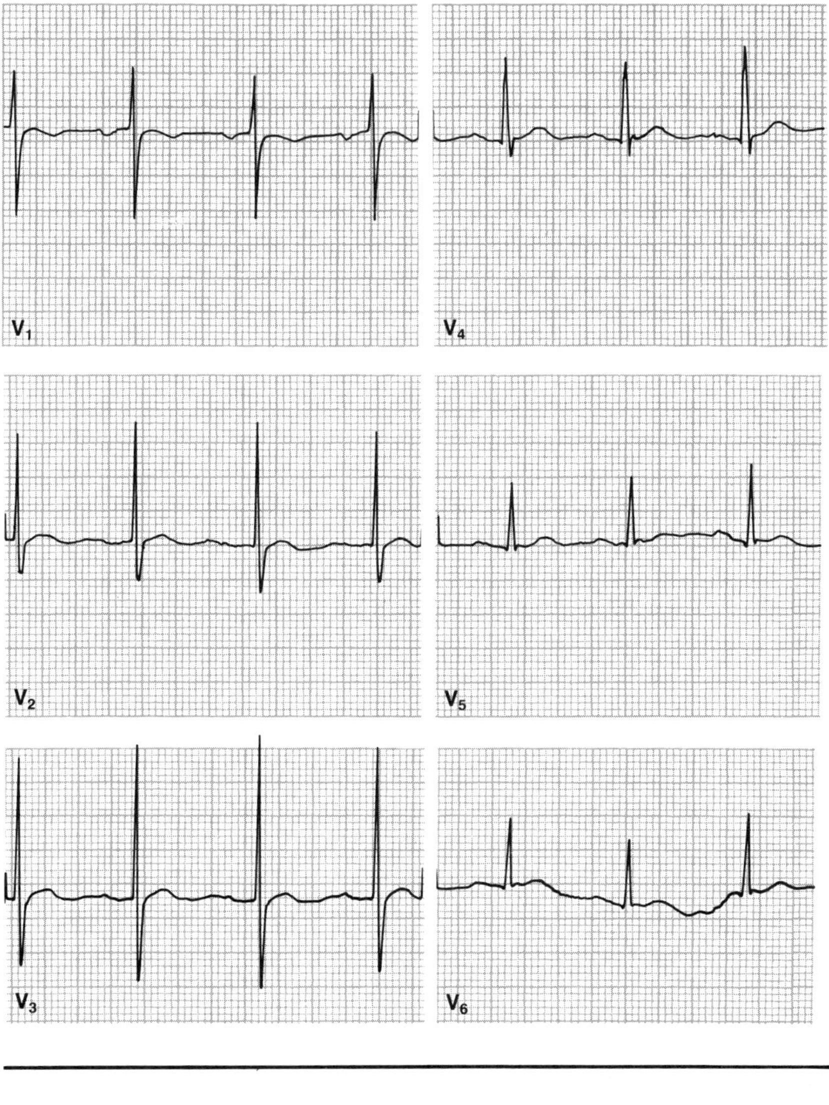
V1
V4
V2
V5
V3
V6

Figure A-5. ECG from a 60-year-old man who was found unresponsive at home.

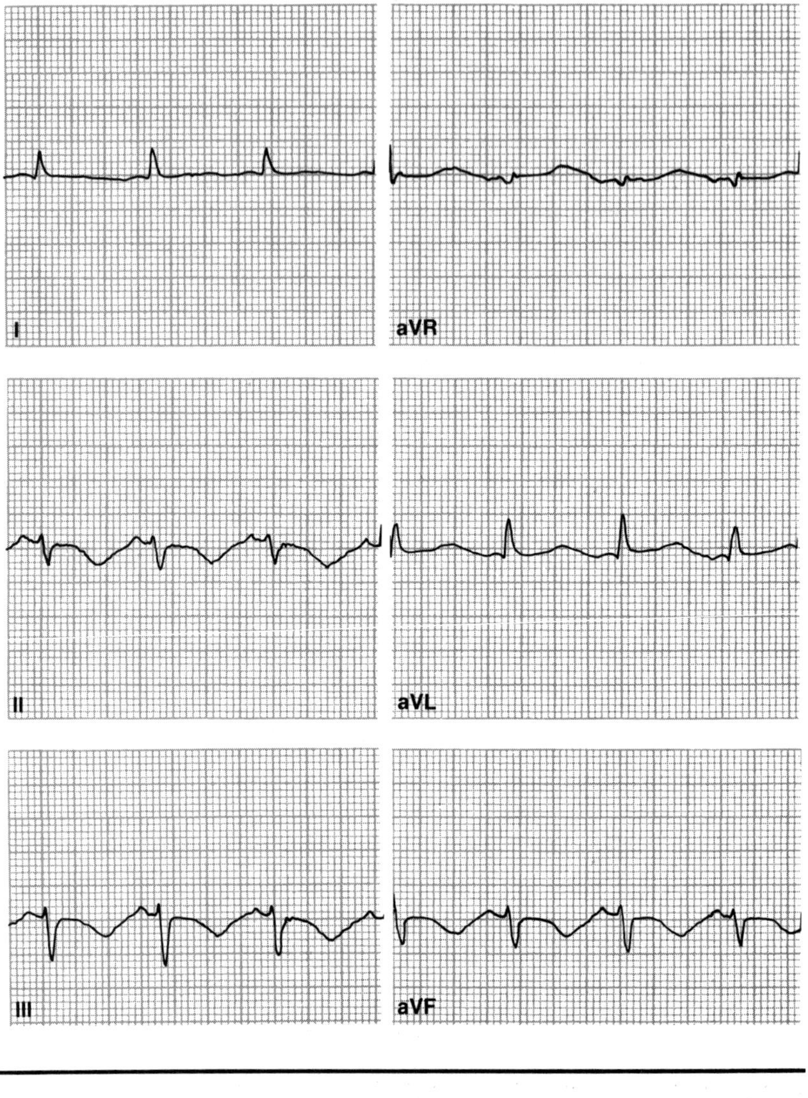

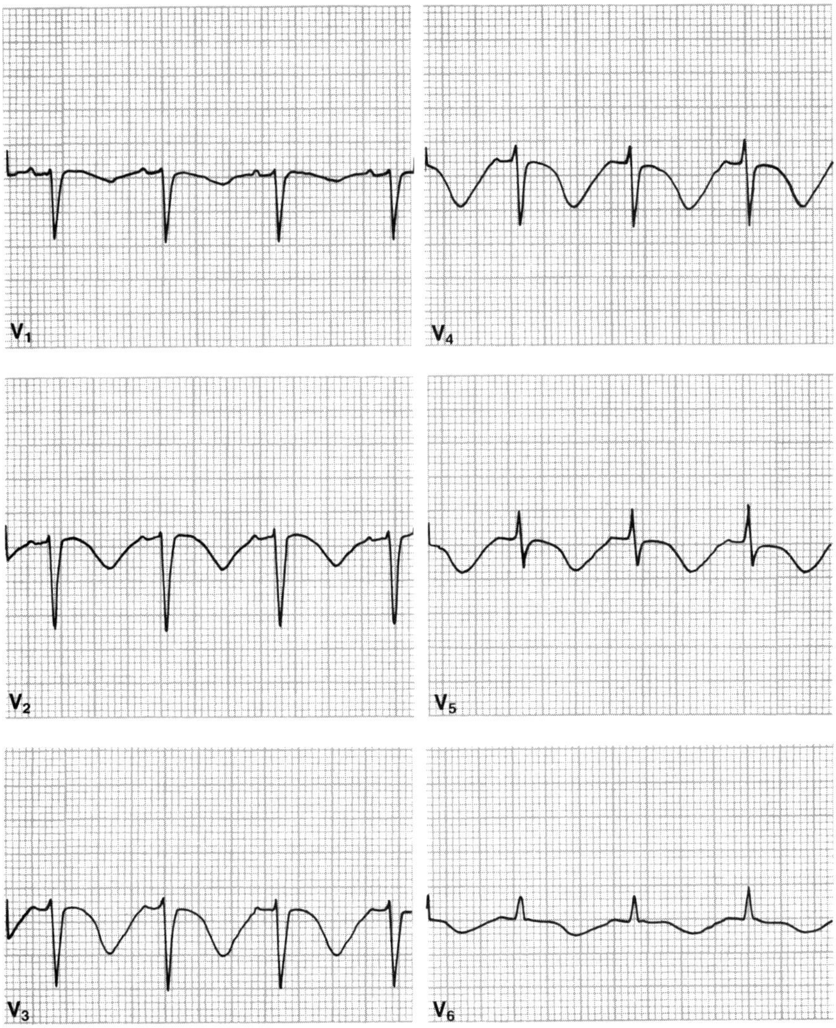
V1
V4
V2
V5
V3
V6

Figure A-6. ECG from a healthy, asymptomatic 31-year-old woman. No medications.

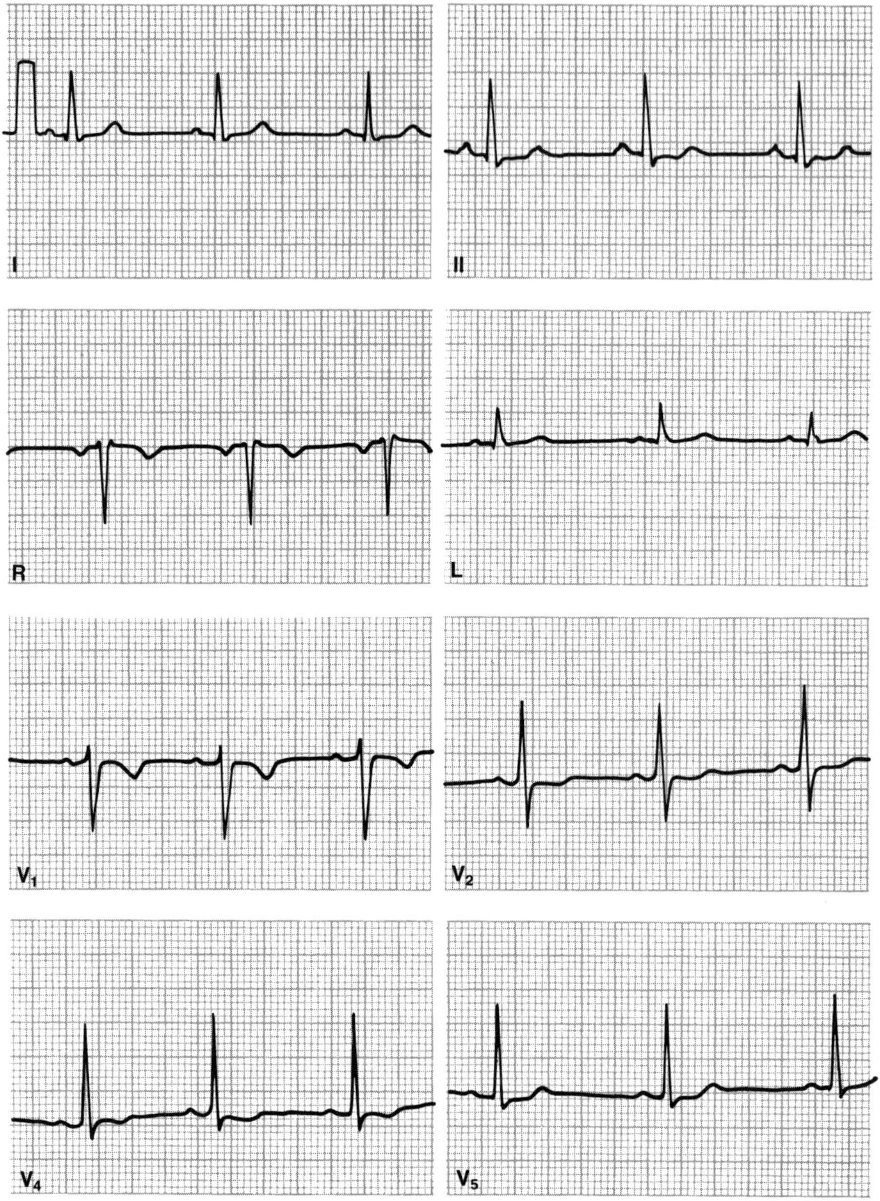

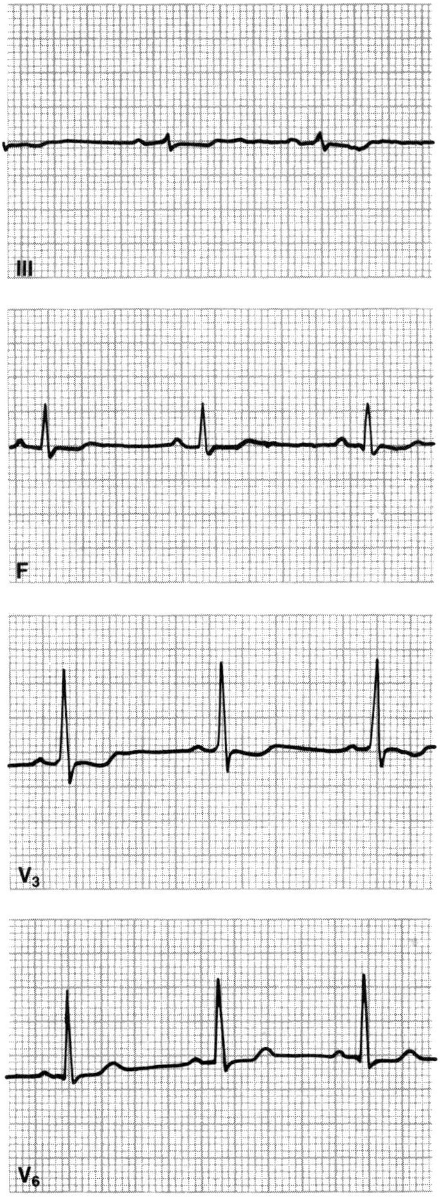
III
F
V_3
V_6

INTERPRETATION of Fig. A-1

Sinus rhythm at 70 beats/min. Axis $\approx +75°$. LVH with strain and/or ischemia. U waves are present in leads V_2 and V_3, suggesting possible *hypokalemia.*

Voltage is markedly increased in this tracing. While T waves are not inverted, they are decreased in amplitude. When considered in conjunction with the scooped ST-segment depression that is particularly well seen in leads with prominent R-wave voltage, these ST-T wave changes should qualify as a "strain-equivalent." Confidence in the diagnosis of LVH would therefore be high.

The history notes that the patient has hypertension and is on multiple medications. Two of these might be digitalis and a diuretic. If she were on digitalis, the scooped ST-segment depression would be consistent with "digitalis effect." Prominent U waves as are seen in lead V_2 suggest possible hypokalemia in a patient on a diuretic (although U waves may simply be the result of LVH or digitalis).

Finally, while none of the ST-T wave changes appear acute, the diffuse ST-T segment depression seen here may represent ongoing ischemia. Comparison with prior tracings would be helpful in clarifying this concern.

INTERPRETATION of Fig. A-2

Sinus tachycardia at 110 beats/min. Axis $\approx +65°$. T waves are tall and peaked in multiple leads. In addition, the QT interval appears to be prolonged.

In a patient with renal failure, this picture suggests *hyperkalemia* and *hypocalcemia.* Clinically, this patient's serum potassium was over 7.0 mEq/L, and her ionized serum calcium was decreased.

INTERPRETATION of Fig. A-3

Sinus rhythm at 60 beats/min. Axis $\approx +45°$. J-point ST-segment elevation with an upward concavity in leads V_3 to V_6, probably due to *early repolarization.*

Although T waves are tall and peaked in the precordial leads, this is probably *not* due to hyperkalemia. Clinically, there would be little reason to suspect hyperkalemia in an otherwise asymptomatic 39-year-old man. (Since the patient did have a history of hypertension, however, one might inquire as to whether he was taking a potassium-sparing diuretic.) Far more likely to produce this ECG picture than an electrolyte abnormality would be early repolarization. The "squiggle" at the J-point is extremely characteristic of this entity, and the T waves themselves, though peaked, are not really symmetric—the ascent of the T wave is more gradual than the descent. In addition, its base is broader than one would expect with hyperkalemia. Thus there is *no* metabolic disorder in this case, and this ECG is *normal.*

A final incidental point to make about this tracing is that one should *not* assume a previous anterior infarction on the basis of the QS complexes seen in leads V_1 and V_2. Lack of an r wave in lead V_2 may simply be the result of faulty precordial lead placement, especially since a predominantly positive QRS complex appears in lead V_3. In general, the electrocardiographer should probably *not* indicate previous anterior infarction unless r waves are completely lacking in leads V_1, V_2, *and* V_3.

INTERPRETATION of Fig. A-4

Sinus rhythm at 85 beats/min. Axis $\approx +20°$. Early transition. Although ST-T wave changes in general appear to be nonspecific, the QT interval in the anterior precordial leads appears to be markedly *shortened.* The metabolic disturbance that should come to mind in an unresponsive patient who has this ECG picture is *hypercalcemia.*

Although the ECG will usually *not* be of much assistance in determining the cause of coma, this example illustrates one instance when it did supply the answer long before the laboratory. Actual serum calcium level at the time of this tracing was 15.4 mg%. Hypercalcemia of this degree is a *medical emergency,* and requires immediate treatment.

In this case, the patient's hypercalcemia was attributed to extensive bony metastases from her breast cancer. The QT interval normalized after her serum calcium level was corrected.

INTERPRETATION of Fig. A-5

Sinus rhythm at 85 beats/min. Axis $\approx -40°$ (LAHB). Poor R-wave progression. *Marked QT-interval prolongation.* T waves are extremely broad and diffusely inverted.

While diffuse T-wave inversion as is seen here may be the result of cardiac ischemia, the marked prolongation in the QT interval should suggest a number of other possibilities (see Table 1-4).

- Drug effect (quinidine, phenothiazines, tricyclic antidepressants, etc.)
- Electrolyte disturbance (hypokalemia or hypocalcemia)
- CNS catastrophe (intracerebral bleed or stroke)

All three of these possibilities would have to be strongly considered in an unresponsive patient. In this case there was no history of drug ingestion, and blood chemistries were essentially normal. Serial ECGs and CPK isoenzymes did not suggest infarction. Instead, the patient was found to have a large intracerebral hemorrhage.

INTERPRETATION of Fig. A-6

Sinus arrhythmia. Axis $\approx +40°$. Early transition. *Nonspecific ST-T wave abnormalities.*

This ECG is *not* normal. However, the ST-T wave changes that are present are entirely *nonspecific,* making it difficult to say much more about this tracing other than it is not normal. In an older patient with heart disease, these changes might represent ischemia or underlying coronary artery disease. They might also be caused by drug effect (digitalis or quinidine) or an electrolyte disturbance (hypokalemia). None of these really apply in the case of an otherwise healthy, asymptomatic 31-year-old woman.

Table 1-3 listed a number of additional factors that may influence ST-T wave morphology. Which ones are operative in this instance cannot be determined from inspection of this tracing. Again, not much can be said other than that the ECG is not normal and that nonspecific ST-T wave abnormalities are present.

EXERCISE B

ATYPICAL ECGS IN HEALTHY, ASYMPTOMATIC SUBJECTS

As part of the pre-employment physical examination, many companies require an ECG. This results in a lot of ECGs being performed on otherwise healthy, asymptomatic young adults. All of the following subjects have atypical ECG findings.

- Can you identify the atypical finding(s)?
- What is its clinical significance?

Figure B-1. ECG from a healthy, asymptomatic 24-year-old man.

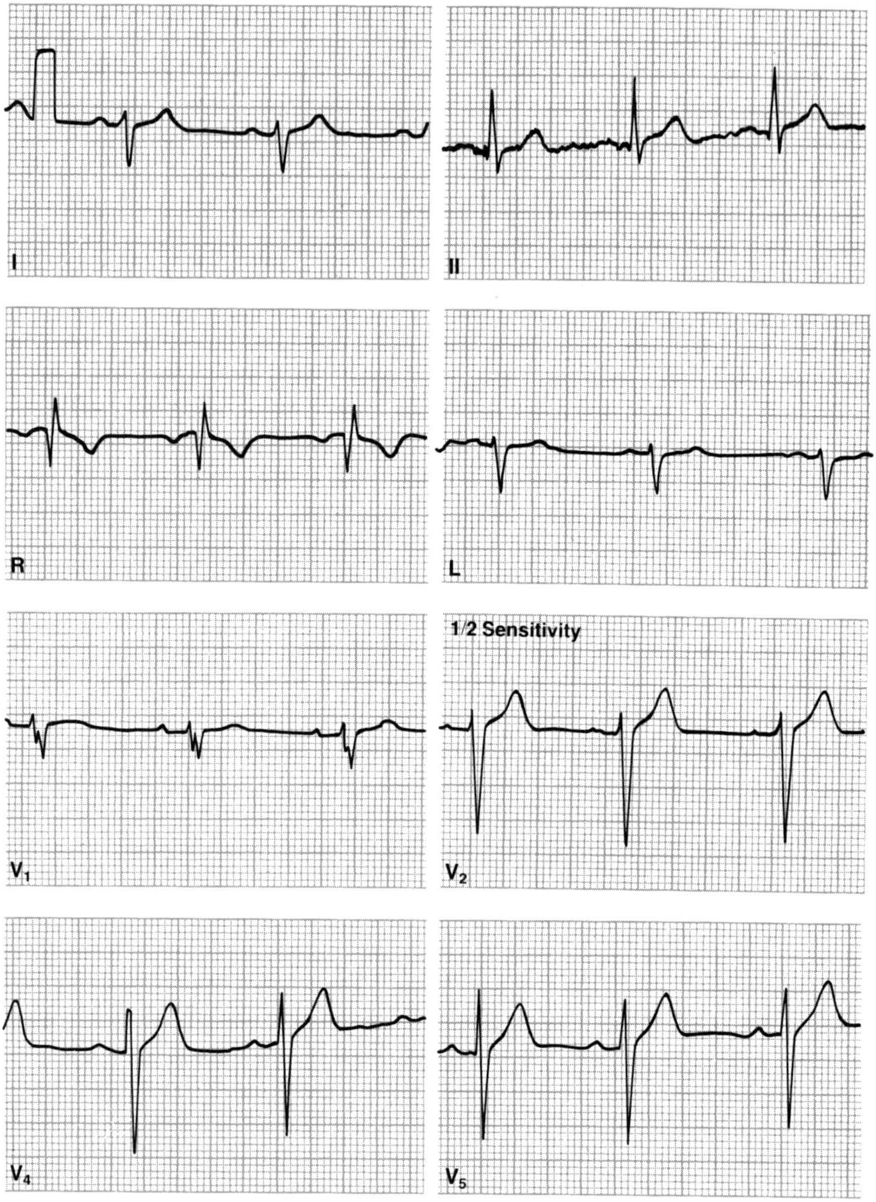

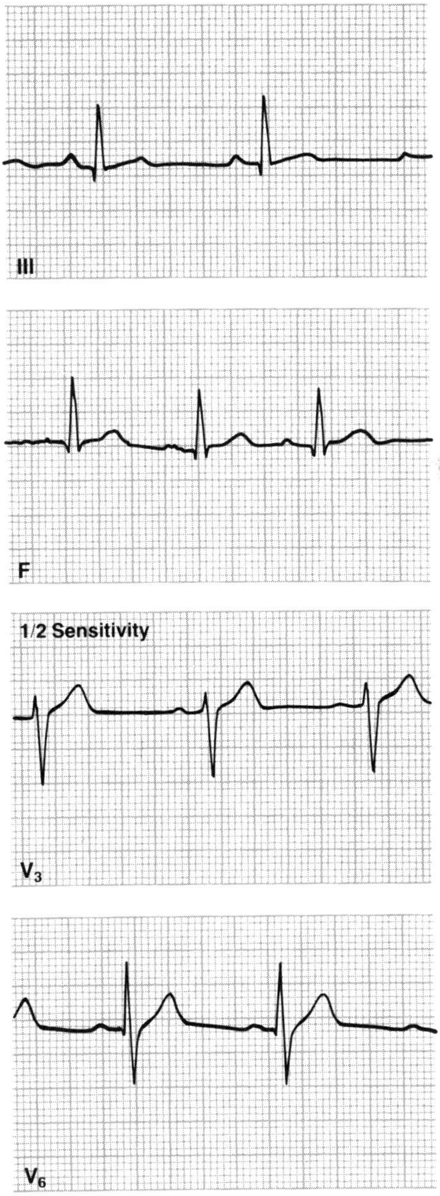
III
F
1/2 Sensitivity
V3
V6

Figure B-2. ECG from a healthy, asymptomatic 19-year-old man.

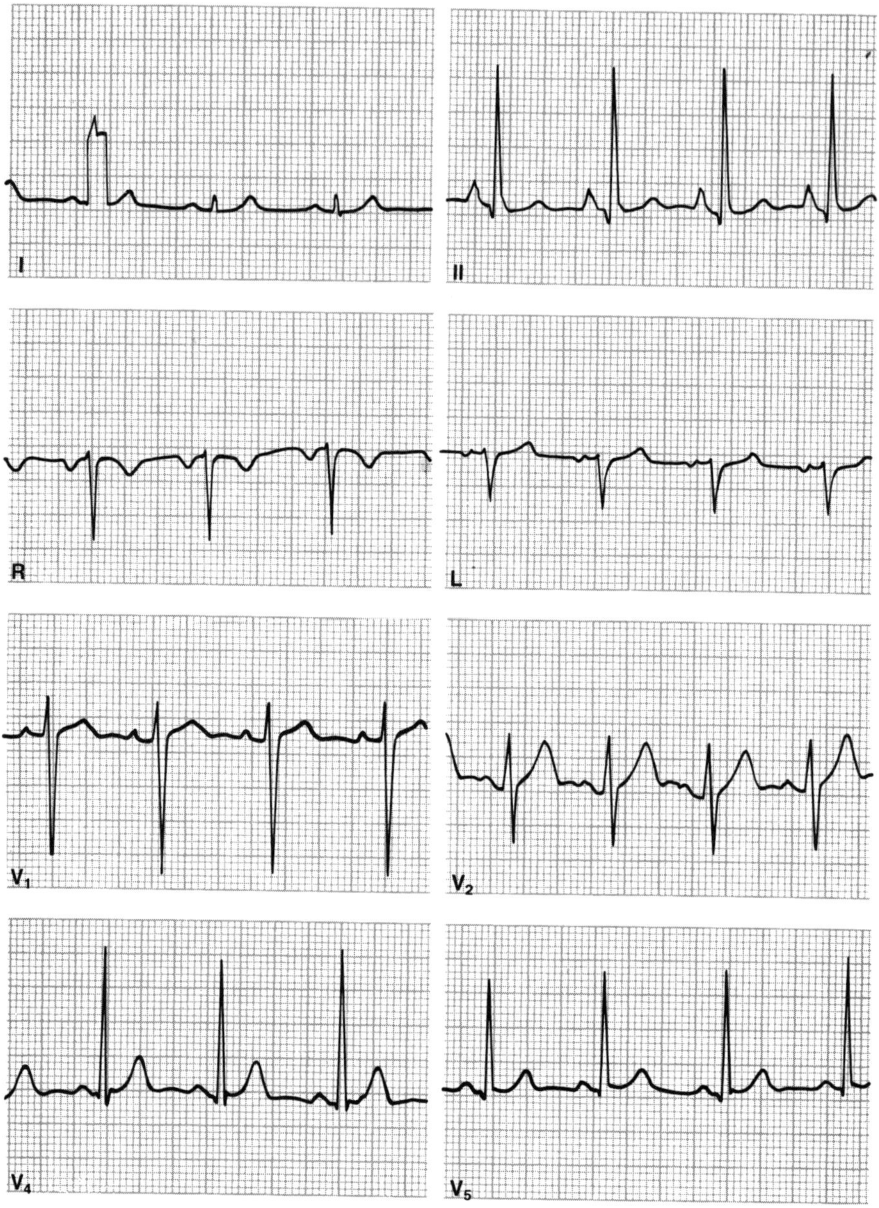

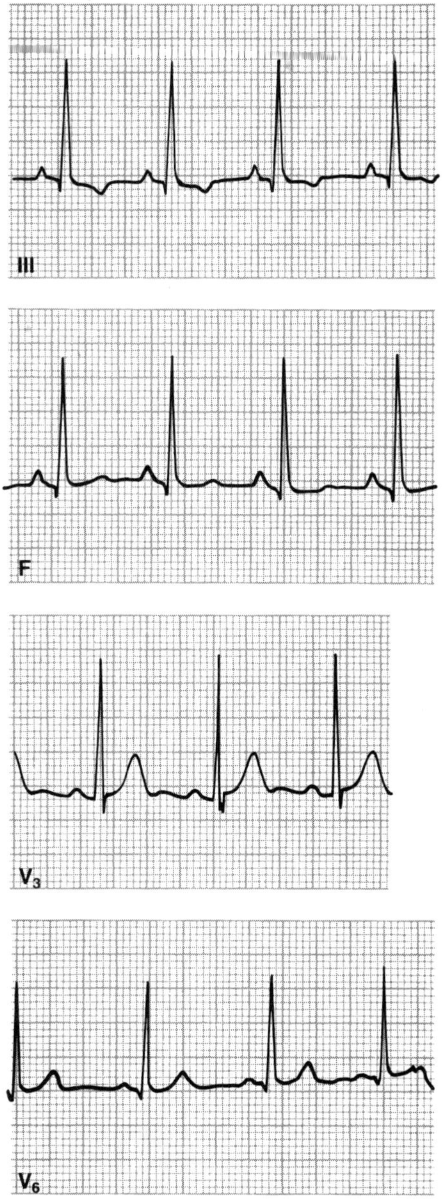
III
F
V3
V6

Figure B-3. ECG from a healthy, asymptomatic 32-year-old man.

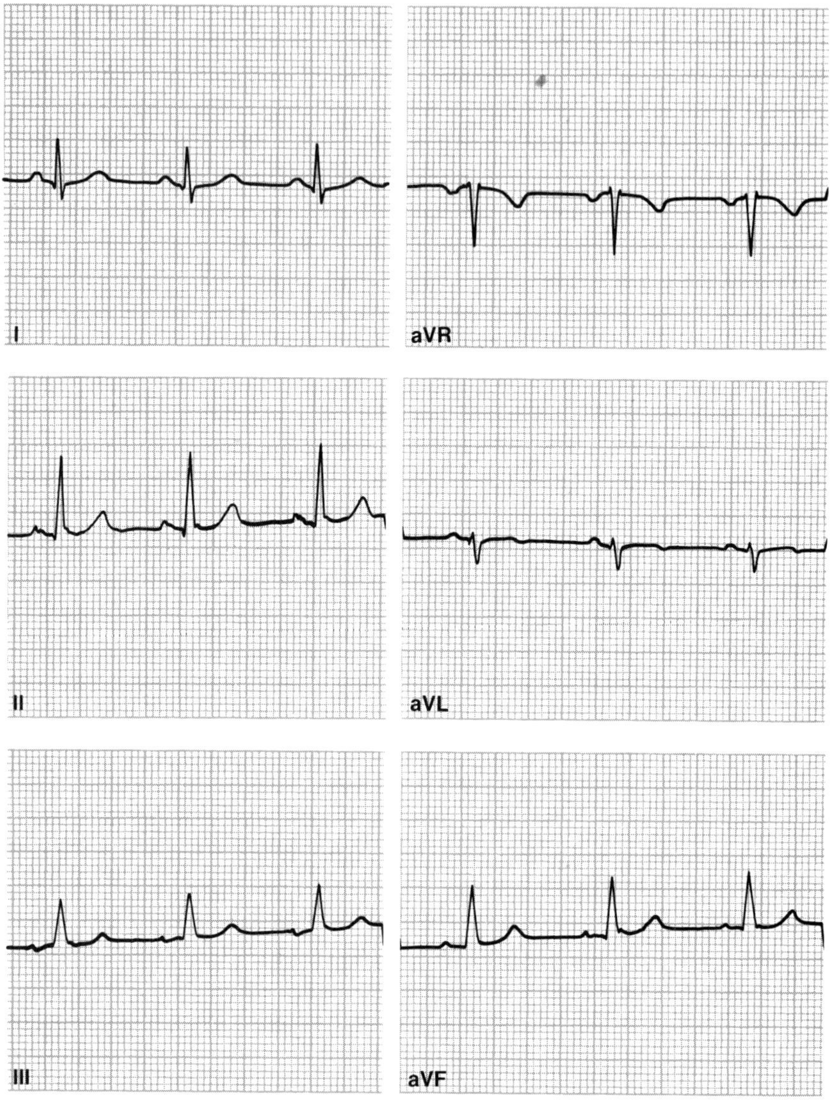

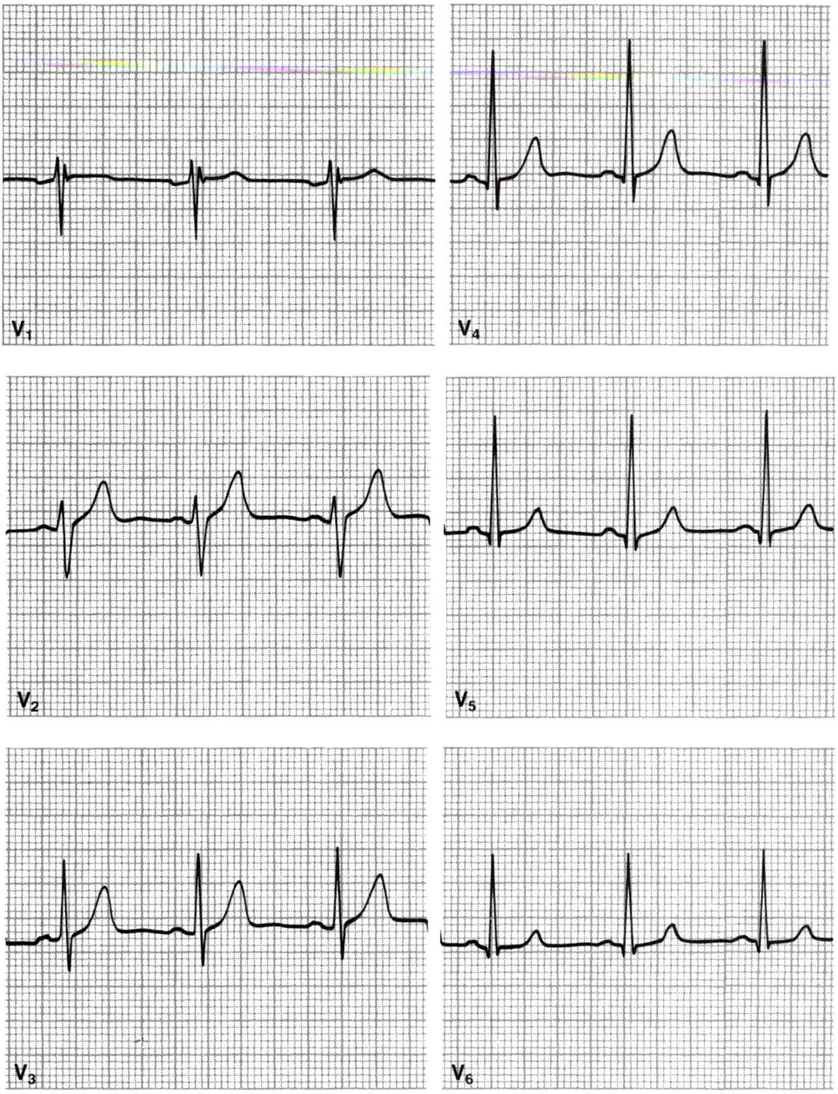
V1
V4
V2
V5
V3
V6

Figure B-4. ECG from a healthy, asymptomatic 40-year-old man.

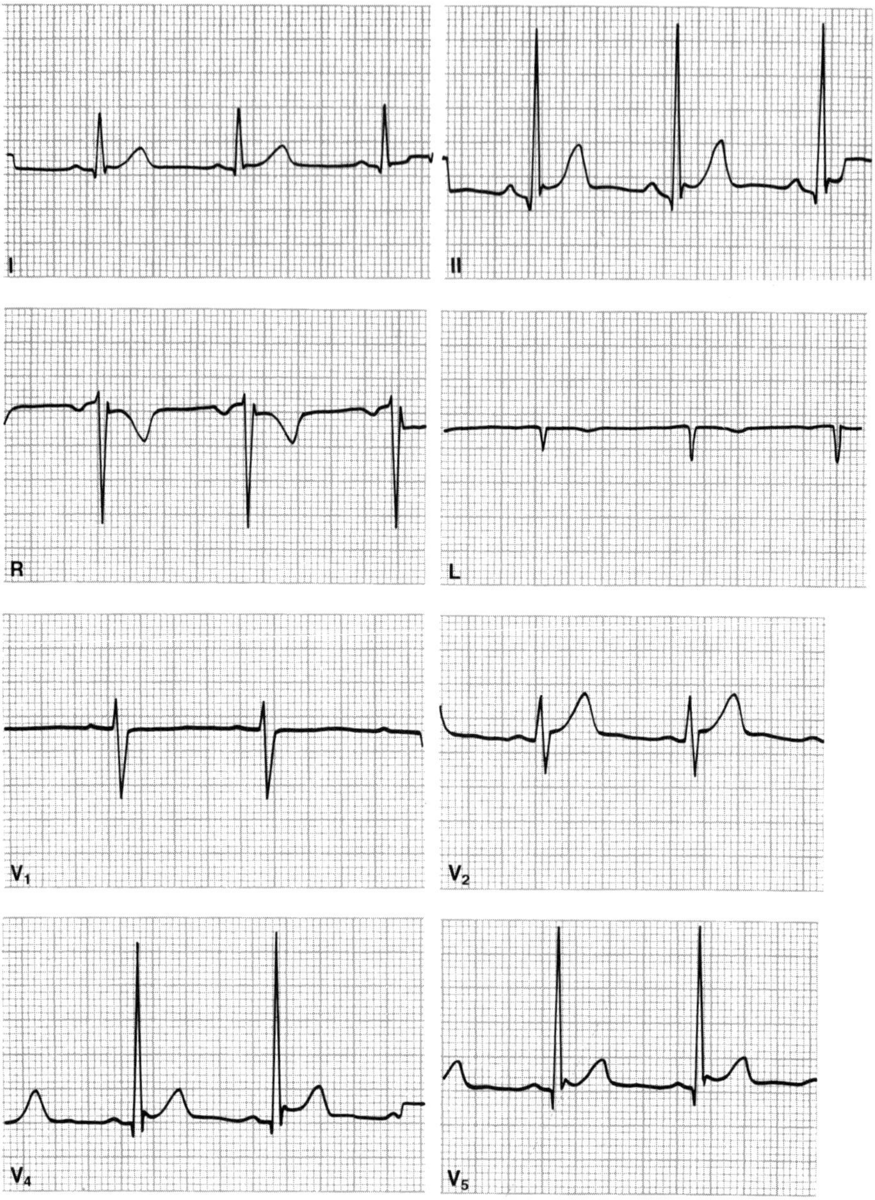

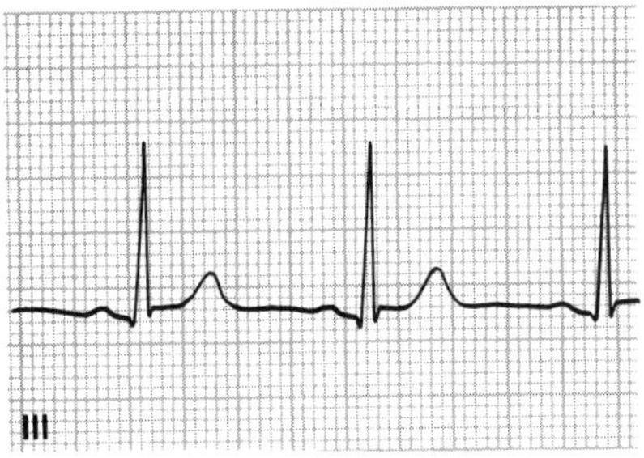
III

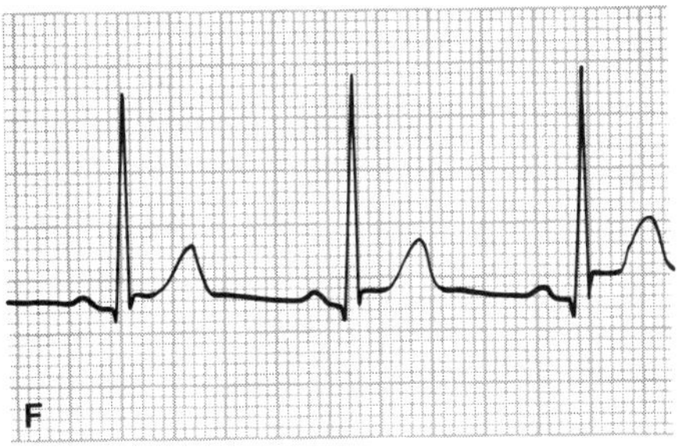
F

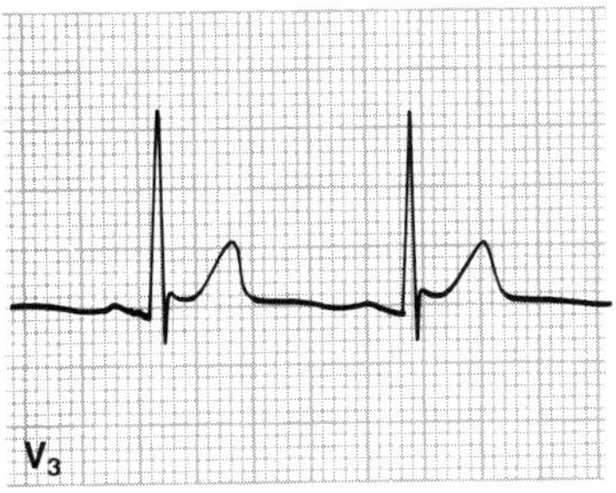
V_3

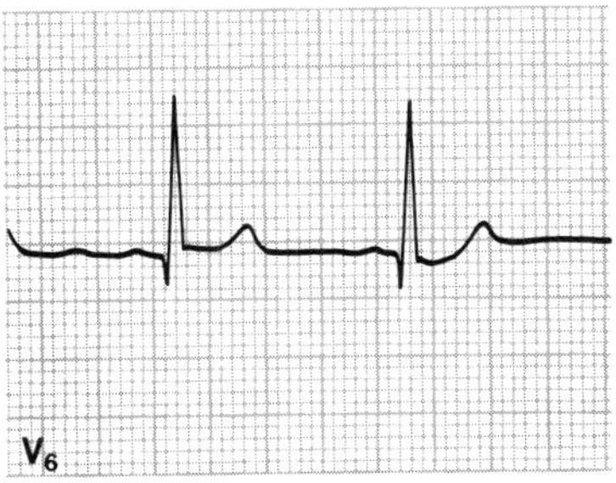
V_6

Figure B-5. ECG from a healthy, asymptomatic 46-year-old man.

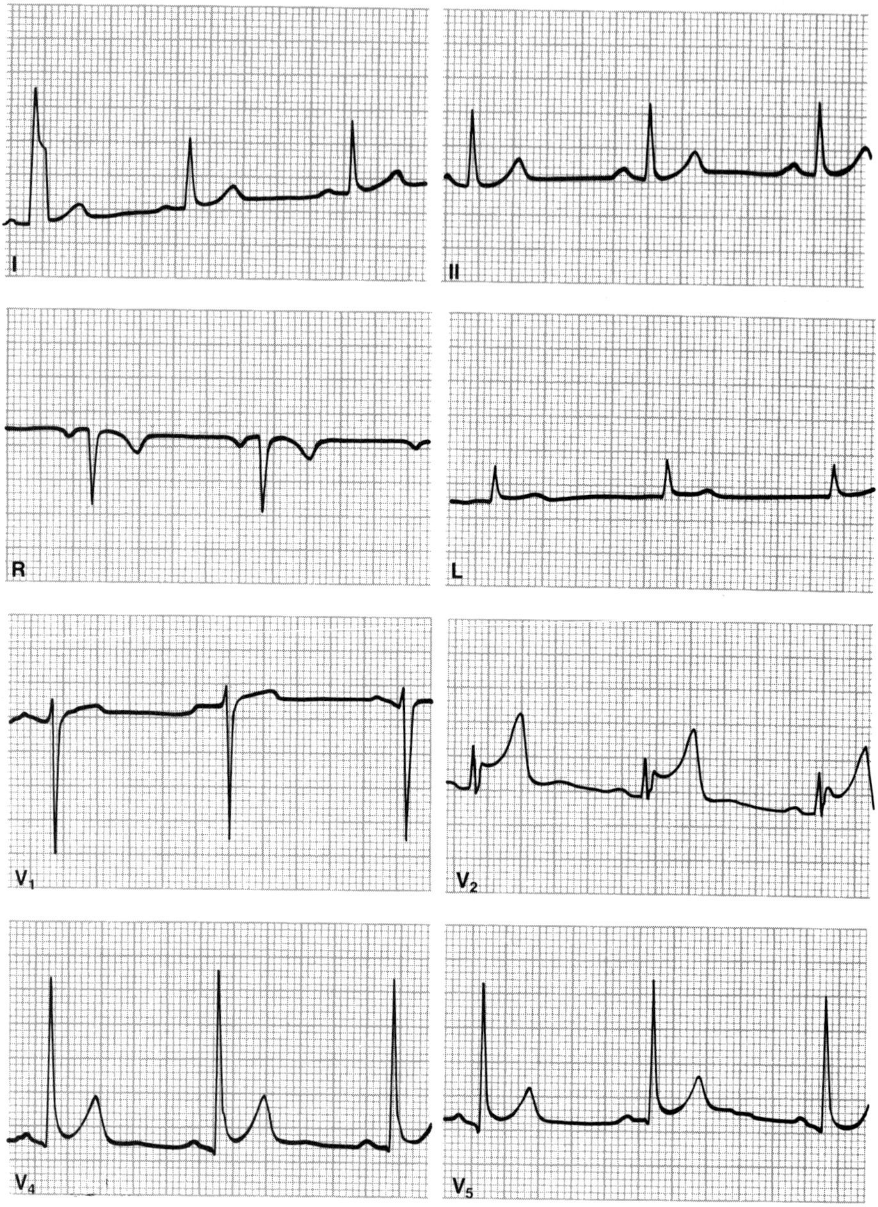

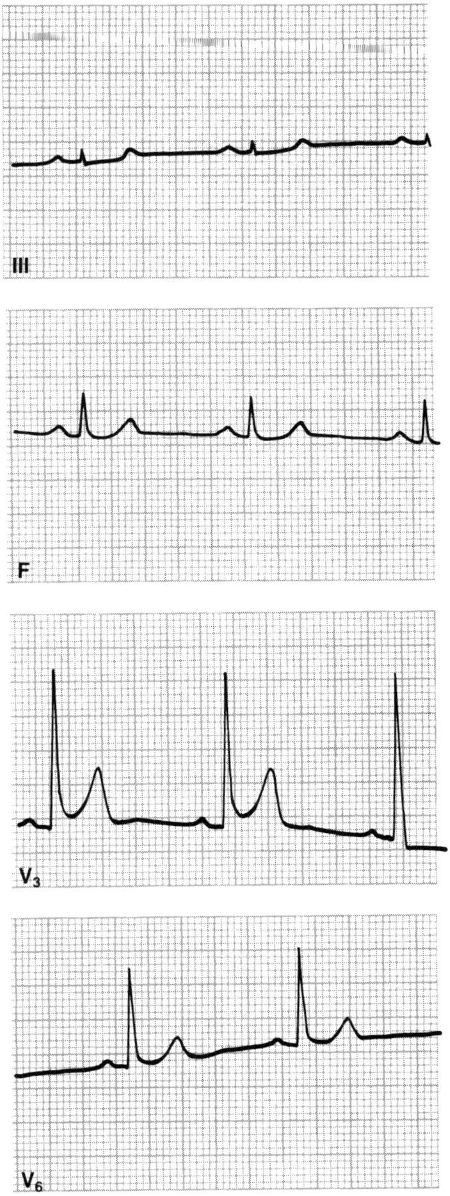
III
F
V3
V6

Figure B-6. ECG from a healthy, asymptomatic 35-year-old man obtained as part of his preemployment physical examination.

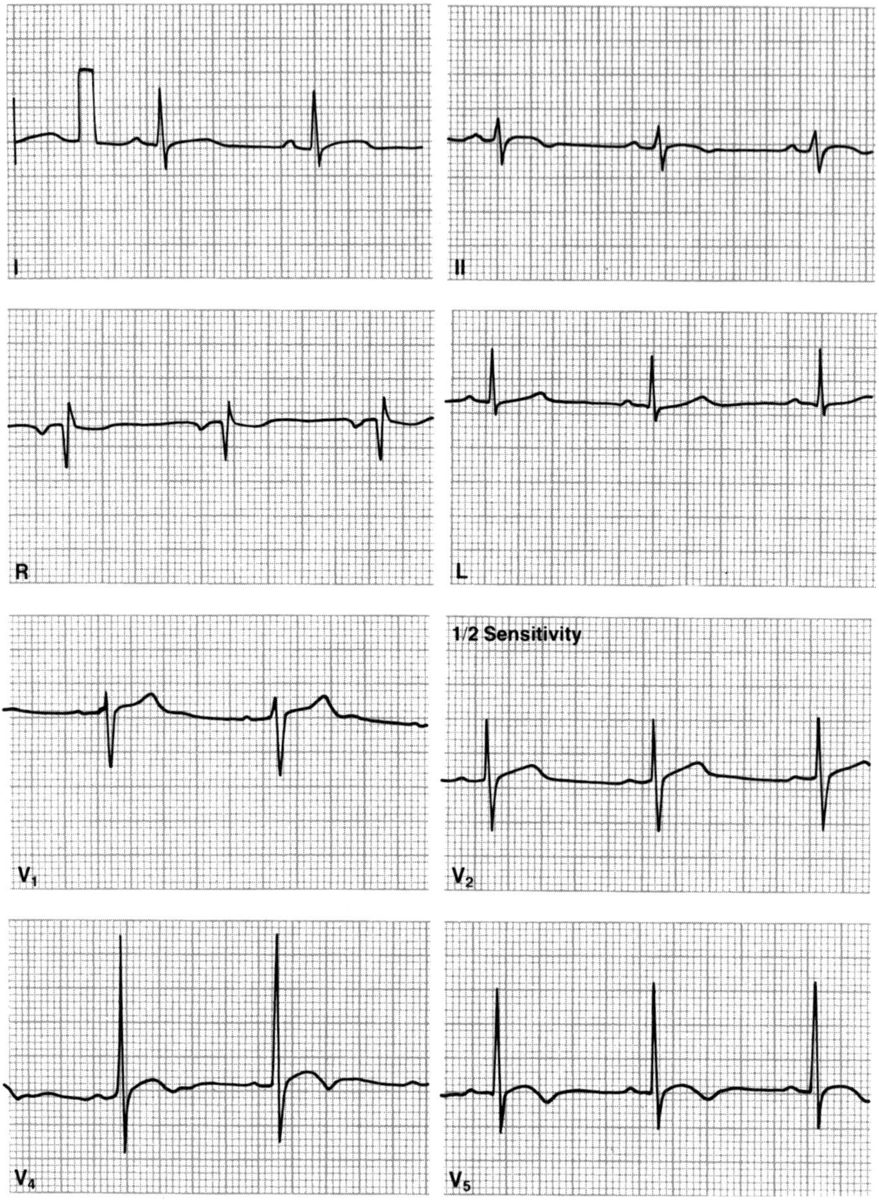

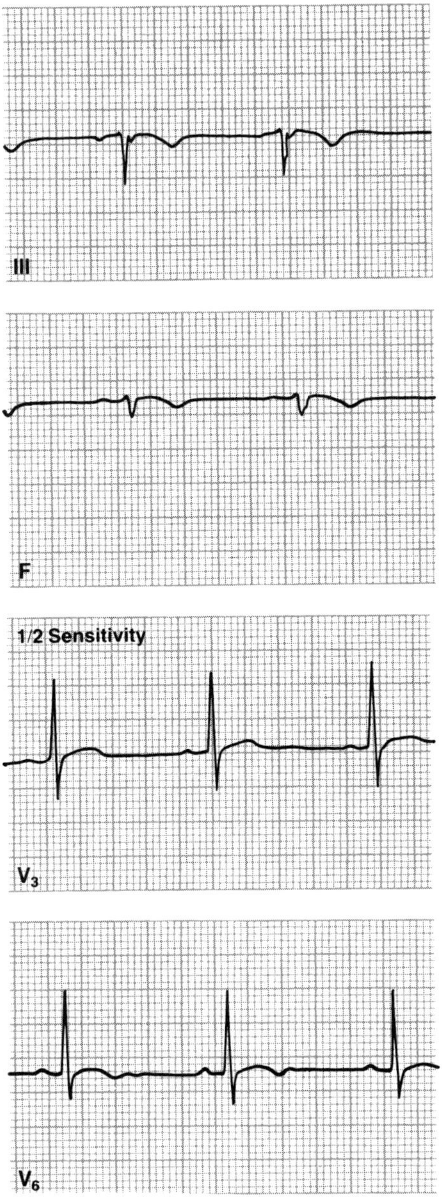
III
F
1/2 Sensitivity
V3
V6

Figure B-7. Exercise test on the 35-year-old man.

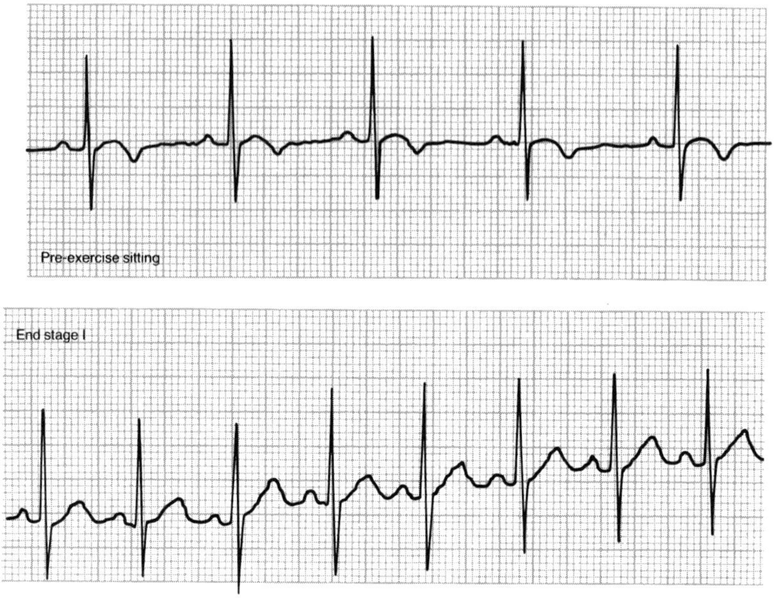

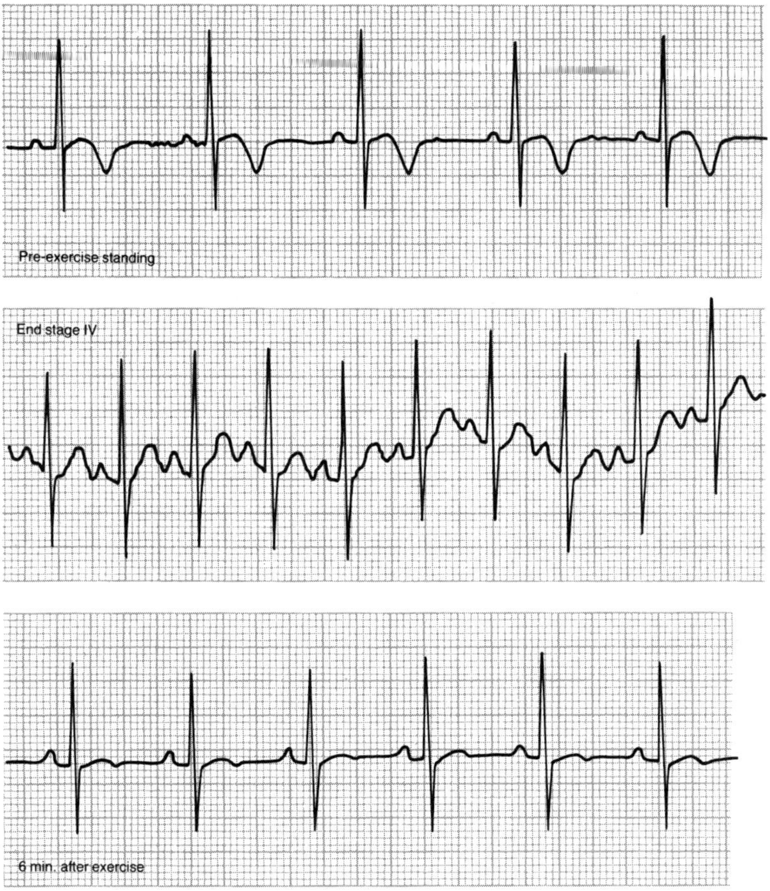
Pre-exercise standing
End stage IV
6 min. after exercise

Figure B-8. ECG from a previously healthy 37-year-old man complaining of epigastric pain.

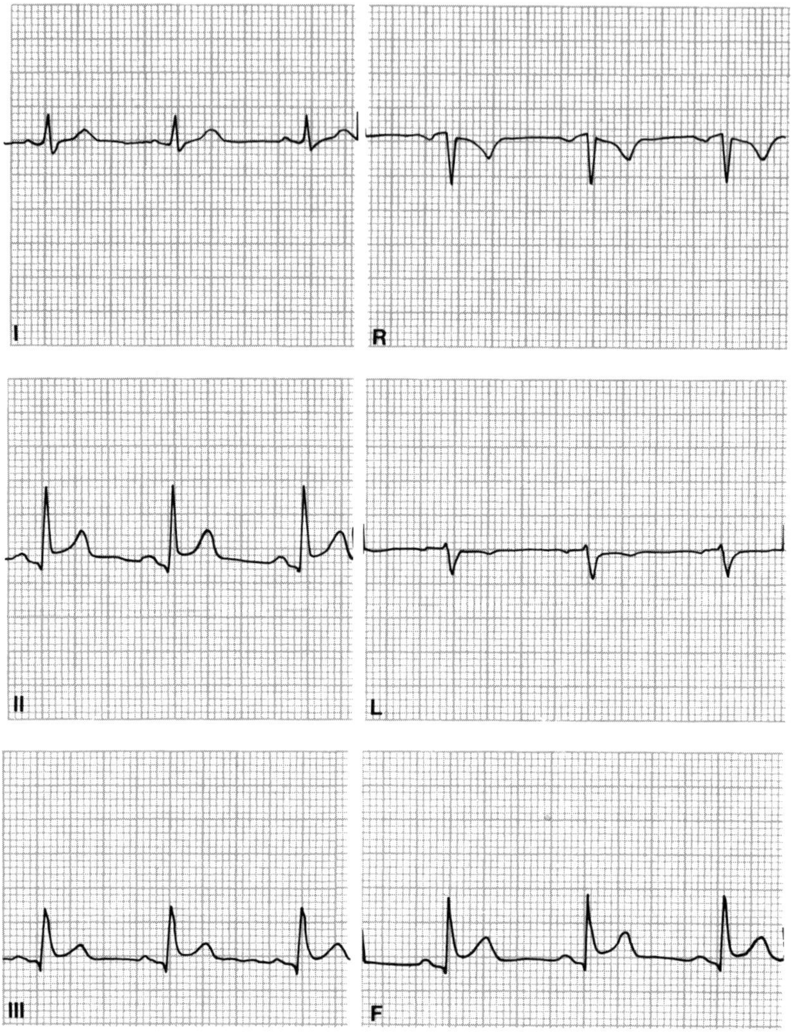

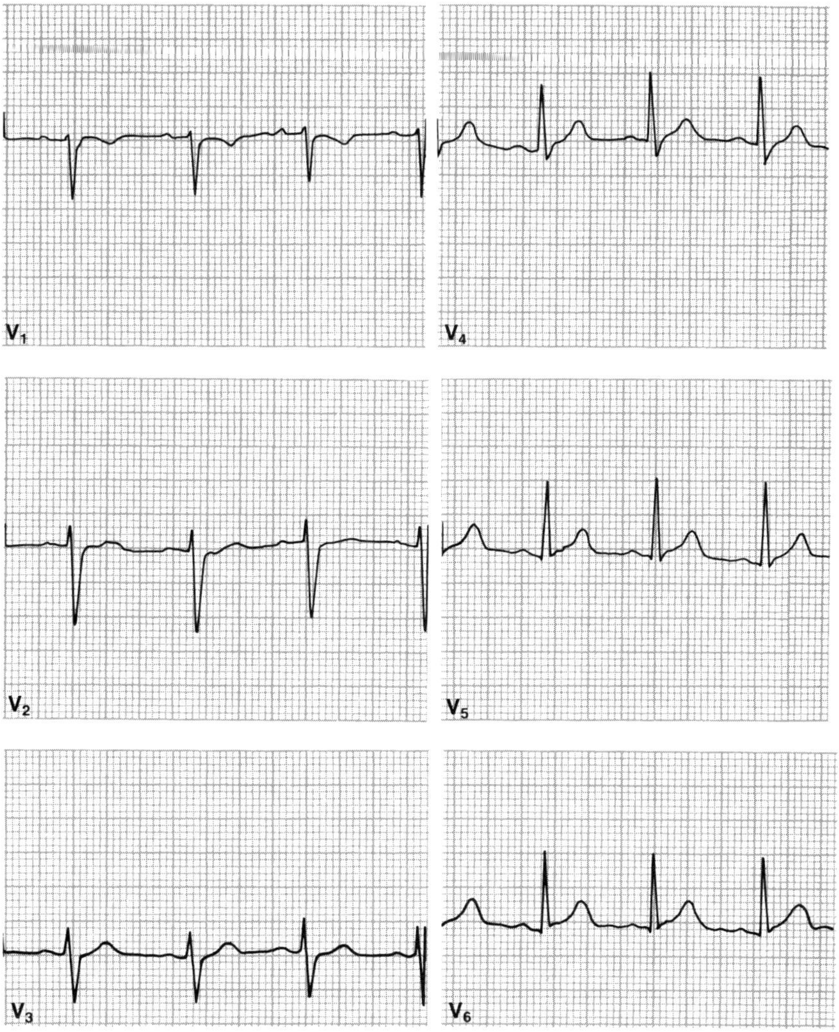
V1
V4
V2
V5
V3
V6

Figure B-9. Follow-up ECG obtained the next day on the 37-year-old man.

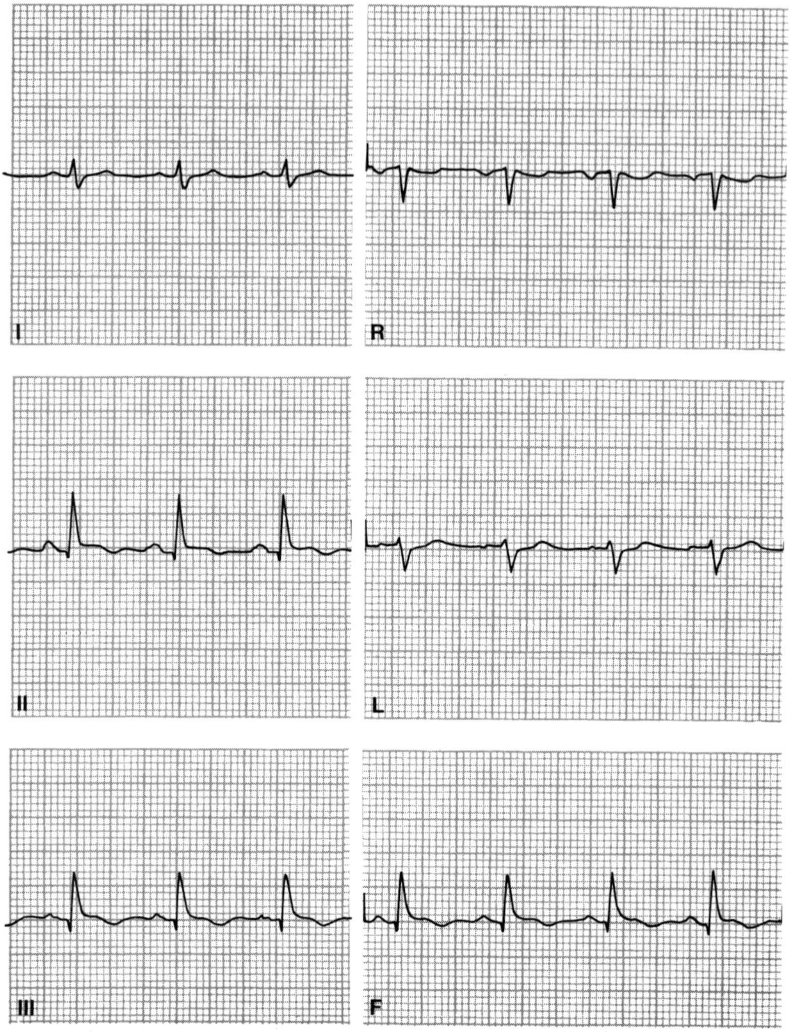

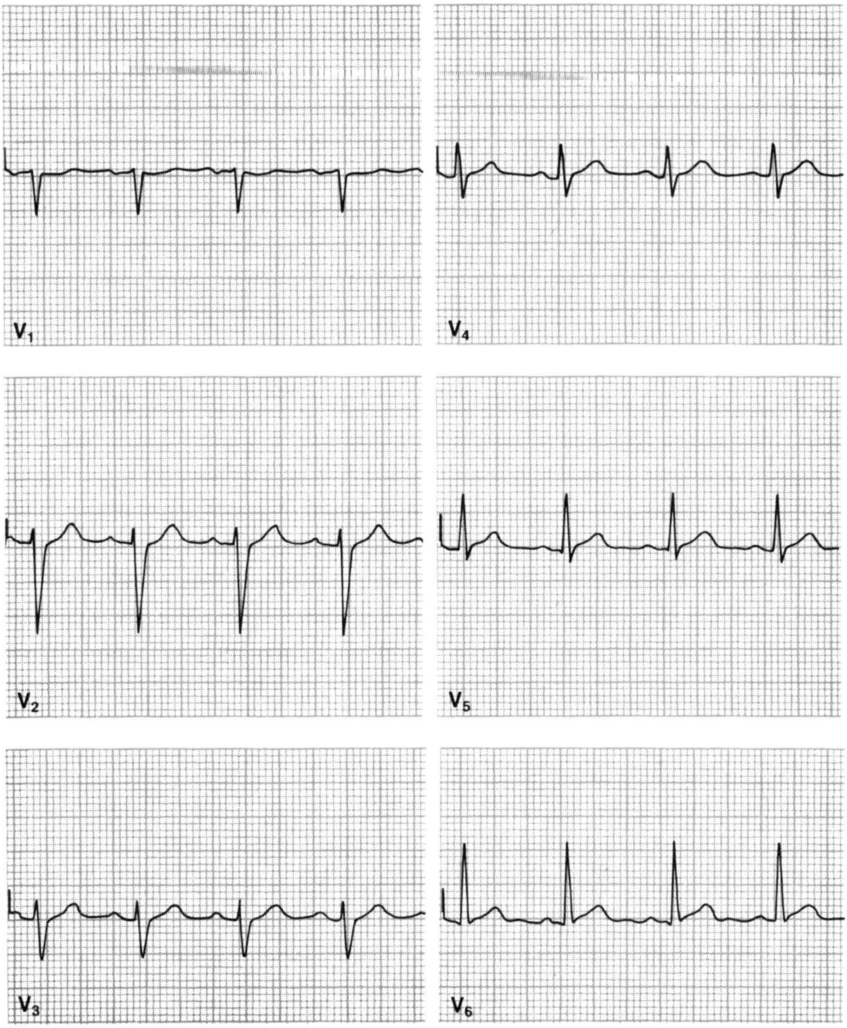
V1
V4
V2
V5
V3
V6

Figure B-10. ECG from a healthy, asymptomatic 47-year-old man.

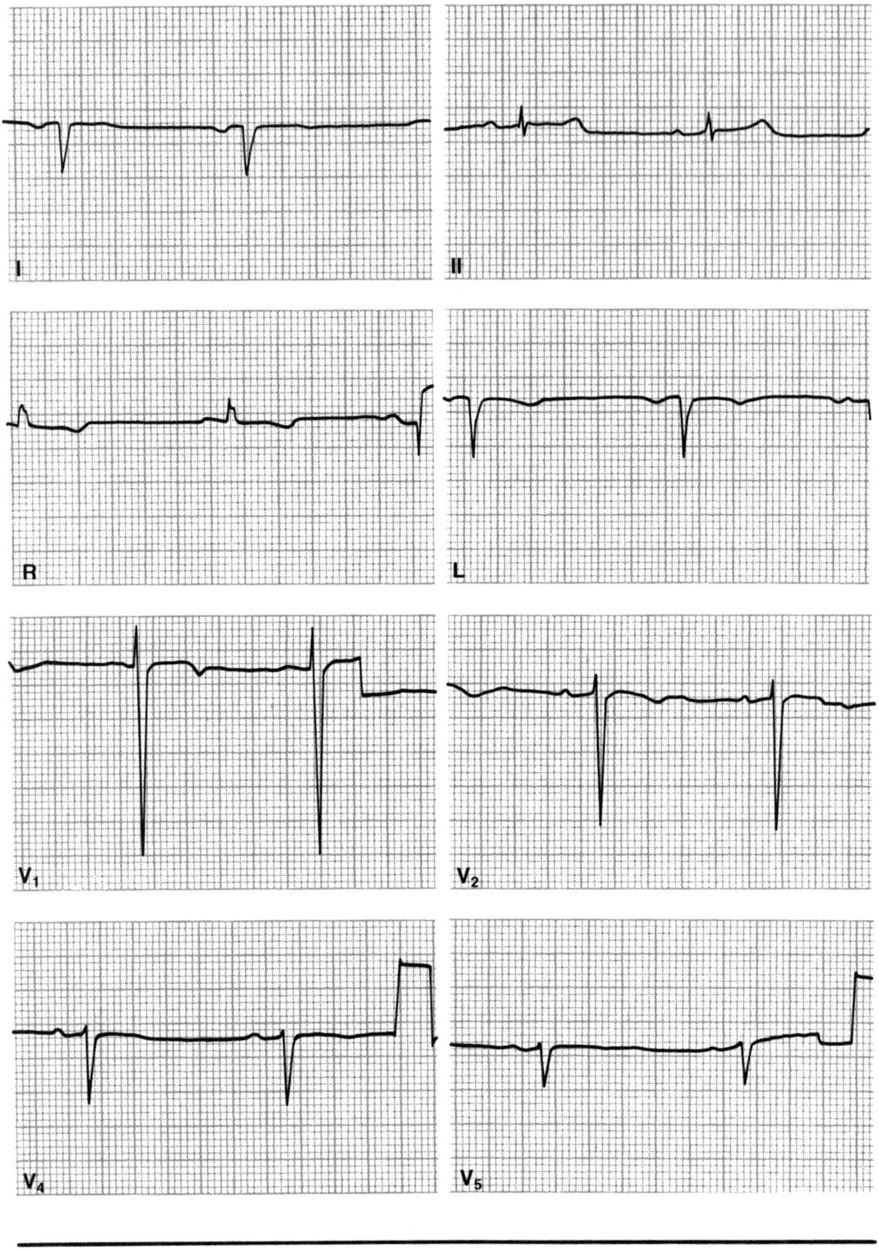

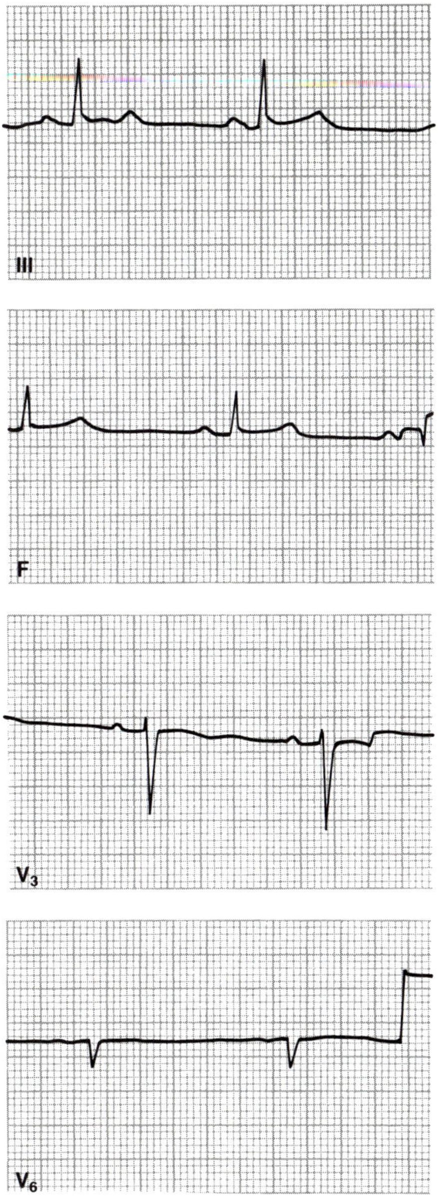
III
F
V_3
V_6

Figure B-11. ECG from the 47-year-old man with the precordial leads mounted on the *right* side of the chest.

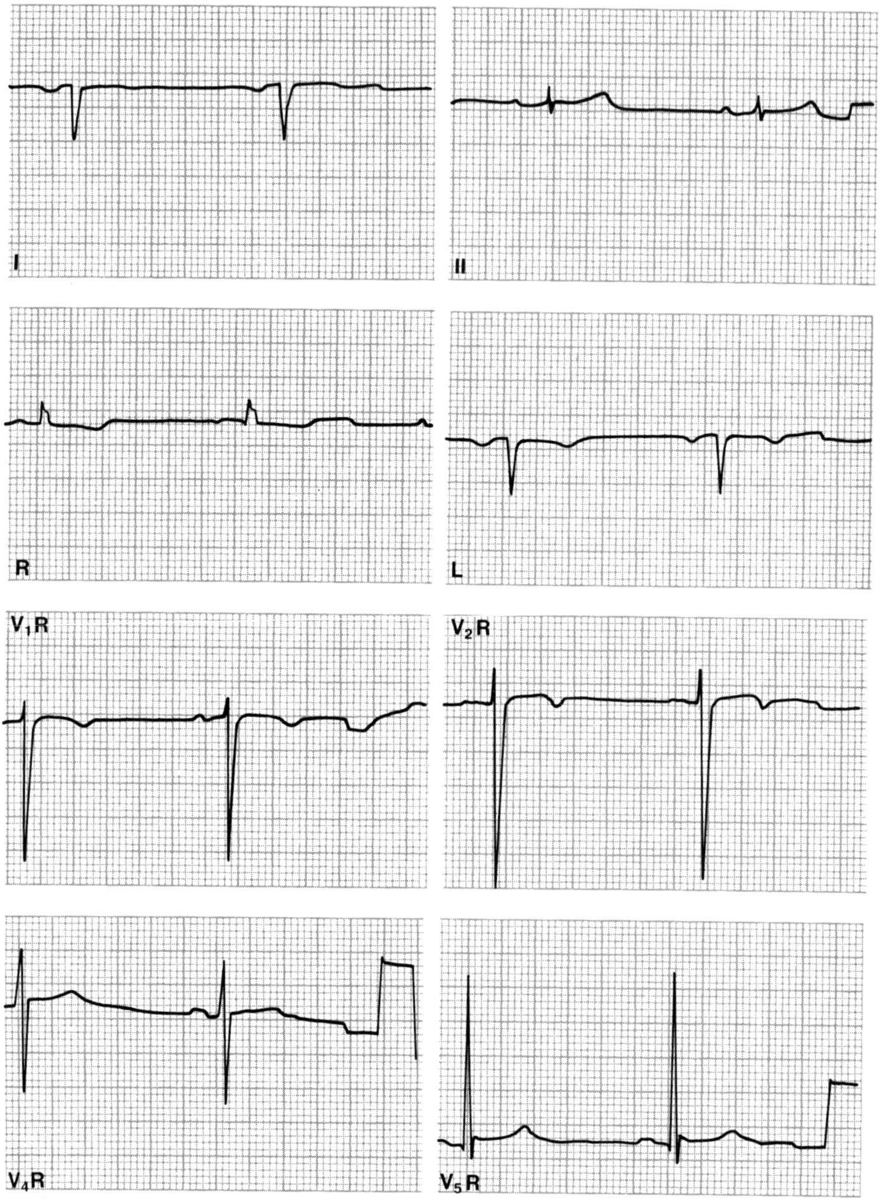

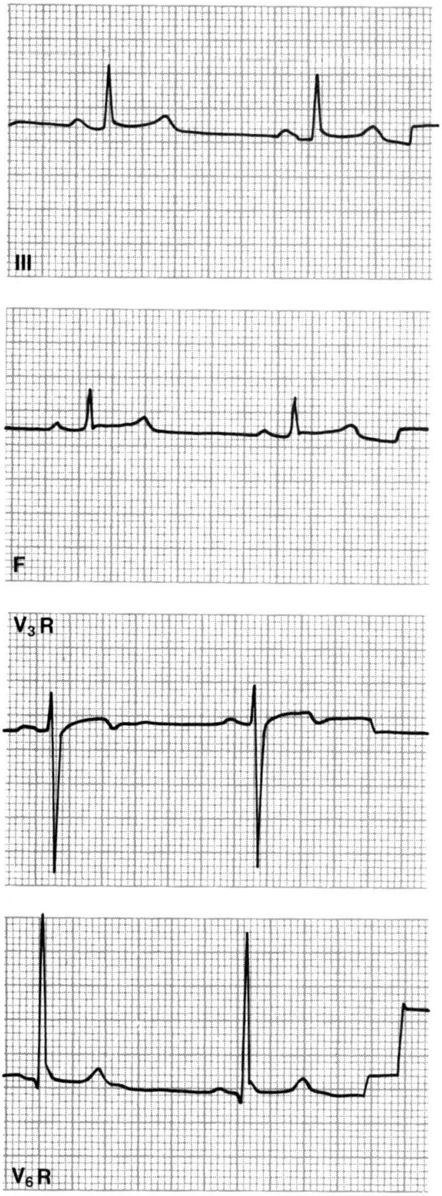
III
F
V3R
V6R

INTERPRETATION of Fig. B-1

Sinus arrhythmia. Axis $\approx +105°$ *(RAD)*. Poor R-wave progression. Persistence of S waves across the precordial leads. No acute changes.

Definite RAD is present in a pattern that resembles left posterior hemiblock (LPHB). However, it is quite uncommon for LPHB to present as an isolated conduction defect, particularly in this age group. Although RAD is one of the signs of RVH, this diagnosis is unlikely in the absence of RAA, prominent anterior forces, and right ventricular strain.

This subject had never noted any symptoms, despite leading a very active lifestyle. Physical examination was entirely normal. Stress testing did not reveal any abnormality through 15 minutes of vigorous exercise. The chest X-ray did not suggest cardiac enlargement. In summary, the patient was felt to have an atypical ECG without any evidence of underlying heart disease. He was encouraged to resume full activity.

Distribution of mean QRS axis in the general population follows a bell-shaped curve. Consequently, a number of otherwise healthy, asymptomatic subjects will have axis deviations at either extreme of distribution (LAD or RAD). In the absence of symptoms or evidence of underlying heart disease, such findings are usually of no clinical significance.

INTERPRETATION of Fig. B-2

Sinus rhythm at about 85 beats/min. Axis $\approx +80°$. *RAA*. Otherwise within normal limits (WNL).

Although definite criteria for RAA *are* present in this tracing, the subject had absolutely no underlying cardiac disease. Instead, the prominent, peaked P waves in the inferior leads were most likely the result of his relatively vertical mean QRS axis. Designating such atypical P-wave morphology by RAA instead of RAE is our acknowledgment that factors other than true atrial enlargement may affect P waves. (The vertical axis also explains the small and almost certainly insignificant inferior q waves, as well as inversion of the T wave in lead III, which as an isolated finding is *not* abnormal.)

Voltage for LVH would be present in this tracing (sum of S wave in lead V_1 + R wave in $V_5 > 35$ mm), except for the fact that the patient is under 35 years old.

INTERPRETATION of Fig. B-3

Sinus rhythm at 75 beats/min. Axis $\approx +70°$. *Incomplete RBBB.* Otherwise WNL.

Incomplete RBBB is an extremely common finding among young adults. It occurs in up to 5 percent of the general population, and is usually of no clinical significance.

A pearl to remember is that, on occasion, incomplete RBBB may be a tipoff to the presence of atrial septal defect (ASD). Careful auscultation (listening for a fixed split-second heart sound) is therefore warranted among subjects with this finding. In the absence of an abnormal cardiac exam, isolated incomplete RBBB should be viewed as an incidental finding without need for further investigation.

Electrocardiographic features such as RAD, RAA, and incomplete RBBB should really be thought of as atypical rather than abnormal when they occur in otherwise healthy, asymptomatic young individuals. Saying that an ECG feature is *abnormal* implies that the feature has a significantly greater prevalence among diseased individuals than in a healthy population. In contrast, although an *atypical* finding is unusual for a healthy population, it still occurs more commonly in healthy individuals than among those with disease.

INTERPRETATION of B-4

Sinus rhythm at 72 beats/min. Axis $\approx +75°$. *Voltage for LVH.* Small, probably insignificant q waves in the inferolateral leads. J-point ST-segment elevation with an upward concavity in the same leads—probably caused by *early repolarization.*

This tracing most likely represents a normal variant. All of the q waves are small and narrow, and probably due to septal depolarization. The ST-segment elevation has the characteristic appearance of early repolarization, and no reciprocal changes are evident. Yet if this person presented to the emergency department with new-onset chest pain, this ECG, and no comparison tracing, one would be hard pressed to exclude infarction.

Of note, *voltage* for LVH is present since the R wave in a limb lead is ≥ 20 mm and the patient is over 35. Amplitude of the R wave in lead V_5 looks as if it would also exceed voltage criteria (R in $V_5 \geq 25$ mm) if it weren't cut off by the edge of the paper.

INTERPRETATION of Fig. B-5

Sinus rhythm at about 60 beats/min. Axis $\approx +35°$. *Voltage for LVH.* ST segment elevation with an upward concavity in leads V_2 to V_5, most likely due to *early repolarization.* Suggest clinical correlation and comparison with prior tracings.

Once again, *voltage* criteria for LVH are present (sum of deepest S wave in leads V_1 or V_2 + tallest R wave in leads V_5 or $V_6 \geq 35$ mm), though the specificity of this sign for LVH in the absence of strain is limited.

Impressive ST-segment elevation is noted in the precordial leads, particularly in lead V_2, where the ST segment is elevated by 4 mm. The contour of these ST segments, the prominent notch at the J point in lead V_2, and the history of the patient are all most consistent with this being early repolarization. Given a different clinical setting, the same ECG picture might represent acute pericarditis or acute infarction.

INTERPRETATION of Fig. B-6

Sinus rhythm at about 65 beats/min. Axis $\approx -30°$ (LAD). ST-segment coving and symmetric T-wave inversion in the inferior and lateral precordial leads.

What does this most likely represent?

One's final interpretation of this ECG would depend to a large extent on the clinical setting. In this particular case, the patient was a healthy, athletic, asymptomatic 35-year-old man. In this context, the ECG most probably represents a *normal* repolarization variant. On the other hand, if this patient had presented to the emergency department with a history of chest pain and a similar ECG, prompt hospitalization in an coronary care unit would be in order.

Chest X-ray films and physical examination of the patient were entirely normal. Fig. B-7 shows the results of maximal exercise testing. Note that although T-wave inversion actually *deepens* when he arises from a sitting position, the ST segments *normalize* during the first stage of exercise —walking 1.7 mph on a 10 percent graded incline. ST segments remain normal *throughout* exercise (in this case through stage IV = 4.2 mph on a 16 percent graded incline), but pre-exercise ST-segment coving returns in recovery. This is an entirely *normal* response to exercise and supports the clinical impression that the ST-T wave abnormalities in this subject are more than likely benign.

Although not often seen in a typical primary-care practice, repolarization variants similar to the type shown in Fig. B-6 are surprisingly common among young, healthy *athletic* individuals, particularly blacks. One study detected them in greater than 10 percent of professional football players (see Balady, Cadigan, Ryan, 1984). Another study demonstrated that when athletes continue to exercise on a regular basis, ST-T wave repolarization changes may persist into middle age (see Nishimura, Kambara, Chen, et al, 1981).

The etiology for these repolarization changes is unknown, but it is thought to relate to alterations in resting autonomic tone (either increased resting parasympathetic tone or decreased resting sympathetic tone). Other atypical findings attributed to alterations in resting autonomic tone that are commonly found in well-trained athletes include sinus bradycardia, sinus arrhythmia, wandering atrial pacemaker, ectopic atrial rhythm, 1° AV block, and Wenckebach 2° AV block. All of these rhythm changes tend to normalize with exercise.

This patient was given a wallet-sized reproduction of his resting ECG and told to be sure to present it should anyone ever want to repeat an ECG on him.

INTERPRETATION of Fig. B-8

Sinus arrhythmia. Axis $\approx +70°$. Small q waves in the inferolateral leads. ST-segment elevation with an upward concavity in the inferior leads. This most likely represents early repolarization, but *can't rule out* acute injury. Strongly suggest clinical correlation.

Lest one become too complacent, we have included this example. Examine Fig. B-9, taken from the same patient the next day.

A number of changes in the *inferior* leads can be noted in the follow-up tracing. Q waves appear to have deepened slightly, the benign-appearing upward concavity of ST segments in these leads has been replaced by upward *convexity* (coving), and T-wave inversion is beginning to occur. This represents *acute inferior infarction.*

The point to emphasize is that although early repolarization is exceedingly common, the picture it produces is sometimes *indistinguishable* from acute infarction. While history remains the most important factor to consider in deciding whether to admit a patient with chest pain to the hospital, equivocal ECG findings such as those shown in Fig. B-8 are sometimes suspicious enough to warrant hospital admission. When in doubt, it is probably better to err on the side of *caution* (admission to the hospital) than to send home someone who may be having an infarction. In effect, the patient in this case was *not* entirely asymptomatic, but instead was complaining of epigastric abdominal pain. This may sometimes be the presenting complaint of patients with inferior infarction (due to the fact that the inferior surface of the heart sits on top of the diaphragm).

INTERPRETATION of Fig. B-10

Sinus bradycardia and arrhythmia. Global negativity in lead I! This suggests *either* limb-lead reversal or dextrocardia.

Although at first glance one might be tempted to presume lateral infarction from the QS complex in leads I and aVL, close inspection reveals the P wave and T wave, also, to be inverted in these leads. Global negativity should *not* normally be seen in lead I. In addition, the QRS complex in lead aVR, which usually *does* manifest global negativity, is positive.

PROBLEM: The answer to the differential diagnosis of global negativity (limb-lead reversal or dextrocardia) can usually be suspected from evaluating R-wave progression in the precordial leads. What does R-wave progression (or *lack* of it) suggest in this case?

ANSWER: There is *reverse R-wave progression* in the precordial leads (R waves diminish in amplitude as one progresses from lead V_1 to lead V_6, suggesting dextrocardia. With *limb*-lead reversal, R-wave progression is normal, since the heart lies in its normal position within the thoracic cavity and placement of precordial leads has *not* been affected.

Fig. B-11 is this patient's ECG repeated with the precordial leads mounted in their appropriate positions on the *right* side of the chest.

Note that R-wave progression is now *normal,* as one would expect with dextrocardia. Clinically, heart sounds were heard on the right side of the chest. Chest X-ray provided final confirmation. In practice, limb-lead reversal is a *much* more common cause of global negativity in lead I than is dextrocardia.

Knowledge of the position of abdominal organs is important in determining the likelihood that cardiac malformations will be associated with dextrocardia. With complete situs inversus, the heart and abdominal contents form a mirror-image of normal (heart and stomach on the right side, liver on the left). Aside from dextrocardia, these patients usually do *not* have additional cardiac abnormalities. On the other hand, cardiac malformations are much more common when dextrocardia occurs without situs inversus of the viscera.

References

Balady GJ, Cadigan JB, Ryan TJ: Electrocardiogram of the athlete: An analysis of 289 professional football players. *Am J Cardiol* 1984; 53:1339–1343.

Nishimura T, Kambara H, Chen CH, Yamada Y, Kawai C: Noninvasive assessment of T-wave abnormalities on precordial electrocardiograms in middle-age professional bicyclists. *J Electrocardiol* 1981; 14:357–364.

EXERCISE C

ECGS IN PATIENTS WITH CARDIOMEGALY ON CHEST X-RAY

The patients presented in this section all have cardiomegaly on chest X-ray. Can you correlate this information with their ECGs and the brief histories given above each tracing?

Figure C-1. ECG from a 68-year-old woman with a history of congestive heart failure. Taking digitalis.

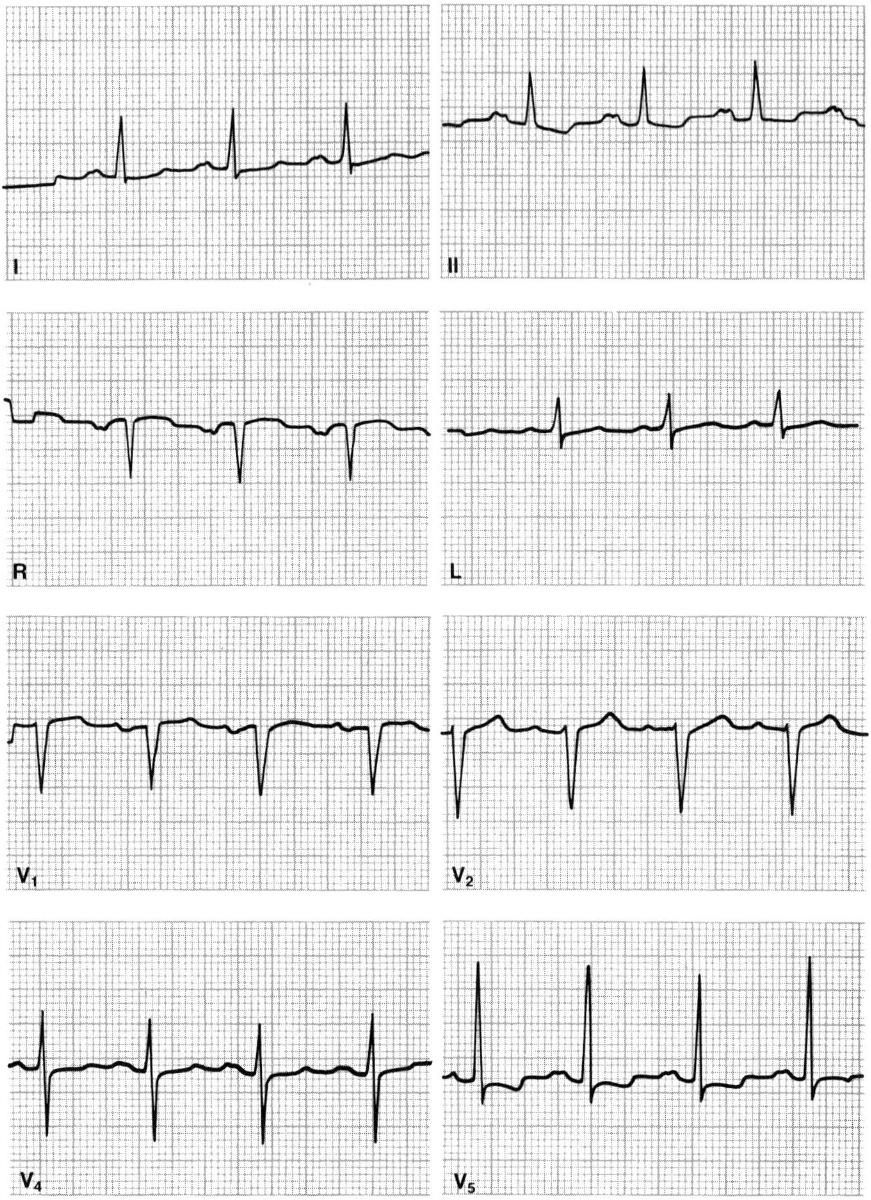

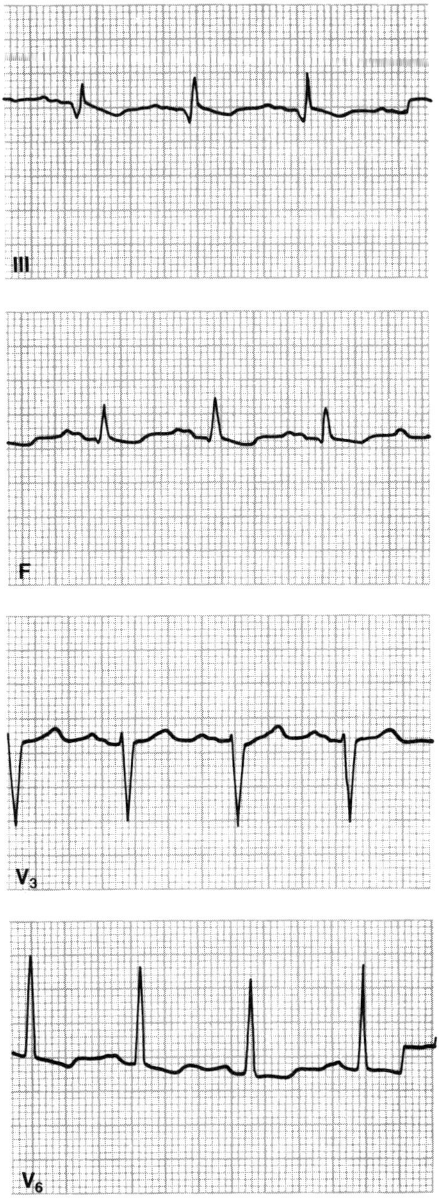
III
F
V3
V6

Figure C-2. ECG from a 62-year-old woman with a systolic heart murmur. No prior history of infarction.

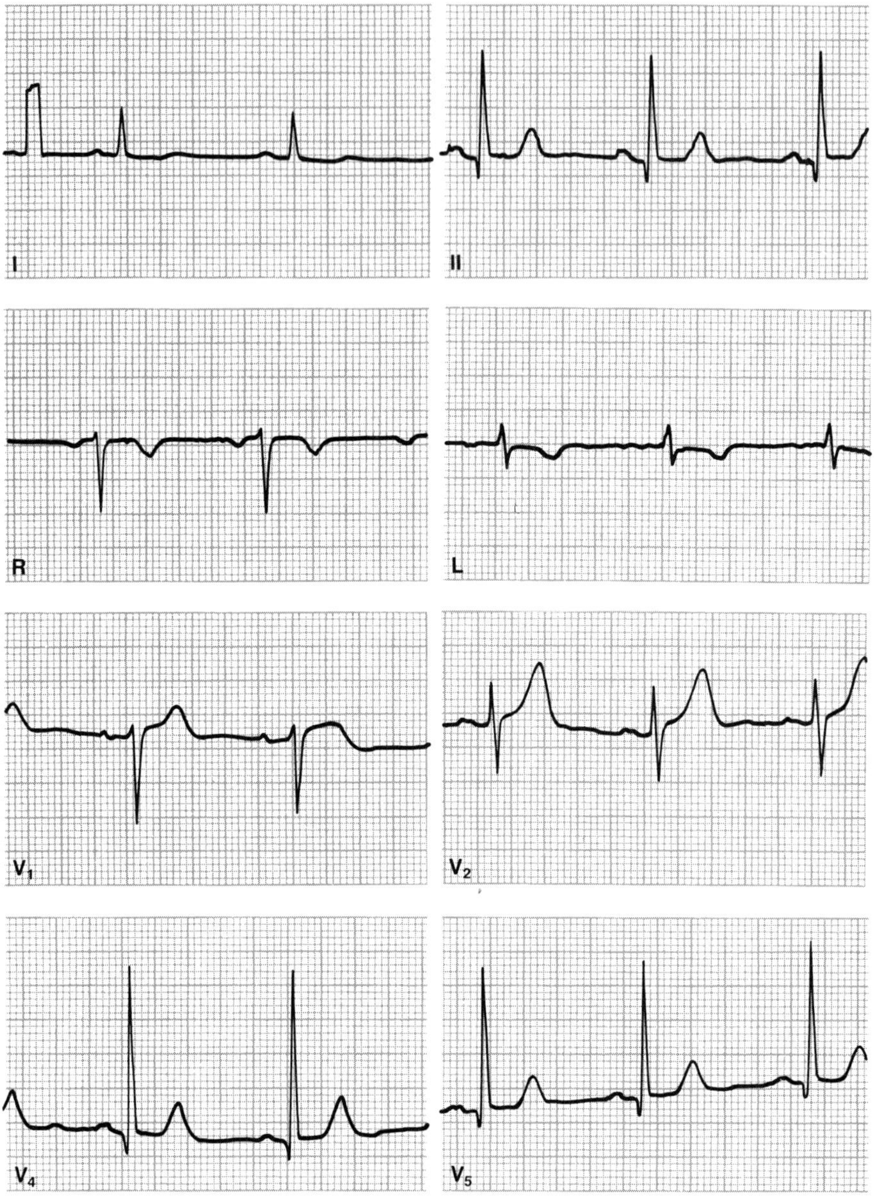

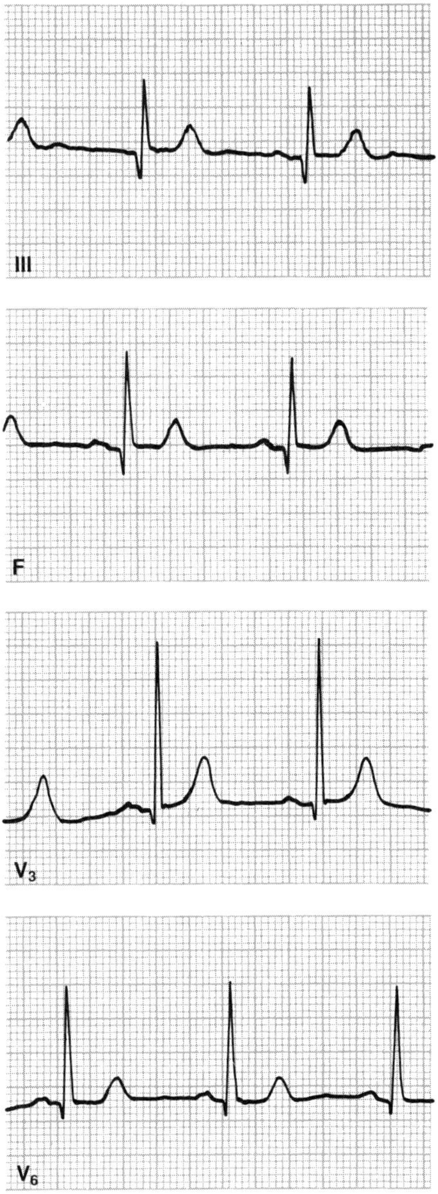
III
F
V3
V6

Figure C-3. ECG from a 68-year-old man presenting with shortness of breath and a globular heart on chest X-ray film.

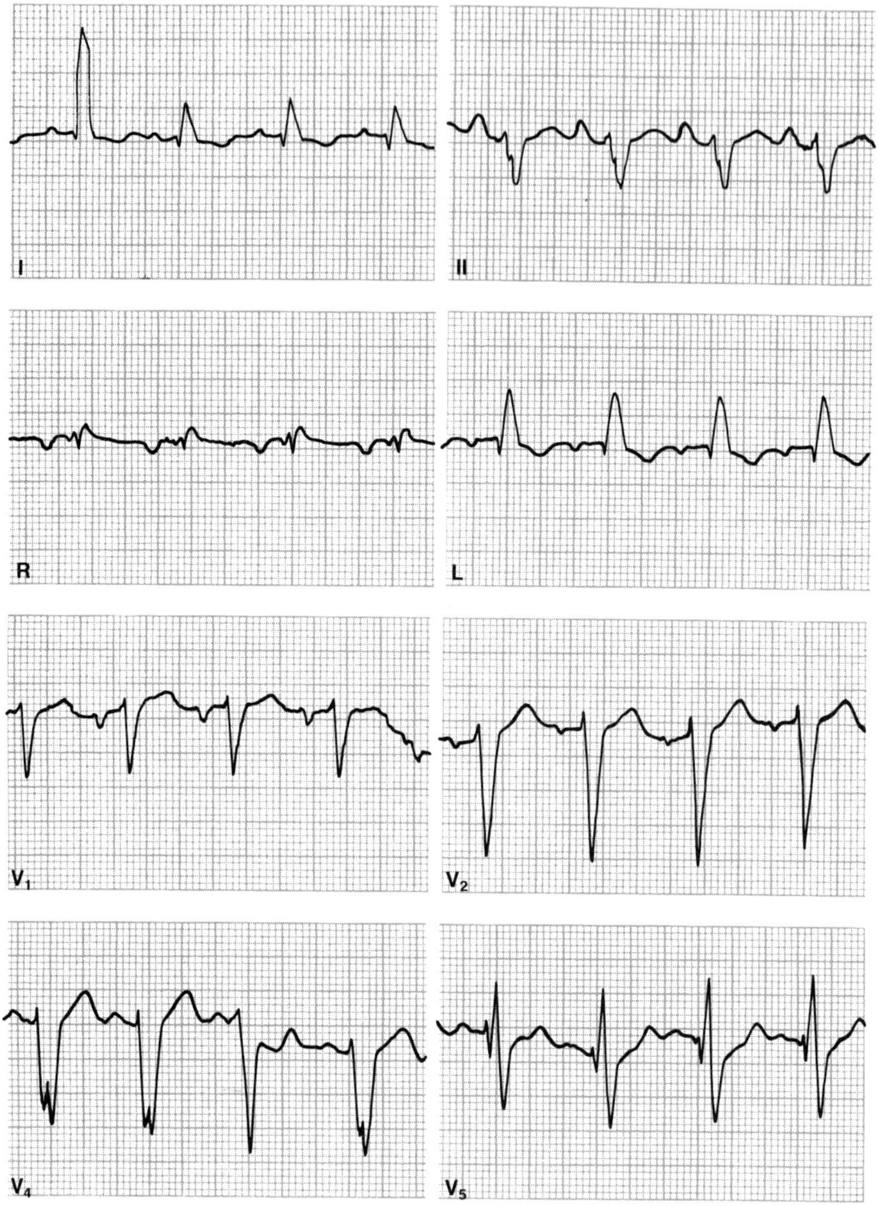

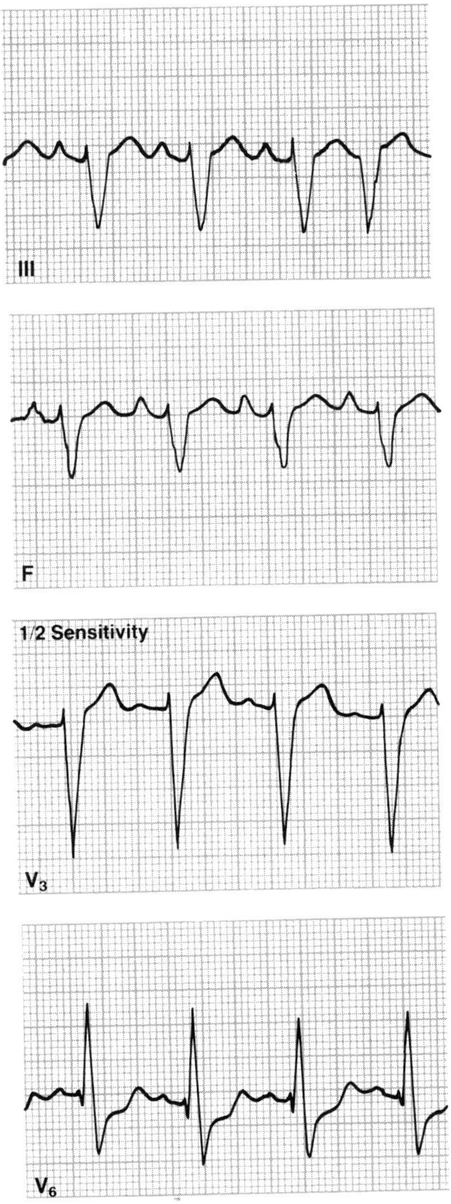
III
F
1/2 Sensitivity
V3
V6

Figure C-4. ECG from a 29-year-old woman presenting with shortness of breath and a globular heart on chest X-ray film.

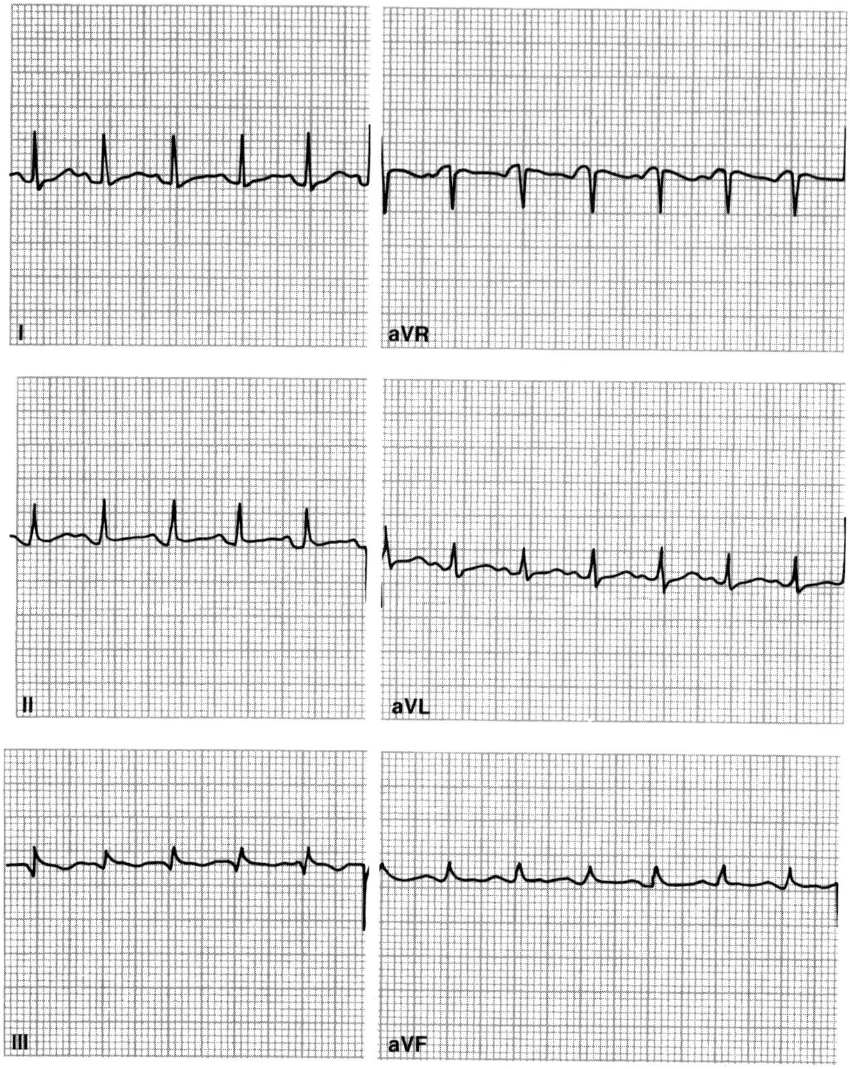

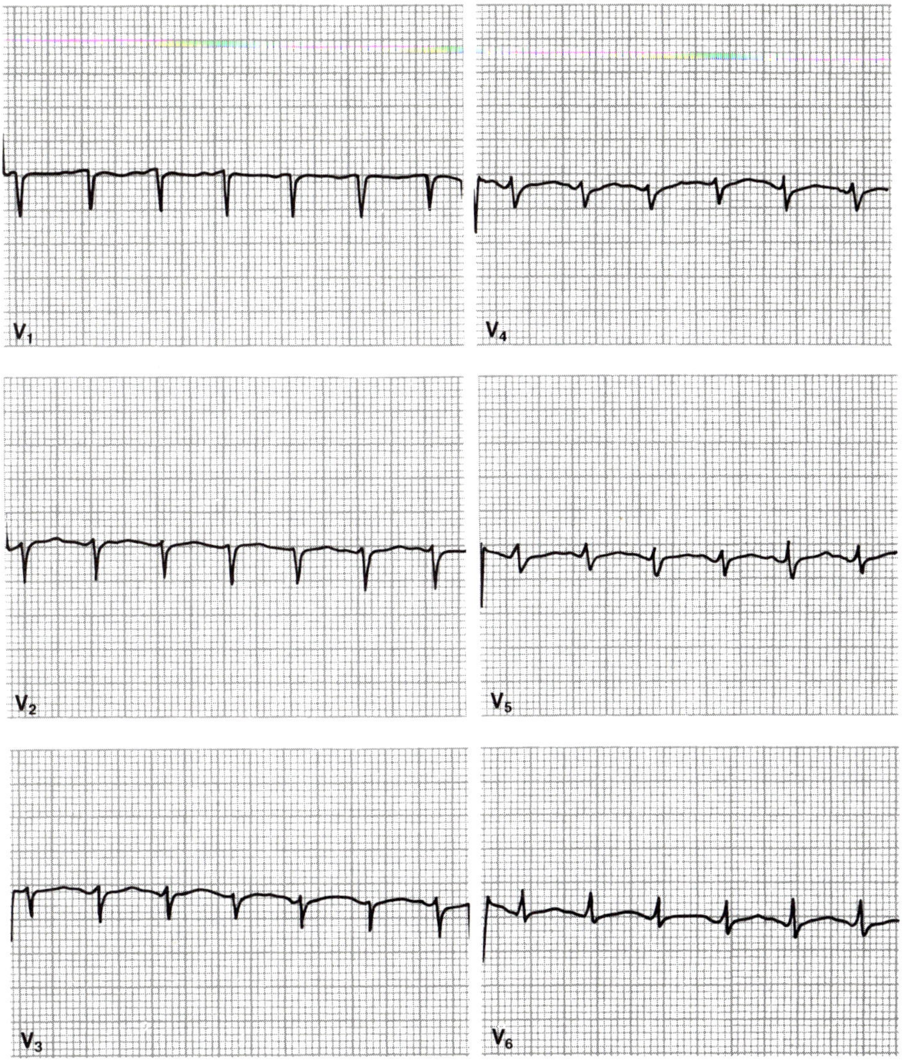
V1
V4
V2
V5
V3
V6

Figure C-5. ECG from a 79-year-old man with congestive heart failure. The heart was markedly enlarged on chest X-ray film.

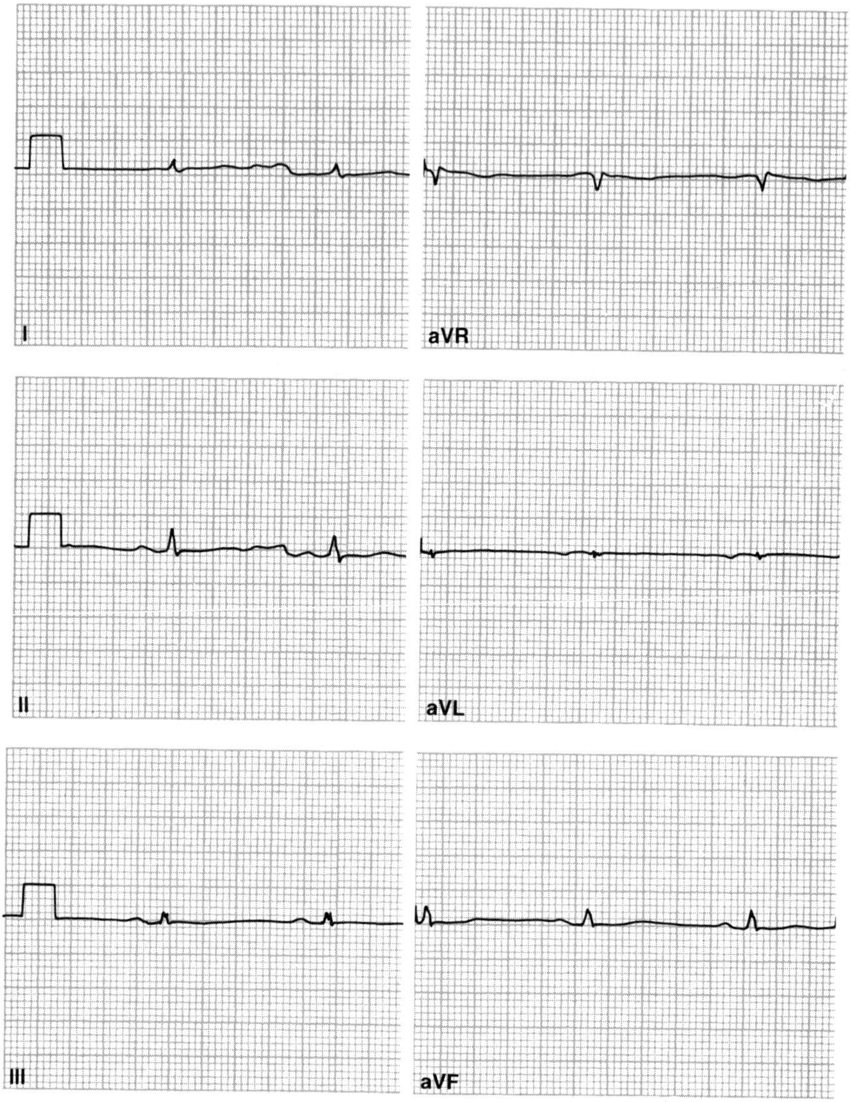

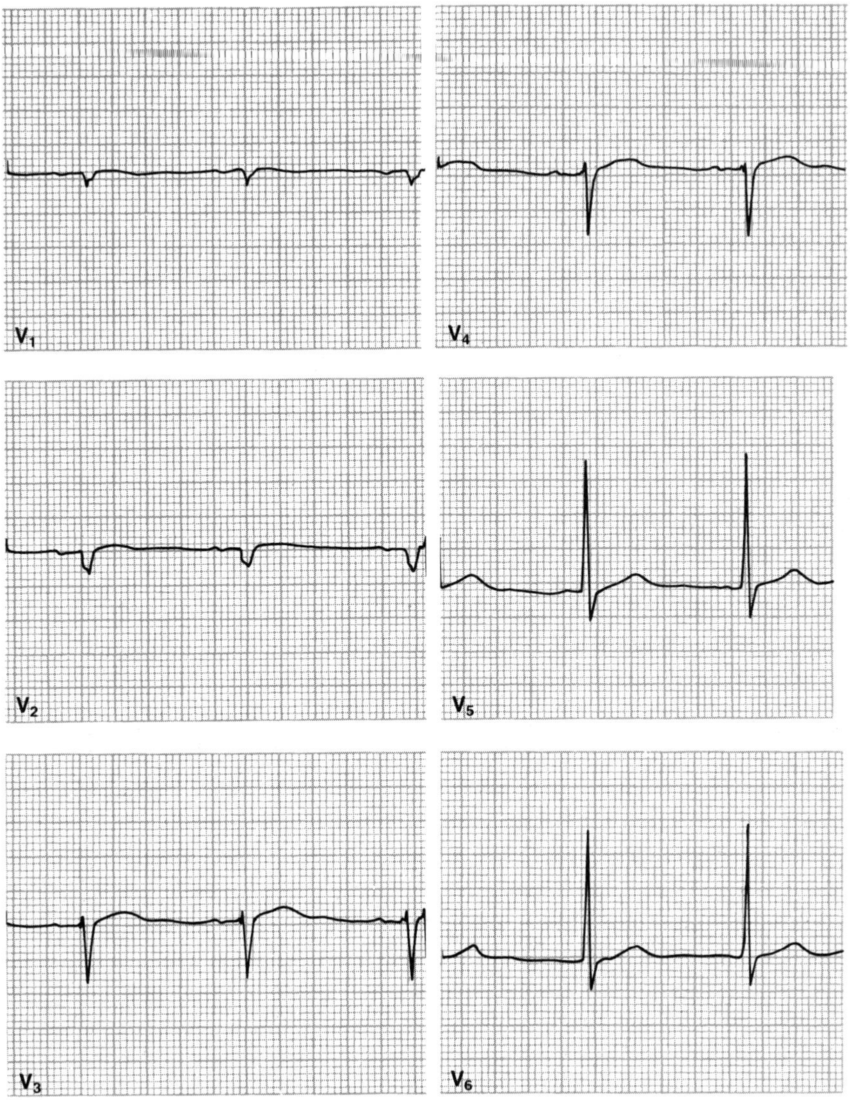
V1
V4
V2
V5
V3
V6

Figure C-6. ECG repeated on the 79-year-old man with normal standardization.

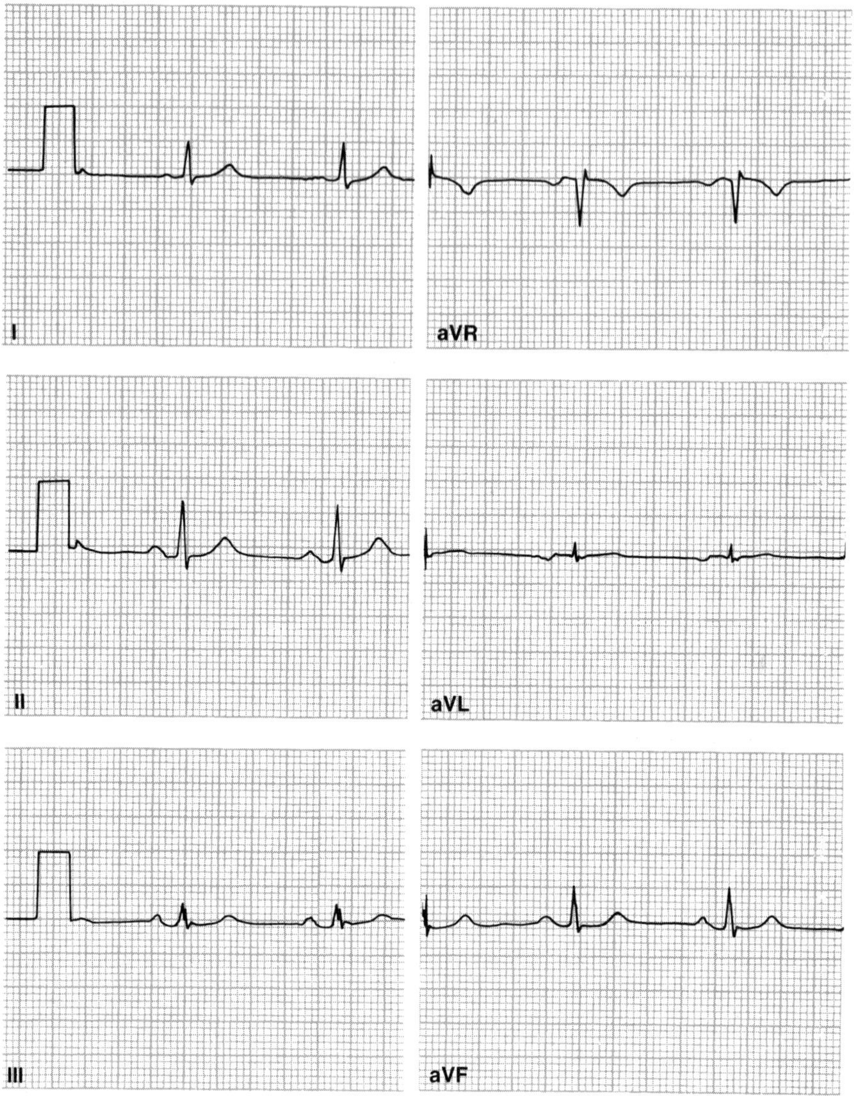

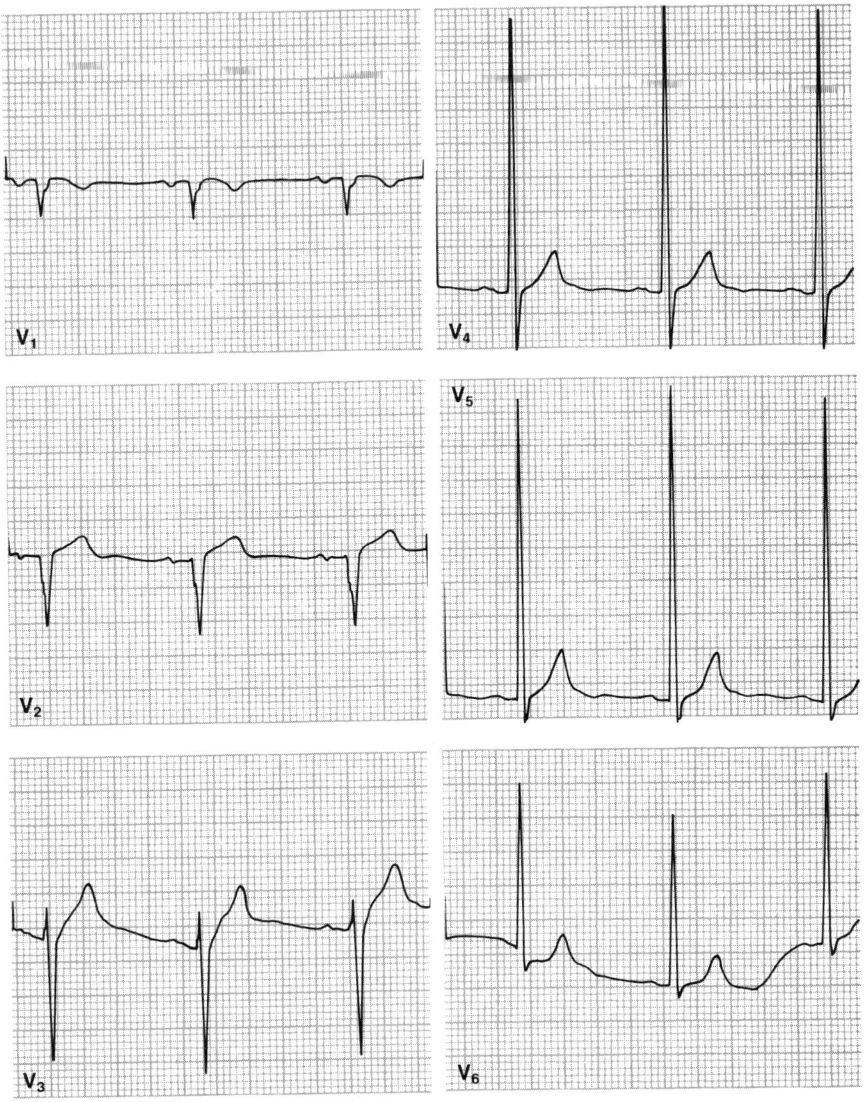
V1
V2
V3
V4
V5
V6

Figure C-7. ECG from a healthy, asymptomatic, 30-year-old long-distance runner. Short systolic heart murmur on exam. Borderline cardiac enlargement on chest X-ray film.

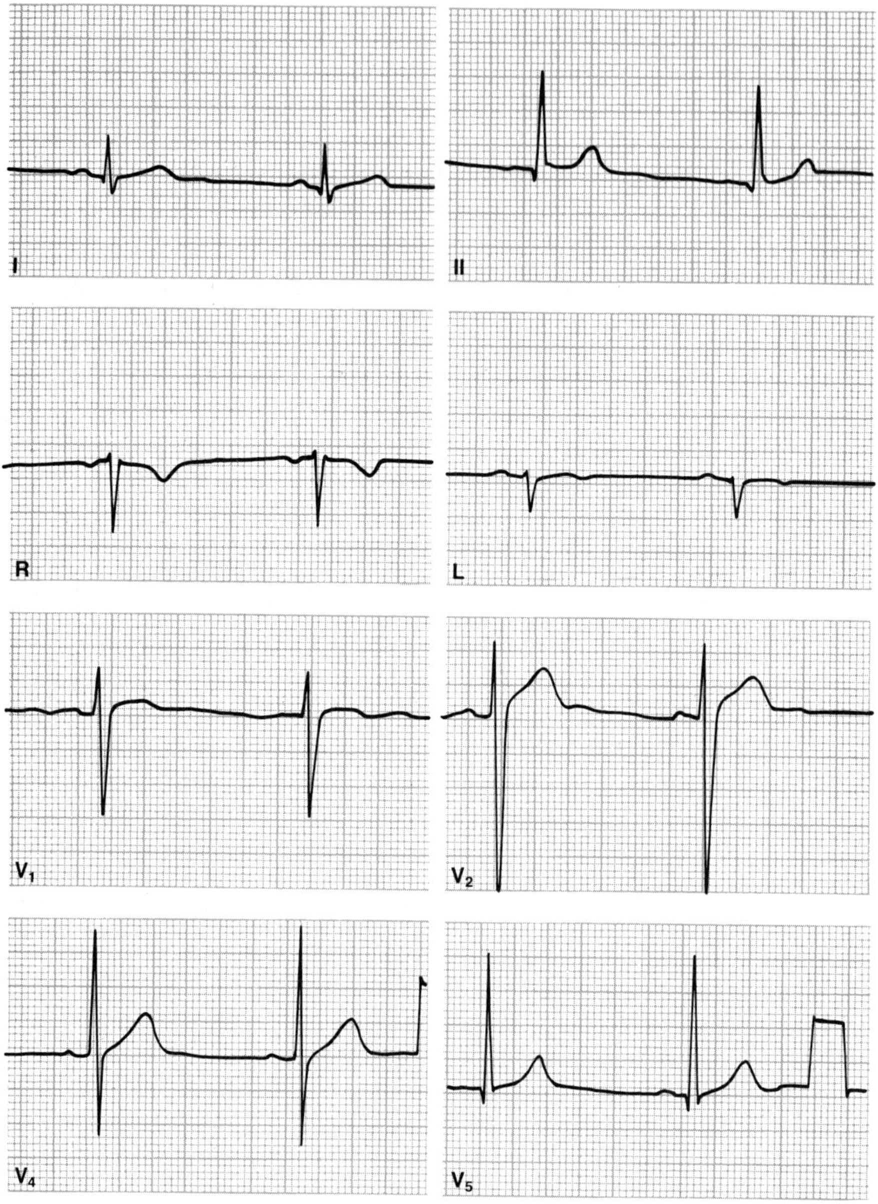

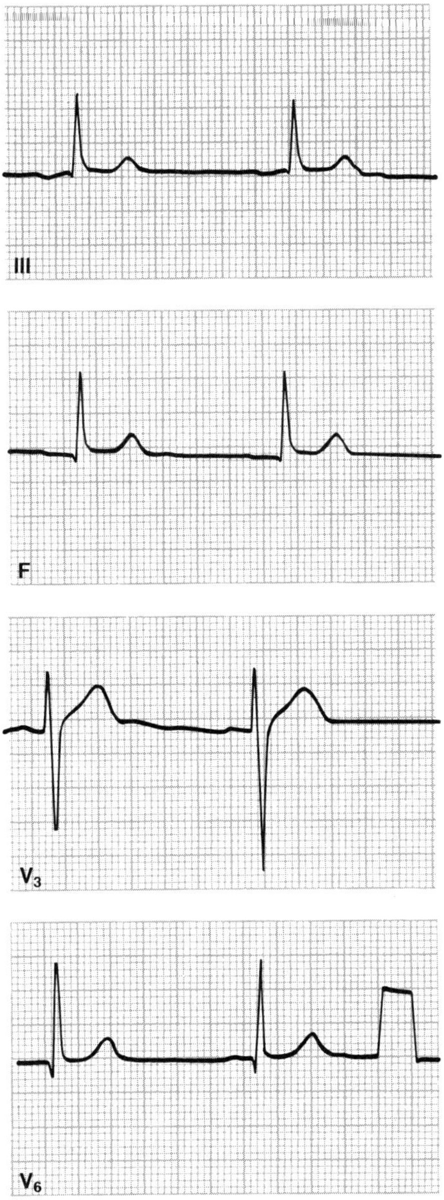
III
F
V_3
V_6

Figure C-8. ECG from a 44-year-old woman with shortness of breath.

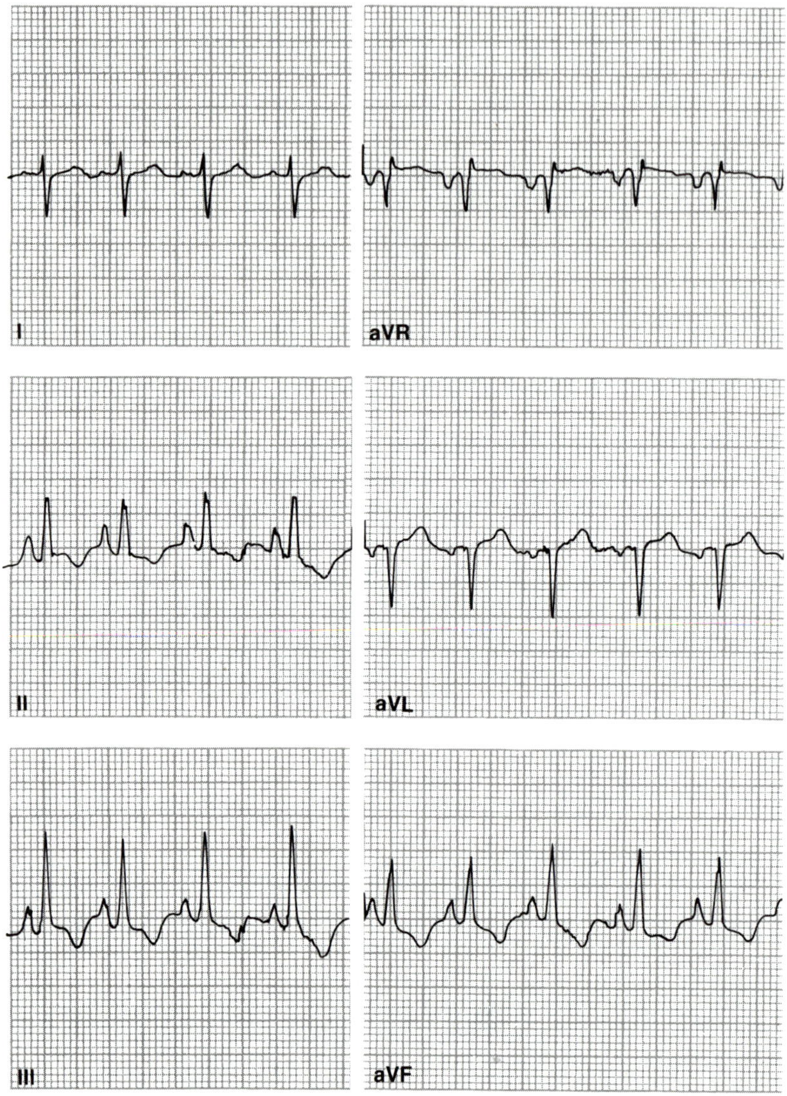

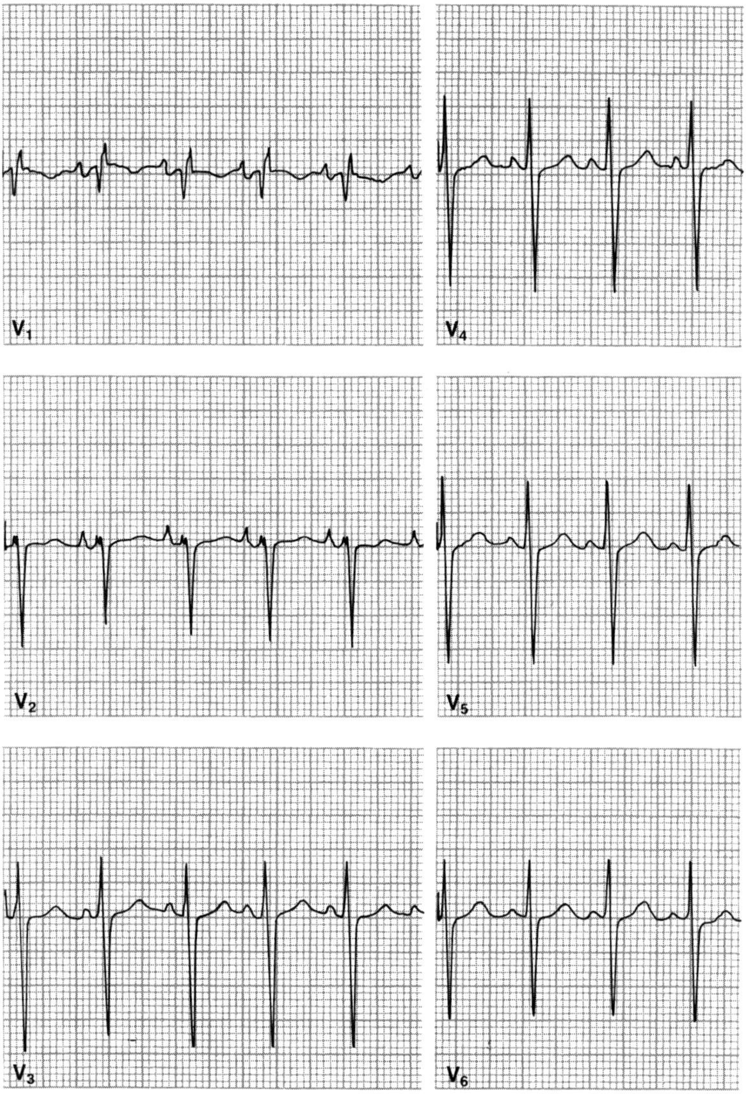
V1
V4
V2
V5
V3
V6

Figure C-9. ECG from a 10-year-old child with a systolic heart murmur. Heart appeared to be slightly enlarged on chest X-ray film.

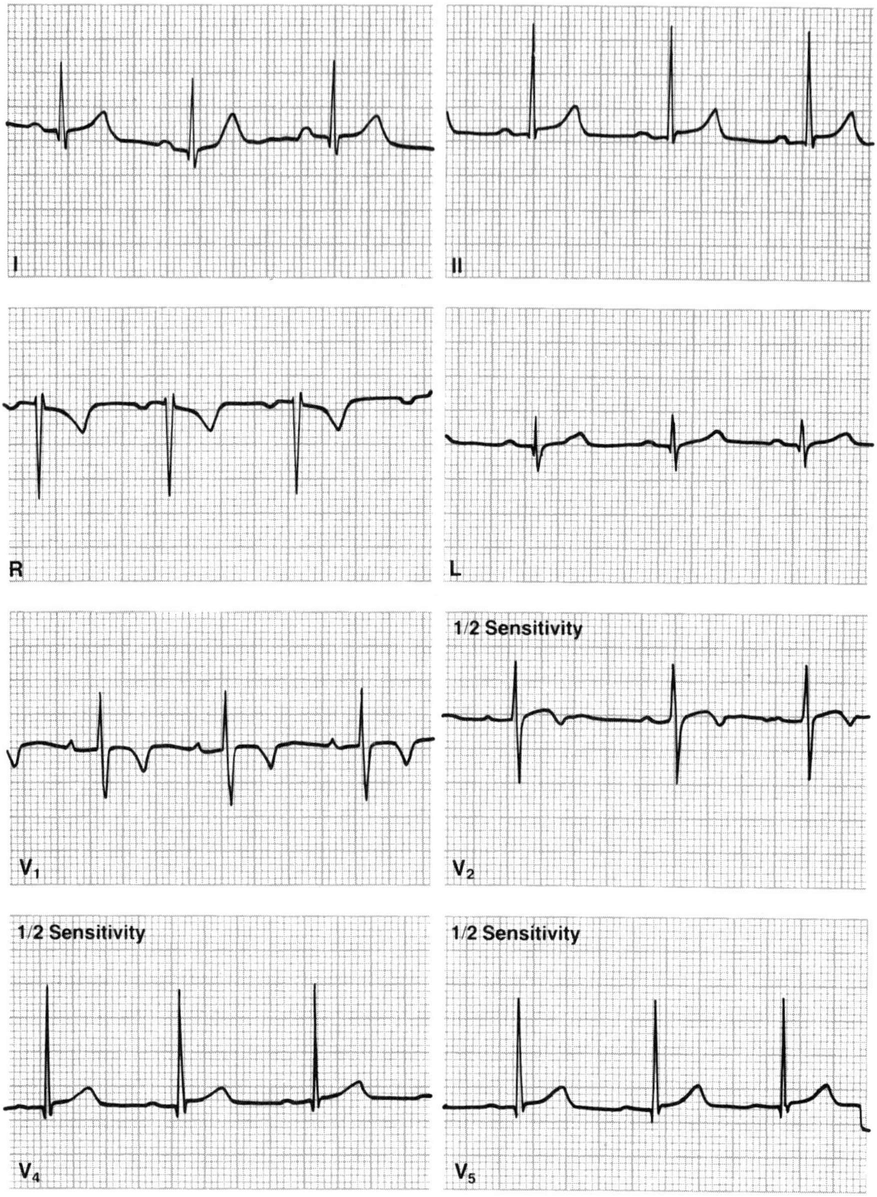

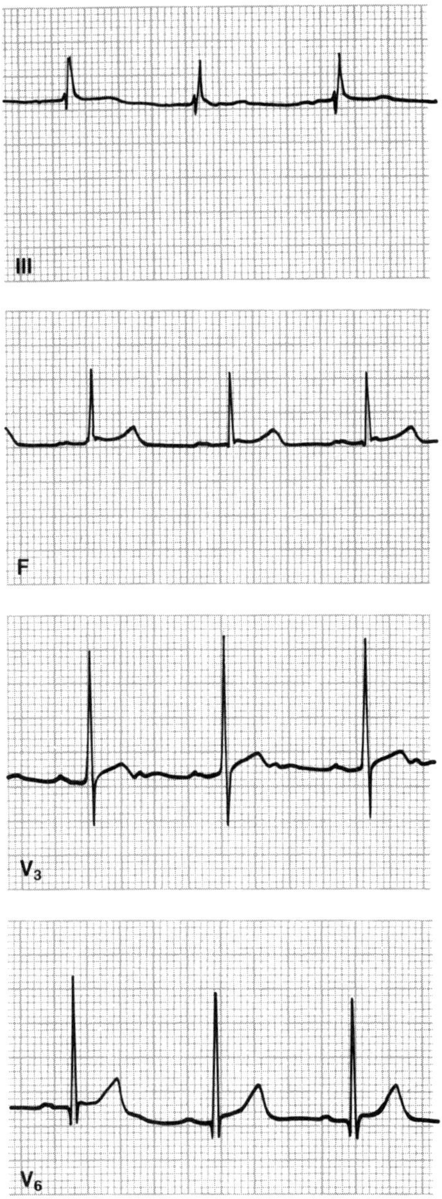
III
F
V_3
V_6

INTERPRETATION of Fig. C-1

Sinus rhythm at 90 beats/min. Axis ≈ +35°. LAA. A Q wave of unknown significance is present in lead III. ST-T wave changes consistent with *strain, digitalis effect,* or both.

The typical configuration of LAA is present in lead II: notching of the P wave with prolongation of P-wave duration (to 0.12 second). Yet despite the presence of LAA, ST-T wave changes consistent with strain, digitalis effect, or both, and a clinical history of congestive heart failure, *none* of the voltage criteria for LVH are satisfied on this tracing, and LVH *cannot* be diagnosed by ECG.

INTERPRETATION of Fig. C-2

Sinus rhythm at 65 beats/min. Axis ≈ +60°. Deep Q waves are evident in the inferior and anterolateral leads, suggestive of prior infarction. Changes do not appear acute. Suggest clinical correlation and comparison with previous tracings.

Although small and narrow q waves reflecting normal *septal* depolarization are frequently seen in the inferolateral leads of normal subjects, the Q waves present in this tracing are much deeper than one would usually expect. While they certainly are consistent with prior inferolateral infarction, another clinical entity should come to mind because the patient has a systolic murmur but no history of infarction.

PROBLEM: What disorder that produces prominent septal Q waves might the patient have?

ANSWER: This patient has *idiopathic hypertrophic subaortic stenosis (IHSS),* also known as hypertrophic cardiomyopathy. At cardiac catheterization she was found to have normal coronary arteries and a markedly hypertrophied interventricular septum.

IHSS is characterized by *asymmetric* septal hypertrophy (see Fig. 8-3C). The ECG picture with this entity is quite varied. Up to 50 percent of patients demonstrate prominent, abnormal Q waves in the inferior and/or lateral leads (as occurs in this case). Abnormal Q waves are felt to be due to *septal hypertrophy,* septal fibrosis, or an altered sequence of septal activation. Other patients demonstrate LAA, LVH and strain, or intraventricular conduction defects. In some, the ECG is entirely normal.

Long before an ECG is obtained, IHSS will usually be suspected clinically from a characteristic heart murmur or positive family history. Yet maintaining a high index of suspicion for typical ECG findings in patients without infarction will occasionally provide a helpful clue to the existence of this disorder. Diagnosis is most readily confirmed noninvasively by echocardiography.

INTERPRETATION of Fig. C-3

Sinus tachycardia at 100 beats/min. IVCD with LAD (axis $\approx -60°$). Biatrial abnormality.

This patient has *congestive cardiomyopathy*. In the full-blown form of this disorder, there is four-chamber cardiac enlargement (see Fig. 8-3E) and a globular heart on chest X-ray film. Left ventricular function is extremely poor. In addition to these findings, this patient had suffered a recent myocardial infarction.

Electrocardiographic findings of congestive cardiomyopathy vary. There may be RAA, LAA, LVH, biventricular hypertrophy, and intraventricular conduction defects (RBBB, LBBB, or IVCD). The ECG in Fig. C-3 is typical. One might argue that instead of "IVCD," QRS morphology is more consistent with the pattern of a LBBB that has been altered by prior infarction—septal Q waves *are* present in leads I and aVL.

INTERPRETATION of Fig. C-4

Sinus tachycardia at 150 beats/min. Axis $\approx +30°$. Low voltage is seen diffusely. Poor R-wave progression. Nonspecific ST-T wave abnormalities.

Although one might be tempted to diagnose anterior infarction from the poor R-wave progression seen in the precordial leads, another diagnosis seems more likely in a 29-year-old woman presenting with shortness of breath and a *globular* heart on chest X-ray.

PROBLEM: Other than congestive cardiomyopathy, which was discussed in the previous case, what clinical entity might produce a *globular* heart and markedly *diminished* QRS voltage?

ANSWER: This patient was found to have a large *pericardial effusion*. With removal of several-hundred milliliters of fluid, QRS voltage increased and R-wave progression normalized.

"Low voltage" is usually a nonspecific finding. Although most commonly associated with chronic obstructive pulmonary disease, low voltage in limb or precordial leads may also be seen with pericardial effusion, pneumothorax, and alterations in body habitus (obesity and muscular chest wall)—anything that dampens QRS voltage or increases the distance between the heart and the chest wall.

INTERPRETATION of Fig. C-5

Sinus rhythm at 65 beats/min. Axis $\approx +60°$. *Low voltage* in the limb leads. Nonspecific ST-T wave abnormalities.

PROBLEM: Is there any finding on this ECG that might explain why QRS voltage is so markedly diminished in the limb leads despite a markedly enlarged heart on chest X-ray? (Hint: The patient does *not* have a cardiomyopathy or a pericardial effusion.)

ANSWER: The answer is given at the very beginning of the ECG before the first QRS complex. This tracing was recorded at *half-standardization.*

Standardization of the ECG machine should *always* be carried out by the technician before taking an ECG. When the machine is set at normal standardization, a 1-mV recording produces a 10-mm deflection on ECG paper. A rectangular *standardization mark* 10 mm high indicates this to the electrocardiographer. Such a mark precedes the first QRS complex in lead I of Fig. C-2. If by chance a QRS complex occurs simultaneously with the recording of the standardization mark, it will be *superimposed* on the rectangle. This has happened with the first QRS complex in lead I of Fig. C-3.

If, as so often happens, no standardization mark is evident on the ECG, the electrocardiographer is left to *assume* that normal standardization is being used. This is the practice we have followed throughout this book. Unfortunately, this may sometimes be a *false* assumption.

Fig. C-6 shows the repeat ECG on this 79-year-old patient with *normal standardization.* Due to slight variation in precordial lead placement, transition occurs between leads V_3 and V_4 of this tracing, whereas it occurred between leads V_4 and V_5 in Fig. C-5. It is now apparent why half-standardization was used to record the ECG in this patient — QRS voltage is so markedly increased that the recording stylus goes off the paper! Despite the tremendously increased R-wave amplitude in the lateral precordial leads, repolarization changes are absent. Thus the correct *electrocardiographic* interpretation of this finding is *voltage for LVH.*

(Of note — standardization for Fig. C-4 was rechecked and found to be correct. The low voltage demonstrated on this tracing was a real finding due to the pericardial effusion.)

INTERPRETATION of Fig. C-7

Bradycardia is present at a rate of 48 beats/min. The P wave is of extremely low amplitude in lead II. It appears to have a slightly *negative* initial component. This suggests a *low atrial* rather than sinus rhythm. Axis $\approx +70°$. Small (probably insignificant) q waves in the inferolateral leads. Prominent septal forces and ST-segment elevation with an upward concavity in the inferolateral leads — most likely due to *early repolarization.*

This tracing demonstrates many of the findings of "runner's heart" — bradycardia, increased voltage despite the patient being under 35 years of age (sum of S wave in lead V_2 + R wave in lead V_5 is at least 45 mm, and possibly more, since the S wave in lead V_2 is cut off), and ST-T wave changes of early repolarization. In addition, there are *prominent septal forces,* as evidenced by the relatively tall R waves in the anterior precordial leads.

PROBLEM: Is there any clinical entity that one should consider in a long-distance runner with a systolic murmur and prominent septal forces on ECG?

ANSWER: One should strongly consider IHSS. Instead of demonstrating deep Q waves (as did the patient in Fig. C-2 who had IHSS), septal hypertrophy may sometimes manifest itself by prominent R waves in leads V_1 and V_2. Clinically, the importance of discovering IHSS in athletes is the increased incidence of sudden death if the disorder goes undetected.

In this particular case, full evaluation was performed. Left ventricular thickness was increased (as might be expected in a long-distance runner), but IHSS was not present. The heart murmur was felt to be of no clinical significance, and the subject was allowed to continue running in an unsupervised manner.

INTERPRETATION of Fig. C-8

Sinus tachycardia at 115 beats/min. Incomplete RBBB. Axis $= +105°$ (RAD). RAA. Persistence of deep S waves across the precordium. Taken together, these findings suggest RVH.

The cardiomegaly on chest X-ray in this case was the result of RVH that had developed as a manifestation of this patient's *end-stage pulmonary disease.*

INTERPRETATION of Fig. C-9

Sinus arrhythmia. Axis $\approx +55°$. R = S in lead V_1. Considering that leads V_2 and V_5 were recorded at half-standardization, the S wave in lead V_2 is relatively deep (≈ 20 mm), and the R wave in lead V_5 relatively tall (≈ 30 mm). Finally, the T wave is inverted in leads V_1 and V_2, and notched in lead V_3.

The principal role of the ECG in evaluating children with heart murmurs is to determine whether there is evidence of ventricular hypertrophy. The findings of concern here are the relatively tall R wave in lead V_1, the deep S wave in V_2, and the tall R wave in V_5.

Guidelines for evaluating ECGs of children for chamber enlargement were discussed in Chapter 8. Although by the age of 10, the R wave in lead V_1 is usually *less* prominent than the S wave in this lead, *none* of the other associated findings that one would expect to see with RVH are present. Mean QRS axis is normal, there is no RAA, and there are only *shallow* S waves in leads V_5 and V_6. Referral to Table 8-9 reveals that R-wave amplitude in lead V_1 may go up to 18 mm in this age group and *still* be normal!

Detection of LVH in children is particularly difficult because unlike adults, a strain pattern *rarely* develops. Referral to a table of norms for the various pediatric age groups is essential when making this diagnosis. Although the R wave in lead V_5 of Fig. C-9 approaches 30 mm, up to 36 mm is normal in this age group.

Finally, persistence of T-wave inversion in the anterior precordial leads ("juvenile T-wave pattern") is an extremely common *normal* variant of childhood. (See Chapter 5.) In summary, this ECG is entirely normal for age.

EXERCISE D

TALL R WAVE IN LEAD V_1

In Chapter 8 the common causes of a tall R wave in lead V_1 were discussed. Can you determine the cause(s) responsible for the tall R waves that are seen in the following examples?

Figure D-1. ECG from a 73-year-old woman.

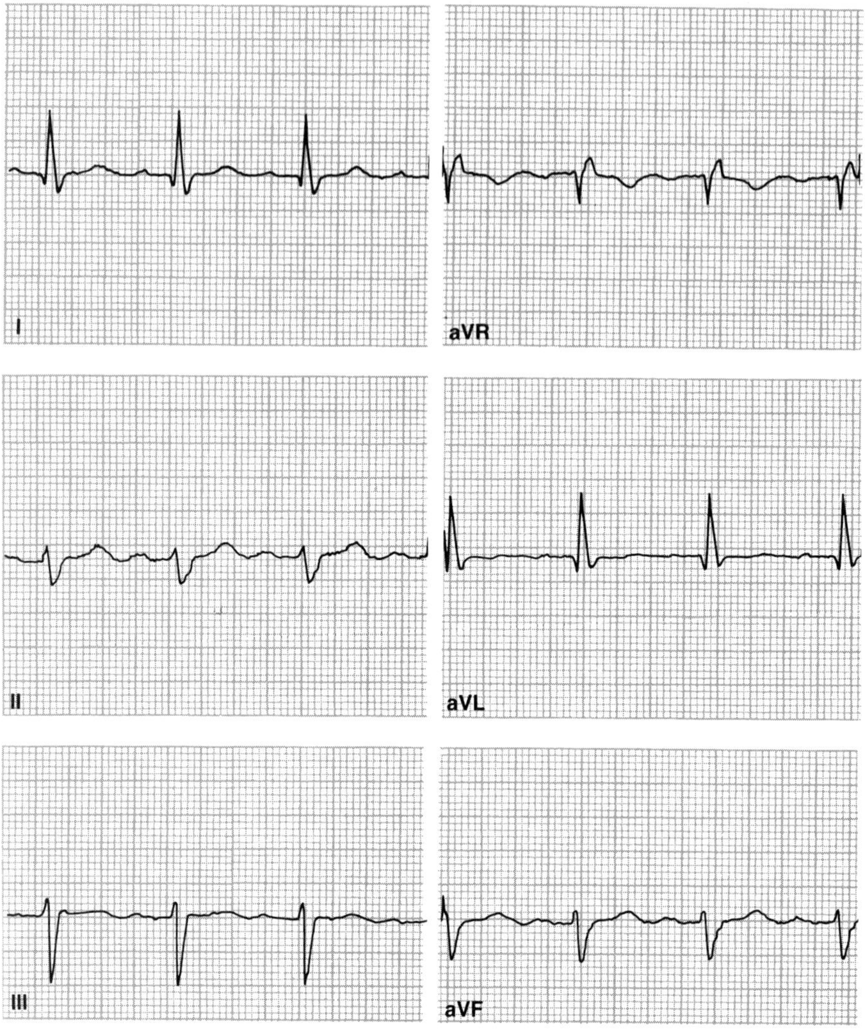

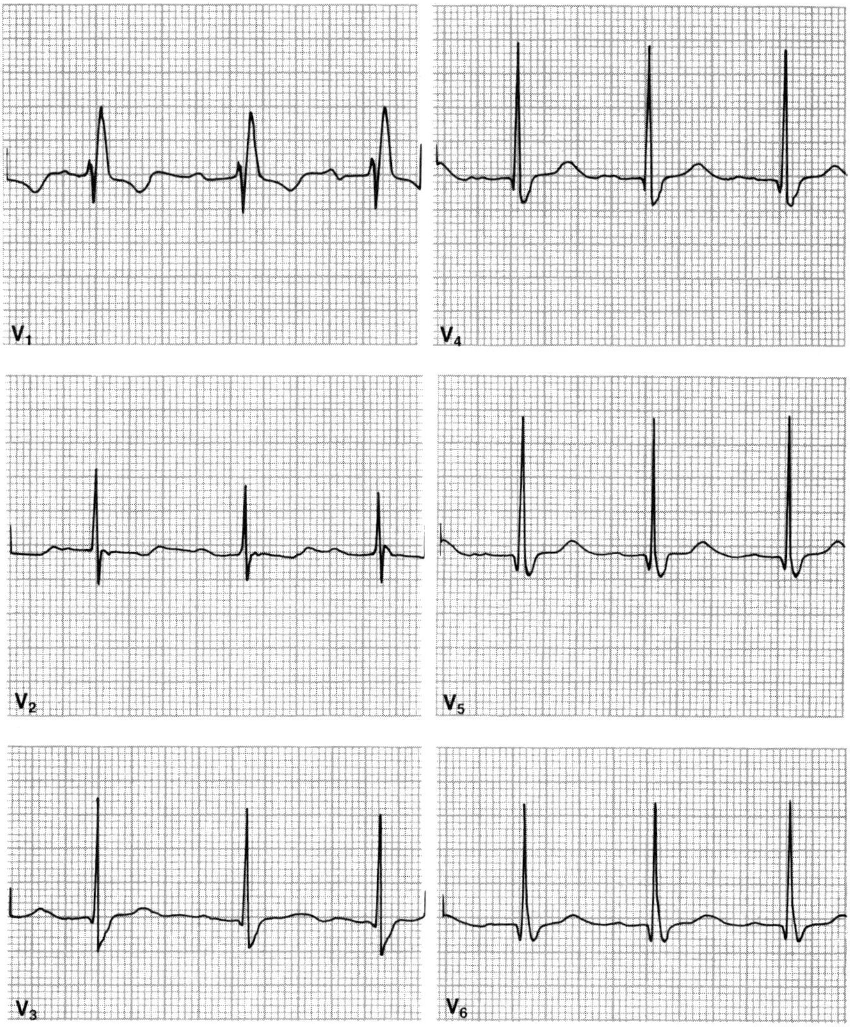

V_1
V_4
V_2
V_5
V_3
V_6

Figure D-2. ECG from a 47-year-old woman with a history of a systolic murmur and new onset chest pain.

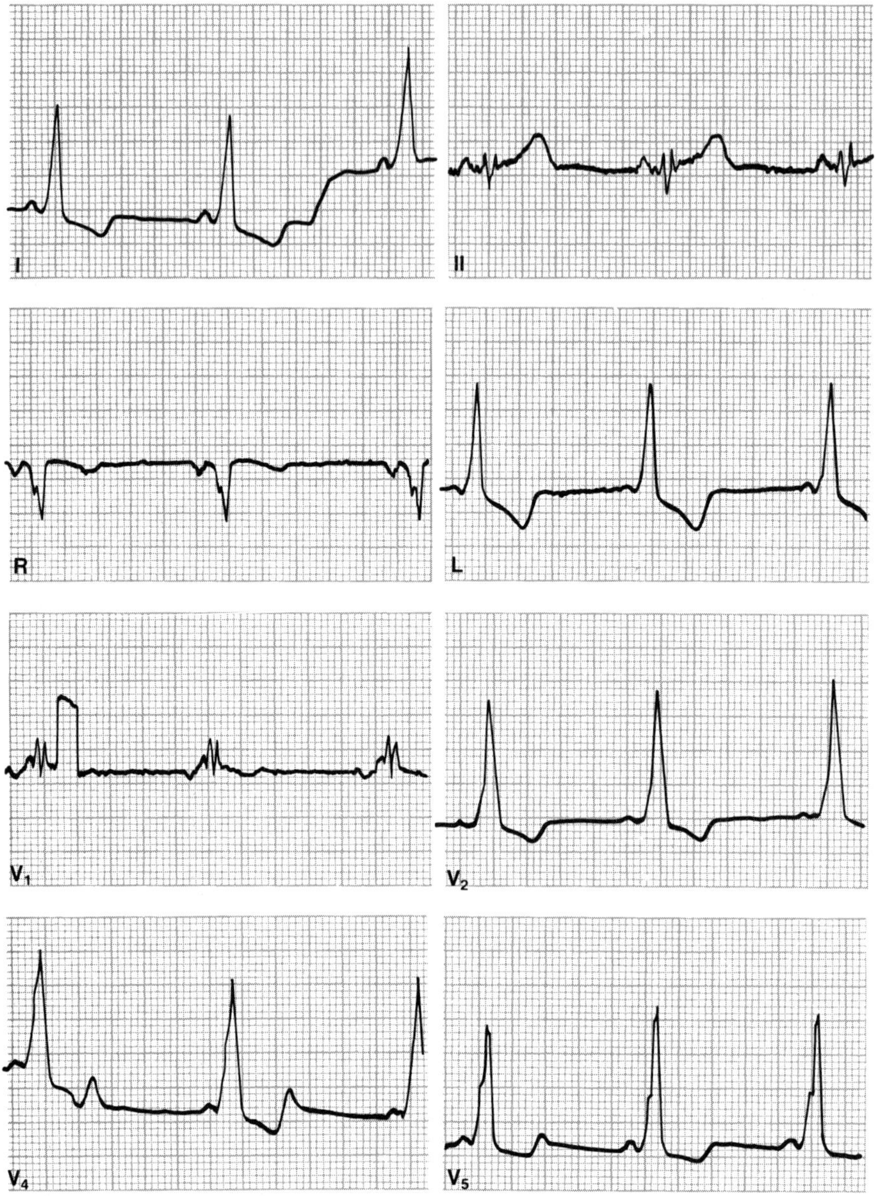

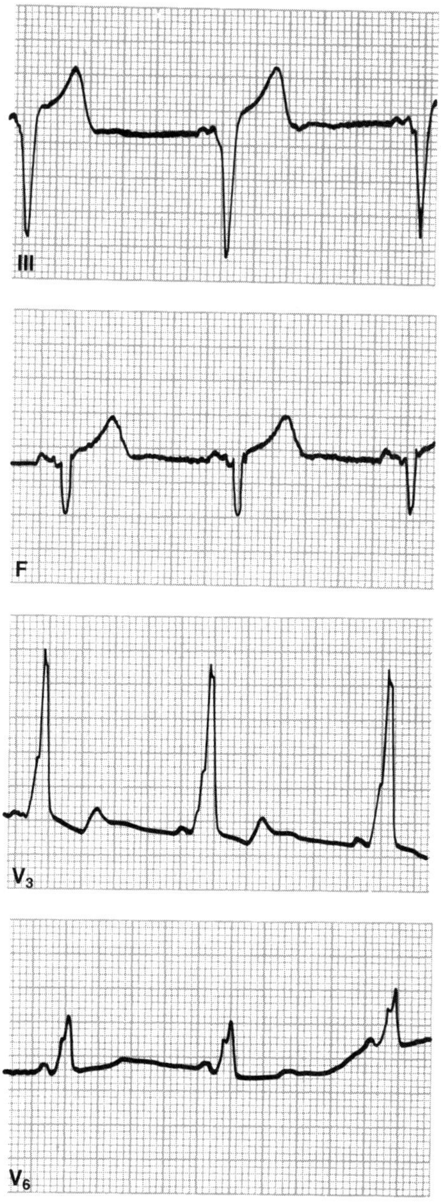
III
F
V3
V6

Figure D-3. ECG from a 60-year-old man with new-onset chest pain.

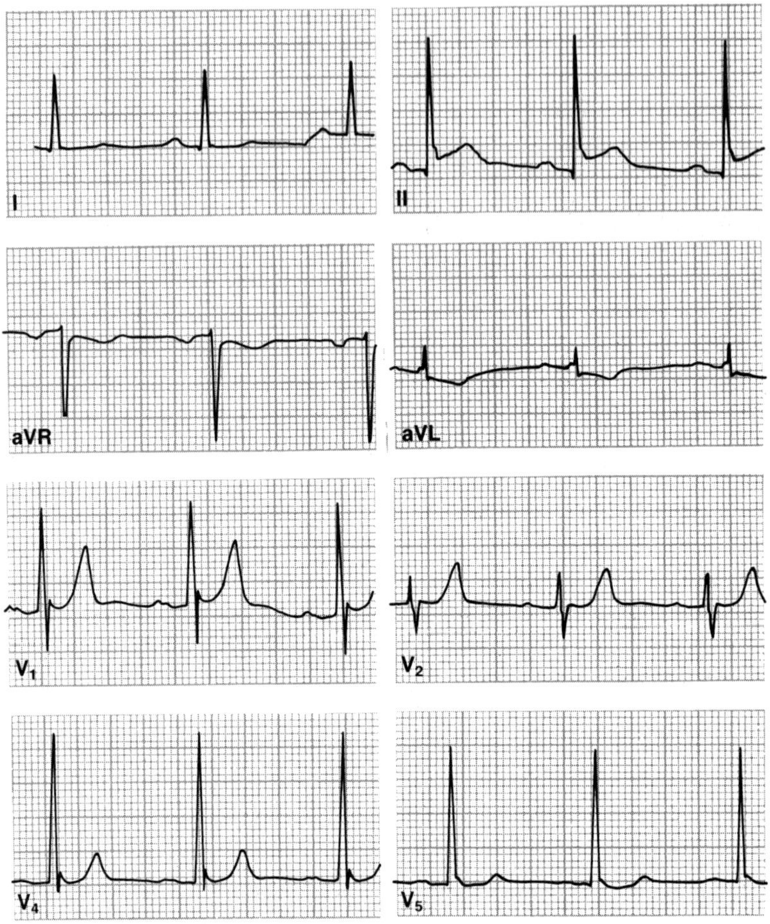

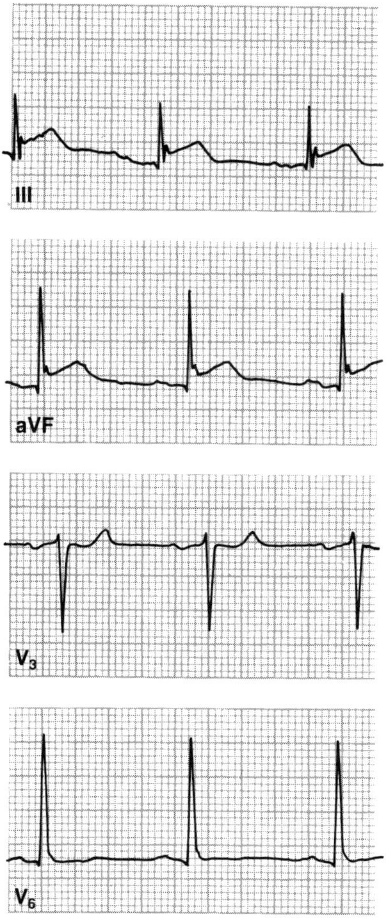
III
aVF
V3
V6

Figure D-4. Admission ECG on the 60-year-old man obtained four days prior to Fig. D-3.

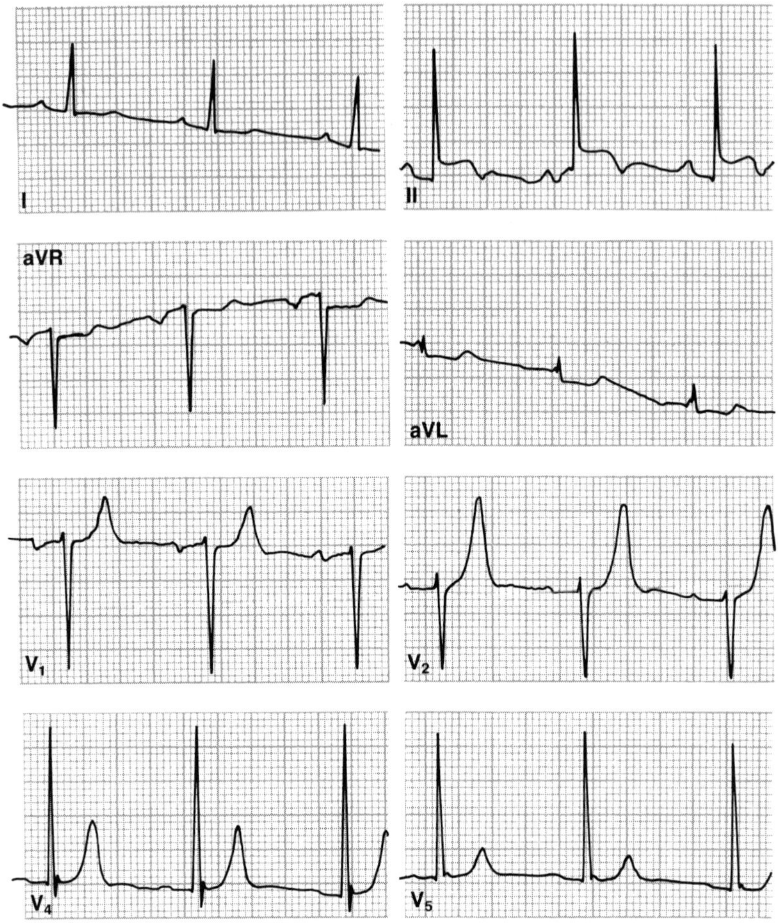

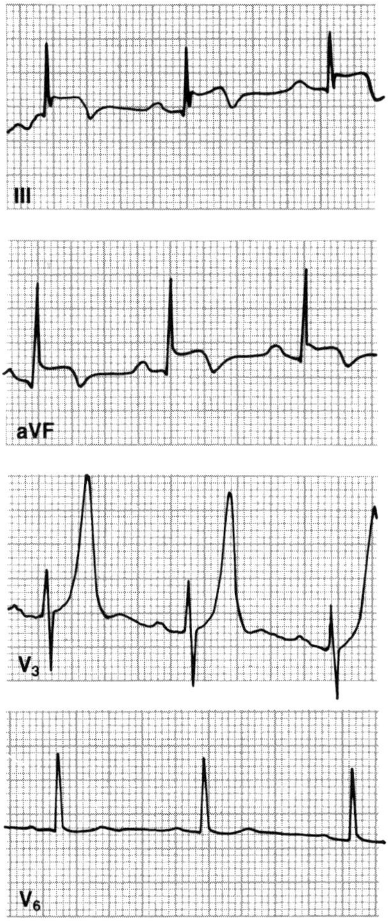
III
aVF
V3
V6

Figure D-5. ECG from a 60-year-old woman with a history of ischemic heart disease.

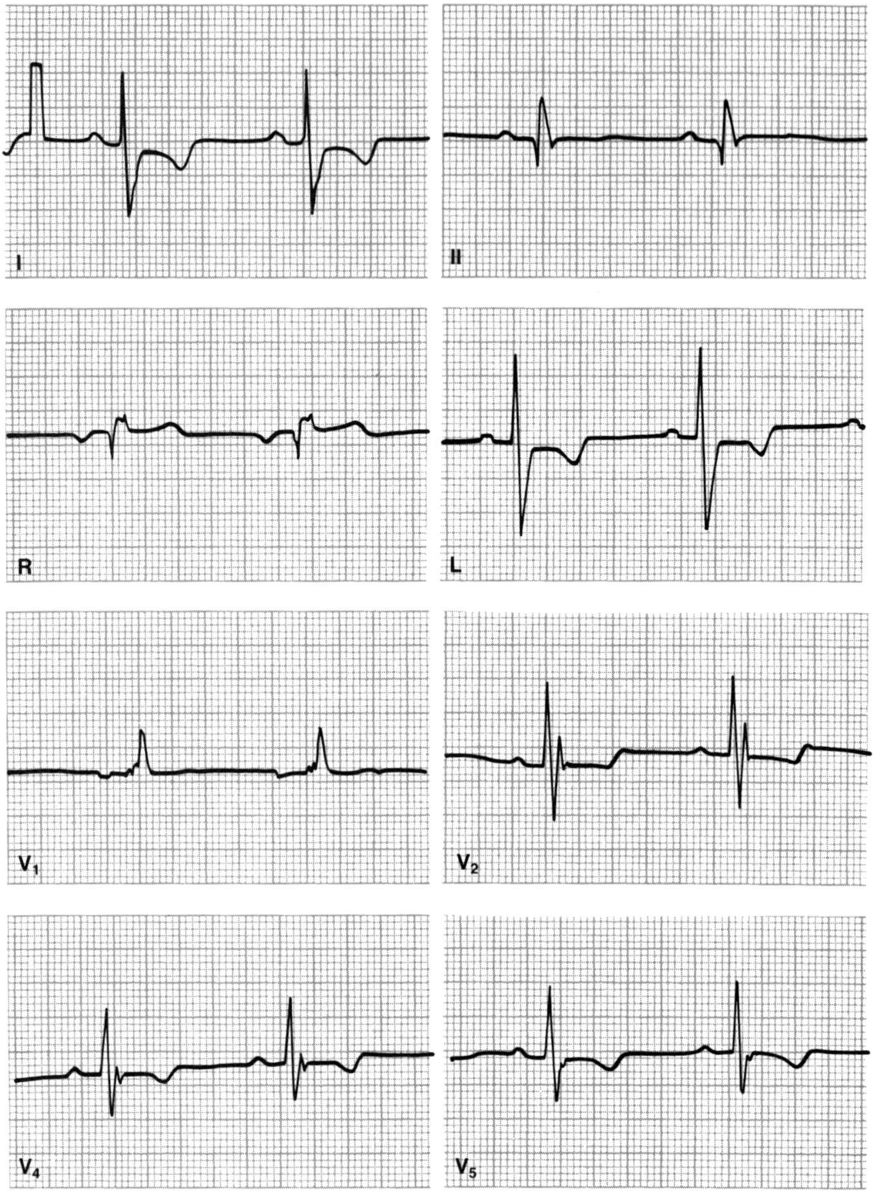

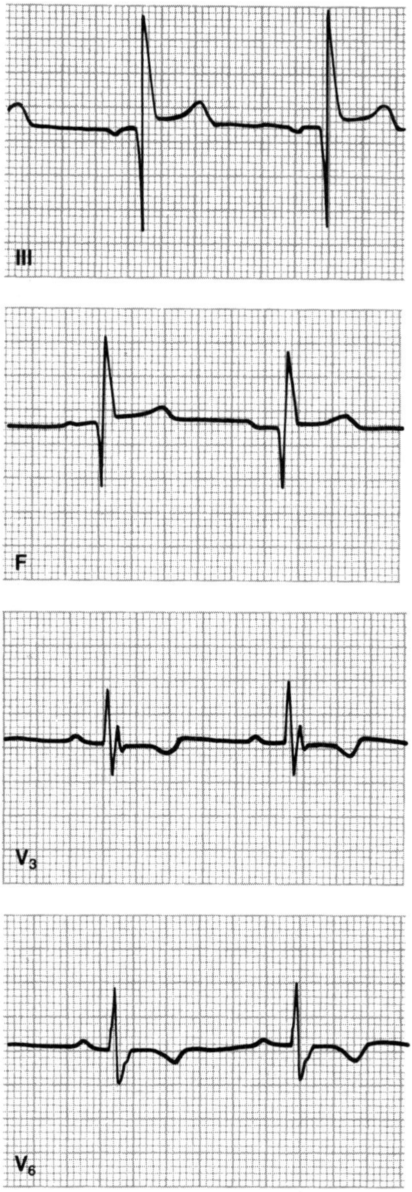
III
F
V3
V6

Figure D-6. Routine ECG from a 60-year-old man with hypertension.

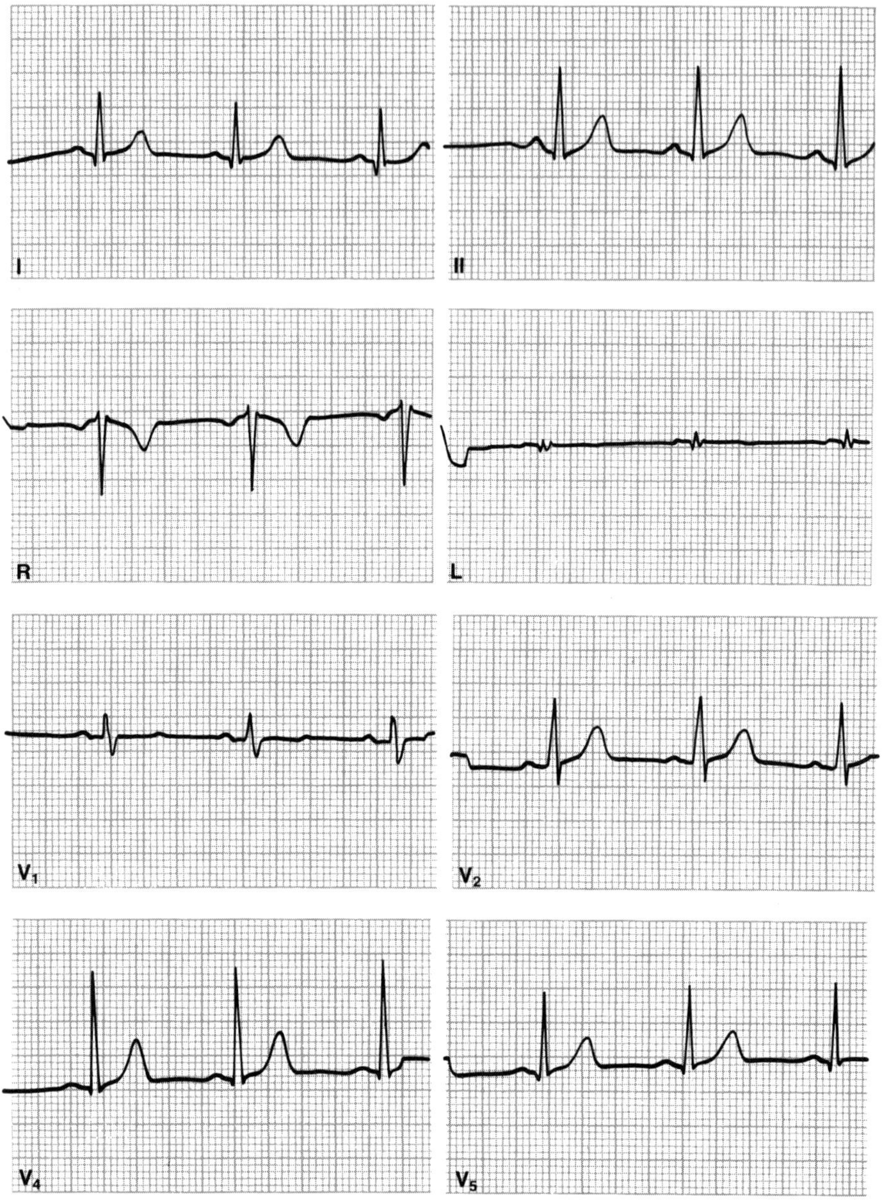

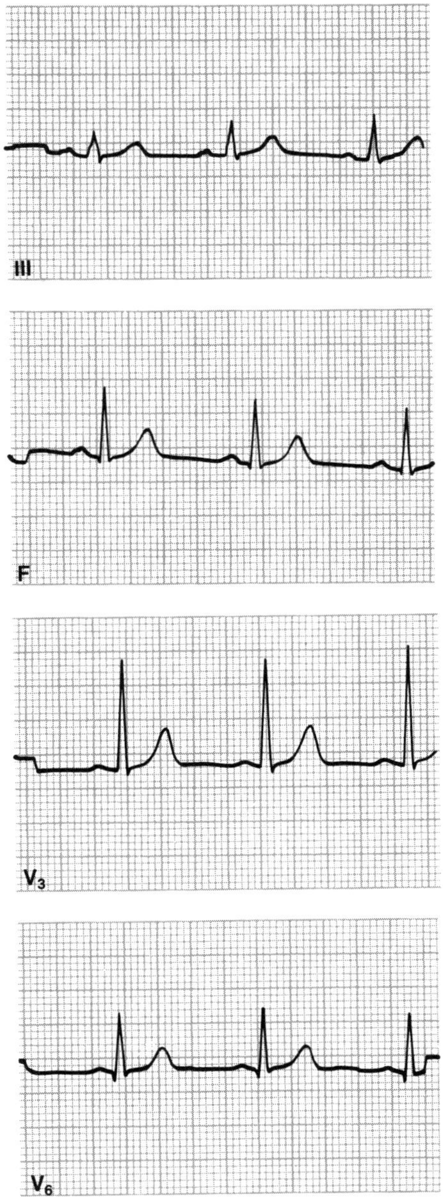
III
F
V_3
V_6

INTERPRETATION of Fig. D-1

Sinus rhythm at 70–80 beats/min. First-degree AV block. LAHB/RBBB. Previous anterolateral infarction.

The cause of the tall R wave in lead V_1 for this example is relatively straightforward. *Complete RBBB* is diagnosed by QRS widening, an rSR′ in lead V_1, and wide terminal S waves in leads I and V_6.

The conduction system defects in this tracing suggest *trifascicular* disease. In addition to RBBB, LAHB is also present as the QRS deflection is markedly negative in lead II. In the setting of bifascicular block, PR-interval prolongation (here to 0.24 second) implies disease along the one remaining conduction pathway.

Fairly wide q waves in the anterolateral leads suggest previous infarction. (Remember that unlike the situation for LBBB, infarction *can* often be diagnosed despite the presence of RBBB).

INTERPRETATION of Fig. D-2

Sinus bradycardia at 55–60 beats/min. Axis $\approx -30°$. The QRS complex is widened, and the tall R wave in lead V_1 appears at first glance to be due to RBBB. In addition, LVH is suggested (R in lead aVL ≥ 12 mm), as is inferior infarction of unknown age (QS complexes in leads III and aVF).

PROBLEM: Do you see why this ECG is *not* really representative of any of these findings?

ANSWER: The reason one cannot say that any of these findings are present is that the patient has *WPW (type A)*. In addition to QRS widening, the PR interval is shortened, and delta waves are present in multiple leads. The *negative* delta waves in leads III and aVF simulate infarction.

INTERPRETATION of Fig. D-3

Sinus rhythm at 65 beats/min. Axis $\approx +50°$. *Acute inferior infarction.* Probable *posterior* extension.

When confronted with a tall R wave in lead V_1 of an *adult,* it is well to keep in mind the differential diagnosis of common causative conditions (See Fig. 8-17):

- WPW
- Posterior myocardial infarction
- Right ventricular hypertrophy
- RBBB
- Normal variant

WPW and RBBB can be eliminated from consideration because the QRS complex is not prolonged in this tracing. None of the associated findings of RVH (RAA, RAD, or deep S waves in V_5, V_6) are present. This ECG is certainly not a normal variant. One is left with *posterior myocardial infarc-*

tion, which is consistent with the coexistent evidence of inferior infarction on this tracing.

Fig. D-4 is the admission ECG of this 60-year-old man, recorded four days prior to Fig. D-3. Note that the prominent R wave in lead V_1 was not present at the time of admission.

An additional interesting finding on this earlier tracing is the marked peaking and increase in amplitude of anterior precordial T waves. Although bearing a striking resemblance to the T waves of hyperkalemia, serum potassium was entirely normal in this case. The tall, peaked T waves shown here instead represent posterior *ischemia.* Performing the mirror test (turning the ECG over while holding it up to the light) produces the more familiar picture of ischemia (deep, symmetric T-wave inversion).

INTERPRETATION of Fig. D-5

Sinus bradycardia at 55 beats/min. Axis is *indeterminate.* Inferior infarction of unknown age. Tall R wave in lead V_1. Deep, symmetric T-wave inversion in the lateral leads, suggesting ischemia.

Two conditions should be strongly considered in this case as the explanation for the tall R wave in lead V_1:

- *RBBB* (widened QRS complex, "RBBB-equivalent" pattern in lead V_1, and wide terminal S waves in leads I and V_6)
- *Posterior infarction* (evidence of associated inferior infarction)

Although it is hard to be sure from inspection of the ECG alone, *both* of these conditions are probably present. Obtaining a vectorcardiogram might be helpful in confirming this suspicion.

While RBBB commonly produces ST-segment depression and T-wave inversion in the anterior precordial leads (secondary ST-T wave changes of RBBB), T-wave inversion does *not* usually extend to the lateral precordial leads, and it is normally *not* seen in the lateral limb leads when only RBBB is present. Thus, one might suspect that in addition to inferoposterior infarction and RBBB, *laterial ischemia* is also present.

INTERPRETATION of Fig. D-6

Sinus rhythm at about 70 beats/min. Axis $\approx +50°$. R = S in lead V_1—most likely a *normal variant.*

The diagnosis of normal variant for the relatively tall R wave in lead V_1 is made by exclusion. The QRS complex is not widened, excluding RBBB and WPW. There are no associated findings of RVH, and no evidence of inferior infarction (making posterior infarction much less likely). One is left with the sole remaining possibility—a normal variant.

EXERCISE E

ECGS IN PATIENTS WITH CHEST PAIN

The patients in this section all presented with chest pain. In which of them would you be concerned about acute infarction?

Figure E-1. ECG from a 46-year-old woman who presented with a two-day history of chest pain. No prior tracing available.

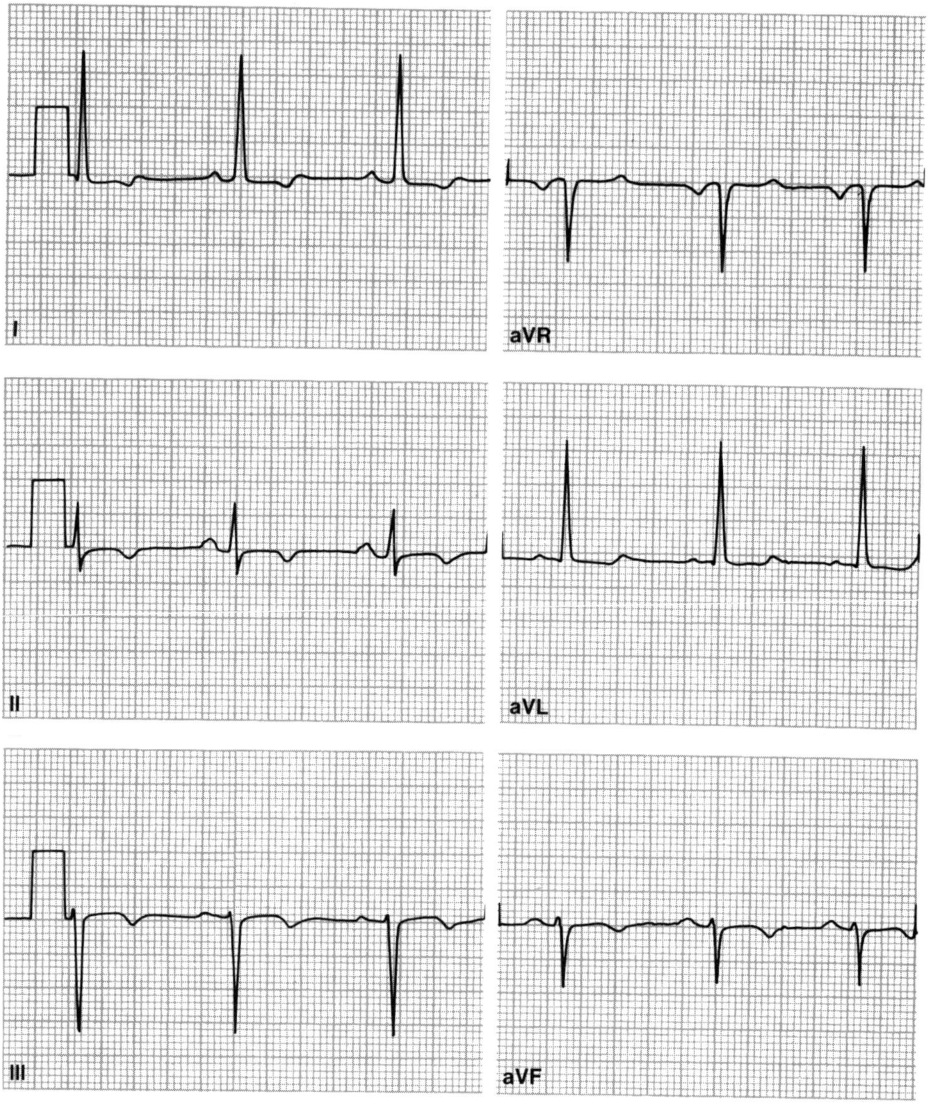

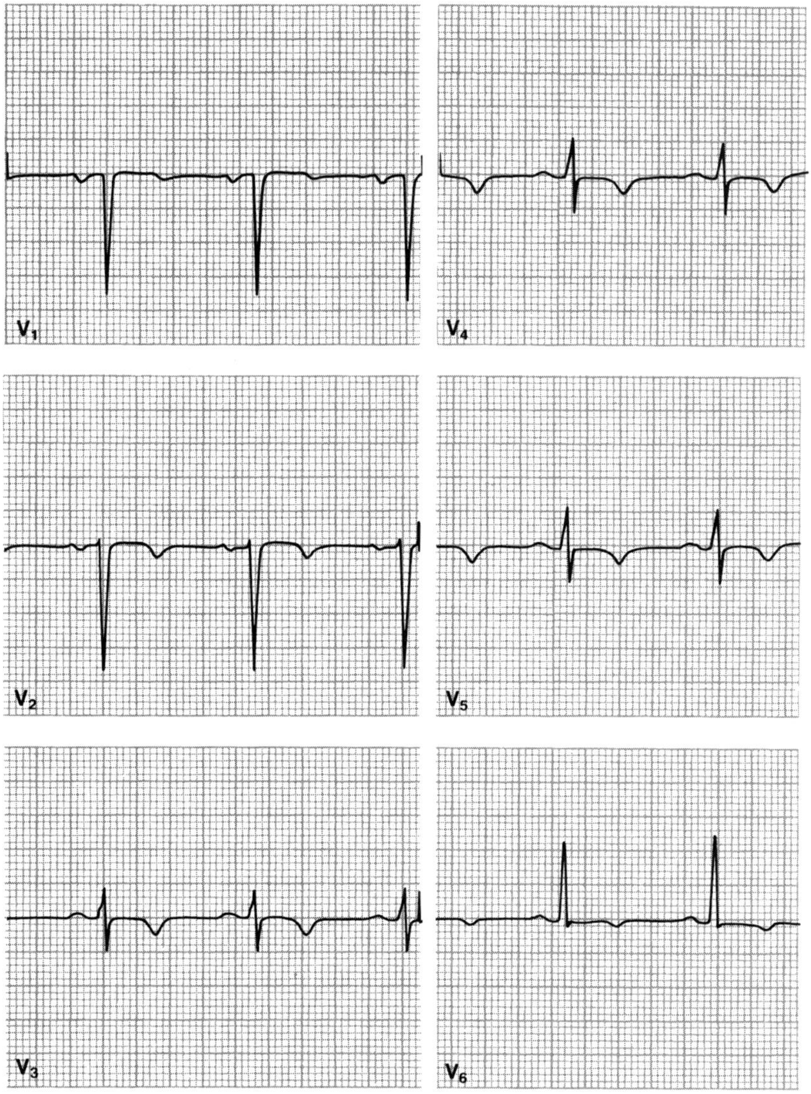
V1
V4
V2
V5
V3
V6

Figure E-2. ECG from a 46-year-old woman who presented with new-onset chest pain.

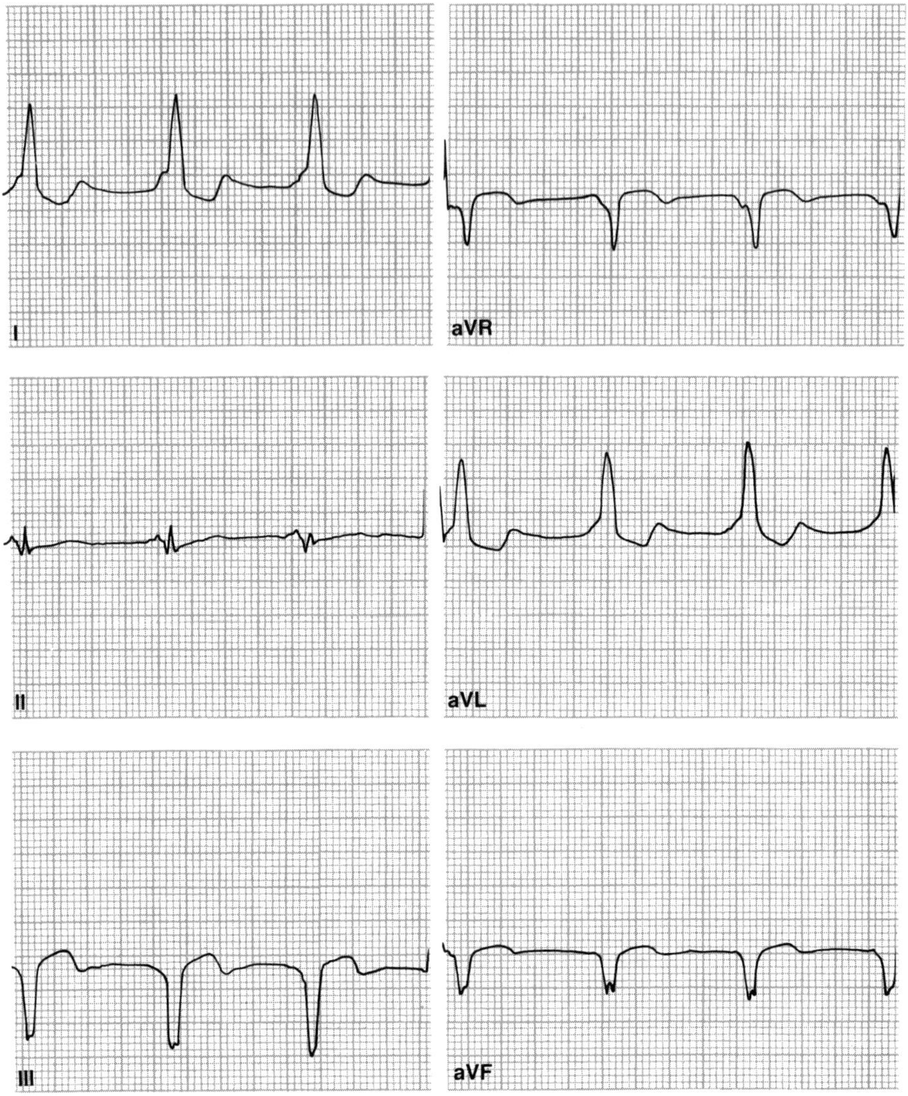

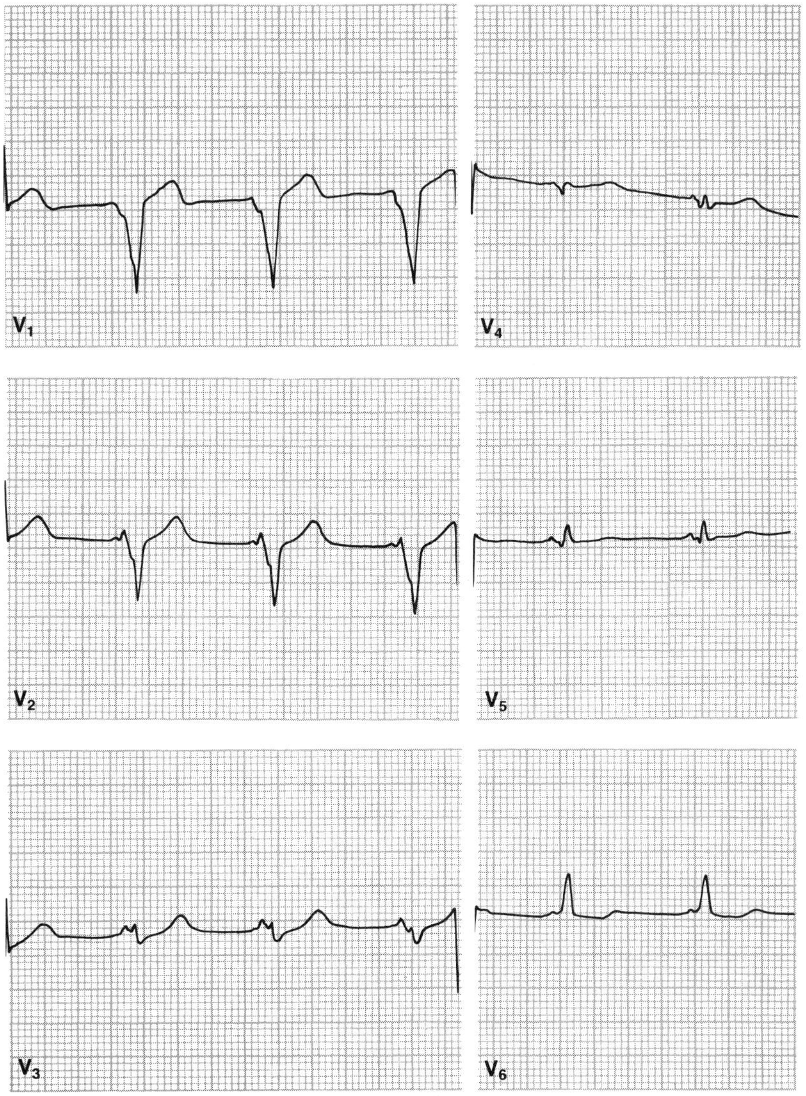
V1
V4
V2
V5
V3
V6

Figure E-3. ECG from a 78-year-old woman with a history of chest pain over several days.

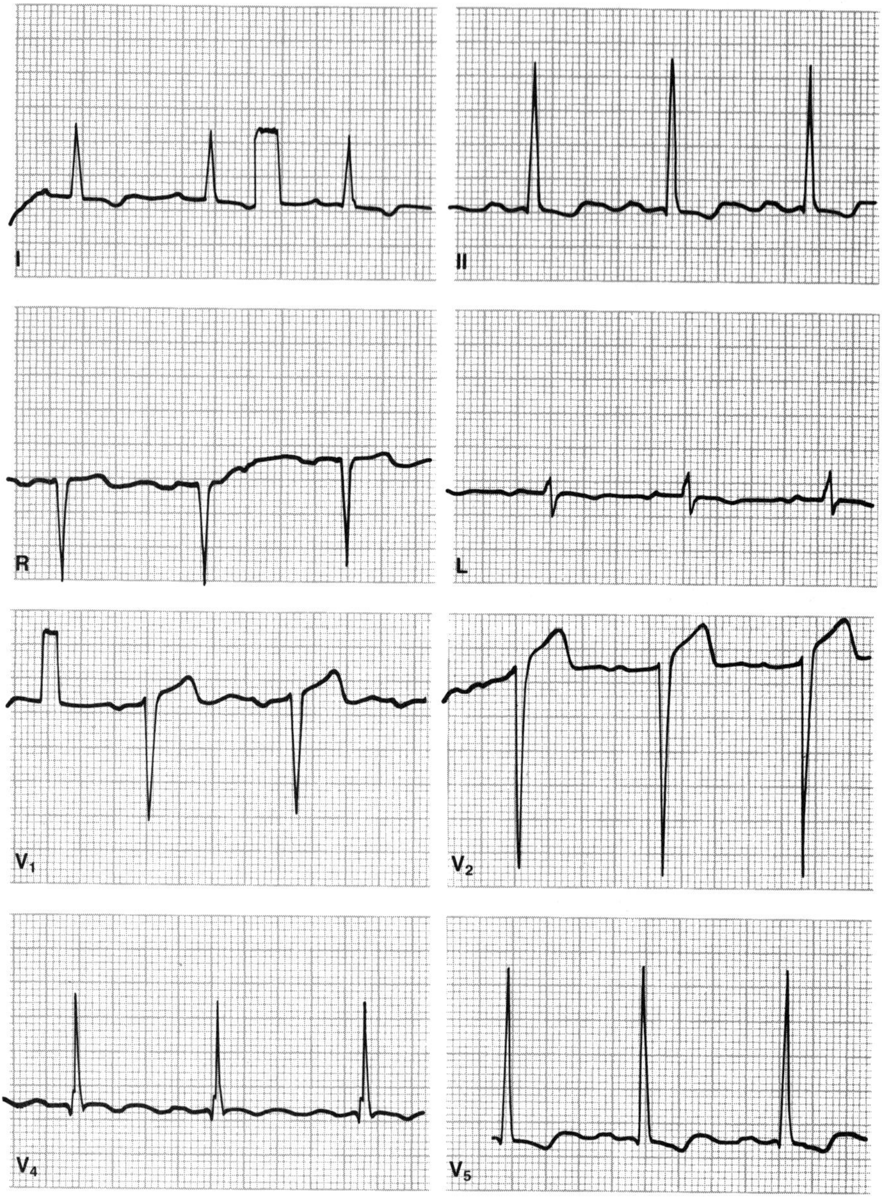

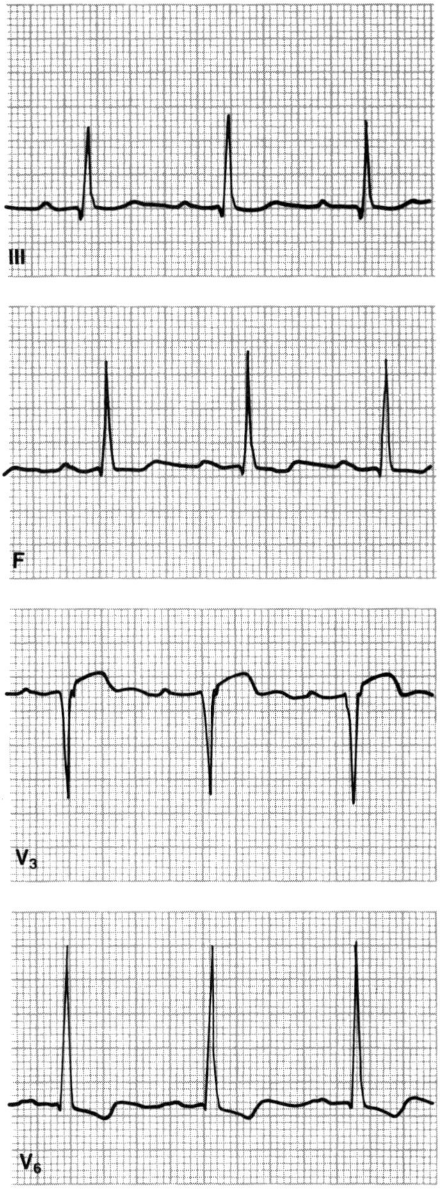
III
F
V3
V6

Figure E-4. ECG (1984 tracing) from a 37-year-old man with chest pain. History of a prior infarction a year ago.

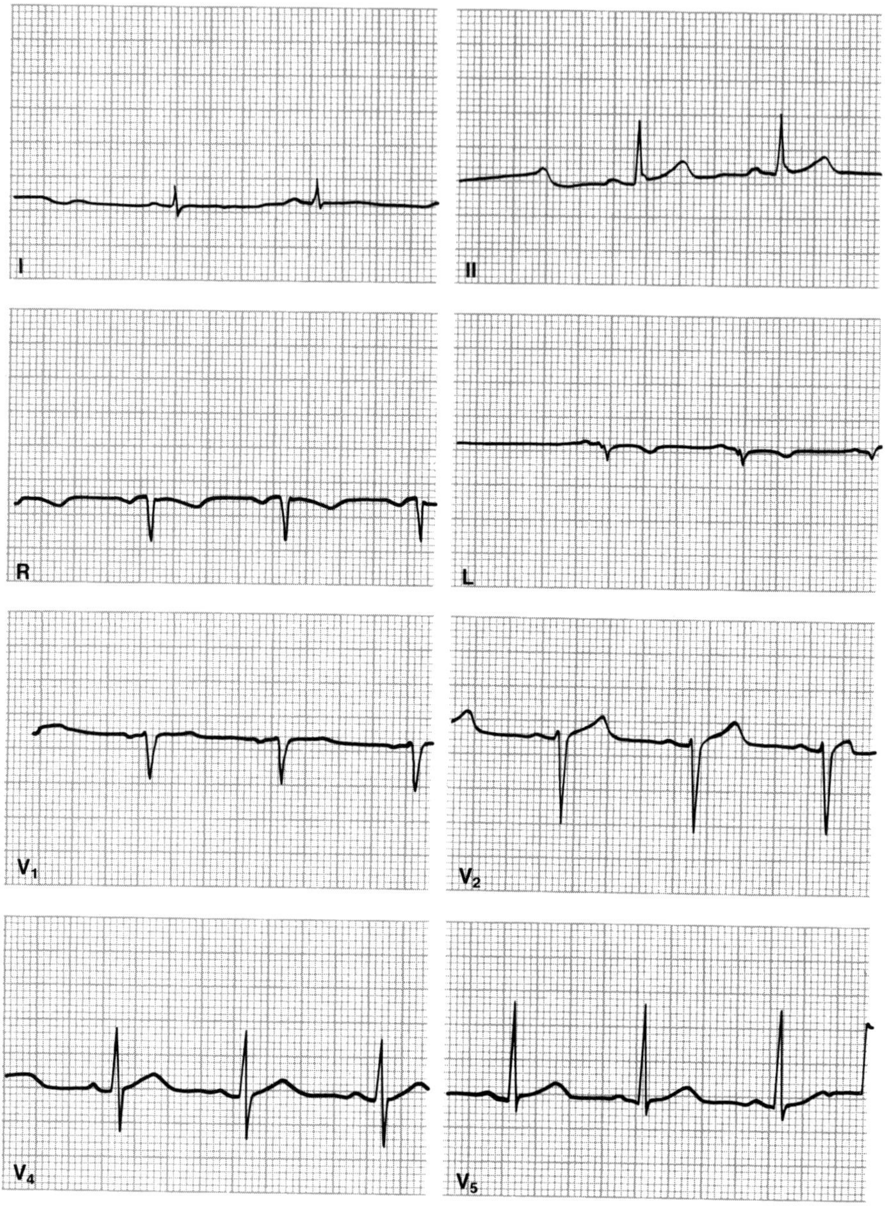

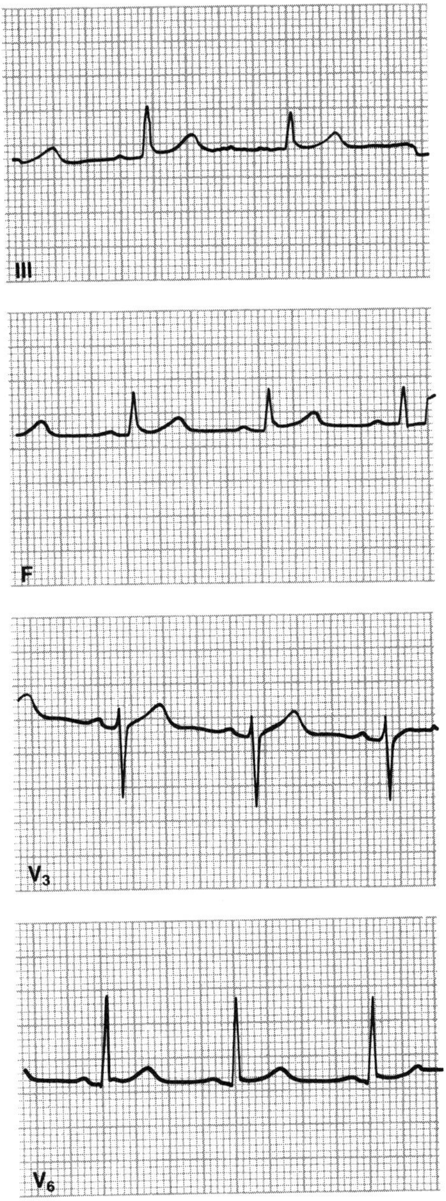
III
F
V3
V6

Figure E-5. ECG from the 37-year-old man a year earlier (1983) at the time of his infarction.

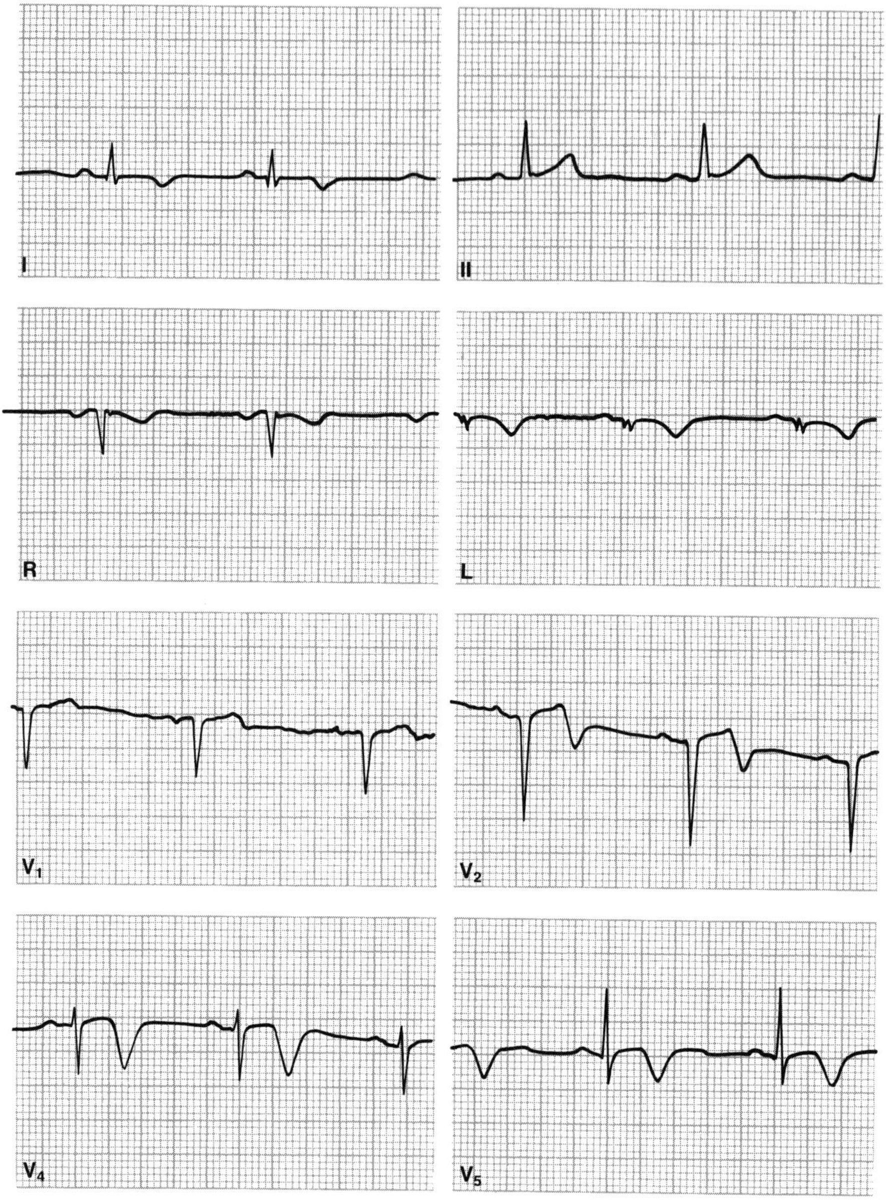

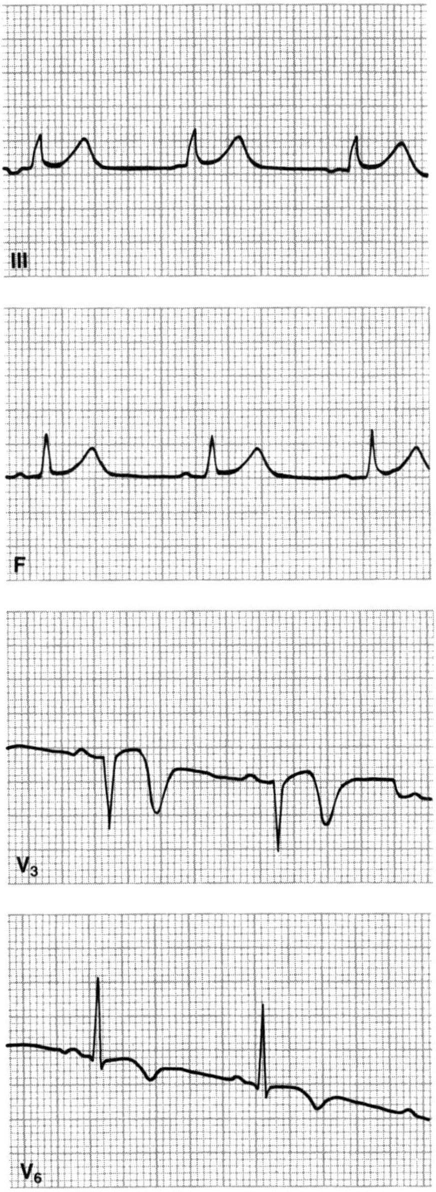
III
F
V_3
V_6

Figure E-6. ECG from a 47-year-old woman with a one-day history of chest pain.

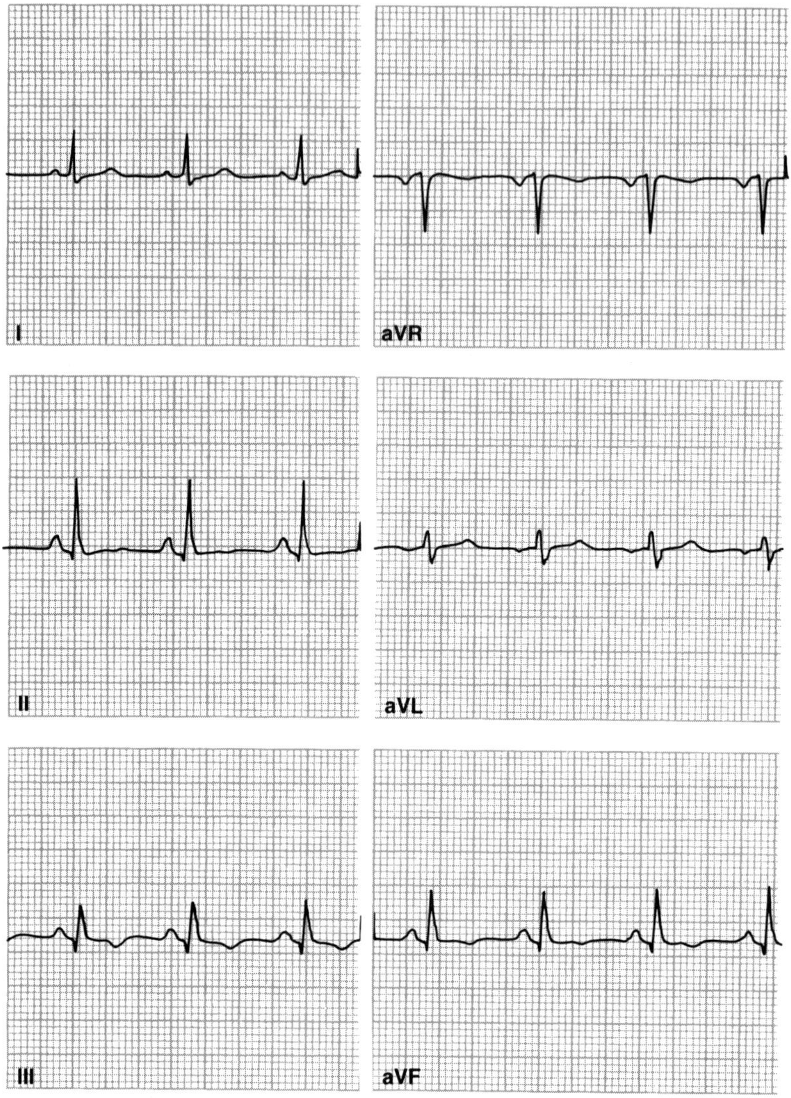

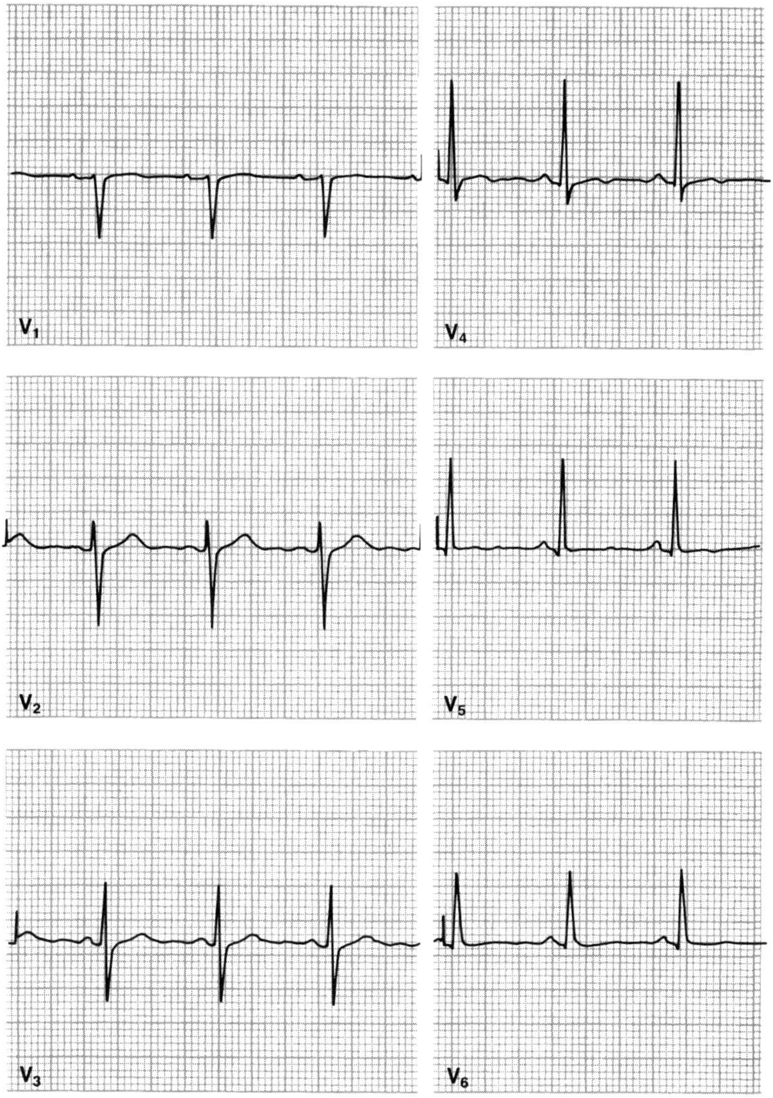
V_1
V_4
V_2
V_5
V_3
V_6

Figure E-7. ECG from 63-year-old woman with a 10-hour history of chest pain. There is neck vein distension, but no sign of left-sided heart failure.

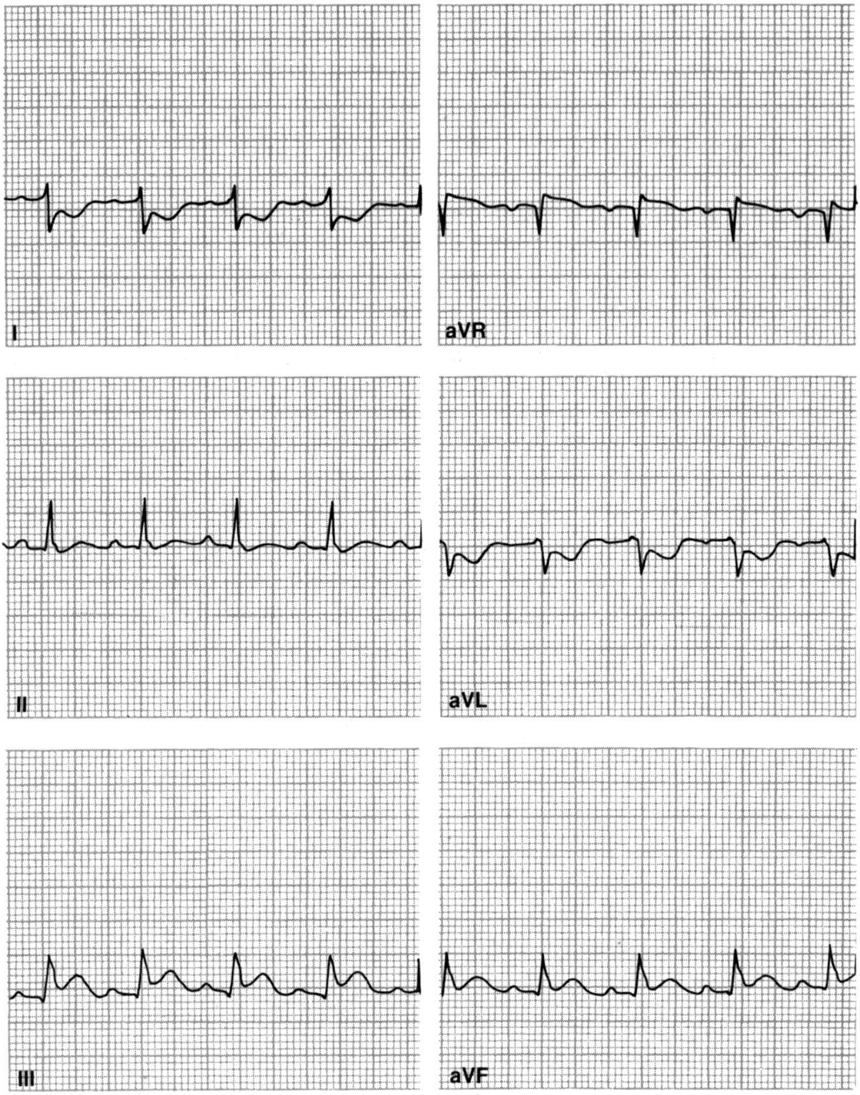

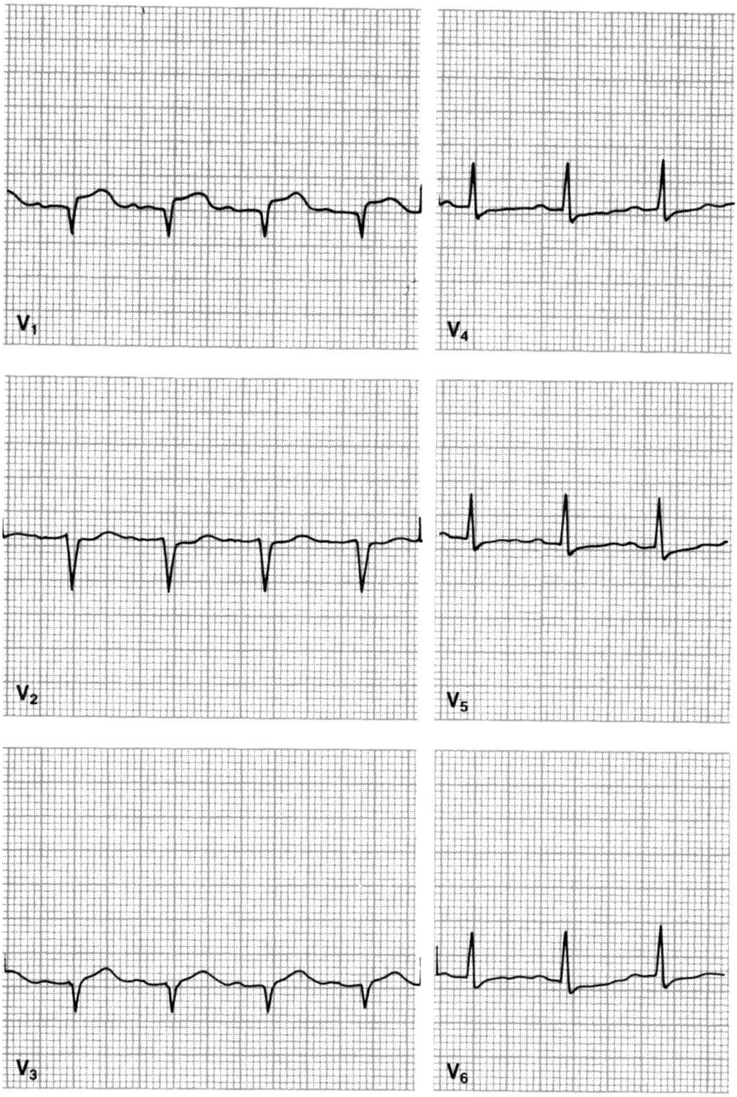
V1
V4
V2
V5
V3
V6

Figure E-8. ECG from a 71-year-old man with stabbing right-sided chest pain that increased on inspiration.

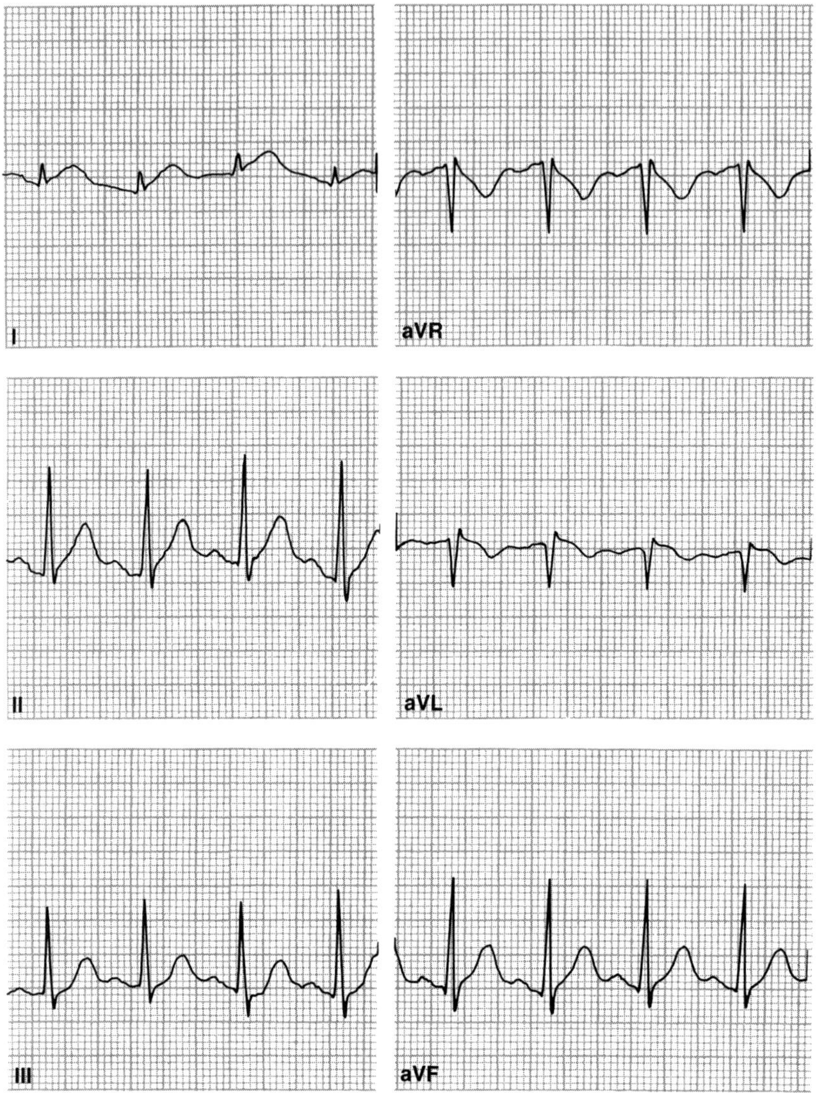

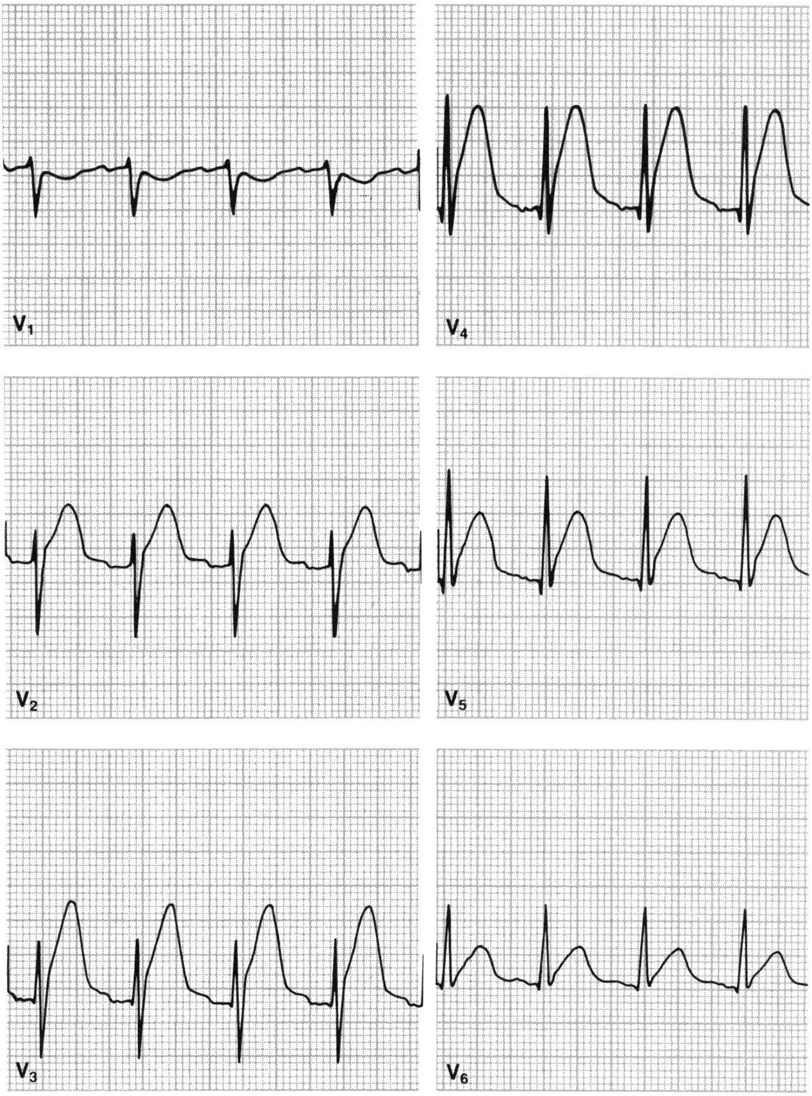
V1
V4
V2
V5
V3
V6

Figure E-9. ECG from an 82-year-old man with a history of IHSS. Now complaining of new-onset chest pain.

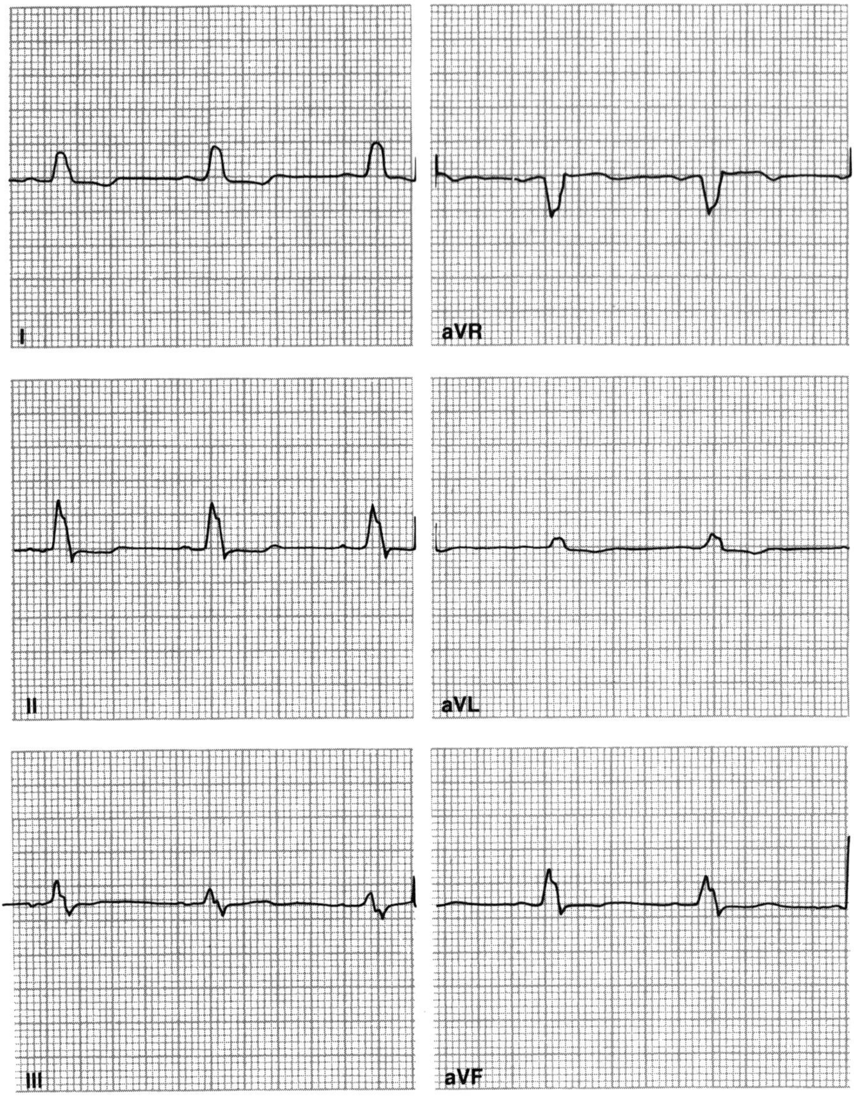

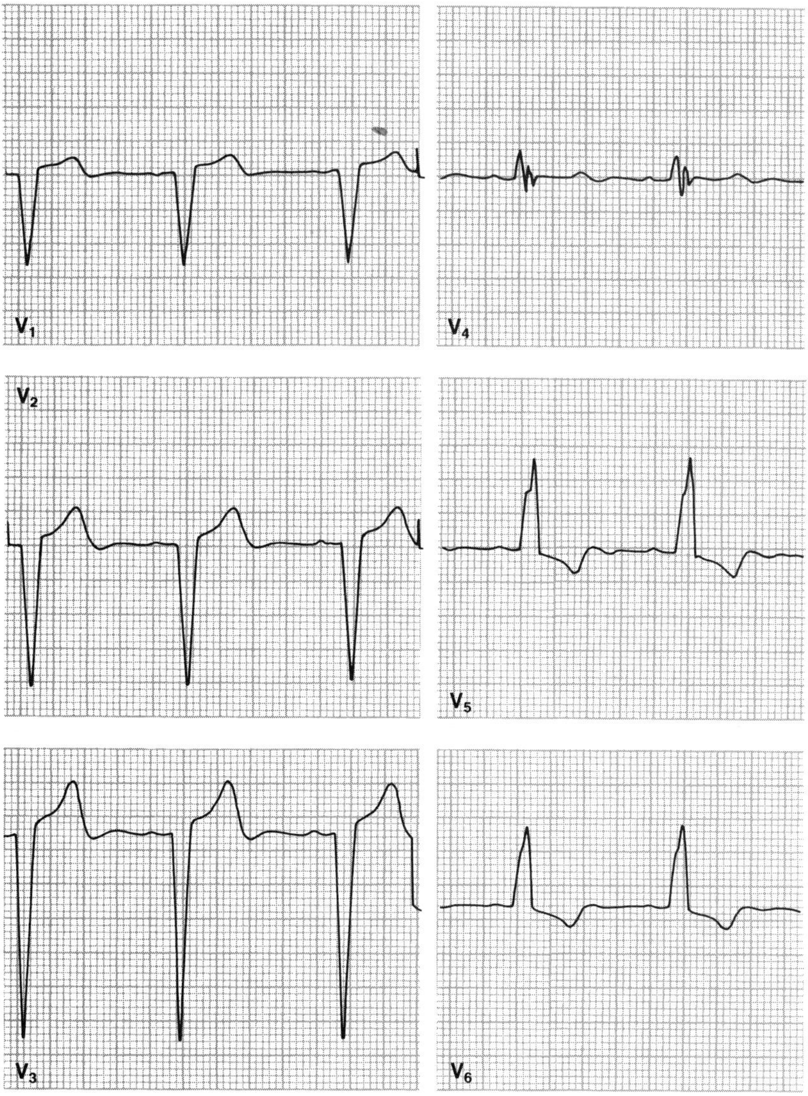
V1
V2
V3
V4
V5
V6

Figure E-10. ECG from a 67-year-old woman who presented with new-onset chest pain.

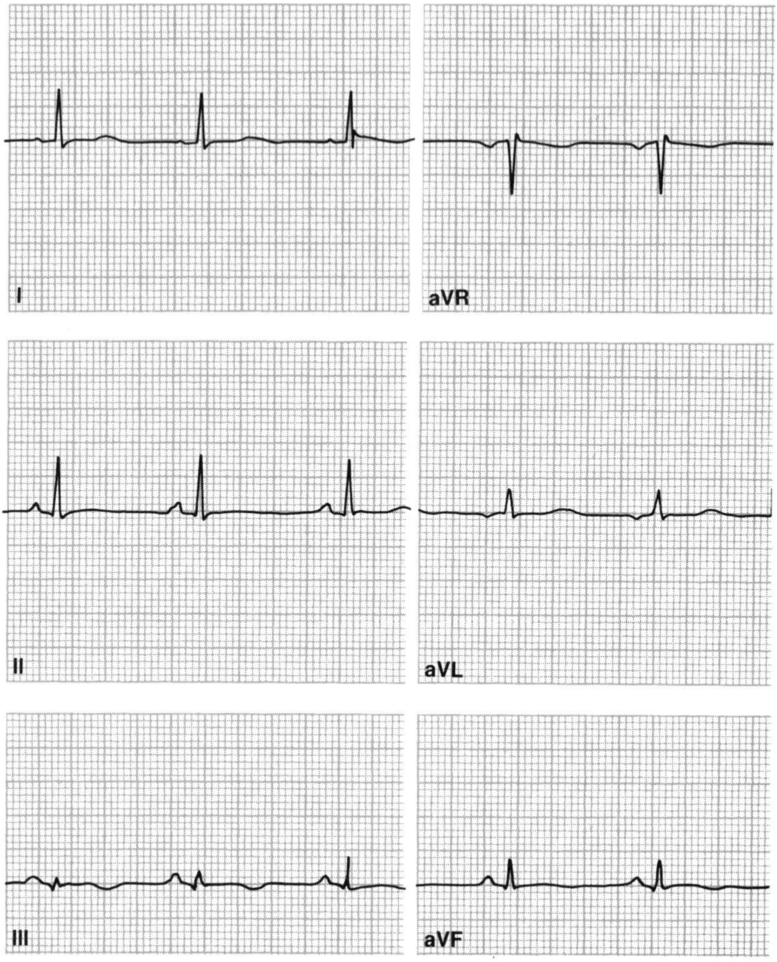

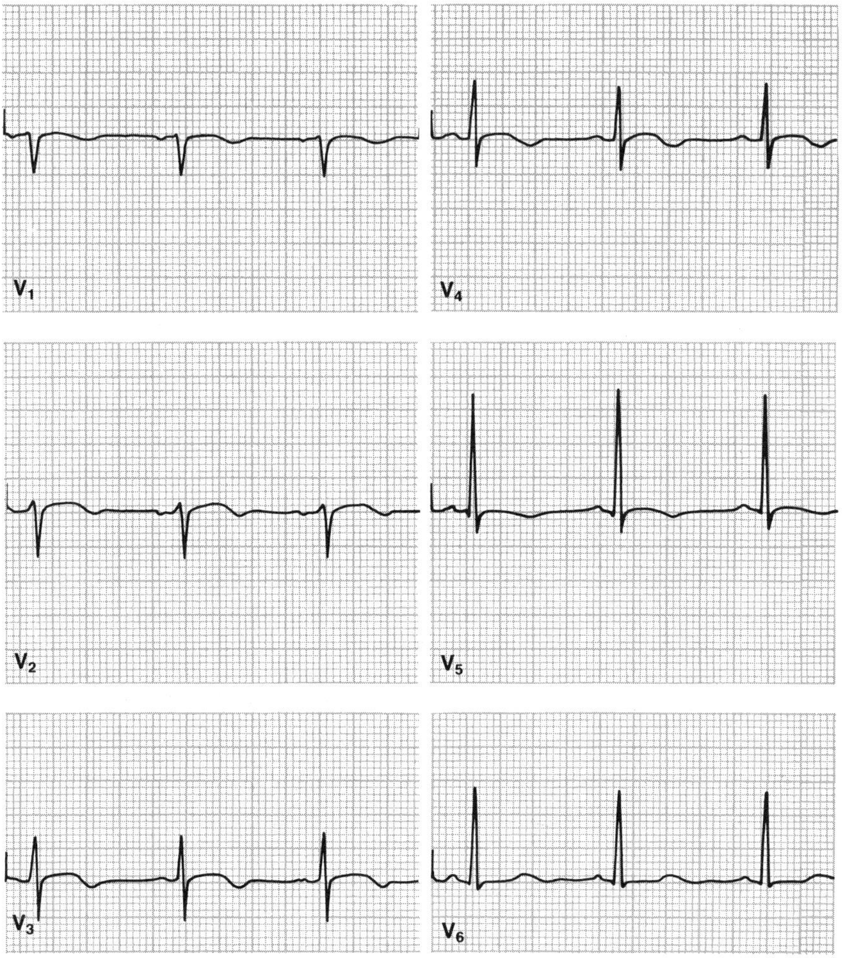
V1
V4
V2
V5
V3
V6

Figure E-11. Follow-up ECG on the 67-year-old woman taken one day after Fig. E-10.

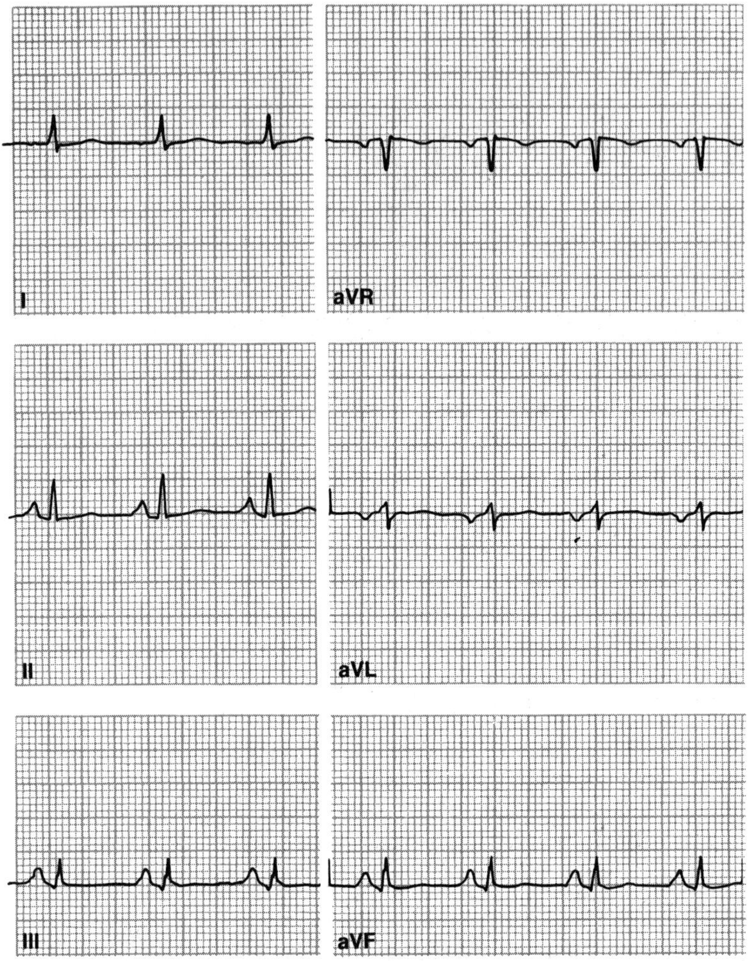

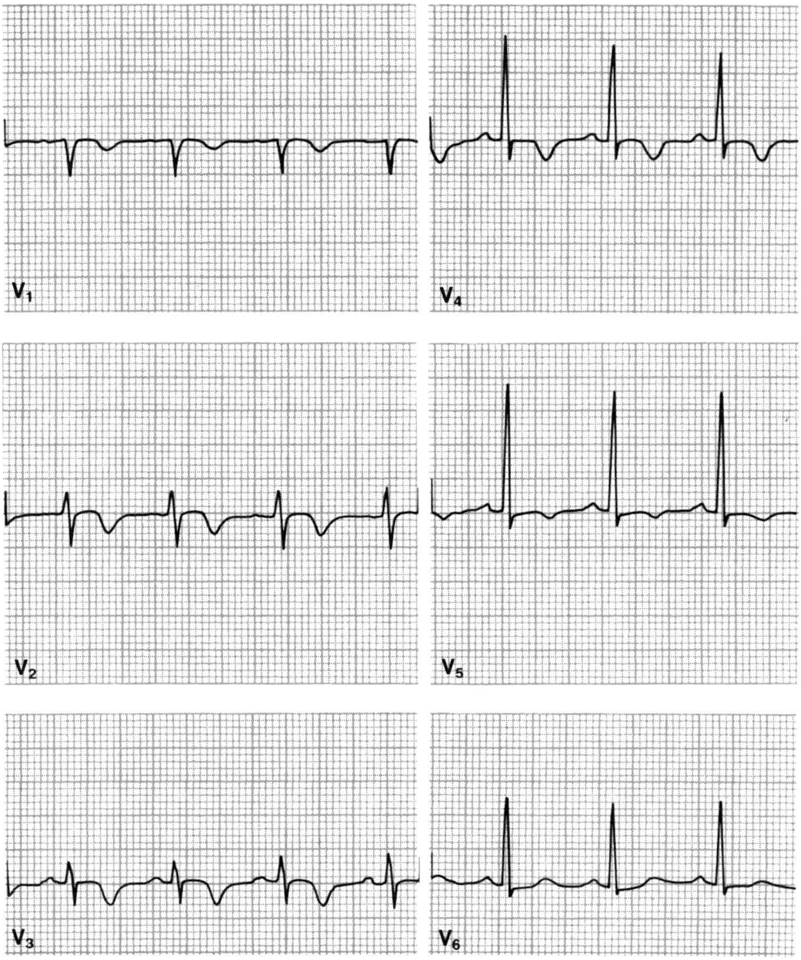
V1
V2
V3
V4
V5
V6

Figure E-12. Third ECG on the 67-year-old woman taken two days after Fig. E-11.

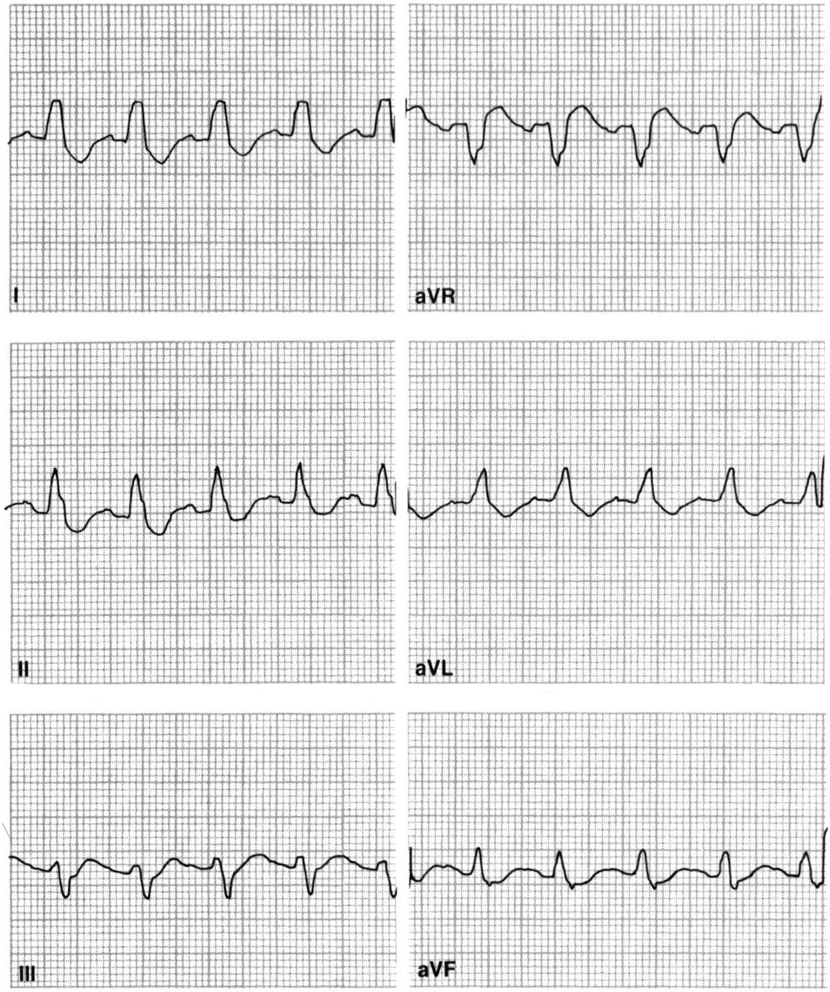

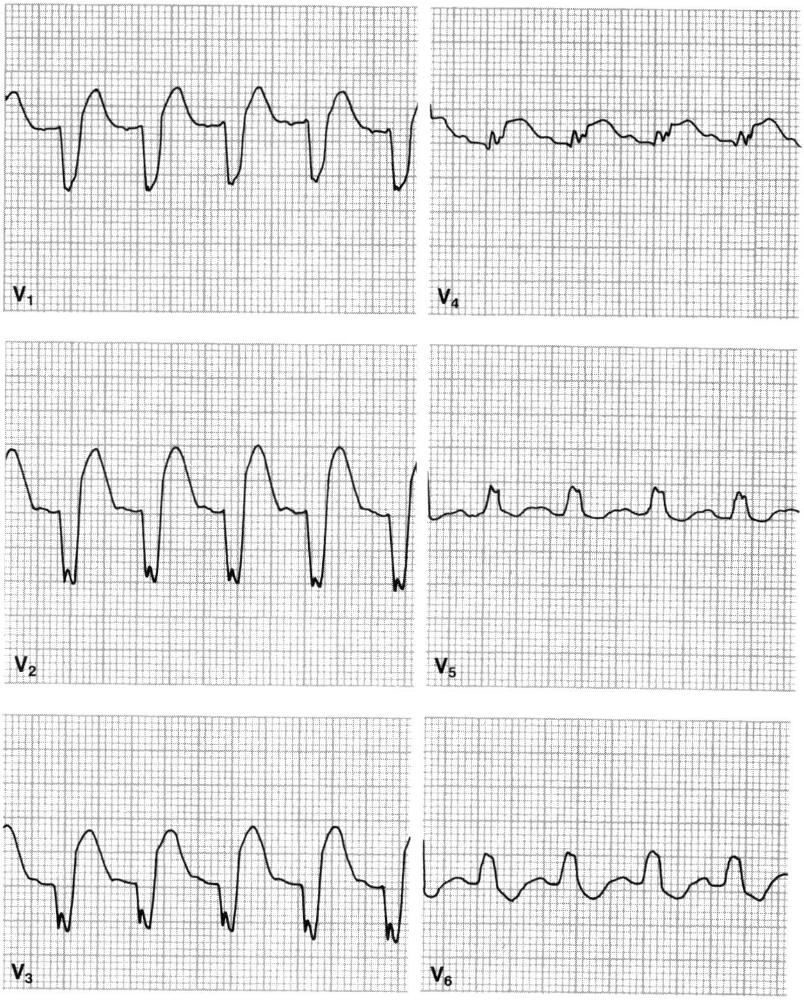
V1
V2
V3
V4
V5
V6

Figure E-13. Fourth ECG on the 67-year-old woman taken one day after Fig. E-12.

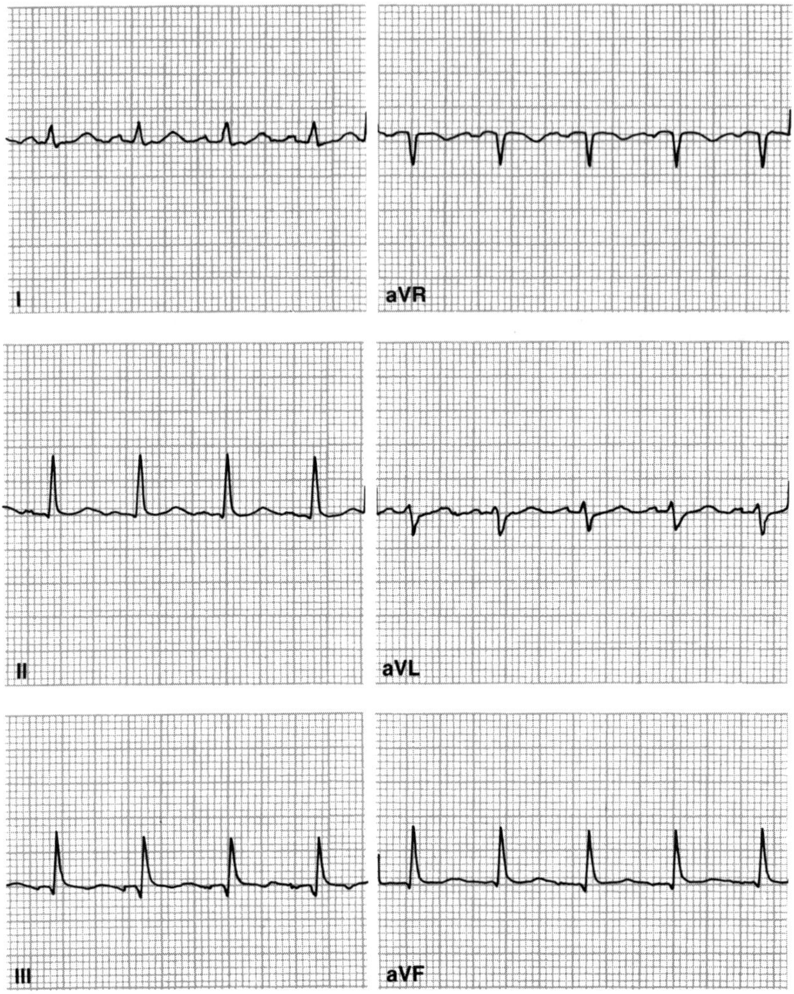

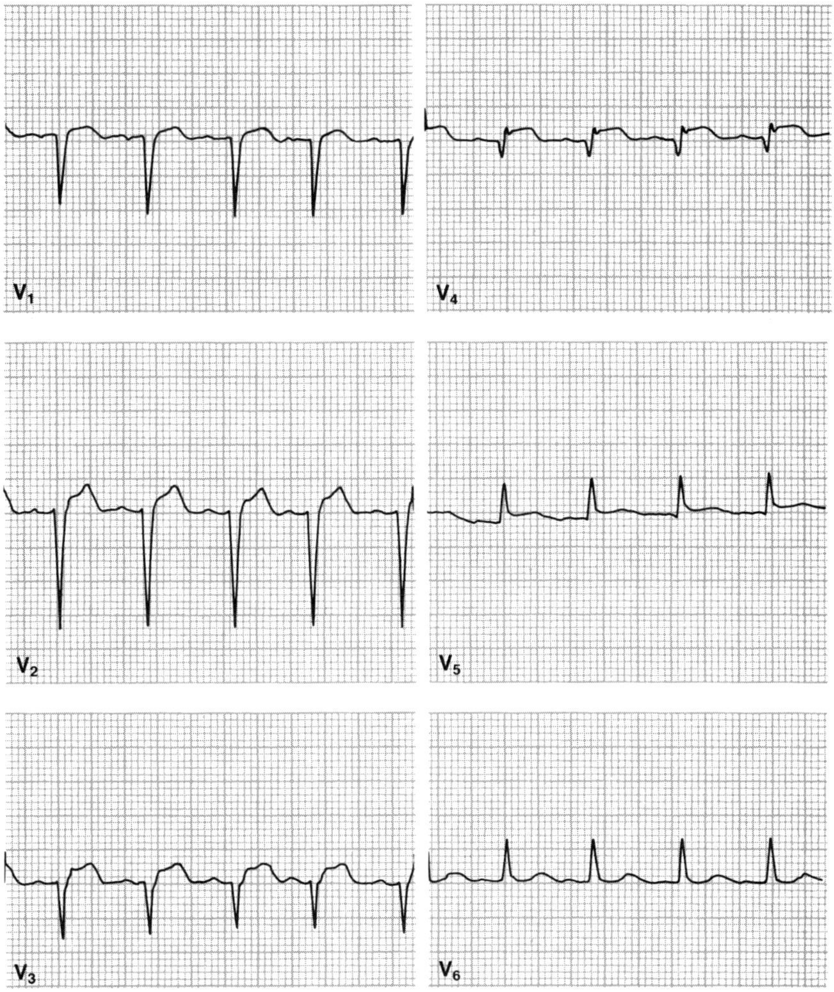
V1
V4
V2
V5
V3
V6

Figure E-14. ECG from a 56-year-old man with new-onset chest pain.

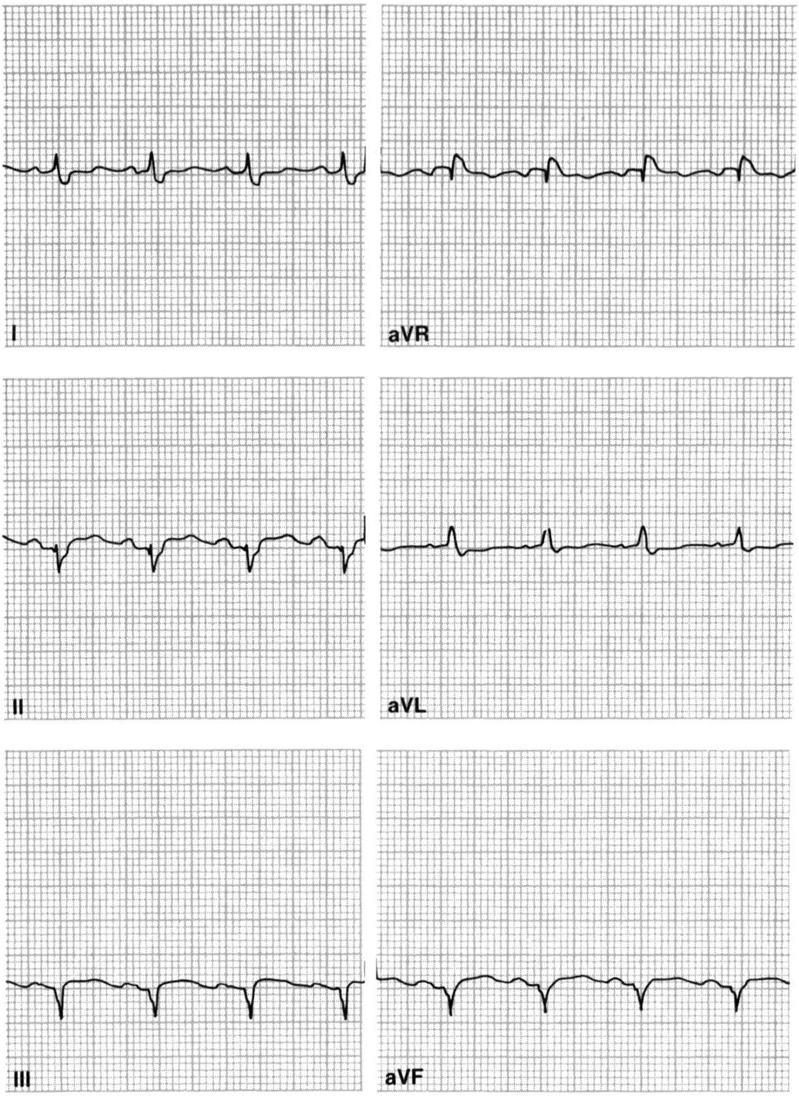

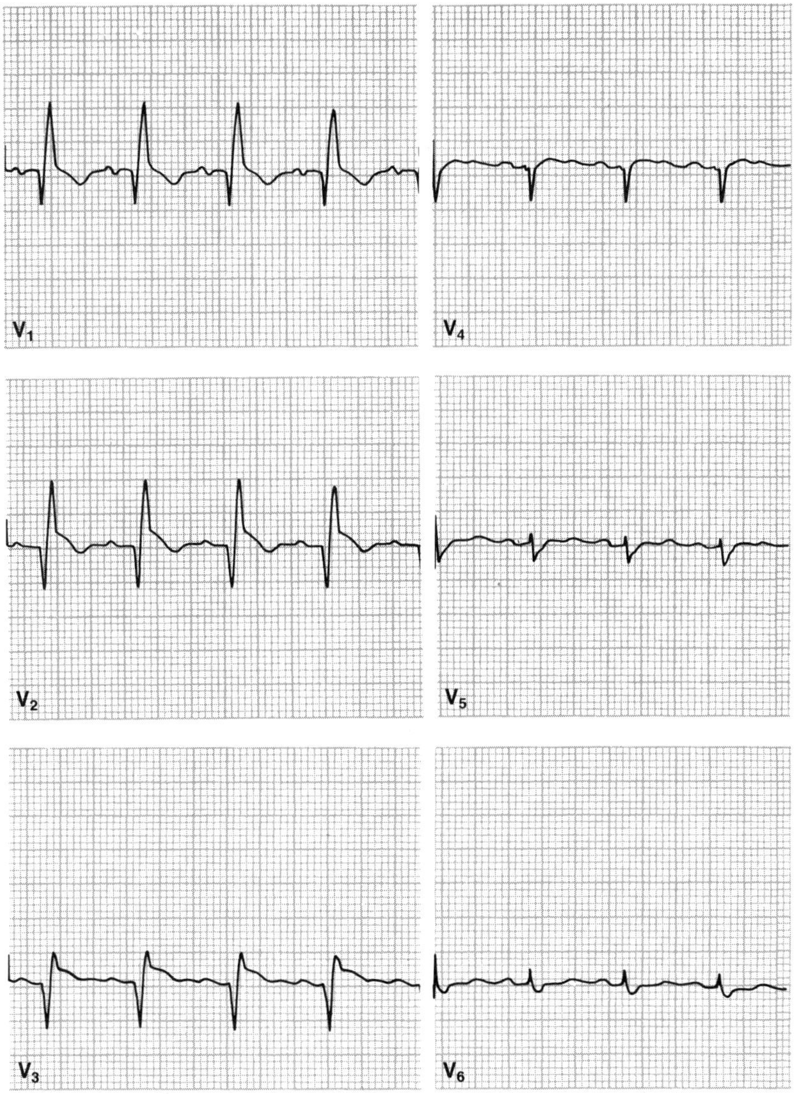
V1
V4
V2
V5
V3
V6

Figure E-15. ECG from a 49-year-old man with new-onset chest pain.

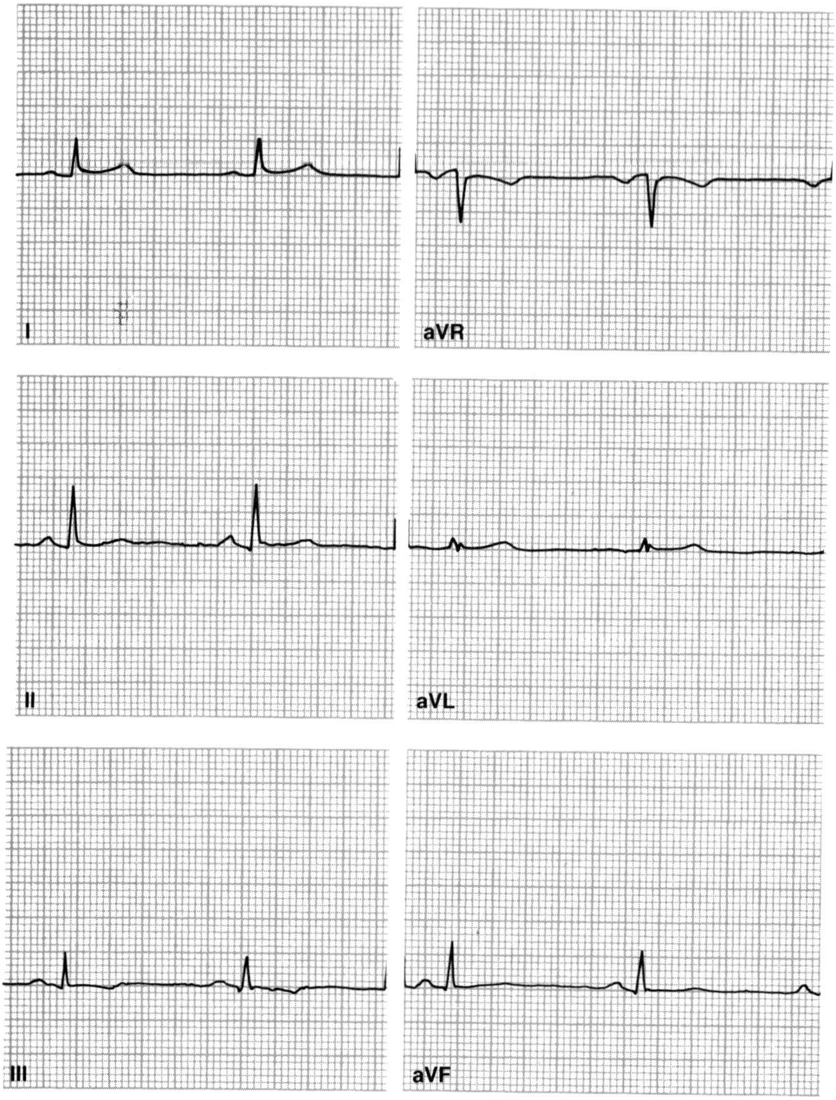

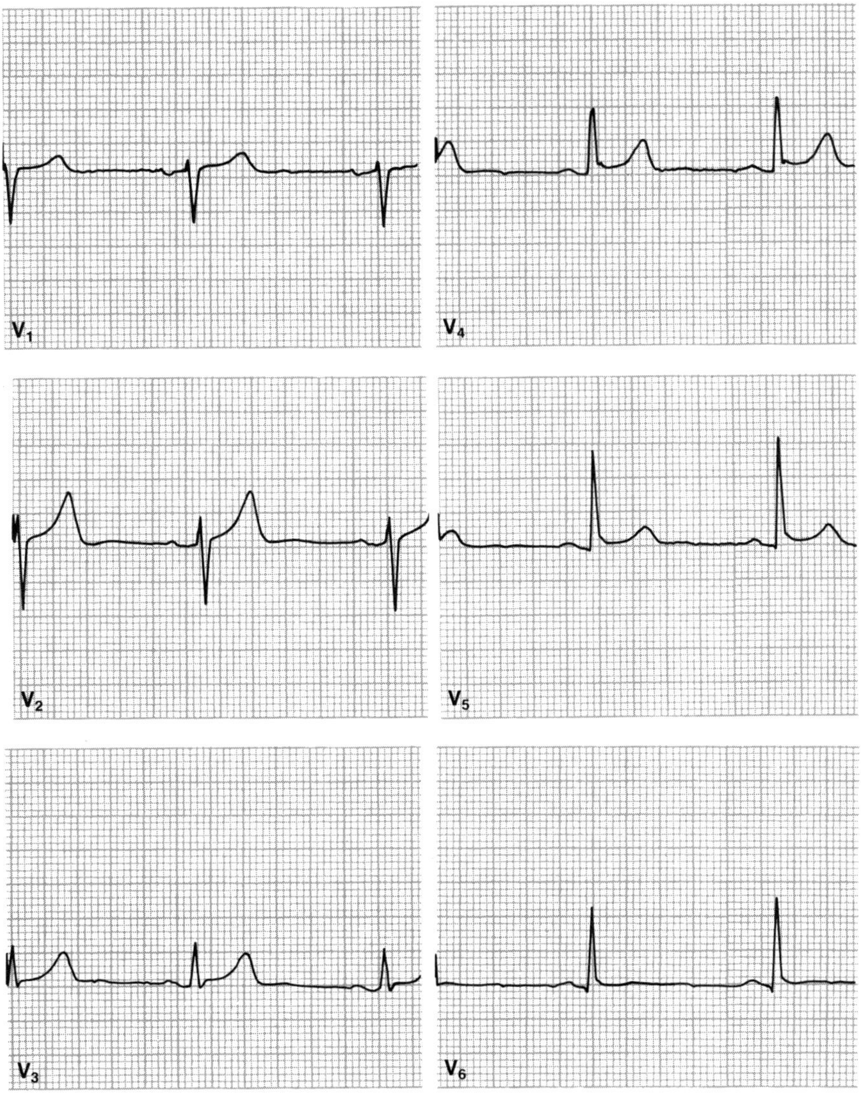
V1
V4
V2
V5
V3
V6

Figure E-16. Follow-up ECG on the 49-year-old man taken the next day.

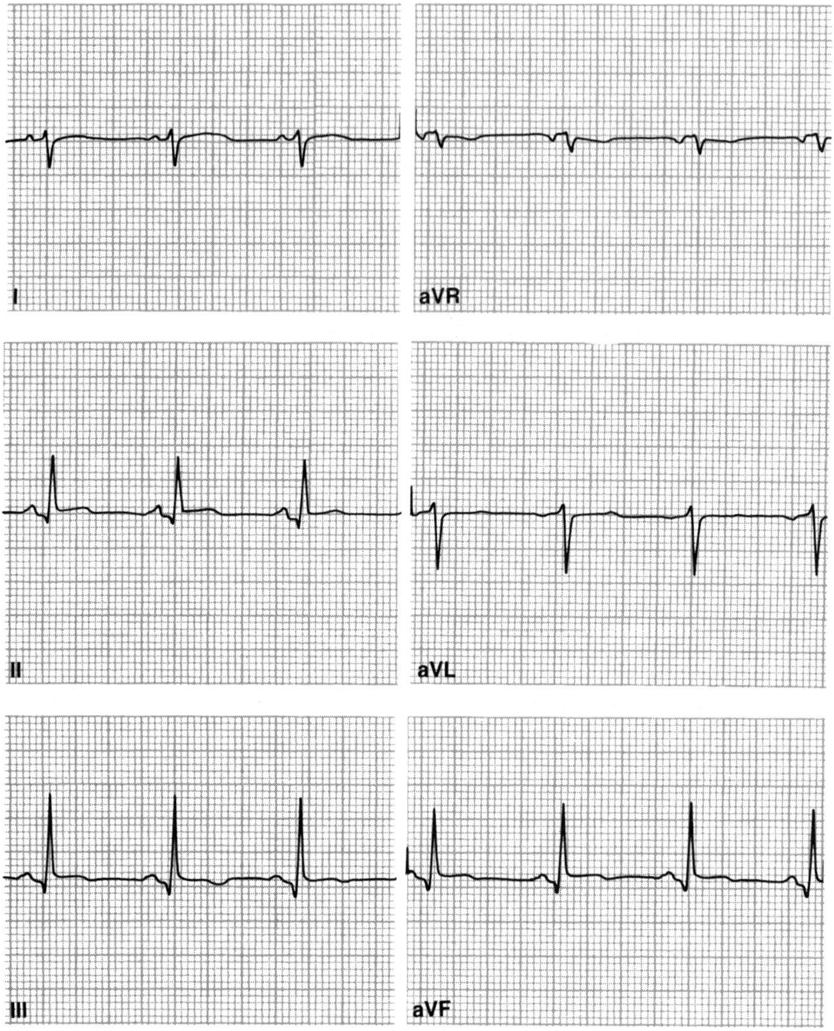

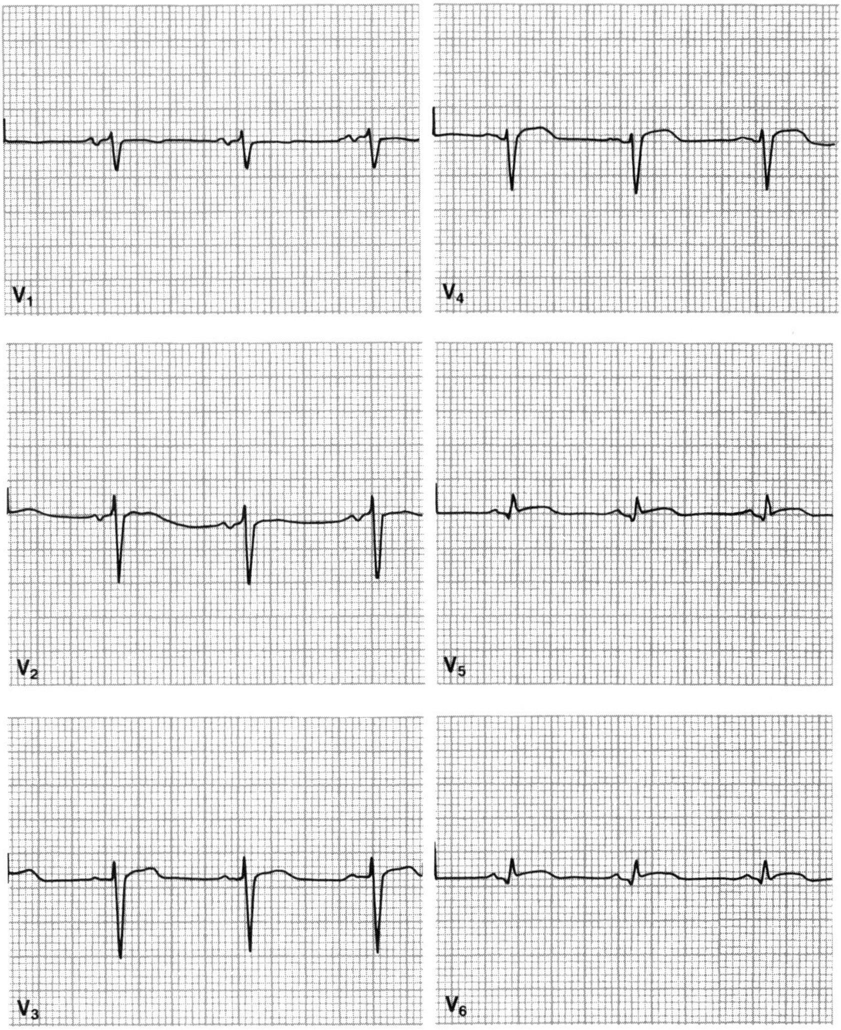
V1
V4
V2
V5
V3
V6

Figure E-17. ECG from a 67-year-old woman complaining of atypical chest pain.

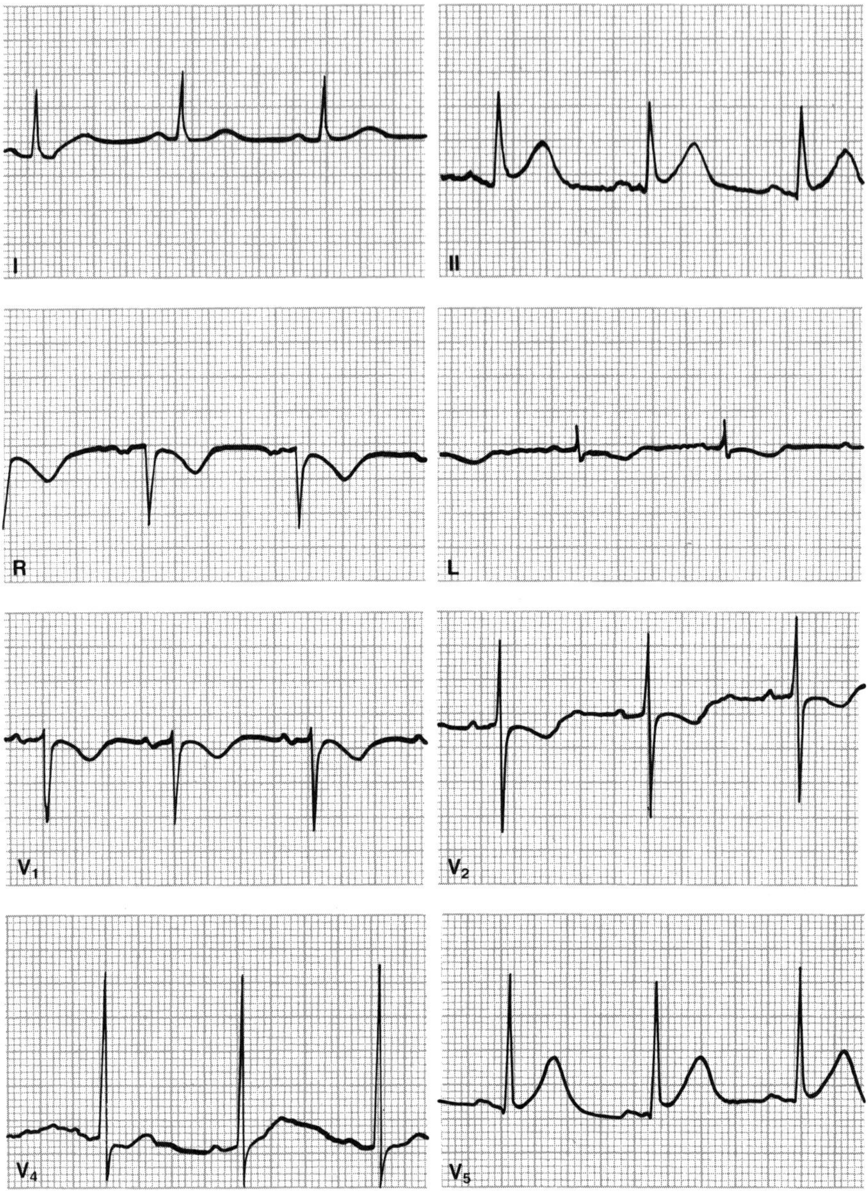

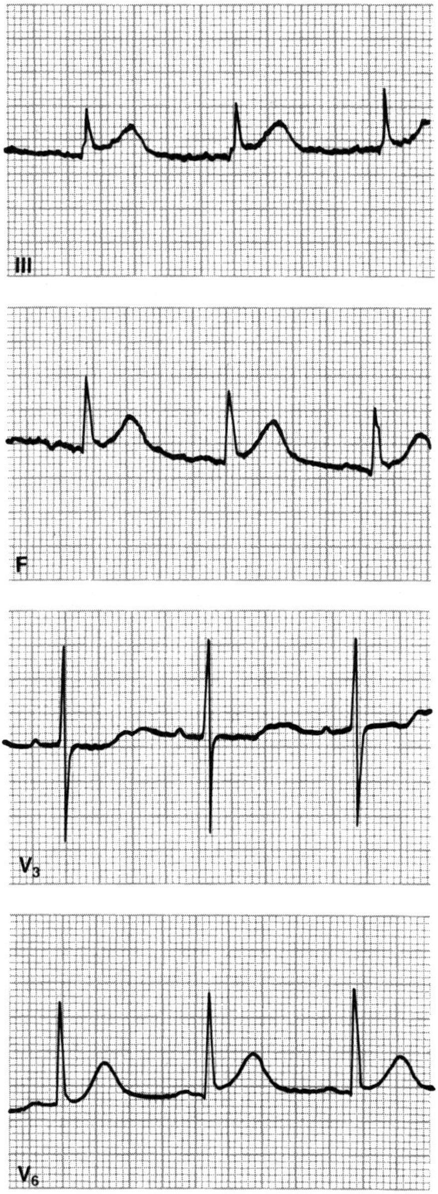
III
F
V_3
V_6

INTERPRETATION of Fig. E-1

Sinus rhythm at 65 beats/min. Axis $\approx -15°$. LAE. LVH and strain. Symmetric T-wave inversion in the inferior leads and across the precordium, suggesting *ischemia.*

With a two-day history of chest pain and no prior ECG available for comparison, the findings on this tracing would certainly be of concern. The ischemic T-wave changes could definitely be new, and the patient should be admitted to a monitored unit.

Prominent voltage in this tracing is only evident in the limb leads due to the leftward axis. Voltage criteria for LVH are satisfied (R in aVL ≥ 12 mm; sum of R wave in lead I + S wave in lead III ≥ 25 mm), and the typical ST-T wave changes of strain are evident in the leads I and aVL.

INTERPRETATION of Fig. E-2

Sinus rhythm at 70 beats/min. Axis $\approx -30°$. The QRS complex is widened. QS complexes are seen in leads III and aVF, and there is poor R-wave progression.

PROBLEM: Can you explain all of these findings?

ANSWER: This ECG does *not* represent inferior infarction, but instead is another example of *WPW (type B).* In addition to QRS widening, note how short the PR interval is in lead II. Positive delta waves are readily apparent in leads I and aVL as an initial slurring of the upstroke of the QRS complex. Inferior infarction is simulated by the negative delta waves in leads III and aVF.

It is of interest that the QRS complex in leads V_4 to V_6 does *not* appear widened. This is because the delta wave is primarily *isoelectric* in these leads.

INTERPRETATION of Fig. E-3

Sinus rhythm at 70 beats/min. Axis $\approx +60°$. LAE. LVH and strain. *Anterior infarction* of *unknown age, possibly acute.*

There are a number of interesting findings on this tracing. QRS amplitude is markedly increased both in limb and precordial leads, and ST-T wave changes consistent with strain are evident in virtually all limb leads as well as in leads V_5 and V_6. Considering this degree of increased voltage, the P-wave notching and prolongation in lead II, together with the somewhat deepened terminal negative component to the P wave in lead V_1 more than likely represent *true* left atrial enlargement.

Small (probably insignificant) q waves are evident in the inferior leads. R-wave progression is *poor,* and there is *loss of R wave* between leads V_2 and V_3. This suggests *anterior infarction.* Since the initial small r wave in lead V_1 is still present, the septum is probably intact.

Associated with loss of R wave in the anterior precordial leads is ST-segment elevation with a *coved* appearance, particularly in leads V_3 and V_4. This suggests that the anterior infarction may be *acute.*

In Chapter 4 (R-Wave Progression), we discussed the difficulty LVH might pose to the diagnosis of anterior infarction. As illustrated in Fig. 4-9, the transverse-plane vector loop becomes oriented more posteriorly with LVH. Increased *posterior* forces from the enlarged left ventricle may thus overshadow normal anterior forces, resulting in poor R-wave progression that simulates anterior infarction. Similarly, loss of anterior forces (as occurs with anterior infarction) results in unopposed posterior forces. Thus, with anterior infarction, S waves in the anterior precordial leads may deepen, sometimes to a extent great enough to satisfy voltage criteria for LVH. It should be apparent that whenever LVH *or* anterior infarction is present on an ECG, diagnosis of the other condition must be made with extreme caution.

In Fig. E-3, diagnosis of LVH should be secure from the tremendous QRS amplitude present in *both* limb and precordial leads in association with secondary repolarization changes. In this setting, *loss* of r wave (between leads V_2 and V_3) and ST-segment coving in the anterior precordial leads strongly suggest anterior infarction *regardless* of the coexistent LVH.

A final clinical point to derive from this tracing regards the ST-segment elevation. When this patient's old records were found, it was discovered that she had had a previous anterior infarction several months earlier, and that an ECG at the time of discharge looked identical to the one shown in Fig. E-3.

PROBLEM: Considering this new information, how would you interpret the ST-segment elevation in the anterior precordial leads?

ANSWER: Persistent ST-segment elevation this long after infarction suggests development of *ventricular aneurysm.*

INTERPRETATION of Fig. E-4 (1984 tracing)

Sinus rhythm at 70–75 beats/min. Axis $\approx +70°$. Nonspecific ST-segment flattening in lead I, and a qrS′ complex in lead aVL with shallow, symmetric T-wave inversion in this lead. These findings are of unknown significance. Suggest clinical correlation and comparison with prior tracings.

One really does *not* see definitive evidence of this patient's prior myocardial infarction on this ECG. The ST-segment flattening in lead I is entirely nonspecific. The predominantly negative QRS complex and accompanying T-wave inversion in lead aVL could represent *high lateral infarction* of unknown age. However, when such findings are isolated to this one lead in a patient with a relatively vertical axis, they are much more commonly of no clinical significance.

In the precordial leads, R-wave progression is normal, transition occurs as expected between leads V_3 and V_4, and the ST-T waves do not suggest any acute changes.

PROBLEM: Now examine Fig. E-4—this patient's ECG from a year earlier at the time of his infarction (Fig. E-5 obtained in 1983). How has the 1984 ECG (Fig. E-4) changed since the infarction tracing (Fig. E-5)?

INTERPRETATION of Fig. E-5 (1983 tracing)

Sinus rhythm at about 60 beats/min. Axis ≈ +65°. *Acute anterolateral ischemia, infarction,* or both is suggested by QS complexes and ST-segment coving in the anterior precordial leads, a q wave in lead I, and a QrS complex in lead aVL, and deep, symmetric T-wave inversion in the high lateral leads and across the precordium.

By 1984 (Fig. E-4), most of the abnormalities seen in the 1983 tracing have resolved. The small q wave in lead I has disappeared, and r waves have returned to the anterior precordial leads (R-wave progression has normalized). With the exception of the nonspecific ST-segment flattening in lead I and the shallow T-wave inversion in lead aVL, the 1984 ECG is almost a *normal* tracing!

Cardiac catheterization performed in 1984 revealed near total occlusions of the left anterior descending and circumflex arteries, corresponding to this patient's previous anterolateral infarction. One would never suspect these findings from simple inspection of Fig. E-4. Thus, this example emphasizes that an ECG does *not* always indicate evidence of a previous infarction. Even when changes of infarction do develop (as they did in the 1983 tracing), they may totally resolve with time!

INTERPRETATION of Fig. E-6

Sinus rhythm at 90 beats/min. Axis ≈ +60°. Probable *inferior infarction,* possibly *acute.* Nonspecific ST-T wave flattening in leads V_4 to V_6.

Narrow Q waves are present in the inferior leads. As an isolated finding, such Q waves would *not* necessarily be pathologic. Of particular concern is the associated slight coving to the ST segments in leads III and aVF, and the hint of T-wave inversion in these leads. In a 47-year-old woman with a one-day history of chest pain, this picture may well represent an acute inferior infarction.

INTERPRETATION of Fig. E-7

Sinus tachycardia at about 110 beats/min. Axis ≈ 95° (RAD). Probable *acute inferior infarction.* Possible anterior infarction of unknown age.

The changes indicating acute inferior infarction are small q waves in each of the inferior leads, ST-segment elevation in leads III and aVF, and reciprocal ST-segment depression in leads I and aVL.

Accurate determination of mean QRS axis is difficult in this tracing because of the ST-segment deviations from the baseline. RAD is probably present, since net deflection of the QRS complex in lead I appears to be slightly negative. However, criteria for left posterior hemiblock are *not* met (Table 4-5), and the slight rightward axis (to about +95°) is of unknown clinical significance.

The most interesting finding on this ECG is the ST-segment elevation in lead V_1. Although previous anterior infarction is suggested by the paucity of anterior forces in leads V_1 and V_3, ST-segment elevation is usually seen in *each* of these leads when anterior infarction is acute. Instead, it is only present in lead V_1.

PROBLEM: Considering the clinical history and the occurrence of associated inferior infarction, to what might you attribute the ST-segment elevation in lead V_1?

ANSWER: The ST-segment elevation in lead V_1 of this tracing may represent acute *right ventricular infarction.*

Right ventricular infarctions virtually never occur alone. Instead they are almost always associated with acute inferior infarctions, since both areas of the heart are supplied by the same right coronary artery. Although the right ventricle is involved in up to 25 percent of inferior infarctions, most of the time such involvement is *not* clinically significant. It is nevertheless important to recognize those occasional instances in which right ventricular involvement *does* become important clinically, since treatment differs dramatically from the usual treatment of myocardial infarction.

Clinically significant right ventricular infarction results in acute *right* ventricular failure. Neck veins distend and the liver may become passively congested, but there are no signs of left-sided heart failure—rales don't occur. If the patient is hemodynamically unstable (hypotensive), treatment may include volume infusion, which improves performance of the right ventricle. In contrast, the problem in patients with acute infarction and *left-sided* heart failure tends to be fluid overload. Treatment is often best accomplished with diuretics.

Right ventricular infarction is difficult to recognize electrocardiographically. This is because none of the standard recording electrodes look directly at the right ventricle. Lead V_1 (positioned just to the right of the sternum in the fourth intercostal space) comes the closest. When ST-segment elevation is seen in *only* this lead in association with evidence of acute inferior infarction, *right ventricular infarction* should be suspected. Application of special *right*-sided precordial leads (leads V_{2R} to V_{4R}) should demonstrate characteristic development and evolution of Q waves, ST-segment elevation, and T-wave inversion. Consideration of invasive hemodynamic monitoring (placement of a Swan-Ganz catheter) may be needed to confirm the clinical impression and guide therapeutics.

INTERPRETATION of Fig. E-8

Sinus tachycardia at 105 beats/min. Axis ≈ +80°. Small q waves are present in the infero-anterolateral leads. ST-segment elevation with an abrupt "takeoff" is seen in leads V_2 to V_6. Possibilities include acute injury (myocardial infarction) or *acute pericarditis.*

Stage I of acute pericarditis is characterized by diffuse ST-segment elevation in all leads *except* aVR, and occasionally leads III, aVL, or V_1 (see Fig. 7-23). In addition, PR-segment depression (seen here in leads II, V_2, and V_3) is commonly seen with acute pericarditis. The ECG shown in Fig. E-8 and the clinical history of this 71-year-old man would be typical except for the presence of q waves. Strong consideration of acute myocardial infarction would have to be given if these q waves were known to be new. Confirmation of the diagnosis requires comparison with a previous ECG, careful auscultation for a pericardial friction rub, serial tracings, and cardiac enzyme studies.

INTERPRETATION of Fig. E-9

Sinus rhythm at 65 beats/min. Axis $\approx +40°$. *Complete LBBB.*

Although deep QS complexes are seen in leads V_1 to V_3, this picture is typical of LBBB. Anterior myocardial infarction may be present, but it *cannot* be diagnosed by this ECG. Similarly, ST-segment depression and T-wave inversion in the lateral leads, and ST-segment elevation in the anterior precordial leads, represent characteristic *secondary* ST-T wave changes of LBBB rather than injury, ischemia, or strain. Thus, the correct ECG interpretation of this tracing is sinus rhythm with complete LBBB. Nothing more, nothing less. *LBBB is a common ECG manifestation of IHSS.*

INTERPRETATION of Fig. E-10

Sinus rhythm at 70 beats/min. Axis $\approx +40°$. Small q waves in the inferior and lateral precordial leads. Slight coving of the ST segments in the inferior and anterior precordial leads with shallow T-wave inversion. *Can't rule out acute injury or ischemia.* Suggest clinical correlation and comparison with prior tracings.

Although the findings on this ECG are nonspecific, they would have to be interpreted with caution considering the clinical history. Availability of a previous ECG from this patient would prove very helpful in determining whether the findings seen in Fig. E-10 were likely to be acute. Without evidence to the contrary, acute infarction should be assumed until proven otherwise.

PROBLEM: Examine the follow-up ECG that was taken the next day on this patient (Fig. E-11). What has happened in the interim?

ANSWER: Since Fig. E-10, the rate has increased, and T waves have become much more deeply and symmetrically inverted in the anterior leads. This suggests *ischemia, evolving subendocardial infarction,* or both.

PROBLEM: The ECG shown in Fig. E-12 was obtained two days after the one in Fig. E-11. What has happened? What therapeutic intervention should be considered?

ANSWER: The QRS complex has now widened (to 0.12 second) and taken on the pattern of complete LBBB (monophasic R wave in leads I and V_6, and deep negative deflection in leads V_1 to V_3). Strong consideration should be given to placement of a prophylactic pacemaker.

PROBLEM: The final ECG in this sequence is shown in Fig. E-13, taken one day after Fig. E-12. Is there now definitive evidence of acute infarction?

ANSWER: Sinus tachycardia persists. R-wave progression has definitely been lost since the initial tracing. Although a tiny r wave appears to be present in lead V_2, and possibly also in lead V_3, a deep and wide Q wave is seen in lead V_4. Associated with this is coved ST-segment elevation in leads V_1 to V_5. This series of tracings is *indicative* of *acute anterior infarction.* Not surprisingly, cardiac enzymes were markedly elevated.

Return for a moment to Fig. E-12. This tracing probably represents an exception to the general rule that determination of acute myocardial infarction is not possible in the setting of complete LBBB. At least in retrospect, the marked degree of ST-segment elevation in leads V_2 and V_3 (of up to 10 mm), and particularly the coved contour of the ST-segment elevation in lead V_4 of this tracing, are distinctly atypical for the usual appearance of complete LBBB. (You may wish to compare Fig. E-12 with a *typical* LBBB, such as the one discussed in Fig. E-9.)

Finally, note that the small q waves that were evident in the inferior leads of Figs. E-10 and 11 are masked by development of LBBB in Fig. E-12, only to return again in Fig. E-13 after the conduction defect resolves. Recognition of myocardial infarction in the presence of complete LBBB is a tricky business. In general (with rare exceptions), one would do perfectly well to follow the easily remembered axiom that *determination of acute infarction is not readily accomplished in the setting of complete LBBB.*

INTERPRETATION of Fig. E-14

Sinus tachycardia at 110 beats/min. Complete RBBB and LAHB (*bifascicular* block). *Anteroseptal infarction,* possibly *acute.* Can't rule out inferior infarction of unknown age.

Unlike the case for LBBB, RBBB does *not* alter the initial vector of ventricular depolarization. Consequently, inscription of Q waves is *not* affected by RBBB, and detection of myocardial infarction can usually be accomplished despite the presence of this conduction defect. Thus, the deep and wide Q waves in leads V_1 to V_3 of this tracing and the QS complex in lead V_4 suggest anterior infarction. Although usual secondary ST-T wave changes of RBBB result in T-wave inversion in the anterior precordial leads, ST-segment elevation such as is seen in leads V_2 and V_3 is atypical, and indicates that the *anteroseptal infarction* may be *acute.*

LAHB is diagnosed from the predominantly negative QRS deflection in lead II. Although a nubbin of an r wave may be present in leads III and aVF, one can't rule out the possibility of associated inferior infarction on the basis of this tracing alone.

Clinically, the presence of bifascicular block in the setting of acute anterior infarction would be an indication for prophylactic pacemaker insertion.

INTERPRETATION of Fig. E-15

Sinus bradycardia at about 55 beats/min. Axis ≈ +55°. Tiny q waves are present in the inferior and lateral precordial leads. The T wave in lead III is inverted. These changes do not appear acute. Suggest clinical correlation.

Physical examination of this patient was unremarkable. Despite this relatively benign-appearing ECG, he was admitted to an observation unit because of his history.

PROBLEM: The ECG shown in Fig. E-16 is the follow-up ECG obtained the next day. Comparing it to Fig. E-15, what has happened?

ANSWER: Compared to Fig. E-15, the heart rate in Fig. E-16 has increased to about 80 beats/min, and the mean QRS axis has shifted markedly to the right. Q waves in the inferior and lateral precordial leads have deepened, and slight but definite coved ST-segment elevation is now evident in these areas. In addition, R-wave amplitude has significantly diminished in the lateral precordial leads. The picture suggests acute inferolateral infarction.

These two tracings offer yet one more example of how an initial ECG of a patient who is having an acute infarction may look relatively benign.

INTERPRETATION of Fig. E-17

Sinus rhythm at about 70 beats/min. Axis ≈ +50°. Suspicious-looking ST-segment elevation in the inferior and lateral precordial leads, with ST-segment depression in lead aVL and leads V_1 to V_3. Can't rule out acute injury. Suggest clinical correlation.

This 67-year-old woman had a cardiac arrest five minutes after this ECG was taken. She was resuscitated, and went on to evolve an acute inferior infarction. Retrospectively, the ST-segment elevation in Fig. E-17 represented a *hyperacute* T-wave change. Although sometimes difficult to differentiate from the ST-segment elevation of early repolarization, the clinical history and associated ST-segment depression (*reciprocal* ST-segment depression) in this case should have alerted the electrocardiographer to the significance of these changes.

EXERCISE F

PSEUDO-INFARCTION PATTERNS

A *pseudoinfarction pattern* is an ECG change that *simulates* myocardial infarction, but has some other cause. We have already discussed a number of causes of pseudoinfarction patterns, including early repolarization and other repolarization variants, ventricular hypertrophy, cardiomyopathy, left bundle branch block and intraventricular conduction defects (IVCD), pericardial effusion, WPW, limb-lead reversal, and dextrocardia.

The patients in this section pose a final (and fairly *difficult*) challenge to you. The ECGs from all but one of them represent a pseudoinfarction pattern.

- Can you deduce the likely cause of the pseudoinfarction pattern in each case?
- Can you determine which of the seven tracings truly reflects an infarction?

Figure F-1. ECG from a 57-year-old man with sudden onset of chest pain. A repeat ECG performed minutes later after his pain subsided was virtually normal.

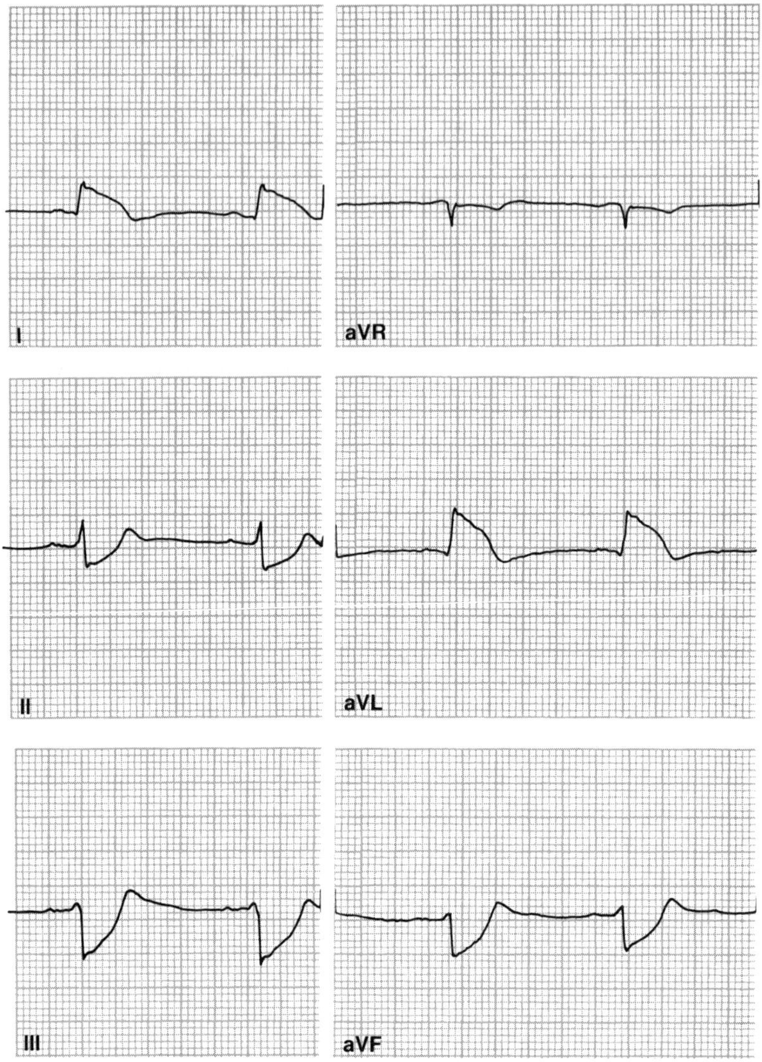

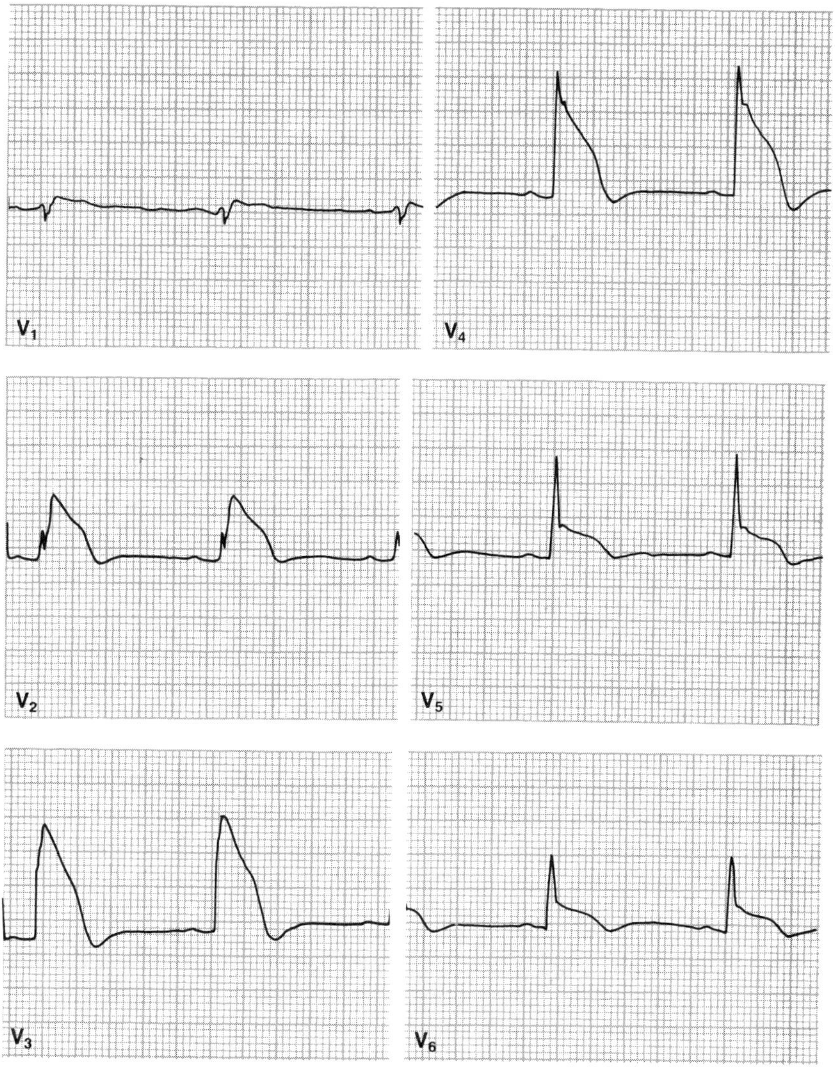
V_1
V_4
V_2
V_5
V_3
V_6

Figure F-2. ECG from a middle-aged woman with chest pain and shortness of breath.

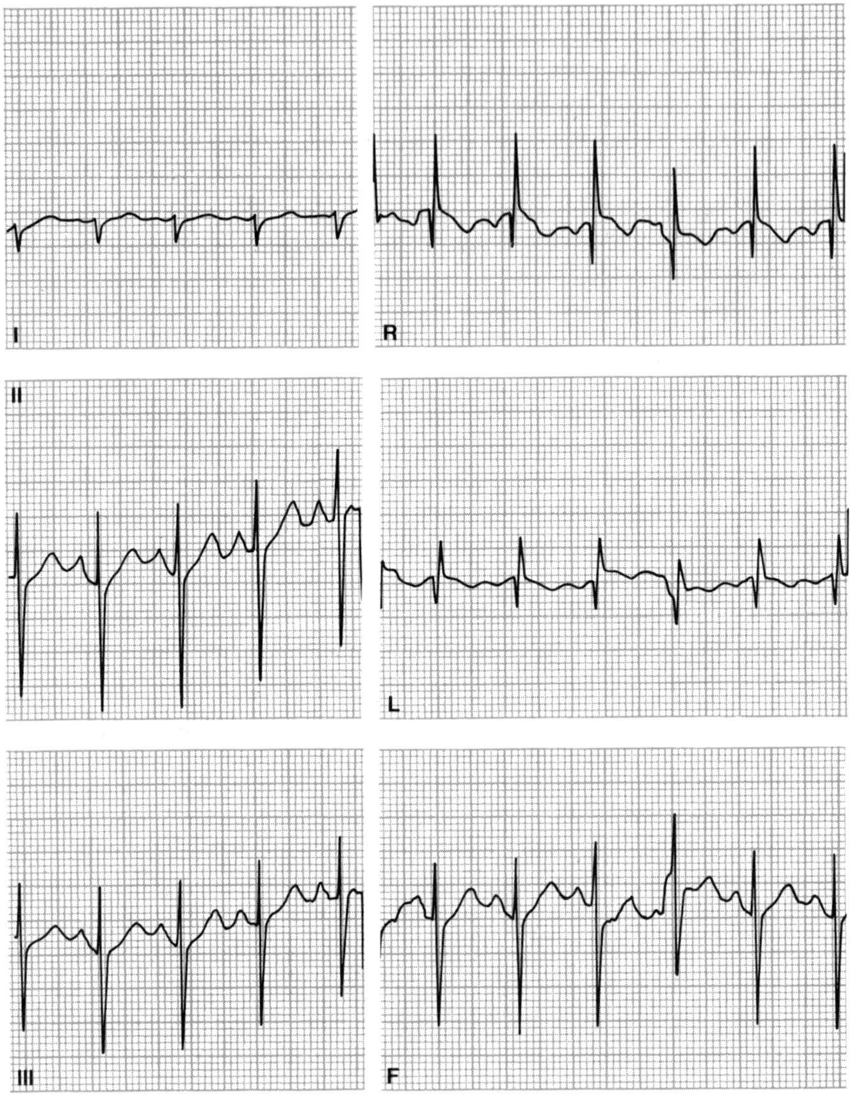

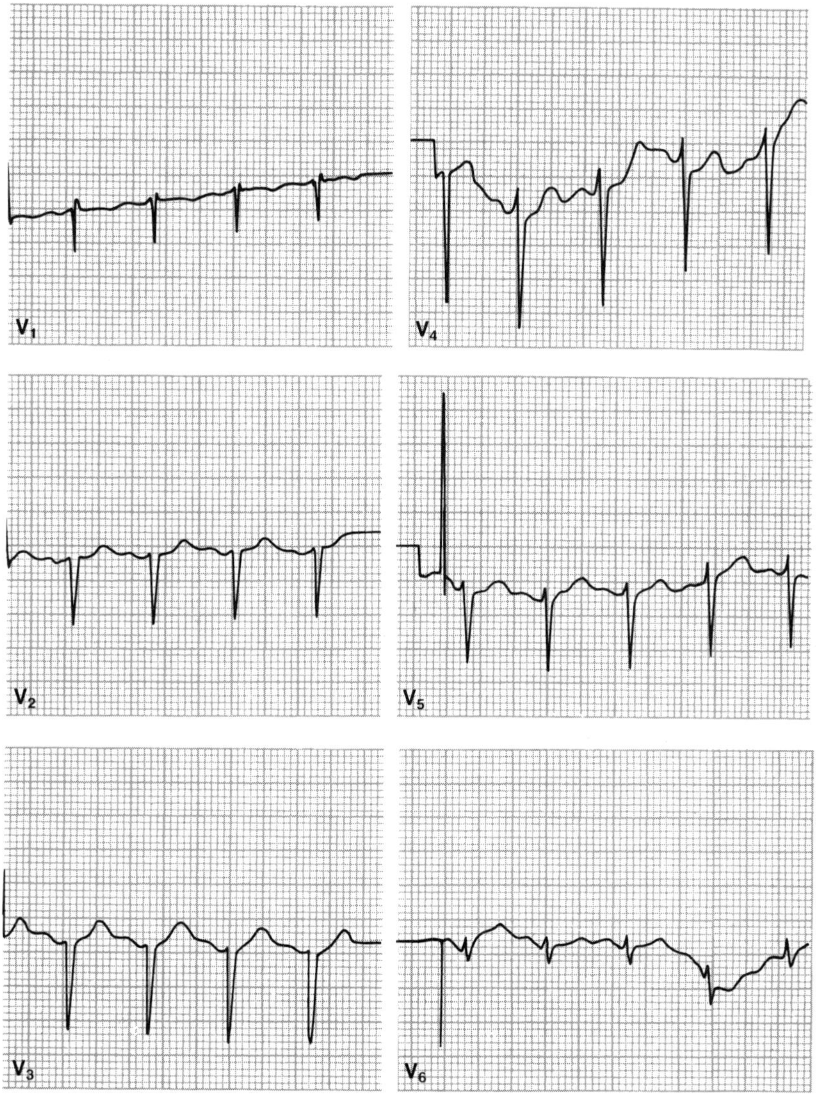
V1
V4
V2
V5
V3
V6

Figure F-3. ECG from a middle-aged man with atypical chest pain.

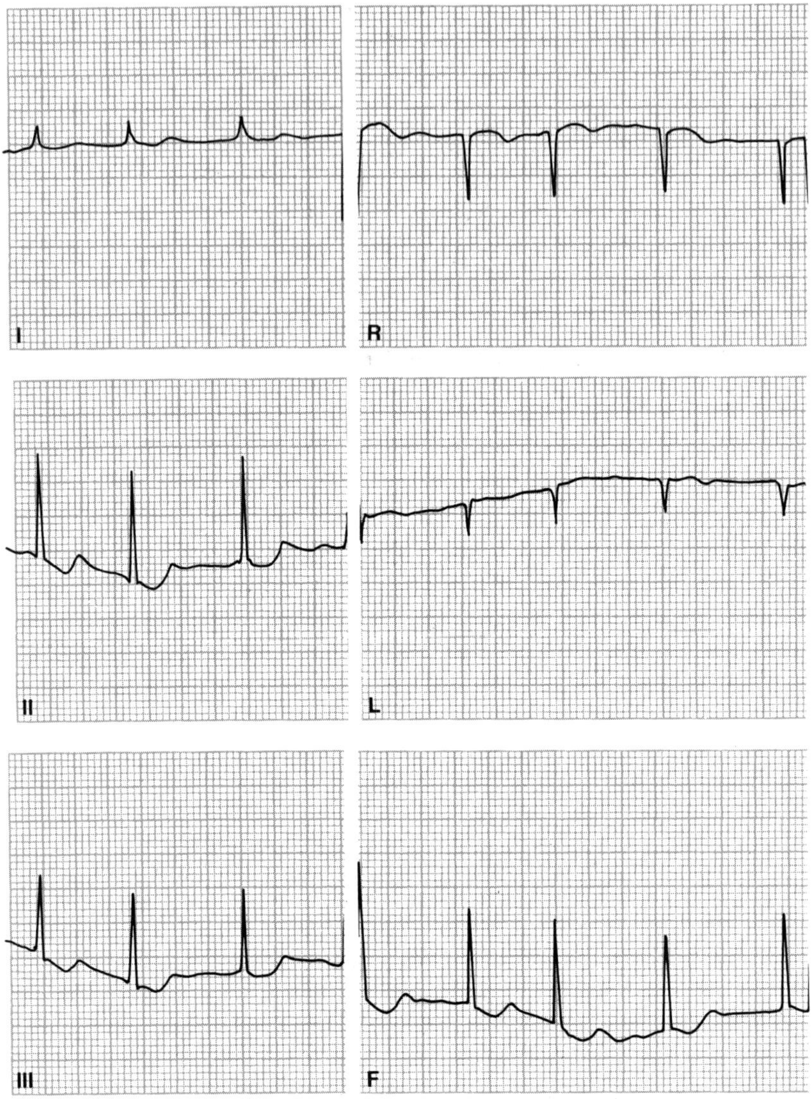

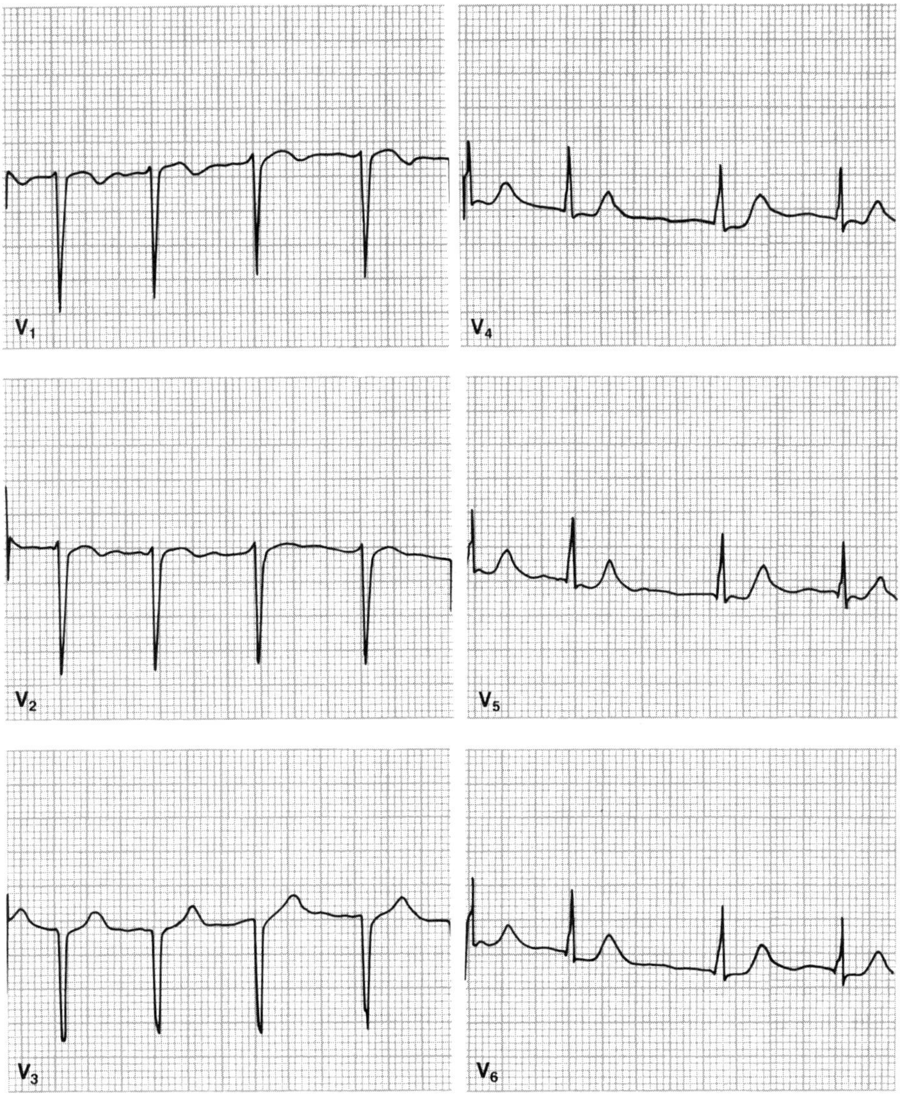
V1
V2
V3
V4
V5
V6

Figure F-4. ECG from an asymptomatic 77-year-old man.

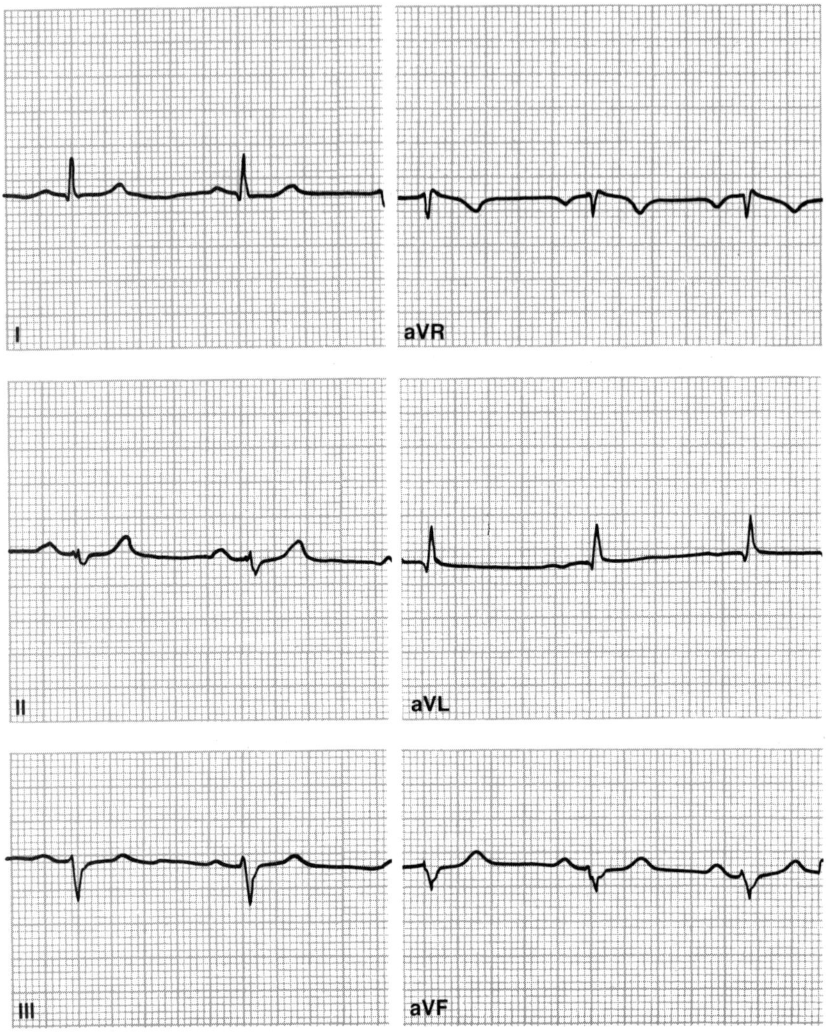

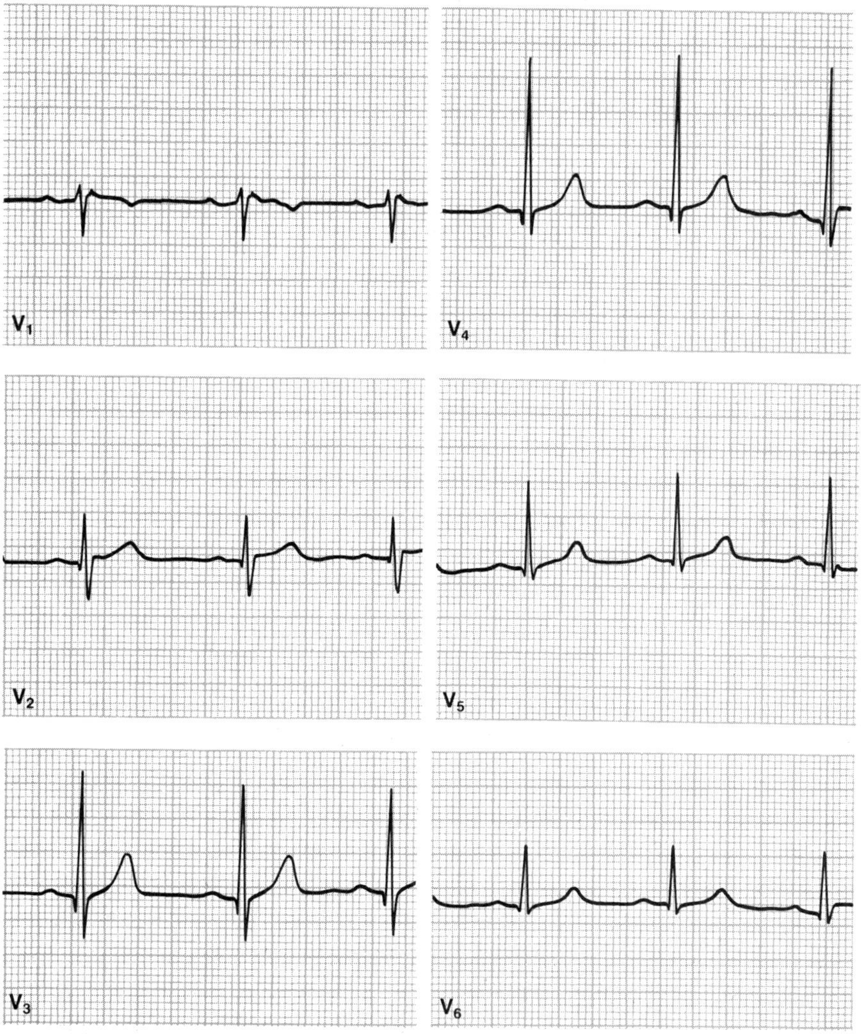
V1
V4
V2
V5
V3
V6

Figure F-5. ECG from a 61-year-old man with shortness of breath and a large, globular heart on chest X-ray film.

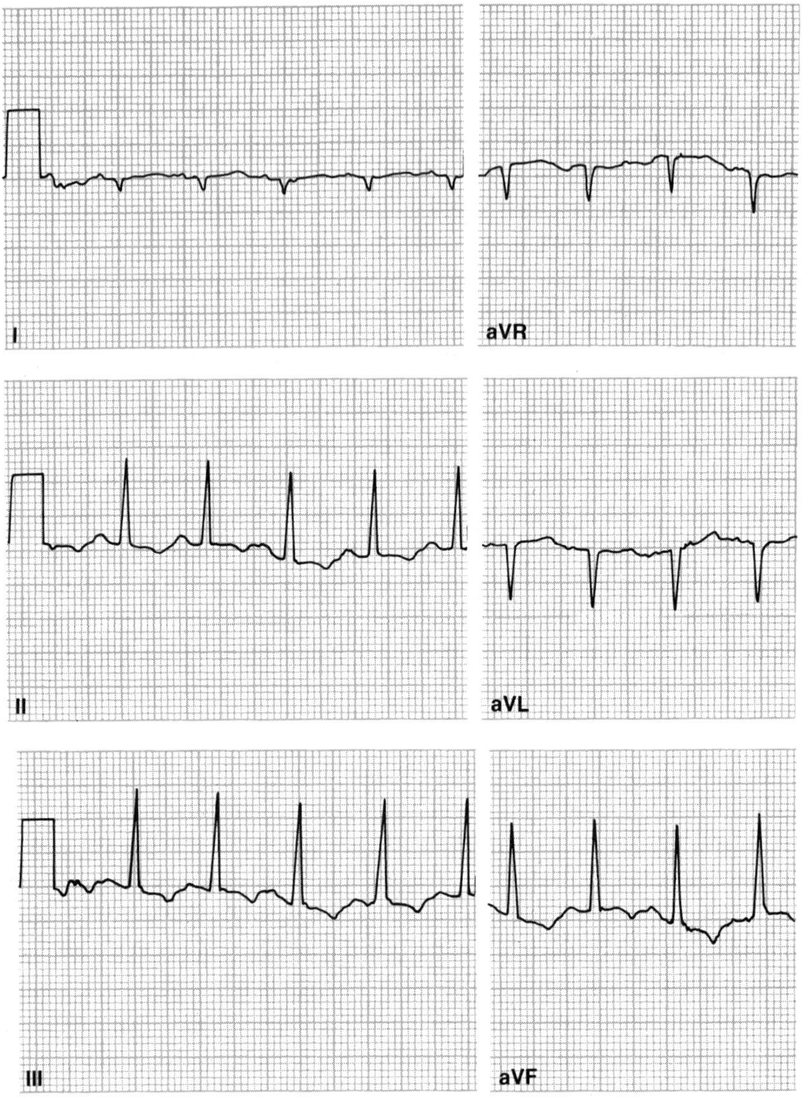

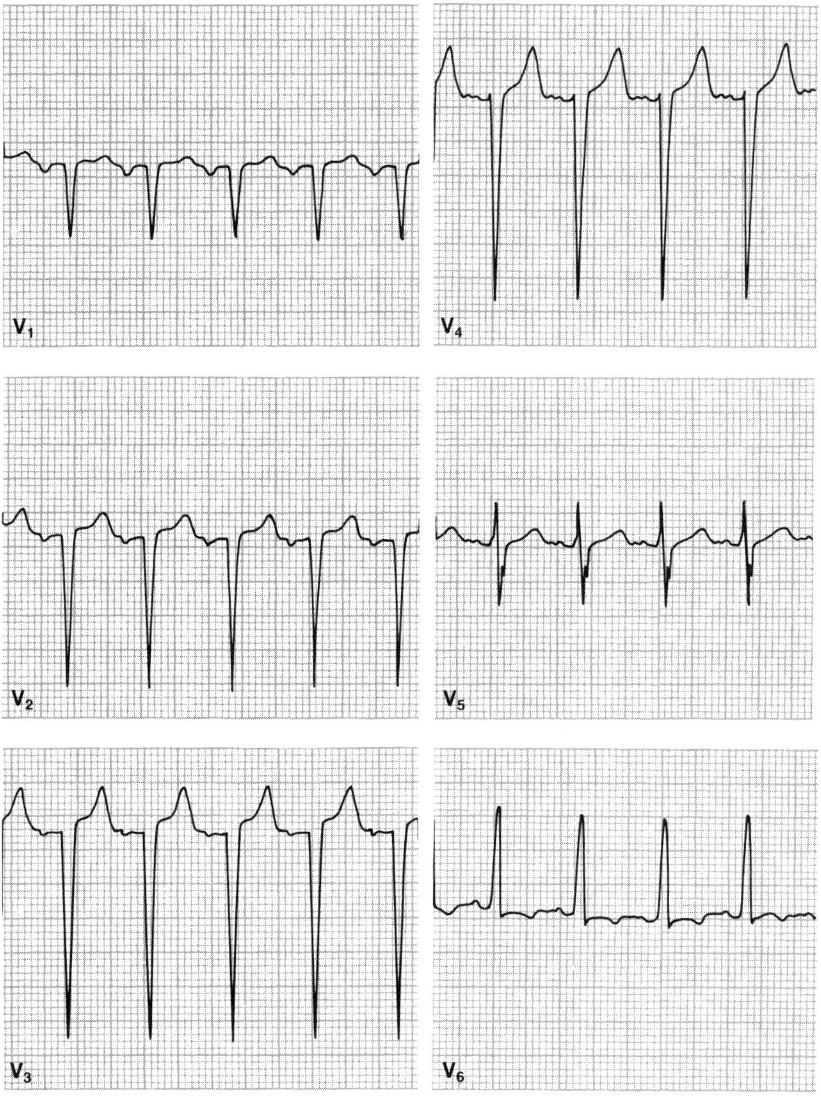
V1
V4
V2
V5
V3
V6

Figure F-6. ECG from a 78-year-old man with a history of chest pain of several days' duration.

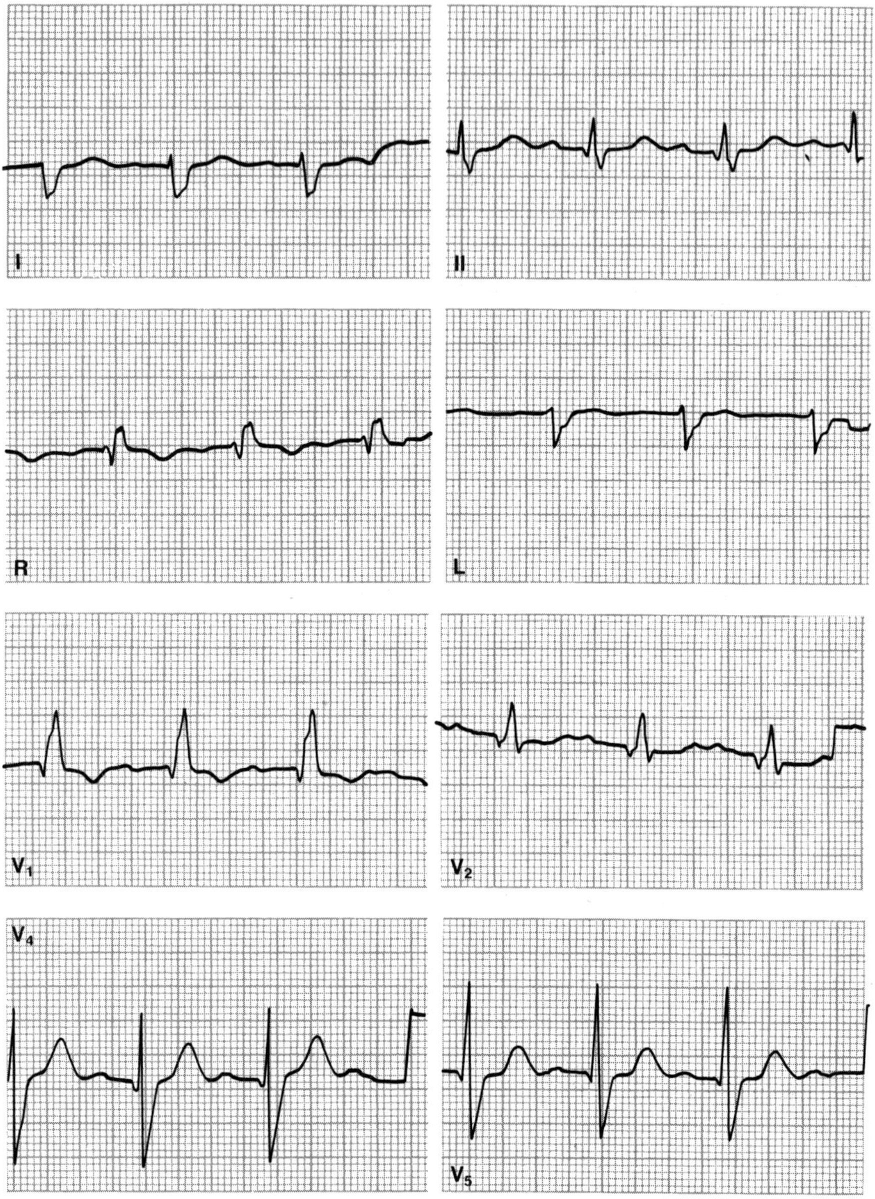

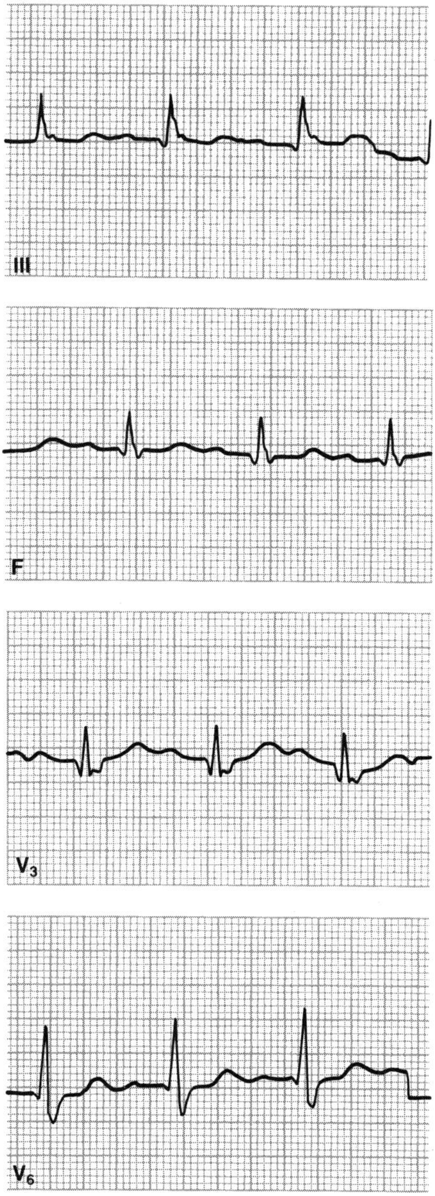
III
F
V_3
V_6

Figure F-7. ECG from a 30-year-old man with cardiomegaly on chest X-ray film and a history of Friedreich's ataxia. The ECG was obtained because the patient was complaining of palpitations.

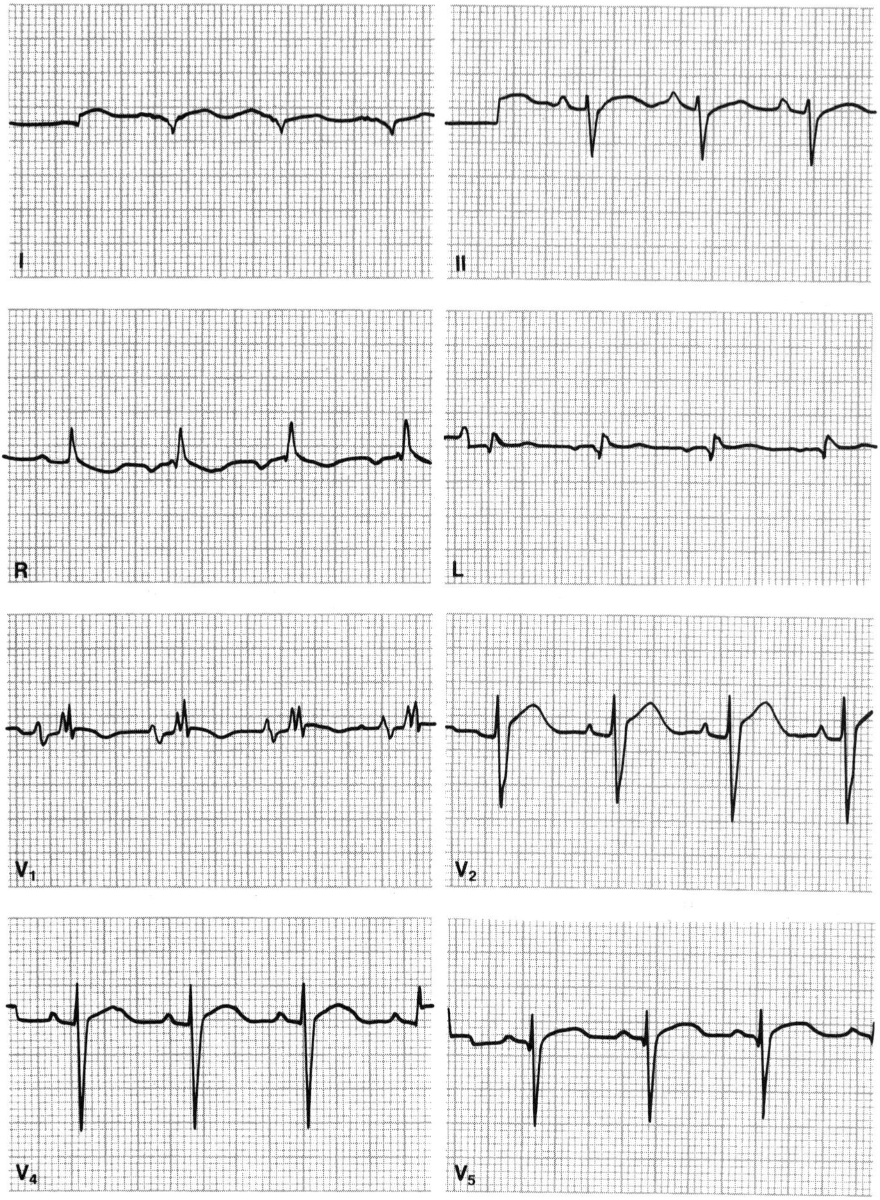

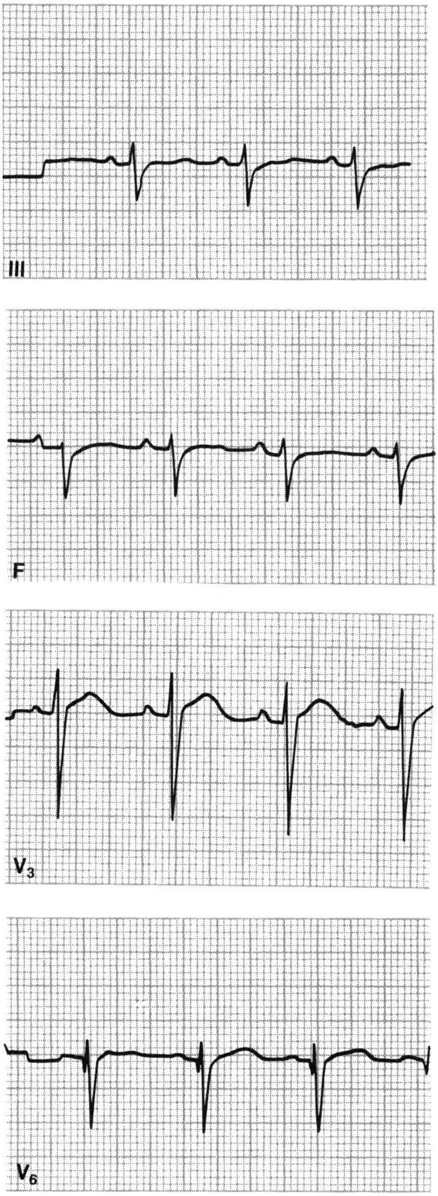
III
F
V_3
V_6

INTERPRETATION of Fig. F-1

Sinus bradycardia at 58 beats/min. Axis $\approx -30°$ (LAD). Dramatic ST-segment elevation in the anterolateral leads, with reciprocal ST-segment depression inferiorly.

As indicated, a repeat ECG on this patient performed only minutes later when his pain had subsided was virtually normal. This strongly suggests that the changes present in Fig. F-1 were *not* the result of acute infarction, but were due to *coronary artery spasm.* Confirmation of this clinical impression would require serial ECGs and cardiac enzyme studies.

Coronary spasm has been defined as a *transient* reduction in coronary artery lumen diameter accompanied by objective evidence of ischemia. This objective evidence may be the angiographic demonstration of coronary artery narrowing, and/or ECG changes (ST-segment elevation or depression) that accompany chest pain and resolve when the chest pain subsides.

Although *pure* coronary spasm exists, most patients with this disorder fit into a spectrum in which spasm is superimposed on a fixed, underlying, atherosclerotic lesion. Overall, coronary spasm has been estimated to play a role in at least 10 percent of all patients with chronic angina pectoris. It is felt to occur in acute myocardial infarction at least as often. Since treatment and prognosis of coronary spasm may differ from that of fixed atherosclerotic disease, identification is important. This may often be accomplished by *immediately* obtaining an ECG at the onset and subsidence of chest pain.

INTERPRETATION of Fig. F-2

Sinus tachycardia at 120 beats/min. Indeterminate axis. Incomplete RBBB. RAE. Persistence of S waves across the precordium.

Although there is poor R-wave progression on this tracing, it more than likely is *not* the result of anterior infarction. Instead, clinical history and the constellation of findings, such as indeterminate mean QRS axis, incomplete RBBB, RAE, and persistence of S waves across the precordium, suggest *type C RVH* as the unifying diagnosis.

The patient in this case had a 20-year history of asthma. Chronic pulmonary disease such as this is a common cause of poor R-wave progression, which may simulate anterior infarction, anterolateral infarction, or both.

INTERPRETATION of Fig. F-3

Atrial fibrillation with a controlled ventricular response. Axis $\approx +75°$. Poor R-wave progression, with *loss* of R wave between leads V_2 and V_3. Nonspecific ST-T wave abnormalities.

Although anterior infarction of unknown age is suggested in Fig. F-3 by loss of R wave between leads V_2 and V_3, R-wave progression *normalized* on the follow-up ECG obtained the next day. Fig. F-8 offers an explanation for this discrepancy.

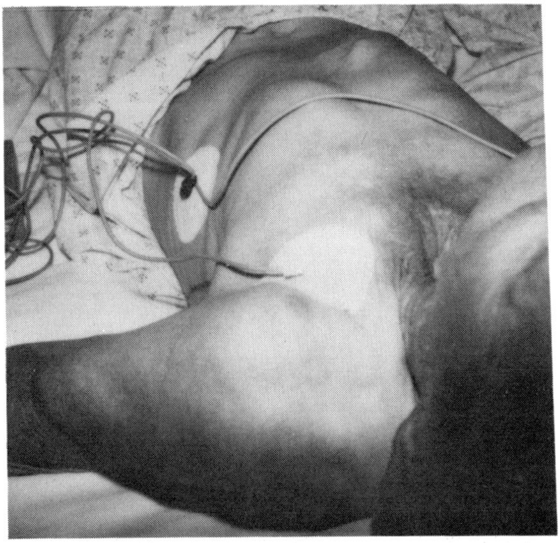

Figure F-8. Chest-wall configuration of the patient whose ECG is shown in Fig. F-3. Pectus carinatum is present, hindering accurate placement of the chest leads.

The patient has *pectus carinatum* (pigeon breast) with undue prominence of the sternum. Accurate placement of precordial chest leads is hindered by the difficulty in determining anatomic landmarks.

Alteration in R-wave progression with serial tracings commonly occurs in patients with *normal* chest-wall configurations as a result of variation in chest-lead *placement* by different technicians on different days. Even the same technician may vary chest-lead placement slightly from one tracing to the next. The problem is magnified in the patient with an *abnormal* chest wall configuration. Consideration should be given to minimizing variation in chest-lead placement by *marking* the chest wall of these individuals.

INTERPRETATION of Fig. F-4

Sinus arrhythmia. Axis $\approx -40°$ (LAHB). Incomplete RBBB (rSr′ in lead V_1). Early transition. *Narrow q waves are present in leads V_2 to V_6.*

The finding of an early transition with narrow q waves in the anterior and/or anterolateral precordial leads is subtle, but quite common in older individuals. Because the q waves in leads V_2 to V_4 are usually very small (as they are in Fig. F-4), they are easily overlooked. Determination of their clinical significance is equally problematic. Three causes have been attributed to this finding:

- Anterior infarction
- *Rotation of the thoracic aorta*
- Pseudoinfarction pattern produced by LAHB

In elderly patients with atherosclerosis, the aorta often becomes tortuous. When it "uncoils," the ascending aorta may rotate to the right in such a manner as to pull the left ventricular outflow tract into a more anterior position. Concomitant rotation of the interventricular septum results in production of a qR complex in the anterior precordial leads.

LAHB may mimic or mask diagnosis of myocardial infarction in a number of ways. The mechanism whereby it may mask inferior infarction was discussed in Chapter 7. In tracings such as Fig. F-4, its presence may mimic anterior infarction. Although primarily a superior and lateral structure, the left anterior hemidivision of the left bundle branch lies relatively more *anterior* than the left posterior hemidivision. Consequently, after the impulse leaves the bundle of His, it will be oriented in a relatively *posterior* direction if the more anterior hemidivision is blocked (as it is in LAHB). This may produce small q waves in the anterior precordial leads.

It is *impossible* to rule out previous anterior infarction from simple inspection of ECGs (such as Fig. F-4) that demonstrate early transition with narrow q waves in the anterior precordial leads. However, it is likely that rotation of the thoracic aorta and/or LAHB are much more frequent causes of this common ECG pattern among asymptomatic elderly patients.

INTERPRETATION of Fig. F-5

Sinus tachycardia at 125 beats/min. Axis $\approx$ 105° (RAD). LAA. *Poor R-wave progression.*

This ECG highlights the dilemma of the differential diagnosis of *poor R-wave progression.* One or more of three entities must be strongly considered:

- LVH
- RVH
- Anterior infarction

Diagnosis of LVH is suggested by prominent voltage (sum of S wave in lead V_2 + R wave in lead $V_6 \geq 35$ mm), the presence of LAA, and ST-T wave changes consistent with strain (ST-segment depression in the inferior leads, T-wave inversion in lead V_6, and reciprocal repolarization changes in the anterior precordial leads).

Diagnosis of RVH is usually hard to make when there is also LVH because increases in left *and* right ventricular mass tend to cancel each other out. However, when RAD is found in association with definite criteria for LVH, biventricular hypertrophy most likely is present.

The question of anterior infarction remains. Although anterior infarction *cannot* be excluded from simple inspection of Fig. F-5, one should remember that LVH and RVH can each produce poor R-wave progression that simulates anterior infarction. Determination of anterior infarction therefore requires independent confirmation (by history, comparison with previous tracings, vectorcardiography, etc.).

As implied by the history, the patient in this case was found to have congestive cardiomyopathy. Echocardiography revealed *biventricular hypertrophy* and enlargement. There was no history of infarction.

INTERPRETATION of Fig. F-6

Sinus rhythm at 80 beats/min. Trifascicular block (1° AV block, RBBB, and LPHB). Evidence of previous *infero-anterolateral infarction.*

This is the one ECG in this section that definitely represents myocardial infarction. Despite trifascicular conduction disease, abnormal Q waves indicative of previous infarction are present in the inferior, anterior, and lateral precordial leads. None of the changes appear to be acute.

INTERPRETATION of Fig. F-7

Sinus rhythm at 90 beats/min. Indeterminate axis. Borderline QRS prolongation (to 0.10 second) with an incomplete RBBB pattern (RSR′ in lead V_1). Biatrial abnormality. Persistence of S waves across the precordium. Probable RVH.

Although RAA is usually identified by the presence of tall, peaked P waves in the inferior leads, this is one instance when the diagnosis is made instead from the finding of a prominent, peaked initial component of the P wave in lead V_1. The deep negative component of this P wave suggests concomitant LAA. Putting together the above findings (RAD, RAA, IRBBB, and persistent S waves), RVH is likely.

Yet even if RVH explains some of the findings, one is still left with the QS complex in lead I and the q waves in leads aVL, V_5, and V_6 that simulate myocardial infarction. This is a bizarre tracing, particularly for an individual who is only 30 years old.

PROBLEM: Can you think of any disorder that might produce cardiomegaly on chest X-ray in a 30 year old in association with cardiac dysrhythmias and a bizarre ECG pattern such as the one shown here?

ANSWER: A *cardiomyopathy* should be suspected when cardiomegaly accompanies cardiac dysrhythmias, an unusual ECG pattern, or both in a young individual. In this case, the patient had the cardiomyopathy that is associated with Friedreich's ataxia. This hereditary neurodegenerative disorder commonly involves the heart, producing interstitial fibrosis of the myocardium. Ventricular hypertrophy, congestive heart failure, cor pulmonale, and/or cardiac dysrhythmias result. The cardiomyopathy is progressive and is often the cause of death.

Other heredofamilial neuromyopathic disorders that involve the heart include the progressive muscular dystrophies (Duchenne's dystrophy) and myotonic muscular dystrophy.

References

Goldberger AL: Recognition of ECG pseudo-infarct patterns. *Mod Concepts Cardiovasc Dis* 1980; 49:13–18.

Grauer K: Recognition of pseudo-myocardial infarction patterns. *Cont Ed Fam Phys* 1983; 18:267–274.

Perloff JK: Neurological disorders and heart disease. In Braunwald E (ed): *Heart Disease—A Textbook of Cardiovascular Medicine.* Philadelphia, WB Saunders Co, 1980.

Yanagisawa N: Counterclockwise rotation of the heart: Correlation of electrocardiography and chest radiography and their clinical significance. *J Electrocardiol* 1981; 14:233–238.

Zema MJ, Kligfield P: Electrocardiographic poor R wave progression: Correlation with the frank vectorcardiogram. *J Electrocardiol* 1979; 12:3–10.

APPENDIX

Abbreviations

This list notes many of the abbreviations used in this book. It includes a number of additional abbreviations that the reader will encounter in the literature on electrocardiography. This list is *not* exhaustive.

AV—Atrioventricular
AV block—Atrioventricular block
AV node—Atrioventricular (or junctional) node
AV nodal rhythm—Atrioventricular (or junctional) rhythm

BBB—Bundle branch block

CW—Clockwise
CCW—Counterclockwise
CNS—Central nervous system
COPD—Chronic obstructive pulmonary disease
CSM—Carotid sinus massage (=CSP)
CSP—Carotid sinus pressure (=CSM)
CVA—Cerebral vascular accident

ECF—Extracellular fluid
ECG—Electrocardiogram
EKG—Electrocardiogram (from the German ElektroKardioGraph)
ENDO—Endocardium
EPI—Epicardium
ETT—Exercise tolerance (stress) test

HIS—Bundle of His

ICF—Intracellular fluid
ILBBB—Incomplete left bundle branch block
IRBBB—Incomplete right bundle branch block
IVCD—Intraventricular conduction delay
IVS—Interventricular septum
J POINT—Junctional point (Point marking the *junction* between the end of the QRS complex and the beginning of the ST segment)

LA—Left atrium
LAA—Left atrial abnormality
LA electrode—Left arm recording electrode
LAD—Left axis deviation
LAD artery—Left anterior descending artery
LAE—Left atrial enlargement
LAFB—Left anterior fascicular block (=LAHB)
LAH—Left anterior hemidivision (of the LBB)
LAHB—Left anterior hemiblock
LAI—Left atrial involvement (=LAA)
LBB—Left bundle branch
LBBB—Left bundle branch block
LCA—Left coronary artery
LGL syndrome—Lown-Ganong-Levine syndrome
LL electrode—Left leg recording electrode
LPFB—Left posterior fascicular block (=LPHB)
LPH—Left posterior hemidivision (of the LBB)
LPHB—Left posterior hemiblock
LV—Left ventricle
LVE—Left ventricular enlargement (=LVH)
LVH—Left ventricular hypertrophy

MAT—Multifocal atrial tachycardia (=chaotic atrial mechanism)

NS ST-T Abns—Nonspecific ST-T wave abnormalities

PA—Pulmonary artery
PAC—Premature atrial contraction
PAT—Paroxysmal atrial tachycardia
PJC—Premature junctional contraction
PJT—Paroxysmal junctional tachycardia
PSVT—Paroxysmal supraventricular tachycardia
PVC—Premature ventricular contraction

QT interval—Period from onset of Q wave until end of T wave
QTc—QT interval *corrected* for heart rate

RA—Right atrium
RA electrode—Right arm recording electrode
RAA—Right atrial abnormality
RAD—Right axis deviation
RAE—Right atrial enlargement

RAI—Right atrial involvement (=RAA)
RBB—Right bundle branch
RBBB—Right bundle branch block
RCA—Right coronary artery
RV—Right ventricle
RVE—Right ventricular enlargement (=RVH)
RVH—Right ventricular hypertrophy

SA block—Sinoatrial block
SA node—Sinoatrial node
SSS—Sick sinus syndrome
SVT—Supraventricular tachycardia
SVC—Superior vena cava

Ta wave—Atrial T wave (wave of atrial repolarization)

WNL—Within normal limits
WPW syndrome—Wolff-Parkinson-White syndrome

Handy Reference Guide

Systematic Approach to ECG Interpretation

RATE
RHYTHM
- Regularity of rhythm?
- Presence of P waves?
  - —Upright P wave in lead II?
- Width of QRS complex?
  - —INTERVALS: PR/QRS/QT intervals
  - —Is bundle branch block present?
- Relation of P waves to QRS complex?
- —Is each QRS "married" to a preceding P wave?

AXIS
CHAMBER ENLARGEMENT
- LAE/RAE?
- LVH/RVH?

QRST CHANGES
- Presence of **Q** waves?
- Is there normal **R**-wave progression?
- Is there **ST**-segment elevation or depression?
- Is there **T**-wave inversion?

Calculation of Heart Rate

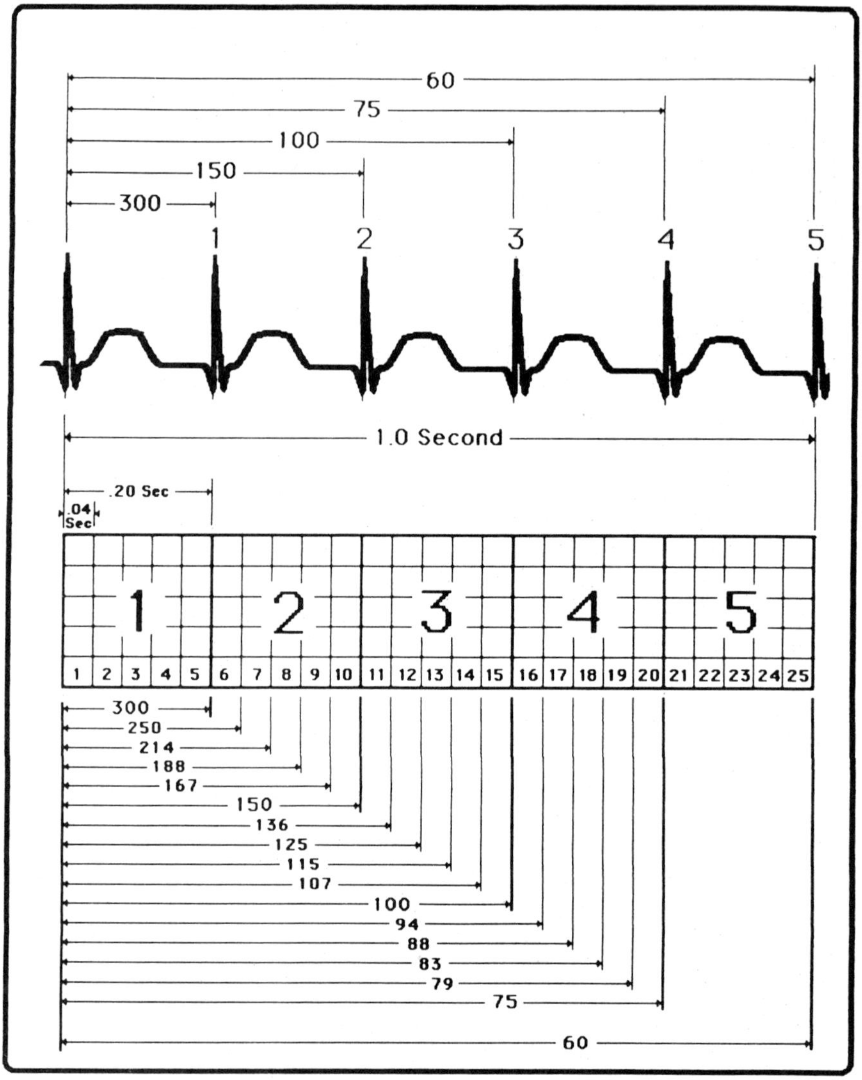

QT-Interval Determination and Clinical Significance

Simplified Table for Determination of QT Interval Prolongation

Heart Rate (beats/min)	Approximate upper normal limit of the QT interval (sec.)
50	0.47
60	0.43
70	0.41
80	0.39
90	0.37
100	0.35
110	0.33

Normal QT Interval

-should be less than 1/2 the R-R interval (this method is only accurate if HR <100/min)

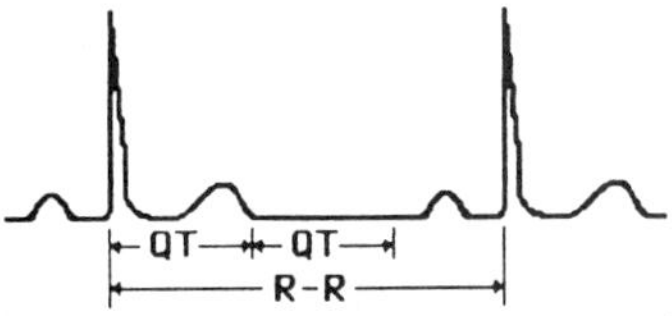

QT Prolongation

-QT interval is greater than 1/2 R-R interval

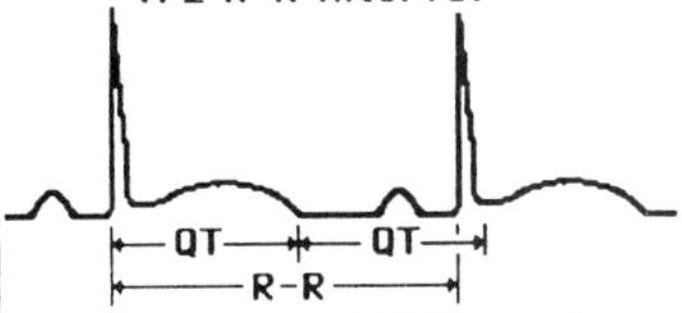

Common Causes of QT Interval Prolongation

CONDITIONS IN WHICH QT PROLONGATION MAY BE THE ONLY ECG CLUE:

- Drugs (quinidine, procainamide, phenothiazines, tricyclic antidepressants, etc.)
- Electrolytes (hypokalemia, hypocalcemia)
- Central nervous system catastrophe (Subarachnoid or subdural bleed, CVA, etc.)

CONDITIONS IN WHICH QT PROLONGATION IS USUALLY SECONDARY TO THE UNDERLYING ELECTROCARDIOGRAPHIC DISORDER:

- Myocardial ischemia or infarction
- Intraventricular conduction abnormalities (LBBB, RBBB, IVCD)

Axis Determination and Clinical Significance

AXIS

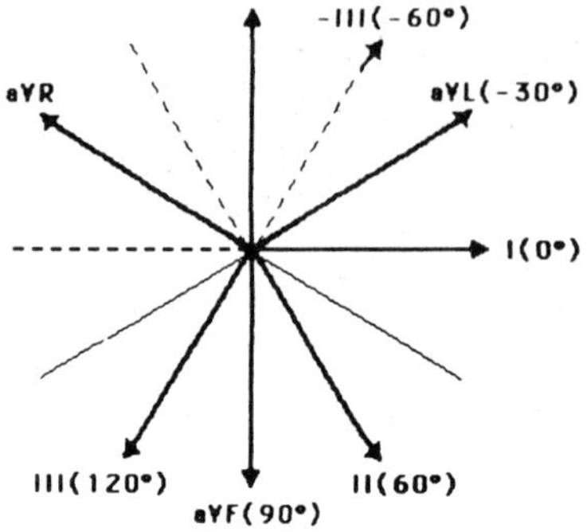

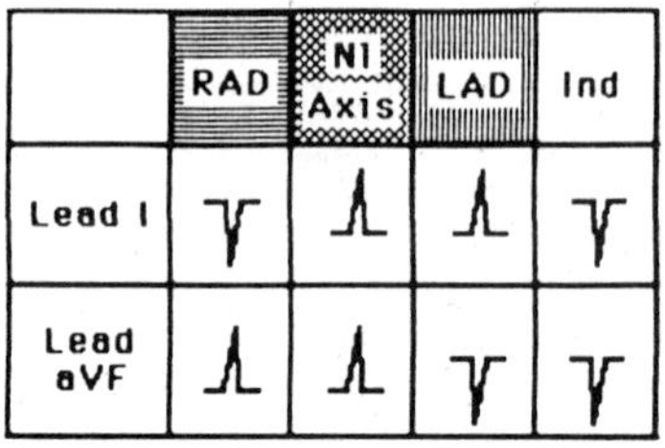

Causes of LAD
- Nl variant
- LAHB
- LBBB
- LVH
- Elevated diaphragm (pregnancy, ascites)
- Obesity
- Inferior infarction

Causes of Ind
- Nl variant
- COPD
- RVH

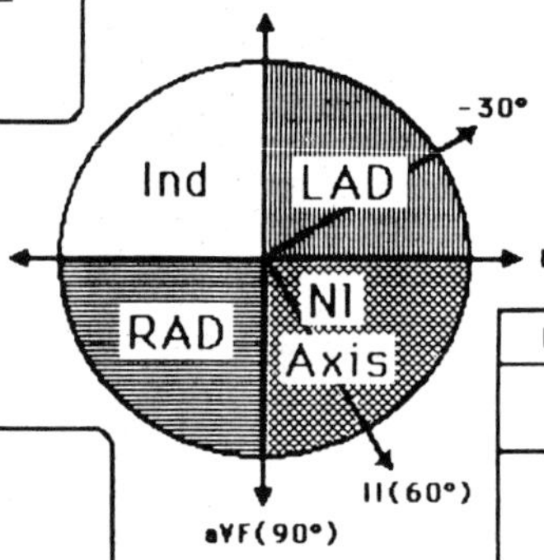

Lead II	Axis	
	<−30°	Nonpathologic LAD
	−30°	An isoelectric QRS complex in lead II (at 60°) ⇒ axis is 90° away (at −30°)
	>−30°	Pathologic LAD (LAHB)

Causes of RAD
- Nl variant
- LPHB
- RVH and/or cor pulmonale
- Limb-lead reversal
- Dextrocardia
- Childhood
- Lateral infarction

Ind — Indeterminate axis
RAD — Right axis deviation
LAD — Left axis deviation
Nl axis — Normal axis

LAHB — Left anterior hemiblock
LPHB — Left posterior hemiblock
LVH — Left ventricular hypertrophy
RVH — Right ventricular hypertrophy
COPD — Chronic obstructive pulmonary disease

Bundle Branch Blocks and Hemiblocks

RBBB

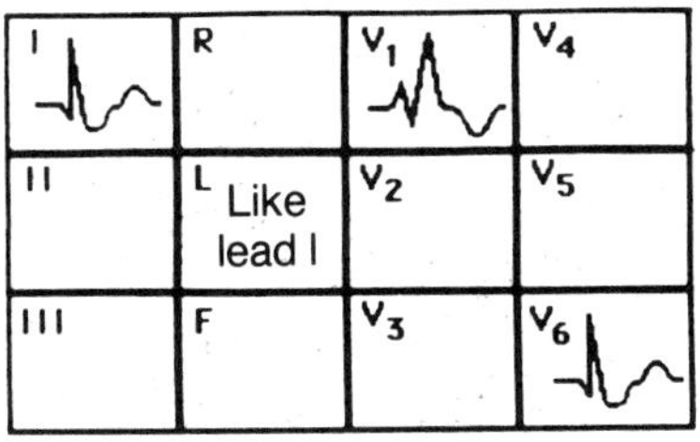

RECOGNITION:

—rSR′ or "RBBB-equivalent" in lead V_1
—Wide terminal S wave in leads I and V_6
—QRS ≥0.11 second for complete RBBB

CLINICAL SIGNIFICANCE:

—Does not affect initial vector of depolarization → infarction can usually be diagnosed
—RVH suggested by very tall R′ (≥15 mm) in lead V_1 and associated RAA
—LVH suggested by R≥25 mm in leads V_{5-6} or R≥12 mm in lead aVL

LBBB

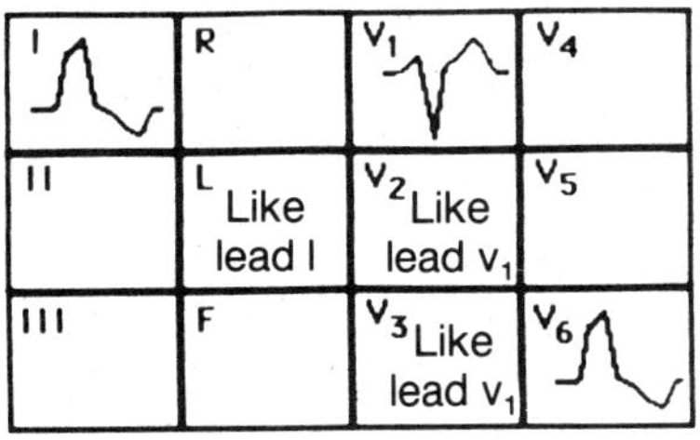

RECOGNITION:

—Monophasic R wave (sometimes with notching) and absence of septal q wave in leads I and V_6
—QS or rS complex in leads V_{1-3}
—QRS ≥0.12 second for complete LBBB

CLINICAL SIGNIFICANCE:

—Altered direction of depolarization vector → hard to diagnose infarction
—Can't diagnose RVH
—LVH suggested by very deep S wave (≥30 mm) in leads V_{1-2} and/or associated LAA

Typical ST-T Wave Changes:

ST-T wave in typical BBB is normally directed opposite terminal portion of QRS

IVCD: QRS is wide, but does not manifest typical pattern of RBBB or LBBB in key leads (I, V_1, and V_6)

LAHB

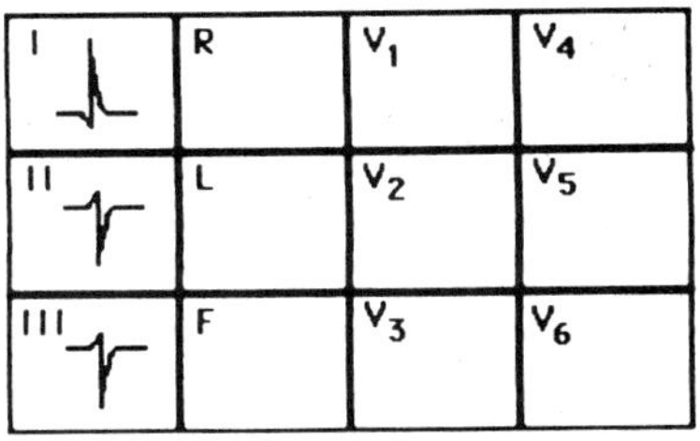

RECOGNITION: —Much more common

—Lead II has net negative deflection (axis >−30°)

CLINICAL SIGNIFICANCE:

—May mask inferior infarction and simulate anterior infarction

LPHB

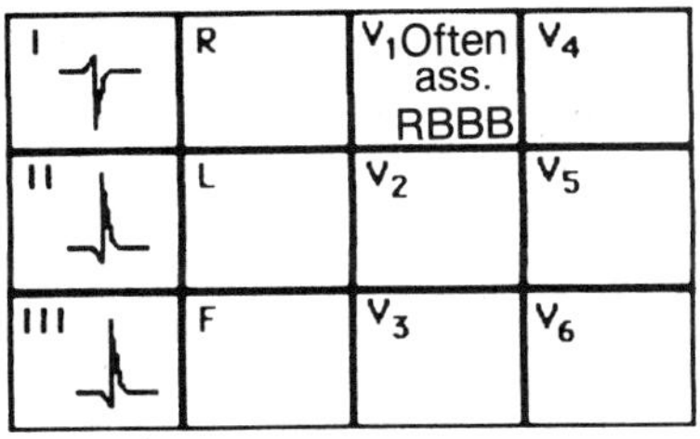

RECOGNITION: —Uncommon

—QRS axis ≥+ 105°

CLINICAL SIGNIFICANCE:

—Often associated with RBBB
—Implies much more extensive disease

ST-T Wave Abnormalities

Normal

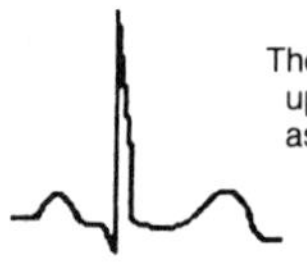

There is a smooth and gradual upsloping of the ST segment as it melts into the T wave

Nonspecific ST-T Wave Abnormalities

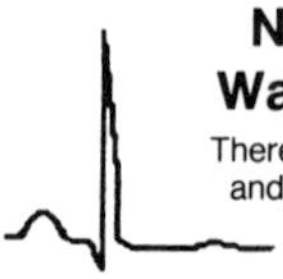

There is flattening of the T wave and/or the ST segment. This type of nonspecific change may be produced by multiple causes.

Ischemia

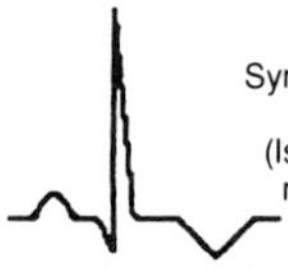

Symmetric T-wave inversion

(Ischemia may also be manifest by ST-segment depression)

Strain

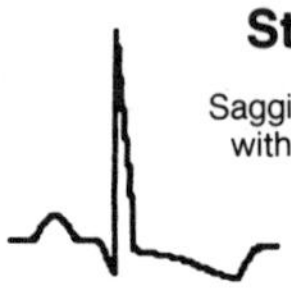

Sagging ST segment depression with asymmetric T wave inversion Usually best seen in the lateral leads (I, aVL, V_5, V_6)

Digitalis Effect

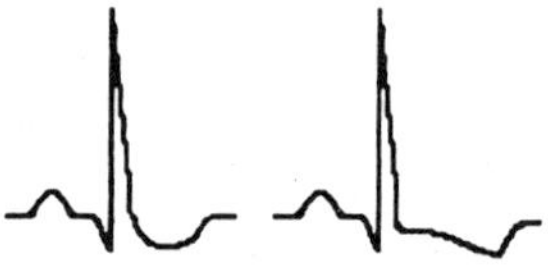

May present as either scooping ST-segment depression with shortening of the QT interval or as slowly descending ST-segment depression with asymmetric T-wave inversion (that is identical in appearance to strain)

There is a poor correlation between digitalis effect on the ECG and serum digoxin levels

Hypokalemia

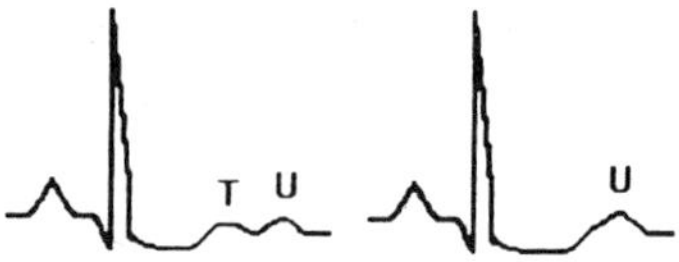

Earliest change is flattening of the T wave. This is followed by ST-segment depression that is often diffuse, and development of U waves that may eventually become taller than the T wave. A pseudo-P pulmonale pattern may be seen.

ECG changes of hyperkalemia are often nonspecific.

Hyperkalemia

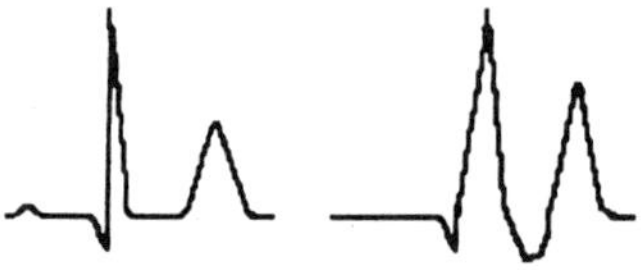

Earliest and most characteristic change is peaking of the T wave. The P-wave amplitude becomes less and eventually disappears as the QRS complex widens.

ECG changes of hyperkalemia correlate much better with serum potassium levels than do ECG changes of hypokalemia.

Hypercalcemia

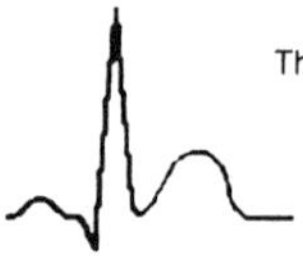

There is shortening of the QT interval

This effect is usually not seen until serum calcium levels are ≥12 mg/dL.

Hypocalcemia

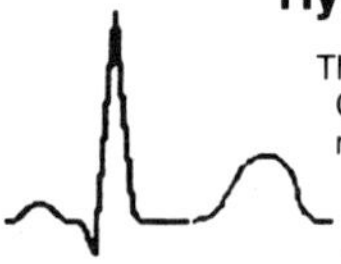

There is lengthening of the QT interval, with a relatively normal-appearing T wave occurring at the end of a long isoelectric segment.

ST-Segment Elevation

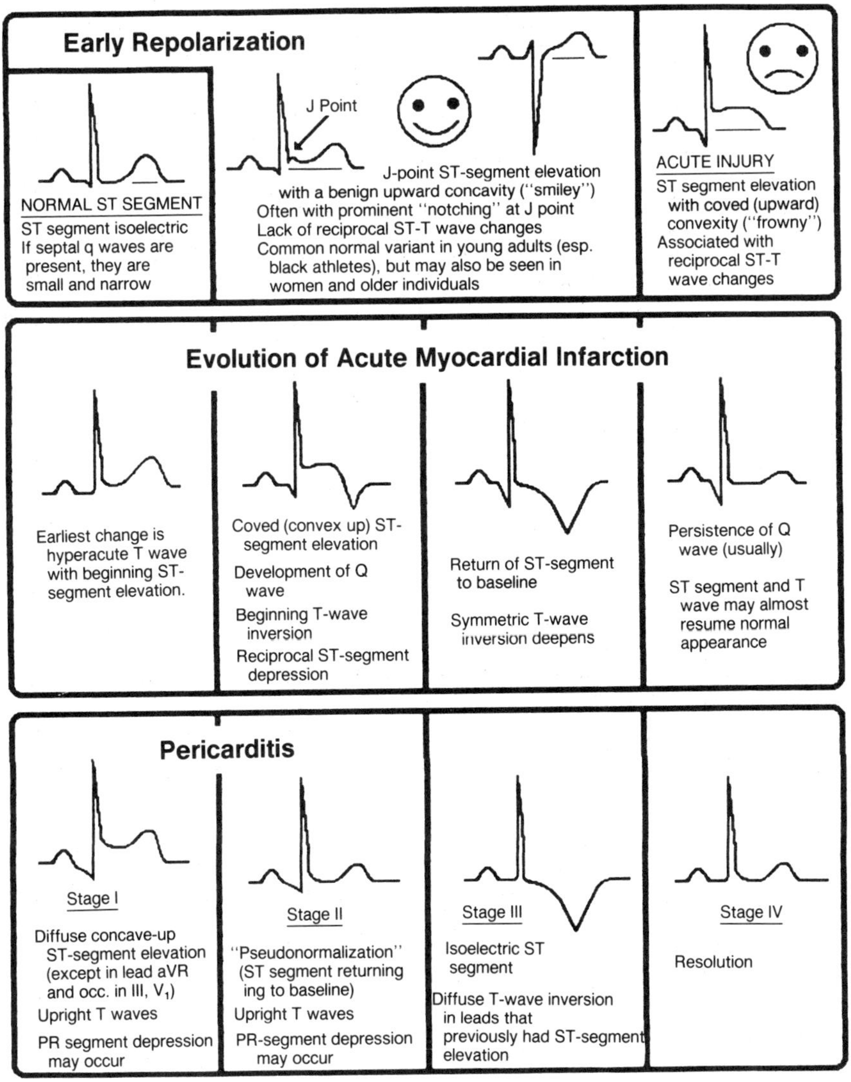

Miscellaneous Tables

Lead Localization

Septal leads—V_{1-2}
Anterior leads—V_{2-4}
Lateral precordial leads—V_{4-6}
High lateral leads—I, aVL
Inferior leads—II, III, aVF
Posterior leads—V_{1-3} (mirror image)
Apical leads—II, III, aVF, V_{2-4}
Right ventricular leads—V_1, $V_{2-4}R$

Common Causes of Poor R Wave Progression

—Anterior or anteroseptal infarction
—Left ventricular hypertrophy
—Right ventricular hypertrophy (Type C)
—Chronic obstructive pulmonary disease
—Left bundle branch block
—Left anterior hemiblock
—Cardiomyopathy
—Lead misplacement
—Normal variant

Common Causes of ST Segment Elevation

—Acute myocardial infarction
—Coronary spasm
—Acute pericarditis
—Repolarization variants
—Left ventricular hypertrophy (ie, anterior leads)
—Ventricular aneurysm
—Hyperkalemia

Common Causes of Pseudo-Infarction Patterns

—Repolarization variants
—Left ventricular hypertrophy
—Right ventricular hypertrophy
  —Chronic obstructive pulmonary disease
  —Pulmonary embolism
—Cardiomyopathy
  —Idiopathic hypertrophic subaortic stenosis
  —Congestive cardiomyopathy
—Interventricular conduction defects
  —Left bundle branch block
  —IVCD
  —Left anterior hemiblock
—Wolff-Parkinson-White syndrome
—Pericardial effusion
—CNS catastrophe
—Chest wall deformity
  —Pectus excavatum
  —Pectus carinatum
Technical mishaps
  —Limb-lead reversal
  —Malpositioned chest leads

Common Causes of ST Segment Depression

—"Strain" from LVH
—Ischemia
—Reciprocal changes
—Rate-related ST-segment depression
—Digitalis effect
—Hypokalemia
—Secondary ST-T wave changes from BBB

Ventricular Hypertrophy

LVH

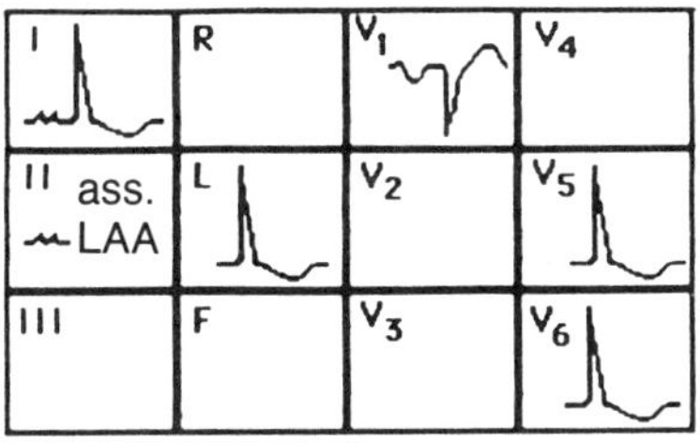

AGE OF PATIENT:

≥35 years of age

REPOLARIZATION CHANGES:

"Strain" in the left-sided leads (leads I, aVL, V_{5-6})

Strain equivalent

VOLTAGE CRITERIA:

—Sum of deepest S wave in lead V_{1-2} + tallest R wave in lead V_{5-6} ≥35 mm
—R wave in lead aVL ≥12 mm

—Deep S waves in V_{1-2} ≥25 mm
—Tall R waves in V_{5-6} ≥25 mm
—Sum of tallest precordial lead R wave + deepest precordial lead S wave ≥45 mm

—R wave in V_6 > R wave in V_5
—Sum of R wave in lead I + S wave in lead III ≥25 mm
—R wave or S wave in any limb lead ≥20 mm

ASSOCIATED MINOR CRITERIA:

LAE
Left axis deviation

Type A RVH

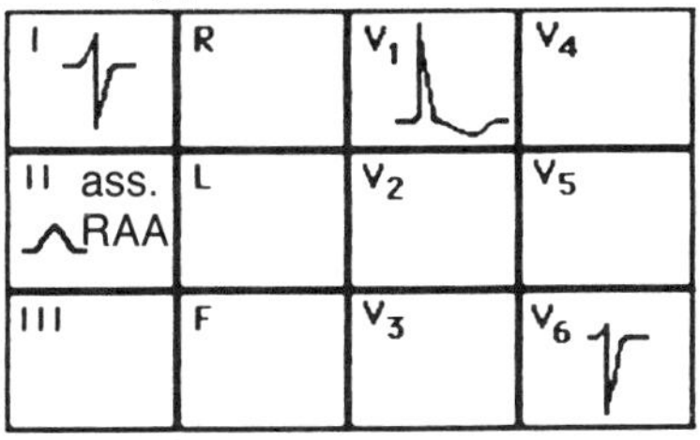

RECOGNITION:

—Predominant R wave in lead V_1
—"Strain" pattern in inferior and/or anterior precordial leads
—RAA
—Right axis deviation
—Deep S waves in leads V_{5-6}

TYPE B RVH is a less common intermediate form. Distinction of it from type A RVH may be difficult without a vectorcardiogram.

Type C RVH

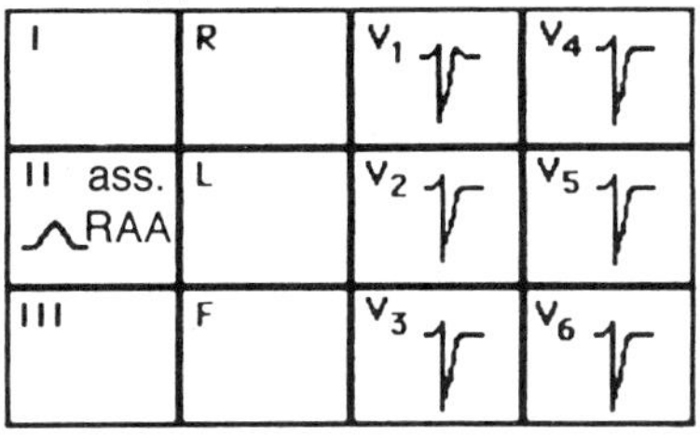

RECOGNITION:

—Low voltage in the limb leads
—IRBBB
—RAA
—Right axis deviation or indeterminate axis
—Persistence of S waves across the precordium
—S waves in leads I, II, and III

Atrial Abnormality—Tall R Wave in Lead V_1

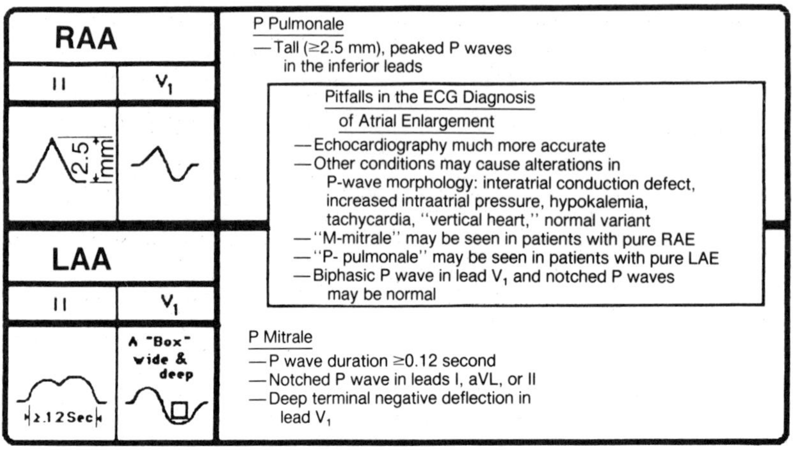

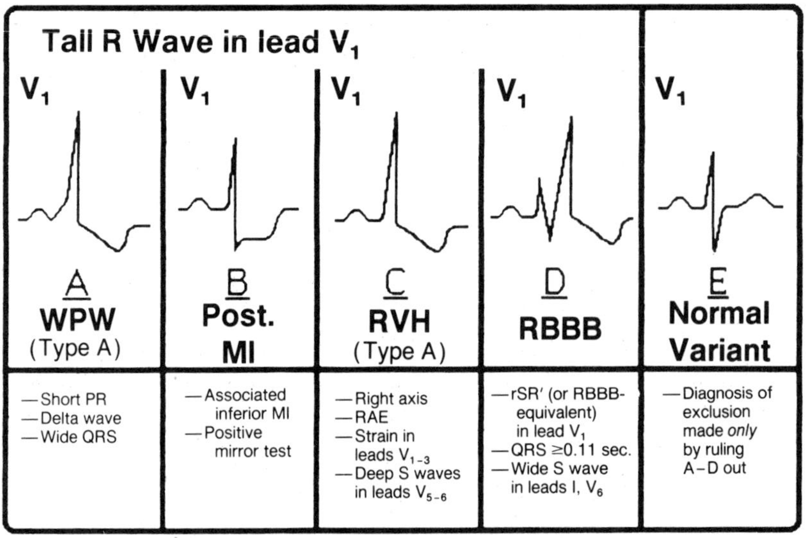

Bibliography

1. Chung EK: *Electrocardiography: Practical Applications with Vectorial Principles.* Harper & Row, Publishers, Hagerstown, Md, 1980.

2. Dubin D: *Rapid Interpretation of EKGs: A Programmed Course.* Cover Publishing Company, Tampa, Fla, 1981.

3. Garson A: *The Electrocardiogram in Infants and Children: A Systematic Approach.* Lea & Febiger, Philadelphia, 1983.

4. Goldberger AL, Goldberger E: *Clinical Electrocardiography: A Simplified Approach.* The C.V. Mosby Company, St. Louis, 1981.

5. Goldschlager N, Goldman MJ: *Electrocardiography: Essentials of Interpretation.* Lange Medical Publications, Los Altos, Calif, 1984.

6. Grauer K, Curry RW: *Interpreting ECGs: A Workbook.* Monograph #47 in the AAFP Home Study Self-Assessment Program, Kansas City, 1983.

7. Lipman BS, Dunn M, Massie E: *Clinical Electrocardiography.* Year Book Medical Publishers, Inc, Chicago, 1984.

8. Marriott HJL: *Practical Electrocardiography.* Williams & Wilkins Co, Baltimore, 1982.

9. Marriott HJL: *Workshop in Electrocardiography.* Tampa Tracings, Oldsmar, 1974.

10. Mudge GH: The Resting Electrocardiogram. In Cohn PF, Wynne J. (eds): *Diagnostic Methods in Clinical Cardiology.* Little, Brown, and Company, Boston, 1982.

11. Silverman ME, Myerburg RJ, Hurst JW: *Electrocardiography: Basic Concepts and Clinical Application.* McGraw-Hill Book Company, New York, 1983.

12. Wharton JM, Goldschlager N: *Guide to Interpreting 12-Lead ECGs.* Medical Economics Books, Oradell, NJ, 1984.

INDEX